1001
HEART
HEALTHY
RECIPES

1001 HEART HEALTHY RECIPES

Quick, Delicious Recipes High in Fiber and Low in Sodium & Cholesterol That Keep You Committed to Your Healthy Lifestyle

Dick Logue

Author of the best-selling *500 Low Sodium Recipes*

FAIR WINDS
PRESS
BEVERLY, MASSACHUSETTS

Text © 2009 Dick Logue
First published in the USA in 2013 by
Fair Winds Press, a member of
Quayside Publishing Group
100 Cummings Center
Suite 406-L
Beverly, MA 01915-6101
www.fairwindspress.com

17 16 15 14 13   1 2 3 4 5

ISBN: 978-1-59233-540-4

Digital edition published in 2013
eISBN: 978-1-61058-610-8

This book is a compilation of two previously published books, *500 High-Fiber Recipes* (2009) and *500 Low-Cholesterol Recipes* (2009).

Library of Congress Cataloging-in-Publication Data available

Printed and bound in USA

The information in this book is for educational purposes only. It is not intended to replace the advice of a physician or medical practitioner. Please see your health care provider before beginning any new health program.

This book is dedicated to all the people who have helped me reach this point in my writing life, from my mother who taught me to cook, to my wife and kids who dealt with the failed experiments in addition to the successes, the people at Fair Winds Press and the Quayside Publishing Group, and all the loyal newsletter subscribers who have provided inspiration and suggestions.

Contents

What Do We Mean By Heart Healthy?

First let's define exactly what we mean by heart-healthy recipes and how this collection is different from other cookbooks you may have or have seen. Heart-healthy diets are aimed at preventing or reducing a number of risk factors that can lead to heart attacks and heart disease. Among the more important ones are coronary artery disease, high cholesterol and high blood pressure.

The American Heart Association lists seven key items for maintaining cardiovascular health. They are:

- Don't smoke

- Maintain a healthy weight

- Engage in regular physical activity

- Eat a healthy diet

- Manage blood pressure

- Take charge of cholesterol

- Keep blood sugar, or glucose, at healthy levels.

You can easily see that while they list diet as a separate factor, what you eat affects everything on the list except smoking and exercise. If you start digging into the details of dietary recommendations for staying a healthy weight, maintaining a healthy blood pressure and cholesterol level, and managing blood sugar levels you immediately find that the same recommendations are key to many or all of them. Common themes at such diverse web sites as the Centers for Disease Control and Prevention, the U.S. Department of Agriculture, the American Heart Association, the Mayo Clinic and WebMD include:

- Limit the amount of unhealthy fats such as saturated fats and trans fats that you eat

- Choose lean sources of protein

- Eat more whole grains

- East more fruits and vegetables

- Limit your sodium intake

- Limit your cholesterol intake.

We'll go into more detail on what these recommendations mean and how to follow them in the next chapter.

Given the importance of the topic, there are of course a number of heart-healthy cookbooks available. I have quite a few myself and some of them have a number of really good recipes. But what I've found in looking at them is that most of them focus on one or another aspect of heart healthy cooking and tend to ignore the others. So you'll find a book that has pages of great information on lower fat substitutions, but still includes a number of high sodium ingredients for which there are equally easy-to-find substitutions. Another book may focus on including more whole grains, but have recipes that are high in saturated fat. Or they give you a small number of recipes. It seemed to me that what was needed was one book that took all the aspects of heart-healthy cooking into consideration and gave you enough recipes that you could always find what you were looking for: a one stop shop for heart-healthy cooking. That is what this book is. It contains healthy versions of some things that may already be family favorites like fried chicken, meatloaf, and pizza as well as things that you may not have thought about, such as roasted chickpeas and bean pie.

Why Is Heart-Healthy Cooking Important?

According to the U.S. Department of Health and Human Services' Centers for Disease Control and Prevention, heart disease is the number one cause of death in the United States among both men and women. A few statistics from their website show:

- In 2008, over 616,000 people died of heart disease, almost 25% of deaths in the United States.

- In that same year, 405,309 people died from coronary heart disease.

- Every year about 785,000 Americans have a first coronary attack. Another 470,000 who have already had one or more coronary attacks have another attack.

- In 2010, coronary heart disease alone was projected to cost the United States $108.9 billion. This total includes the cost of health care services, medications, and lost productivity.

- More than 27 million adults in the United States have been diagnosed with heart disease.

Clearly heart health is a major problem. Statistics in other parts of the world vary, but in many countries heart disease is also the number one cause of death.

A Little Bit about Me

Some of you may already know me from my Low-Sodium Cooking website and newsletter or from my other books focused on low-sodium and other heart-healthy recipes. For those who don't, perhaps a little background information might be useful.

I started thinking about heart-healthy cooking after being diagnosed with congestive heart failure in 1999. One of the first, and biggest, things I had to deal with was the doctor's insistence that I follow a low-sodium diet . . . 1,200 mg a day or less. At first, like many people, I found it easiest to just avoid the things that had a lot of sodium in them. But I was bored. And I was convinced that there had to be a way to create low-sodium versions of the foods I missed. So I learned all kinds of *new* cooking things. I researched where to get low-sodium substitutes for the things that I couldn't have anymore, bought cookbooks, and basically redid my whole diet. And I decided to share this information with others who may be in the same position I had been in. I started a website, www.lowsodiumcooking.com, to share recipes and information. I sent out an email newsletter with recipes that now has more than 20,000 subscribers. And I wrote my first book, *500 Low Sodium Recipes*.

Perhaps the best way to start telling you who I am is by telling you who I'm not. I'm not a doctor. I'm not a dietician. I'm not a professional chef. What I *am* is an ordinary person just like you who has some special dietary needs. I have enjoyed cooking most of my life. I guess I started it seriously about the time my mother went back to work when I was twelve or so. In those days, it was simple stuff like burgers and hot dogs and spaghetti. But the interest stayed. After I married my wife, we got pretty involved in some food-related pursuits—growing vegetables in our garden, making bread and other baked goods, canning and jelly making, that kind of thing. She always said that my "mad chemist" cooking was an outgrowth of the time I spent in college as a chemistry major, and she might be right. So creating the kind of food that people said couldn't be done, low in sodium and high in taste, was a fun challenge for me.

Along the way, I also learned about other things that make a diet heart healthy. I became more aware of cholesterol, fiber, and other things that make some foods better for your heart than others. I began incorporating what I'd learned into the recipes. So you will find that the recipes here are not only low in sodium, but they also tend to be low in saturated fat, contain whole grains and other high-fiber foods, and tend to focus on fresh ingredients. This all actually comes together nicely, because in many cases the same foods that fit one of those requirements also support others.

How Is the Nutritional Information Calculated?

The nutritional information included with these recipes was calculated using the AccuChef program. It calculates the values using the latest U.S. Department of Agriculture National Nutrient Database for Standard Reference. I've been using this program since I first started trying to figure out how much sodium was in the recipes I've created. It's inexpensive, easy to use, and has a number of really handy features. For instance, if I go in and change the nutrition figures for an ingredient, it remembers those figures whenever I use that ingredient. AccuChef is available online from www.accuchef.com. They offer a free trial version if you want to try it out and the full version costs less than twenty dollars.

Of course, this implies that these figures are estimates. Every brand of tomatoes, or any other product, is a little different in nutritional content. These figures were calculated using products that I buy here in southern Maryland. If you use a different brand, your nutrition figures may be different. Use the nutritional analysis as a guideline in determining whether a recipe is right for your diet.

1

What Does Eating Heart Healthy Mean (And How Can You Do It)?

In this chapter I'm going to take a more in-depth look at the aspects of heart-healthy cooking that we identified in the introduction. For each one I'll talk about how the recipes in this book support that dietary guideline. Then I'll give you a list of suggested foods to include and food to avoid.

Eat the Right Amount of the Right Kinds of Fats

Fats are one of the big factors in heart-healthy cooking. There are several areas that we want to be aware of here.

Reduce Saturated Fats

Saturated fats have been shown by a number of studies to be one of the major contributors to high cholesterol and arterial disease.

In general, saturated fats are fats that are solid at room temperature. There are several categories of saturated fats. In each case there are better alternatives or things we can do to reduce the fat. The recipes in this book are designed with that in mind.

- Red meats—Beef, pork and lamb have been mentioned often as being the worst in terms of saturated fat. It's true that they tend to have more than fish or poultry. How much they have is very dependent on which cut you choose. Some high-fat cuts of beef may contain 5 times the amount of saturated fat as a lean cut. This book contains recipes using lean cuts of beef and pork such as extra lean ground beef and pork loin.

- Poultry skin—While not containing as much saturated fat as red meat, poultry skin does have a significant amount. A chicken thigh with the skin has more than 2 grams additional saturated fat, compared to the meat only. And this is a case where eliminating that fat is really easy, just don't eat the skin. We also have many recipes here which use low fat boneless, skinless chicken breasts.

- Whole fat dairy products—Dairy products are another area where making smart choices can significantly reduce the amount of saturated fat you ingest. Avoid using products made from whole milk or cream. Choose skim milk, reduced fat cheeses, and fat free versions of sour cream and cream cheese. Use fat free evaporated milk in place of cream.

- Tropical oils—Some plant oils in the category typically called tropical oil also contain saturated fats. These include palm, palm kernel, and coconut oils and cocoa butter. They are generally easy to avoid.

Reduce Trans Fats

Trans fats are also called trans-fatty acids. They are produced by adding hydrogen to vegetable oil through a process called hydrogenation. This makes the fat more solid and less likely to spoil. Commonly found trans fats include:

- Margarine and other hydrogenated oils—Avoid margarine and solid shortening containing hydrogenated or partially hydrogenated oils.

- Commercial baked goods and fried foods—Although increased awareness of their health risks have started to reduce their use, trans fats are still a common ingredient in baked goods and fried foods. Food manufacturers are required to list trans fat content on nutrition labels.

Avoid the use of trans fats as much as possible. Use olive oil for cooking and canola oil for baking in place of solid fats.

Reduce the Total Fat Intake

While some fats are healthier than others and do provide benefits, it is still recommended that less than 10 percent of your total calories come from fat. Reduce consumption of fried foods and high fat baked goods. Replace some or all of the fat in baked goods with fruit.

Here also some positive fat choices you can make.

- Olive and canola oils—While we want to limit the amount of fats in our diet, oils like olive and canola oil contain polyunsaturated fat, which is the most healthful kind. Recipes in this book that contain oil specify either olive or canola.

- Fish—The oils contained in fish contain a compound called Omega 3 fatty acids that actually help to reduce blood vessel blockages and clots. It's often recommended that you eat fish at least twice a week.

- Increase consumption of Omega-3 fatty acids. Again, eat more fish. Adds nuts to baked goods and salads for an extra Omega-3 boost.

Eat More Whole Grains and High Fiber Foods

There have been a number of studies showing the benefits of increasing our fiber intake, both to heart health and other areas. A few key findings were:

- A study published in the May 11, 2000 issue of *The New England Journal of Medicine* reported that diabetic patients who maintained a very high fiber level in their daily diet lowered their glucose levels by 10%.

- A 1976 by the Veterans Administration Medical Center, Lexington, Kentucky, showed that fiber is useful in treating diabetes, high blood pressure and obesity, and in reducing cholesterol levels.

- Two studies published in *The Lancet* showed that people with high fiber diets suffered from fewer incidents of colon polyps and colon cancer.

So there are a lot of good reasons to add more fiber to your diet. There are several key areas for increasing fiber.

- Add more whole grains to the diet. Eat whole grain breads and other baked goods. Replace white rice with brown. Choose whole grain pastas over regular. In many cases you'll find that the whole grain version is not only healthier, but better tasting.

- Increase the amount of other water soluble fiber in the diet, such as oat bran and barley.

- Eat more legumes. Beans and other legumes are the poster child for high fiber foods. A single serving can provide 15 grams or more of fiber. They also have been proven to be one of the foods that is effective at keeping you from feeling hungry the longest and have been linked to reduced risk of heart disease, diabetes and certain kinds of cancer.

Eat Minimally Processed Foods

There has been an increased focus on avoiding processed foods in recent years. It has resulted in things like the caveman diet and Paleolithic diet. I'm not going to go so far as to suggest that, but I will say that I believe processing reduces natural nutrients and replaces them with chemicals, some of questionable safety. The Canyon Ranch Spa cookbook I own suggests "don't eat anything your great-grandmother didn't," and that seems like a reasonable approach to me. To do this, follow these guidelines.

- Eat foods as close to the way they grow as possible. Fresh is better than frozen. Whole is better than juice. Real potatoes are better than fried chips. It's really a simple rule that can make a lot of difference.

- Avoid refined and processed food as much as possible. Eat whole grains rather than white flour. Eat natural sweeteners rather than white sugar and high fructose corn syrup.

- Avoid things that contain added chemicals as much as possible.

- Increase your use of colorful fruits and vegetables. I know it sounds funny, but a key to the nutritional value of fruits and vegetables seems to be bright colors. Red peppers contain an incredible amount of vitamin A. Greens such as spinach, kale, and Swiss chard contain more nutrients per ounce than any other food. Brightly colored fruits tend to be high in antioxidants. Eating a variety of fruits and vegetables and eating at least the recommended five servings a day is one of the best things you can do for your health. There's truth in that old saying that an apple a day keeps the doctor away.

Reduce Your Sodium Intake

As many of you who are familiar with my other books or my website may know, reducing sodium was the first goal of my heart-healthy cooking journey. To me this is now obvious and second nature. After 11 years on a low sodium diet I can't imagine eating any other way. The fact that I feel so much better now than I did when I first started it is enough proof for me. But you don't have to rely on my word alone:

- The United States Food and Drug Administration recommends 2300 milligrams (mg) of sodium daily for healthy adults.

- The U.S. Department of Agriculture recommends that individuals with hypertension, African Americans and adults 50 and above should consume no more than 1500 mg of sodium per day.

- The United Kingdom Recommended Nutritional Intake (RNI) is 1600 mg daily.

- The National Research Council of the National Academy of Sciences recommends 1100 to 1500 mg daily for adults.

- Many experts recommend less than 1500 mg daily for anyone with a history of heart trouble, high blood pressure or other risk factors for heart disease.

- It's estimated that the average daily intake in the United States and Western Europe is 3 to 5 times these recommendations.

Given these figures, it's pretty safe to say that many of us consume more sodium than is good for us. If you already have a history of heart disease, or have a family history of it, it's even worse. I know I sound a bit like a zealot on this, but I can honestly say that I'm in a better position now medically than I was 11 years ago. All I can say is it's worked for me and lots of other people I've talked to.

I've tried not to be a fanatic about sodium content in these recipes. There are a couple that have more sodium than I would typically eat. There are recipes with foods I rarely or never use, such as Cheddar cheese and regular sodium-based baking powder. I'm not going to tell you that you have to be as strict as I am. But I honestly believe you'll be healthier and feel better if you watch your sodium.

Reduce Dietary Cholesterol

Although there has been some disagreement about how significant the role of eating foods high in cholesterol is in increasing your blood cholesterol, most experts still recommend reducing it. Common sources of dietary cholesterol are:

- Egg yolks—Personally I almost never use whole eggs, preferring to use an egg substitute like Egg Beaters that is made from egg whites. I can't tell the difference. The recipes in this book do contain eggs, but you can substitute $1/4$ cup egg substitute per egg and save a lot of cholesterol.

- Organ meats—Good news for everyone who hates liver (I happen to like it, but only eat it once every couple of months).

- Shellfish—Another thing I like but try to limit.

What to Eat and What to Avoid

The following are general guidelines for making heart-healthy food selections. Even when you follow these recommendations, you also need to be a careful label reader; there are big variations within some categories, with specific products being either better or worse than the average.

- Breads
  - Better: Homemade, wheat, pumpernickel, and other types of whole grain breads and rolls
  - Avoid: Sweet rolls, breads or rolls with salted tops, packaged cracker or bread crumb coatings unless unsalted, packaged stuffing mixes, biscuits, cornbread

- Cereals
  - Better: Whole grain cooked cereals such as oats, cream of wheat, rice, or farina; puffed wheat; puffed rice; shredded wheat
  - Avoid: Instant hot cereals, heavily sweetened cereals

- Pasta and carbohydrates
  - Better: Whole grain pastas such as macaroni, spaghetti, rigatoni, ziti; potatoes; brown rice
  - Avoid: Macaroni and cheese mix; seasoned rice, noodle, and spaghetti mixes

- Dried beans and peas
  - Better: Pinto beans, Great Northern beans, black-eyed peas, lima beans, lentils, split peas, etc.
  - Avoid: Any beans or peas prepared with ham, bacon, salt pork, or bacon grease; canned beans unless no-salt-added

- Meat, poultry, and fish
  - Better: Fresh or frozen lean meat, poultry, and fish
  - Avoid: High fat meats; poultry skin; salted, smoked, canned, and pickled meats, poultry, and fish; cold cuts; luncheon meats; hot dogs; breaded frozen meats, fish, and poultry; TV dinners; meat pies

- Fruits and vegetables
  - Better: Fresh, frozen, or low-sodium canned vegetables or vegetable juices; low-sodium tomato products; fresh, canned, or frozen fruits and juices
  - Avoid: Regular canned vegetables and vegetable juices, regular tomato sauce and tomato paste, olives, pickles, relishes, sauerkraut, or vegetables packed in brine

- Dairy products
  - Better: Low fat milk, sour cream, cheese, yogurt, low-sodium cottage cheese
  - Avoid: Full fat dairy products, buttermilk, processed cheese slices and spreads, regular cheese, cottage cheese

- Fats and oils
  - Better: Healthy oils such as canola and olive, unsalted butter when solid shortening is needed
  - Avoid: Margarine and other solid fats

- Soups
  - Better: Salt-free soups and low-sodium bouillon cubes
  - Avoid: Regular commercially canned or prepared soups, stews, broths, or bouillon; packaged and frozen soups

- Condiments
  - Better: Fresh and dried herbs; lemon juice; mustard, vinegar, and hot pepper sauce; low-sodium or no-salt-added ketchup; extracts (almond, lemon, vanilla); baking chocolate and cocoa; seasoning blends that do not contain salt
  - Avoid: Table salt, lite salt, bouillon cubes, regular ketchup, chili sauce; cooking wines, onion salt, garlic salt, meat flavorings, meat tenderizers, steak and barbecue sauce, seasoned salt, monosodium glutamate (MSG), Dutch-processed cocoa

Comments on a Few Specific Ingredients

- Eggs—Even though the recipes call for eggs I often use egg substitute instead. I started this as a way to reduce the amount of cholesterol I was taking in, especially since I have eggs for breakfast fairly often. The brand I use does have 25 mg more sodium than whole eggs, so there is a tradeoff. If cholesterol isn't an issue for you, it's cheaper and easier to just use whole eggs. I use a store brand egg substitute that is similar to Egg Beaters. It's basically colored egg whites with some vitamins and minerals, so it does not contain a lot of unnatural ingredients. You could also just use egg whites in most of the recipes, but I'm the kind of guy whose mother did too good of a job teaching me to clean my plate and I have a tough time just throwing the yolks away. The "real" whites have more sodium than the yolks do, by the way, so you don't save any sodium by doing that.

- Butter vs. margarine—The recipes in this book call for unsalted butter. I've been back and forth over the years about butter or margarine, but my current thinking is that the amount of cholesterol in the butter does not outweigh the possible health effects of the trans fats in margarine.

- Milk—The recipes call for skim milk and nonfat dairy products when they are readily available, reduced fat ones when they are not. This is another area where I thought I couldn't stand the taste of things like skim milk, but found after using it that it really was just fine. I use fat free evaporated milk in place of cream wherever it is called for. This is a great product for reducing fat and calories while still allowing you the taste and feel of the original.

- Baking powder and baking soda—In my humble opinion, this is a no-brainer. If you bake anything that uses baking powder with the regular stuff off your grocer's shelves you are eating sodium that can easily be avoided. Given the amount of sodium in standard baking powder, it's likely to be 100 to 200 mg per serving. Some doctors also believe the aluminum in regular baking powder is bad for you. The simple solution is sodium-free, aluminum-free baking powder. There are several brands available, but they have been difficult to find locally. I've found the Featherweight brand at a health food store. It's also available online at Healthy Heart Market. The price is comparable to regular baking powder. Recently Clabber Girl released a reduced sodium version of their Rumford baking powder. It's not sodium-free like the Featherweight, but it does contain significantly less sodium than regular baking powder and is widely available at Wal-Mart and other grocery chains. Like baking powder, regular baking soda is unnecessary sodium intake. The only brand of sodium-free baking soda I'm familiar with is Ener-G and the only place I've seen it is online at Healthy Heart Market. The manufacturer does recommend doubling the amount of baking soda called for in your favorite recipes when using this product. The recipes in this book already have the amount doubled. I've used both products for more than eleven years. The baking powder has never failed to produce the desired results. The baking soda sometimes doesn't seem to rise as much as I would have expected. I don't know whether that's because mine has gotten old or whether it has to do with particular recipes, but it's something to be aware of.

- Seasoning blends—You'll likely be able to find some salt-free versions of these on your regular grocer's shelves. Mrs. Dash makes a number of different blends that are widely available, and major spice manufacturers like McCormick do also. Many spices come in bottles small enough to be exempt from the usual labeling requirements in the United States, so you'll need to read the ingredient list and look for added salt. Health food stores often stock salt-free spice blends, and there are a number of places to get them online.

- Sauces and condiments—In looking at products like barbecue sauce, Asian sauces, ketchup, mustard, and salsa, you'll find a wide range of nutritional values. Many are very high in sodium. Look for products that are lower in sodium, either on your grocer's shelves or online.

- Canned tomato products, vegetables, and beans—In the United States, most of the large food companies like Hunt's and Del Monte make these low sodium products. I have no trouble finding a good selection of no-salt-added tomato products and a more limited selection of other no-salt-added vegetables in any large supermarket. Beans are less common and are another area where organic food producers are leading the way. With a little more effort you can cook your own dried beans without salt for a fraction of the cost of the canned ones. I usually cook a 1-pound bag at a time and freeze what I don't need for future use.

- Soups, broths, and bouillon—Like other products, low-sodium versions of these are available, but not as widely as we might like. Again, organic food producers are the best bet for finding a truly low-sodium item. There are also some very low-sodium soup bases from companies like Redi-Base available online. These come in a variety of flavors and have a much more natural taste than the sodium-free bouillon cubes.

- Bread—Pick whole grain commercial bread, but be aware of the amount of fat and sodium. I highly recommend a bread machine so you can make your own. The notes in Chapter 21 go into this in detail, and the chapter contains a number of recipes to get you started.

- Meats—Choose lean cuts of meat and preparations that are appropriate for them. Avoid high fat red meats and poultry skin. Also be aware that these days, many fresh meats are "enhanced" by injecting them with a broth solution to make them juicer. Unfortunately, it also increases the sodium level from 75 to 80 mg per serving to more than 300 mg. This is especially true of chicken and turkey and increasingly true of pork. There is still unadulterated meat around, but you have to be careful and look for it.

- Alcohol—There are some recipes in this book that contain beer, wine or other alcohol. I realize that these will not be right for everyone. There are some alternatives that will still let you enjoy the recipes. "Non-alcoholic" beers and wines have had most of the alcohol removed. Typically they contain about one half of one percent alcohol. I've seen it stated that this is about the same as what occurs naturally in orange juice, but I've never seen any conclusive proof of this. You'll have to decide if that is acceptable to you or not. Many of the recipes made with beer or white wine could have chicken broth substituted with no ill effects. For recipes made with red wine, you could replace it with grape juice, adding a few tablespoons of vinegar to counteract the sweetness, although the final flavor may be a little different. In some recipes you may also choose to omit the alcohol. One note . . . if you decide to use wine in cooking, do not buy the cooking wine in the supermarket. It is poor quality and contains added salt, which will affect the taste of the recipe. You'd be better off leaving it out. The rule I heard and follow is if you wouldn't drink it, don't cook with it.

A Final Quick Summary

Based on all of the above it's pretty easy to put together a short list a couple of general guidelines for things that we want to see more of in our diet:

- Fresh whole foods such as produce and fresh lean meats

- Brightly colored fruits and vegetables

- Whole grains

- Legumes, including lentils, soybeans, dried peas, and beans

We can also come up with a high level list of those things that we want to limit:

- Refined, processed foods such as white flour and sugar

- Packaged foods, which often contain ingredients you would be better off without

- Saturated fats and trans fats

And finally, there are a few recommendations for tracking the amount of various foods that would make up a heart healthy diet.

- Eat 6 to 8 daily servings of grain products, with at least half being whole grains.

- Eat 4 to 5 cups of fruits and vegetables each day, in a variety of colors and types.

- Eat 2 to 3 cups of fat-free or low-fat dairy products each day.

- Eat 3 to 6 oz. (cooked) of lean meats, poultry, or seafood per day.

- Limit intake to 2 to 3 servings per day of fats and oils. Use liquid vegetable oils most often to reduce saturated and trans fats.

- Eat 3 to 5 servings per week of nuts, seeds, and legumes.

- Limit cholesterol intake to 300 mg per day for people with no heart disease risk factors or to 200 mg per day for those with heart disease risk factors.

- Eat less than 2300 mg of sodium per day, 1500 mg per day if you have any heart disease history or risk factors.

2

Sauces, Condiments, Mixes, and Spice Blends

It's sometimes hard to find healthy commercial products in this category. Most sauces and dressings and a number of spice blends contain high amounts of sodium. Sauces and mixes tend to contain more fat than you'd want and sometimes still contain trans fats. But these are items that it is easy to create healthy versions of ahead of time so you can just grab them and use them when you need to. We have a wide variety of items in this chapter including Asian sauces, salad dressings and various other sauces and condiments. We also have a few spice blends that are targeted for grilling, but can be used on your favorite meat no matter how you are cooking it. And we end up with some healthy pancake and biscuit mixes.

Dick's Reduced-Sodium Soy Sauce

Soy sauce, even the reduced-sodium kinds, contains more sodium than many people's diets can stand. A teaspoonful often contains at least a quarter of the daily amount of sodium that is recommended for a healthy adult. If you have heart disease or are African American, the recommendation is even less. This sauce gives you real soy sauce flavor while holding the sodium to a level that should fit in most people's diets.

4 tablespoons (24 g) sodium-free beef bouillon

$^1/_4$ cup (60 ml) cider vinegar

2 tablespoons (30 ml) molasses

1$^1/_2$ cups (355 ml) boiling water

$^1/_8$ teaspoon (0.3 g) black pepper

$^1/_8$ teaspoon (0.2 g) ground ginger

$^1/_4$ teaspoon (0.8 g) garlic powder

$^1/_4$ cup (60 ml) reduced-sodium soy sauce

Combine ingredients, stirring to blend thoroughly. Pour into jars. Cover and seal tightly. Keeps indefinitely if refrigerated.

Yield: 48 servings

Per serving: 6 calories (13% from fat, 11% from protein, 76% from carbohydrate); 0 g protein; 0 g total fat; 0 g saturated fat; 0 g monounsaturated fat; 0 g polyunsaturated fat; 1 g carbohydrate; 0 g fiber; 1 g sugar; 3 mg phosphorus; 4 mg calcium; 0 mg iron; 52 mg sodium; 19 mg potassium; 3 IU vitamin A; 0 mg ATE vitamin E; 0 mg vitamin C; 0 mg cholesterol; 10 g water

Dick's Reduced-Sodium Teriyaki Sauce

The story on this recipe is the same as the soy sauce. In this case, you can sometimes find commercial teriyaki sauces that aren't too high in sodium, but this one is much lower and, to my mind, tastes just as good, if not better.

1 cup (235 ml) Dick's Reduced-Sodium Soy Sauce (see recipe on this page)

1 tablespoon (15 ml) sesame oil

2 tablespoons (30 ml) mirin wine

$^1/_2$ cup (100 g) sugar

2 cloves garlic, crushed

two $^1/_8$-inch (31-mm) slices ginger root

Dash black pepper

Combine all ingredients in a saucepan and heat until the sugar is dissolved. Store in the refrigerator.

Yield: 20 servings

Per serving: 37 calories (2% from fat, 0% from protein, 98% from carbohydrate); 0 g protein; 1 g total fat; 0 g saturated fat; 0 g monounsaturated fat; 2 g polyunsaturated fat; 84 g carbohydrate; 0 g fiber; 7 g sugar; 10 mg phosphorus; 7 mg calcium; 0 mg iron; 83 mg sodium; 32 mg potassium; 5 IU vitamin A; 0 mg ATE vitamin E; 0 mg vitamin C; 0 mg cholesterol; 17 g water

Tip: Mirin is a sweet Japanese rice wine; you can substitute sherry or sake.

Lower Fat Peppercorn Dressing

This is my favorite dressing recipe. It's similar to a ranch dressing, but with a little extra pop from the peppercorns.

1 cup (225 g) low fat mayonnaise

1 cup (235 ml) low fat buttermilk

2 teaspoons (0.2 g) dried parsley

1 teaspoon (3 g) onion powder

$^1/_4$ teaspoon (0.8 g) garlic powder

$^1/_4$ teaspoon (0.3 g) dried dill

1 teaspoon (1.7 g) black peppercorns, coarsely cracked

Mix all ingredients together well. Refrigerate overnight before using.

Yield: 16 servings

Per serving: 51 calories (87% from fat, 1% from protein, 12% from carbohydrate); 0 g protein; 5 g total fat; 1 g saturated fat; 0 g monounsaturated fat; 0 g polyunsaturated fat; 2 g carbohydrate; 0 g fiber; 1 g sugar; 10 mg phosphorus; 3 mg calcium; 0 mg iron; 120 mg sodium; 13 mg potassium; 42 IU vitamin A; 0 mg ATE vitamin E; 0 mg vitamin C; 5 mg cholesterol; 8 g water

Tip: You can crack the peppercorns by putting them in a plastic bag and beating on them with a mallet or rolling pin, so you might want to try this recipe on a day when you are feeling a need to release some frustration.

Onion Ranch Dressing

This dressing is better if you make it ahead of time and let it sit at least overnight so the herbs soften and the flavor develops.

$^1/_2$ cup (120 ml) buttermilk

1 cup (225 g) low fat mayonnaise

1 teaspoon (3 g) onion powder

1 teaspoon (0.1 g) dried parsley

$1^1/_2$ teaspoons (6 g) sugar

$^1/_2$ teaspoon (1.5 g) garlic powder

$^1/_2$ teaspoon (1.5 g) dry mustard

$^1/_4$ teaspoon (0.2 g) dried thyme

$^1/_4$ teaspoon (0.2 g) dried basil

$^1/_4$ teaspoon (0.3 g) dried oregano

$^1/_4$ teaspoon (0.3 g) dried rosemary

$^1/_4$ teaspoon (0.2 g) dried sage

$^1/_4$ teaspoon (0.5 g) freshly ground black pepper

Mix all the ingredients together. Store in the refrigerator in a tightly covered jar.

Yield: 12 servings

Per serving: 75 calories (81% from fat, 3% from protein, 16% from carbohydrate); 1 g protein; 7 g total fat; 1 g saturated fat; 0 g monounsaturated fat; 0 g polyunsaturated fat; 3 g carbohydrate; 0 g fiber; 2 g sugar; 22 mg phosphorus; 16 mg calcium; 0 mg iron; 170 mg sodium; 32 mg potassium; 53 IU vitamin A; 1 mg ATE vitamin E; 0 mg vitamin C; 7 mg cholesterol; 20 g water

Reduced-Fat Buttermilk Dressing

I've had a difficult time finding low fat buttermilk around here, but when I can, this is one of the things I make. You can also make this with nonfat buttermilk powder. You can vary the herbs depending on what you like.

$^1/_4$ cup (56 g) low fat mayonnaise

$^1/_2$ cup (120 ml) low fat buttermilk

1 tablespoon (10 g) onion, minced

2 teaspoons (2 g) dried dill

1 teaspoon (0.7 g) dried basil

1 tablespoon (0.4 g) dried parsley

$^1/_4$ teaspoon (0.8 g) garlic powder

$^1/_8$ teaspoon (0.3 g) cayenne pepper

Combine ingredients in a blender or food processor and process until smooth. Refrigerate several hours before serving to allow flavor to develop.

Yield: 6 servings

Per serving: 44 calories (71% from fat, 8% from protein, 21% from carbohydrate); 1 g protein; 4 g total fat; 1 g saturated fat; 0 g monounsaturated fat; 0 g polyunsaturated fat; 2 g carbohydrate; 0 g fiber; 2 g sugar; 28 mg phosphorus; 34 mg calcium; 0 mg iron; 102 mg sodium; 59 mg potassium; 123 IU vitamin A; 1 mg ATE vitamin E; 1 mg vitamin C; 4 mg cholesterol; 26 g water

Tip: Replacing one teaspoon (1 g) of the dill with oregano or Italian seasoning would give you a good ranch-type dressing.

Reduced-Fat Blue Cheese Dressing

I tried a number of recipes for blue cheese dressing when I first started low sodium cooking. The ones that were really low in sodium weren't all that tasty. The key seems to be the use of "real" blue cheese for flavor. Moving from there to a reduced-fat version was easier, by simply using low fat and fat-free products wherever available. This version has 5 total grams of fat per serving, compared to 11 grams in my original recipe.

2 ounces (55 g) blue cheese

1 cup (225 g) low fat mayonnaise

$^1/_2$ cup (115 g) fat-free sour cream

$^1/_2$ cup (120 ml) low fat buttermilk

Combine ingredients and chill overnight.

Yield: 20 servings

Per serving: 61 calories (80% from fat, 8% from protein, 12% from carbohydrate); 1 g protein; 5 g total fat; 1 g saturated fat; 0 g monounsaturated fat; 0 g polyunsaturated fat; 2 g carbohydrate; 0 g fiber; 1 g sugar; 29 mg phosphorus; 29 mg calcium; 0 mg iron; 144 mg sodium; 31 mg potassium; 68 IU vitamin A; 12 mg ATE vitamin E; 0 mg vitamin C; 9 mg cholesterol; 18 g water

Sun-Dried Tomato Vinaigrette

Nice flavor with a little more fat than most recipes here. But it's the good kind from olive oil, so I left it that way.

3 tablespoons (45 ml) white wine vinegar

1/4 cup (28 g) oil-packed sun-dried tomatoes, chopped

1 teaspoon (5 ml) Worcestershire sauce

1 clove garlic, minced

1/2 teaspoon (2 g) sugar

1/2 teaspoon (1 g) white pepper

1/4 cup (60 ml) olive oil

Shake ingredients together in a jar with a tight-fitting lid.

Yield: 8 servings

Per serving: 70 calories (91% from fat, 1% from protein, 8% from carbohydrate); 0 g protein; 7 g total fat; 1 g saturated fat; 5 g monounsaturated fat; 1 g polyunsaturated fat; 1 g carbohydrate; 0 g fiber; 0 g sugar; 6 mg phosphorus; 3 mg calcium; 0 mg iron; 16 mg sodium; 63 mg potassium; 45 IU vitamin A; 0 mg ATE vitamin E; 5 mg vitamin C; 0 mg cholesterol; 7 g water

Reduced-Fat Italian Dressing

This makes an Italian dressing that is every bit as good as the commercial ones, with less fat and fewer calories. It also has a lot less sodium for those who are watching their intake.

2 tablespoons (30 ml) olive oil

1/2 cup (120 ml) cider vinegar

2 tablespoons (30 g) Dijon mustard

1/2 teaspoon (1.5 g) garlic powder

1/2 teaspoon (1 g) black pepper

1/2 teaspoon (2 g) sugar

1 teaspoon (0.7 g) dried basil

1 teaspoon (1 g) dried oregano

1/2 teaspoon (0.6 g) dried rosemary

Combine all ingredients in a jar with a tight-fitting lid. Shake well.

Yield: 6 servings

Per serving: 51 calories (87% from fat, 3% from protein, 10% from carbohydrate); 0 g protein; 5 g total fat; 1 g saturated fat; 3 g monounsaturated fat; 1 g polyunsaturated fat; 1 g carbohydrate; 0 g fiber; 1 g sugar; 9 mg phosphorus; 11 mg calcium; 0 mg iron; 58 mg sodium; 33 mg potassium; 28 IU vitamin A; 0 mg ATE vitamin E; 0 mg vitamin C; 0 mg cholesterol; 23 g water

Creamy Raspberry Vinaigrette

A fresh and fruity creamy salad dressing that is excellent on fruit salads.

1 cup (230 g) plain fat-free yogurt

1/2 cup (55 g) raspberries

1 tablespoon (15 ml) red wine vinegar

2 tablespoons (26 g) sugar

In a blender, combine the yogurt, raspberries, vinegar, and sugar. Blend until smooth and refrigerate until chilled.

Yield: 6 servings

Per serving: 45 calories (3% from fat, 22% from protein, 76% from carbohydrate); 2 g protein; 0 g total fat;

0 g saturated fat; 0 g monounsaturated fat; 0 g polyunsaturated fat; 9 g carbohydrate; 1 g fiber; 8 g sugar; 67 mg phosphorus; 84 mg calcium; 0 mg iron; 32 mg sodium; 121 mg potassium; 6 IU vitamin A; 1 mg ATE vitamin E; 3 mg vitamin C; 1 mg cholesterol; 46 g water

Honey Mustard Cranberry Dressing

Here's a use for the leftover cranberry sauce that always seems to be the last thing left from Thanksgiving. You can use either the jellied or whole berry sauce.

1 1/2 tablespoons (22 g) honey mustard

2/3 cup (185 g) cranberry sauce

1/4 cup (60 ml) rice wine vinegar

1/4 cup (60 ml) olive oil

In a food processor mix together the mustard, cranberry sauce, and the rice wine vinegar. With the machine running, slowly pour in the oil until the dressing is thickened. Store, covered, in the refrigerator.

Yield: 12 servings

Per serving: 65 calories (62% from fat, 1% from protein, 37% from carbohydrate); 0 g protein; 5 g total fat; 1 g saturated fat; 3 g monounsaturated fat; 1 g polyunsaturated fat; 6 g carbohydrate; 0 g fiber; 6 g sugar; 3 mg phosphorus; 2 mg calcium; 0 mg iron; 26 mg sodium; 10 mg potassium; 8 IU vitamin A; 0 mg ATE vitamin E; 0 mg vitamin C; 0 mg cholesterol; 16 g water

Fat-Free Fajita Marinade

Marinate chicken or beef in this, then grill and slice thinly for easy fajitas. You won't miss the fat that is in most marinades at all.

1/4 cup (60 ml) red wine vinegar

2 tablespoons (30 ml) Worcestershire sauce

2 tablespoons (30 ml) lemon juice

2 tablespoons (30 ml) lime juice

1/2 teaspoon (1 g) black pepper

1 tablespoon (4 g) cilantro

1 tablespoon (7 g) cumin

1 teaspoon (3 g) garlic powder

1 teaspoon (1 g) dried oregano

Mix ingredients together and use to marinate beef or chicken at least 6 hours or overnight.

Yield: 8 servings

Per serving: 11 calories (15% from fat, 12% from protein, 73% from carbohydrate); 0 g protein; 0 g total fat; 0 g saturated fat; 0 g monounsaturated fat; 0 g polyunsaturated fat; 2 g carbohydrate; 0 g fiber; 0 g sugar; 11 mg phosphorus; 11 mg calcium; 1 mg iron; 39 mg sodium; 65 mg potassium; 47 IU vitamin A; 0 mg ATE vitamin E; 10 mg vitamin C; 0 mg cholesterol; 15 g water

Enchilada Sauce

You can make your own enchilada sauce that not only tastes better, but also is healthier than any you can buy in a can or jar. Plus, you can make it as mild or hot as you like. Dried chile peppers are available in the fresh food section of larger grocery stores. There are usually several varieties of varying heat levels. The most common are labeled New Mexico (spicy) or California (mild) chiles. The ones I get are 3 ounces (85 g) per bag, and I usually use one bag of each, giving a fairly mild sauce.

6 ounces (170 g) dried chiles

2 quarts (1.9 L) water

1 teaspoon (3 g) garlic, minced

Wash and remove the stems from the chiles, but do not remove the seeds. Placed washed chiles in a pot with just enough water to cover. If the chiles float, just push them down with a wooden spoon. Cook over medium heat for 45 minutes or until softened, adding water if necessary. Allow them to cool to a warm temperature. Remove chiles from the liquid and reserve liquid. Put chiles in a blender, and add a cup of liquid and the garlic. Start the blender on low and increase speed to high. Run the blender on high until the mixture is a smooth consistency (this may take 5 to 10 minutes). When the chiles are completely blended you should not see seeds. If the sauce is too thick, add water for a smoother consistency.

Yield: 32 servings

Per serving: 17 calories (14% from fat, 11% from protein, 75% from carbohydrate); 1 g protein; 0 g total fat; 0 g saturated fat; 0 g monounsaturated fat; 0 g polyunsaturated fat; 4 g carbohydrate; 2 g fiber; 2 g sugar; 9 mg phosphorus; 4 mg calcium; 0 mg iron; 7 mg sodium; 100 mg potassium; 1408 IU vitamin A; 0 mg ATE vitamin E; 2 mg vitamin C; 0 mg cholesterol; 60 g water

Chipotle Marinade

Depending on the peppers you use, this can be hot or not. The ancho chiles are less hot than some. A serving is one tablespoon.

2 ounces (55 g) dried ancho chiles

1 teaspoon (2 g) black pepper

2 teaspoons (4.7 g) cumin

2 tablespoons (8 g) fresh oregano, chopped

1 small red onion, quartered

$^1/_2$ cup (120 ml) lime juice

$^1/_2$ cup (120 ml) cider vinegar

3 cloves garlic, peeled

1 cup (60 g) fresh cilantro

$^1/_2$ cup (120 ml) olive oil

Soak dry chiles in water overnight, or until soft. Remove seeds. Place chiles and remaining ingredients in a food processor or blender and process until smooth.

Yield: 32 servings

Per serving: 39 calories (79% from fat, 3% from protein, 18% from carbohydrate); 0 g protein; 4 g total fat; 0 g saturated fat; 2 g monounsaturated fat; 0 g polyunsaturated fat; 2 g carbohydrate; 1 g fiber; 0 g sugar; 7 mg phosphorus; 8 mg calcium; 0 mg iron; 2 mg sodium; 67 mg potassium; 467 IU vitamin A; 0 mg ATE vitamin E; 2 mg vitamin C; 0 mg cholesterol; 11 g water

Chipotle Sauce

This creamy sauce can be used in a number of dishes and is traditional for fish tacos.

$^1/_2$ cup (115 g) low fat mayonnaise

$^1/_2$ cup (115 g) fat-free sour cream

$^1/_4$ cup (60 ml) Chipotle Marinade (see recipe page 30)

Mix ingredients and chill.

Yield: 10 servings

Per serving: 56 calories (82% from fat, 4% from protein, 14% from carbohydrate); 0 g protein; 4 g total fat; 1 g saturated fat; 0 g monounsaturated fat; 0 g polyunsaturated fat; 2 g carbohydrate; 0 g fiber; 1 g sugar; 18 mg phosphorus; 13 mg calcium; 0 mg iron; 101 mg sodium; 22 mg potassium; 67 IU vitamin A; 12 mg ATE vitamin E; 0 mg vitamin C; 9 mg cholesterol; 16 g water

Spinach Pesto Sauce

A delicious variation on pesto, this makes a perfect sauce for whole wheat pasta.

10 ounces (280 g) frozen spinach, thawed and drained

$^1/_2$ teaspoon crushed garlic

$^1/_4$ cup (25 g) grated Parmesan cheese

$^1/_4$ cup (27 g) almonds

$^1/_2$ cup (30 g) fresh parsley

$^1/_2$ cup (120 ml) olive oil

$^1/_4$ teaspoon black pepper, fresh ground

Process the above ingredients in food processor or blender. Serve over pasta.

Yield: 4 servings

Per serving: 72 g water; 345 calories (85% from fat, 8% from protein, 7% from carb); 7 g protein; 34 g total fat; 5 g saturated fat; 23 g monounsaturated fat; 4 g polyunsaturated fat; 6 g carbohydrate; 4 g fiber; 1 g sugar; 130 mg phosphorus; 209 mg calcium; 2 mg iron; 172 mg sodium; 329 mg potassium; 9209 IU vitamin A; 7 mg vitamin E; 12 mg vitamin C; 6 mg cholesterol

Reduced-Fat Pesto

This makes a fairly typical pesto, but lower in fat and sodium than commercial ones.

2 cups (80 g) packed fresh basil

3 tablespoons (27 g) pine nuts

1 teaspoon (3 g) finely minced garlic

$^1/_4$ cup (25 g) grated Parmesan cheese

$^1/_4$ cup (60 ml) olive oil

Place basil leaves in small batches in food processor and process until well chopped (do about $^3/_4$ cup (30 g) at a time). Add one-third of the pine nuts and garlic and blend again. Add one-third of the Parmesan cheese; blend while slowly adding one-third of the olive oil, stopping to scrape down the sides of the container. Process until it forms a thick, smooth paste. Repeat until all ingredients are used; mix all batches together well. Pesto keeps in the refrigerator one week, or a few months in the freezer.

Yield: 12 servings

Per serving: 77 calories (73% from fat, 9% from protein, 18% from carbohydrate); 2 g protein; 7 g total fat; 1 g saturated fat; 4 g monounsaturated fat; 1 g

polyunsaturated fat; 4 g carbohydrate; 2 g fiber; 0 g sugar; 55 mg phosphorus; 142 mg calcium; 3 mg iron; 34 mg sodium; 208 mg potassium; 535 IU vitamin A; 2 mg ATE vitamin E; 4 mg vitamin C; 2 mg cholesterol; 1 g water

Tip: Serve over pasta or on toasted bread.

Reduced-Fat Sun-Dried Tomato Pesto

Just like the basil pesto, this is a healthier version than you can buy.

$^{1}/_{4}$ cup (40 g) walnuts

$^{1}/_{2}$ cup (55 g) oil-packed sun-dried tomatoes

$^{1}/_{4}$ cup (25 g) grated Parmesan cheese

$^{1}/_{2}$ teaspoon (1.5 g) minced garlic

2 tablespoons (30 ml) olive oil

$^{1}/_{4}$ teaspoon (0.5 g) pepper

Preheat oven to 375°F (190°C, or gas mark 5). Toast the nuts for 7 to 8 minutes; let cool. Drain the oil from the tomatoes. In a food processor, combine all ingredients. Process until smooth.

Yield: 8 servings

Per serving: 82 calories (78% from fat, 12% from protein, 10% from carbohydrate); 3 g protein; 8 g total fat; 1 g saturated fat; 4 g monounsaturated fat; 2 g polyunsaturated fat; 2 g carbohydrate; 1 g fiber; 0 g sugar; 53 mg phosphorus; 41 mg calcium; 0 mg iron; 66 mg sodium; 133 mg potassium; 107 IU vitamin A; 4 mg ATE vitamin E; 7 mg vitamin C; 3 mg cholesterol; 5 g water

Tip: Serve this as a spread for Italian bread, on a sandwich, or (my particular favorite) mixed with warm pasta.

Low Fat White Sauce

Use this recipe to help cut the calories in a variety of dishes calling for a white sauce, such as pastas, rice, casseroles, etc.

6 tablespoons (48 g) flour

3 cups (710 ml) skim milk, divided

$^{1}/_{4}$ teaspoon (0.6 g) ground nutmeg

1 egg

In a heavy medium saucepan, whisk flour to remove any lumps. Gradually add 1 cup (235 ml) milk, whisking until smooth. Add remaining 2 cups (475 ml) of milk and nutmeg. Cook over medium heat, whisking constantly, about 10 minutes, until mixture thickens and boils. Remove from heat. Whisk a little of the mixture into the egg. Then add the egg mixture to the rest of the white sauce mixture, whisking constantly. Season to taste.

Yield: 6 servings

Per serving: 88 calories (8% from fat, 32% from protein, 60% from carbohydrate); 7 g protein; 1 g total fat; 0 g saturated fat; 0 g monounsaturated fat; 0 g polyunsaturated fat; 13 g carbohydrate; 0 g fiber; 0 g sugar; 159 mg phosphorus; 183 mg calcium; 1 mg iron; 91 mg sodium; 85 mg potassium; 287 IU vitamin A; 7 mg ATE vitamin E; 1 mg vitamin C; 35 mg cholesterol; 120 g water

Tip: Can be made ahead, covered, and refrigerated. Reheat before using.

Low Fat Cheese Sauce

A low fat, full-flavored cheese sauce you can use over vegetables or for macaroni and cheese. The cream cheese gives it an extra richness.

2 cups (475 ml) skim milk

2 tablespoons (16 g) cornstarch

1 cup (120 g) low fat Cheddar cheese, shredded

8 ounces (225 g) fat free cream cheese, cubed

Combine the milk and the cornstarch in a saucepan. Bring slowly to almost the boiling point, stirring constantly. Cook at this temperature until the milk begins to thicken. Remove from heat and stir in the cheeses. Let stand until the cheese melts, then stir or whisk until smooth.

Yield: 4 servings

Per serving: 123 calories (20% from fat, 43% from protein, 37% from carbohydrate); 13 g protein; 3 g total fat; 2 g saturated fat; 1 g monounsaturated fat; 0 g polyunsaturated fat; 11 g carbohydrate; 0 g fiber; 0 g sugar; 298 mg phosphorus; 313 mg calcium; 0 mg iron; 275 mg sodium; 246 mg potassium; 318 IU vitamin A; 95 mg ATE vitamin E; 1 mg vitamin C; 9 mg cholesterol; 131 g water

Creamy Lemon Sauce

Another fat-free sauce, this one is great heated over fish or broccoli or as a topping for fruit.

1 cup (230 g) fat-free sour cream

1 teaspoon (1.7 g) grated lemon peel

2 tablespoons (30 ml) lemon juice

$^1/_2$ teaspoon (2 g) sugar

In a medium bowl, combine sour cream, lemon peel, lemon juice, and sugar; mix until well blended.

Yield: 6 servings

Per serving: 57 calories (0% from fat, 32% from protein, 68% from carbohydrate); 1 g protein; 0 g total fat; 0 g saturated fat; 0 g monounsaturated fat; 0 g polyunsaturated fat; 3 g carbohydrate; 0 g fiber; 1 g sugar; 39 mg phosphorus; 43 mg calcium; 0 mg iron; 17 mg sodium; 59 mg potassium; 151 IU vitamin A; 40 mg ATE vitamin E; 3 mg vitamin C; 16 mg cholesterol; 37 g water

Reduced-Fat Creamy Chicken Sauce

An easy white sauce recipe. The chicken broth and onion give it additional flavor.

2 tablespoons (20 g) onion, minced

$^1/_2$ cup (120 ml) low sodium chicken broth

$^1/_3$ cup (40 g) flour

2 cups (475 ml) skim milk

$^1/_2$ cup (120 ml) dry white wine

1 teaspoon (2 g) chicken bouillon

Cook onion and broth in a 1-quart (946-ml) saucepan until liquid is almost all cooked away. In a small bowl, whisk flour with the milk. Add to the onion mixture in the saucepan and continue to cook, whisking, until sauce begins to thicken. Add wine and bouillon and whisk to combine.

Yield: 4 servings

Per serving: 120 calories (6% from fat, 27% from protein, 67% from carbohydrate); 7 g protein; 1 g total fat; 0 g saturated fat; 0 g monounsaturated fat; 0 g polyunsaturated fat; 16 g carbohydrate; 0 g fiber; 1 g sugar; 165 mg phosphorus; 183 mg calcium; 1 mg iron; 91 mg sodium; 289 mg potassium; 250 IU vitamin A; 75 mg ATE vitamin E; 2 mg vitamin C; 2 mg cholesterol; 170 g water

Tip: This makes a good base for an Italian sauce, with the addition of some Italian seasoning and Parmesan cheese.

Cottage Cheese Sauce

This sounds a little strange, but it makes a nice creamy sauce with just a little cheese flavor, and it's fat-free.

1 cup (226 g) nonfat cottage cheese

1 cup (235 ml) skim milk

2 tablespoons (30 ml) water

2 tablespoons (16 g) cornstarch

In blender, blend cottage cheese and milk. Pour into a saucepan and heat almost to a boil. Set aside. Add the water to the cornstarch and mix to a paste. Add to cottage cheese mixture in saucepan and stir well. Cook 10 minutes, stirring constantly until thickened.

Yield: 4 servings

Per serving: 71 calories (4% from fat, 51% from protein, 45% from carbohydrate); 9 g protein; 0 g total fat; 0 g saturated fat; 0 g monounsaturated fat; 0 g polyunsaturated fat; 8 g carbohydrate; 0 g fiber; 1 g sugar; 107 mg phosphorus; 100 mg calcium; 0 mg iron; 42 mg sodium; 124 mg potassium; 136 IU vitamin A; 41 mg ATE vitamin E; 1 mg vitamin C; 4 mg cholesterol; 92 g water

Cabernet Sauce

This sauce is great served over steak. If you pan-fry the steak, you could use the same pan for the sauce, adding extra flavor.

$1/4$ cup (40 g) onion, chopped

$3/4$ cup (53 g) mushrooms, sliced

1 tablespoon (8 g) flour

$1/2$ cup (120 ml) cabernet sauvignon

$1/4$ cup (60 ml) low sodium chicken broth

1 tablespoon (2.7 g) dried thyme

Spray a medium-sized nonstick skillet with olive oil spray. Over medium heat, sauté onions and mushrooms until softened, about 4 to 5 minutes. Add flour to the skillet and mix with vegetables until dissolved. Raise the heat and add the wine. Cook 1 minute. Add the broth and thyme. Cook 4 minutes to reduce liquid and thicken. Add pepper to taste. Spoon sauce over steak.

Yield: 2 servings

Per serving: 87 calories (8% from fat, 19% from protein, 73% from carbohydrate); 2 g protein; 0 g total fat; 0 g saturated fat; 0 g monounsaturated fat; 0 g polyunsaturated fat; 9 g carbohydrate; 1 g fiber; 2 g sugar; 58 mg phosphorus; 40 mg calcium; 3 mg iron; 14 mg sodium; 230 mg potassium; 57 IU vitamin A; 0 mg ATE vitamin E; 3 mg vitamin C; 0 mg cholesterol; 122 g water

Roasted Red Pepper Sauce

I developed this sauce when I had a good crop of red Italian peppers in the garden. It's a simple sauce that is great over pasta or chicken.

4 red bell peppers

$^1/_2$ cup (115 g) fat-free sour cream

$^1/_4$ teaspoon (0.5 g) black pepper

$^1/_2$ teaspoon (1.6 g) garlic powder

Preheat broiler. Place peppers on a baking sheet and broil until the skin blackens and blisters, turning frequently. Place in a paper bag and seal until cooled to loosen skin. Remove skin and place peppers in a blender or food processor and process until smooth. Add remaining ingredients; blend well. May be heated or used cold over meat or pasta.

Yield: 6 servings

Per serving: 48 calories (7% from fat, 18% from protein, 75% from carbohydrate); 1 g protein; 0 g total fat; 0 g saturated fat; 0 g monounsaturated fat; 0 g polyunsaturated fat; 6 g carbohydrate; 2 g fiber; 3 g sugar; 40 mg phosphorus; 27 mg calcium; 0 mg iron; 11 mg sodium; 187 mg potassium; 2408 IU vitamin A; 20 mg ATE vitamin E; 95 mg vitamin C; 8 mg cholesterol; 85 g water

Tofu Mayonnaise

This recipe makes a low fat, almost sodium-free, egg-free mayo—or mayo substitute, I suppose, is more accurate. At any rate, it works well for dishes like potato or tuna salads where there tend to be other flavors that predominate, because it isn't quite the same flavor as real mayonnaise.

$^1/_2$ pound (225 g) firm tofu

$^1/_2$ teaspoon (1.5 g) dry mustard

$^1/_8$ teaspoon (0.3 g) cayenne pepper

2 tablespoons (30 ml) fresh lemon juice

2 tablespoons (30 ml) olive oil

2 tablespoons (30 ml) water

In a food processor or blender, process tofu, mustard, cayenne pepper, and lemon juice until mixed. With machine still running add oil very slowly and then add water. Blend until smooth. Stop the machine a few times during processing and scrape the sides. Keeps up to 3 months when refrigerated in an airtight container.

Yield: 12 servings

Per serving: 32 calories (76% from fat, 16% from protein, 8% from carbohydrate); 1 g protein; 3 g total fat; 0 g saturated fat; 2 g monounsaturated fat; 1 g polyunsaturated fat; 1 g carbohydrate; 0 g fiber; 0 g sugar; 17 mg phosphorus; 6 mg calcium; 0 mg iron; 7 mg sodium; 41 mg potassium; 8 IU vitamin A; 0 mg ATE vitamin E; 1 mg vitamin C; 0 mg cholesterol; 21 g water

Beer Mop

You can use this on any grilled or smoked meat, but it is particularly good on pork.

12 ounces (355 ml) beer

$^1/_2$ cup (120 ml) cider vinegar

$^1/_4$ cup (60 ml) olive oil

$^1/_2$ teaspoon (1.5 g) minced garlic

1 tablespoon (9 g) onion powder

1 tablespoon (15 ml) Worcestershire sauce

1 tablespoon (8 g) The Wild Rub or The Mild Rub (see recipes on this and following pages)

Combine ingredients in a saucepan and heat. Use warm on grilling or smoking meat.

Yield: 24 servings

Per serving: 29 calories (83% from fat, 2% from protein, 15% from carbohydrate); 0 g protein; 2 g total fat; 0 g saturated fat; 2 g monounsaturated fat; 0 g polyunsaturated fat; 1 g carbohydrate; 0 g fiber; 0 g sugar; 4 mg phosphorus; 2 mg calcium; 0 mg iron; 7 mg sodium; 15 mg potassium; 1 IU vitamin A; 0 mg ATE vitamin E; 1 mg vitamin C; 0 mg cholesterol; 18 g water

Smoky Chicken Rub

I recently discovered smoked paprika. It is wonderful to add a smoky flavor to food even if you aren't going to grill it. You should be able to find it in your local grocery store. This rub adds a great flavor to chicken, whether you grill it, smoke it, cook it on a rotisserie or just oven roast it.

3 tablespoons (21 g) smoked paprika

1 tablespoon (6.4 g) freshly ground black pepper

1 tablespoon (6.5 g) celery seed

1 tablespoon (13 g) sugar

1 tablespoon (9 g) dry mustard

1 tablespoon (9 g) onion powder

$1^1/_2$ teaspoons (4 g) poultry seasoning

1 tablespoon (2.7 g) dried thyme

Combine all ingredients, mixing well. Store in an airtight container. Makes enough for one large roasting chicken or two small chickens.

Yield: 8 servings

Per serving: 32 calories (21% from fat, 11% from protein, 68% from carbohydrate); 1 g protein; 1 g total fat; 0 g saturated fat; 0 g monounsaturated fat; 0 g polyunsaturated fat; 6 g carbohydrate; 2 g fiber; 2 g sugar; 23 mg phosphorus; 58 mg calcium; 3 mg iron; 4 mg sodium; 113 mg potassium; 1446 IU vitamin A; 0 mg ATE vitamin E; 3 mg vitamin C; 0 mg cholesterol; 1 g water

The Mild Rub

A sweeter, less spicy rub for grilling and smoking.

$^1/_2$ cup (56 g) paprika

2 tablespoons (13 g) freshly ground black pepper

$^1/_3$ cup (75 g) brown sugar

2 tablespoons (15 g) chili powder

2 tablespoons (18 g) onion powder

2 tablespoons (18 g) garlic powder

Mix well, and store in a cool, dark place.

Yield: 22 servings

Per serving: 28 calories (13% from fat, 9% from protein, 78% from carbohydrate); 1 g protein; 0 g total fat; 0 g saturated fat; 0 g monounsaturated fat; 0 g polyunsaturated fat; 6 g carbohydrate; 1 g fiber; 4 g sugar; 15 mg calcium; 1 mg iron; 10 mg sodium; 105 mg potassium; 1527 IU vitamin A; 0 mg ATE vitamin E; 3 mg vitamin C; 0 mg cholesterol

The Wild Rub

A traditional southern dry rub for barbecue, typically rubbed into the meat and allowed to flavor it overnight in the refrigerator before long, low heat cooking. The main ingredient is paprika, so if you plan to do a lot of grilling or smoking, you may want to get a big bottle at one of the warehouse clubs like Sam's or BJ's. The rub tends to be a bit on the spicy side, so if you don't like your food hot, you may want to try The Mild Rub (see previous page).

$^1/_2$ cup (56 g) paprika

3 tablespoons (19 g) freshly ground black pepper

$^1/_4$ cup (60 g) brown sugar

2 tablespoons (15 g) chili powder

2 tablespoons (18 g) onion powder

2 tablespoons (18 g) garlic powder

2 teaspoons (3.6 g) cayenne pepper

Mix well, and store in a cool, dark place.

Yield: 22 servings

Per serving: 26 calories (15% from fat, 10% from protein, 76% from carbohydrate); 1 g protein; 1 g total fat; 0 g saturated fat; 0 g monounsaturated fat; 0 g polyunsaturated fat; 6 g carbohydrate; 2 g fiber; 3 g sugar; 15 mg calcium; 1 mg iron; 10 mg sodium; 109 mg potassium; 1595 IU vitamin A; 0 mg ATE vitamin E; 3 mg vitamin C; 0 mg cholesterol; 1 g water

Bread and Butter Onions

Okay, I admit there isn't really anything about this recipe that is, by itself, particularly good for you. But I made a batch of these this summer after seeing them at an Amish stand at the local farmer's market, and I've become fond of them as a condiment with a number of things. They just add a nice little extra bit of flavor.

4 onions

$1^1/_4$ cups (300 ml) cider vinegar

$1^1/_4$ cups (250 g) sugar

$^1/_2$ teaspoon (1.1 g) turmeric

$^1/_2$ teaspoon (1.8 g) mustard seed

$^1/_4$ teaspoon (0.5 g) celery seed

Thinly slice onions and separate into rings. In a saucepan, combine vinegar, sugar, turmeric, mustard seed, and celery seed. Heat to boiling. Add onions. Heat 2 to 3 minutes. Chill and serve. May be stored in the refrigerator for one month. For longer storage, sterilize two pint (475 ml) jars. Pack hot pickles to within $^1/_2$ inch (1.3 cm) of the top. Wipe off the rim, screw on the lid, and place in a Dutch oven or other deep pan. Cover with hot water, bring to a boil, and cook 5 minutes.

Yield: 32 servings

Per serving: 41 calories (1% from fat, 2% from protein, 97% from carbohydrate); 0 g protein; 0 g total fat; 0 g saturated fat; 0 g monounsaturated fat; 0 g polyunsaturated fat; 10 g carbohydrate; 0 g fiber; 9 g sugar; 7 mg phosphorus; 6 mg calcium; 0 mg iron; 1 mg sodium; 38 mg potassium; 0 IU vitamin A; 0 mg ATE vitamin E; 1 mg vitamin C; 0 mg cholesterol; 27 g water

Homestyle Pancake Mix

Make up a batch of this mix and you'll always be ready to make pancakes in a flash.

6 cups (720 g) whole wheat pastry flour

1 1/2 cups (210 g) cornmeal

1/2 cup (100 g) sugar

1 1/2 cups (102 g) nonfat dry milk

2 tablespoons (28 g) baking powder

Combine all ingredients and store in tightly covered jar. To cook, add 1 cup water to 1 cup mix; use less water if you want a thicker pancake. Stir only until lumps disappear. Lightly coat a nonstick skillet or griddle with nonstick vegetable oil spray and preheat until drops of cold water bounce and sputter. Drop batter to desired size and cook until bubbles form and edges begin to dry. Turn only once.

Yield: 16 servings

Per serving: 7 g water; 256 calories (4% from fat, 14% from protein, 82% from carb); 9 g protein; 1 g total fat; 0 g saturated fat; 0 g monounsaturated fat; 0 g polyunsaturated fat; 55 g carbohydrate; 6 g fiber; 10 g sugar; 272 mg phosphorus; 196 mg calcium; 3 mg iron; 221 mg sodium; 314 mg potassium; 187 IU vitamin A; 45 mg vitamin E; 0 mg vitamin C; 1 mg cholesterol

Reduced Fat Biscuit Mix

This makes a mix similar to Reduced Fat Bisquick, but mine is even lower in fat. Use it in any recipes that call for baking mix.

6 cups (750 g) flour

3 tablespoons (41.5 g) baking powder

1/3 cup (75 g) unsalted butter

Stir flour and baking powder together. Cut in butter with pastry blender or two knives until mixture resembles coarse crumbs. Store in a container with a tight-fitting lid.

Yield: 12 servings

Per serving: 274 calories (19% from fat, 10% from protein, 72% from carbohydrate); 7 g protein; 8 g total fat; 4 g saturated fat; 1 g monounsaturated fat; 1 g polyunsaturated fat; 49 g carbohydrate; 2 g fiber; 0 g sugar; 146 mg phosphorus; 216 mg calcium; 3 mg iron; 422 mg sodium; 73 mg potassium; 267 IU vitamin A; 61 mg ATE vitamin E; 0 mg vitamin C; 10 mg cholesterol; 9 g water

Reduced-Fat Whole Wheat Biscuit Mix

Similar to the regular baking mix, but with the nutritional boost of whole grain flour. I use this one almost all the time in place of the white flour one.

4 cups (500 g) flour

2 cups (250 g) whole wheat flour

3 tablespoons (41.5 g) baking powder

$^1/_3$ cup (75 g) unsalted butter

Stir flours and baking powder together. Cut in butter with pastry blender or two knives until mixture resembles coarse crumbs. Store in a container with a tight-fitting lid.

Yield: 12 servings

Per serving: 266 calories (19% from fat, 11% from protein, 70% from carbohydrate); 7 g protein; 7 g total fat; 4 g saturated fat; 1 g monounsaturated fat; 1 g polyunsaturated fat; 47 g carbohydrate; 4 g fiber; 0 g sugar; 193 mg phosphorus; 220 mg calcium; 3 mg iron; 422 mg sodium; 132 mg potassium; 268 IU vitamin A; 61 mg ATE vitamin E; 0 mg vitamin C; 10 mg cholesterol; 8 g water

3

Dips and Spreads

This is another category where the commercial products are mostly a heart unhealthy bunch. They are often high in fat and sodium and very weak in anything providing real nutrition. Our solution here is to reconceive them in a healthier form. We have a large selection, something for everyone whether they like creamy dips, Middle Eastern, Southwestern, or just something to give you a nice burst of flavor without overwhelming your heart. Many of them feature fiber-boosting beans and other legumes. All are great when served with healthy fruit or vegetable dippers rather than chips or crackers.

Spinach and Artichoke Dip

This makes a nice dip for entertaining. It's similar to the dip served at a number of restaurants but lower in fat.

6 ounces (170 g) frozen chopped spinach, thawed and drained

7 ounces (210 g) artichoke hearts

2 ounces (55 g) fat-free cream cheese

$^1/_2$ cup (115 g) fat-free sour cream

$^1/_4$ teaspoon (0.8 g) garlic powder

2 tablespoons (10 g) grated Parmesan

$^1/_4$ cup (30 g) shredded low fat Monterey Jack cheese

Preheat broiler. Combine all ingredients in the bowl of a food processor. Process until smooth. Place in an oven-proof dish and broil until the top begins to brown.

Yield: 8 servings

Per serving: 69 calories (35% from fat, 31% from protein, 33% from carbohydrate); 4 g protein; 2 g total fat; 1 g saturated fat; 1 g monounsaturated fat; 0 3g polyunsaturated fat; 5 g carbohydrate; 2 g fiber; 0 g sugar; 82 mg phosphorus; 96 mg calcium; 1 mg iron; 110 mg sodium; 167 mg potassium; 2725 IU vitamin A; 32 mg ATE vitamin E; 2 mg vitamin C; 12 mg cholesterol; 60 g water

Tip: Serve with tortilla chips or French bread slices.

Artichoke Dip

This is the kind of appetizer you can serve to anyone, without any questions about what kind of diet you are on. It also is good just for the family when you want something to nibble on.

1 cup (225 g) low-fat mayonnaise

$^1/_2$ cup (50 g) grated Parmesan cheese

$^1/_4$ teaspoon Worcestershire sauce

$^1/_4$ teaspoon garlic powder

1 can artichoke hearts, chopped

Mix all ingredients but artichoke hearts until well blended. Add chopped hearts and mix. Bake at 350°F (180°C, gas mark 4) until lightly browned.

Yield: 8 servings

Per serving: 44 g water; 141 calories (74% from fat, 10% from protein, 16% from carb); 4 g protein; 12 g total fat; 3 g saturated fat; 1 g monounsaturated fat; 0 g polyunsaturated fat; 6 g carbohydrate; 1 g fiber; 2 g sugar; 82 mg phosphorus; 77 mg calcium; 0 mg iron; 352 mg sodium; 105 mg potassium; 132 IU vitamin A; 7 mg vitamin E; 2 mg vitamin C; 16 mg cholesterol

Tip: Spread warm on crackers.

Spinach Dip

Try this with one of our pita dippers.

8 ounces (225 g) cream cheese, softened

2 cups (300 g) grated Monterey Jack cheese

10 ounces (280 g) frozen spinach, thawed and squeezed dry

$^1/_2$ cup (90 g) finely chopped peeled tomato

$^3/_4$ cup (120 g) chopped onion

$^1/_3$ cup (71 ml) half and half

1 tablespoon finely chopped jalapeño pepper

For the dip, beat together the cheeses, spinach, tomato, onion, half and half and jalapeños in a mixing bowl until very smooth. Spread in a buttered dish and bake at 400°F (200°C, gas mark 6) for 20 to 25 minutes until bubbly. Serve hot, warm, or at room temperature, with dippers.

Yield: 10 servings

Per serving: 73 g water; 204 calories (73% from fat, 19% from protein, 8% from carb); 10 g protein; 17 g total fat; 11 g saturated fat; 5 g monounsaturated fat; 1 g polyunsaturated fat; 4 g carbohydrate; 1 g fiber; 1 g sugar; 168 mg phosphorus; 270 mg calcium; 1 mg iron; 241 mg sodium; 180 mg potassium; 4007 IU vitamin A; 140 mg vitamin E; 4 mg vitamin C; 51 mg cholesterol

Broccoli Dip

Yes, that's what it says: broccoli dip. It's sort of like guacamole with a southwestern flavor, only made with broccoli.

$1^1/_2$ cups (105 g) broccoli, cooked

$1^1/_2$ tablespoons (22 ml) lemon juice

$^1/_4$ teaspoon (0.6 g) cumin

$^1/_8$ teaspoon (0.4 g) garlic powder

$^1/_2$ cup (90 g) diced tomato

2 tablespoons (12 g) sliced scallions

1 tablespoon (7.5 g) canned jalapeno peppers

In a food processor, blend the broccoli with the lemon juice, cumin, and garlic powder until completely smooth. Add the remaining ingredients and mix well by hand. Chill before serving for best flavor.

Yield: 12 servings

Per serving: 6 calories (8% from fat, 22% from protein, 69% from carbohydrate); 0 g protein; 0 g total fat; 0 g saturated fat; 0 g monounsaturated fat; 0 g polyunsaturated fat; 1 g carbohydrate; 0 g fiber; 0 g sugar; 10 mg phosphorus; 7 mg calcium; 0 mg iron; 4 mg sodium; 58 mg potassium; 138 IU vitamin A; 0 mg ATE vitamin E; 12 mg vitamin C; 0 mg cholesterol; 19 g water

Low Fat Scallion Dip

This is not at all like the packaged onion dip mixes, but it's still very tasty, and it has a little more tang.

1 cup (225 g) low fat cottage cheese

$^1/_4$ cup (25 g) scallions, chopped

2 teaspoons (10 ml) lemon juice

Combine all ingredients in a blender or food processor and process until smooth. Refrigerate for at least an hour to give the flavors time to develop.

Yield: 8 servings

Per serving: 27 calories (19% from fat, 60% from protein, 21% from carbohydrate); 4 g protein; 1 g total fat; 0 g saturated fat; 0 g monounsaturated fat; 0 g polyunsaturated fat; 1 g carbohydrate; 0 g fiber; 0 g sugar; 44 mg phosphorus; 22 mg calcium; 0 mg iron; 115 mg sodium; 37 mg potassium; 53 IU vitamin A; 6 mg ATE vitamin E; 1 mg vitamin C; 2 mg cholesterol; 26 g water

Texas Cheese Dip

This dip is a little on the spicy side. You can add or decrease the jalapeños to make it suit your own desired heat.

3 ounces (85 g) cream cheese, room temperature

3 ounces (85 g) blue cheese, room temperature

8 ounces (225 g) sour cream

2$^1/_2$ teaspoons unflavored gelatin

$^1/_4$ cup (60 ml) water

2 tablespoons (28 ml) vinegar

2 jalapeño peppers, minced

1$^1/_4$ cups (138 g) chopped toasted pecans

2 ounces (55 g) pimento, drained and minced

Mix cheeses with sour cream until smooth. Add gelatin that has been softened in water and heated to dissolve. Add vinegar and let stand until slightly thickened. Add jalapeños, pecans, and pimento. Pour into mold that has been sprayed with nonstick vegetable oil spray and chill. Serve with crackers (Ritz are good). Garnish with fresh jalapeños, pimentos, or pecans.

Yield: 12 servings

Per serving: 36 g water; 156 calories (83% from fat, 9% from protein, 8% from carb); 4 g protein; 15 g total fat; 5 g saturated fat; 7 g monounsaturated fat; 3 g polyunsaturated fat; 3 g carbohydrate; 1 g fiber; 1 g sugar; 86 mg phosphorus; 72 mg calcium; 1 mg iron; 129 mg sodium; 112 mg potassium; 370 IU vitamin A; 58 mg vitamin E; 5 mg vitamin C; 20 mg cholesterol

Cheddar Bean Dip

Simple to make and sure to be a hit, this hot bean-and-cheese dip is great with tortilla chips or crispy wedges of pita bread.

$^1/_2$ cup (115 g) mayonnaise

2 cups (342 g) cooked pinto beans, drained and mashed

1 cup (115 g) shredded Cheddar cheese

4 ounces (115 g) chopped green chiles

$^1/_4$ teaspoon Tabasco sauce

Stir all ingredients until well mixed. Spoon into small ovenproof dish. Bake at 350°F (180°C, gas mark 4) for 30 minutes or until bubbly.

Yield: 12 servings

Per serving: 32 g water; 153 calories (64% from fat, 14% from protein, 22% from carb); 5 g protein; 11 g total fat; 3 g saturated fat; 3 g monounsaturated fat; 4 g polyunsaturated fat; 8 g carbohydrate; 3 g fiber; 0 g sugar; 102 mg phosphorus; 97 mg calcium; 1 mg iron; 159 mg sodium; 149 mg potassium; 149 IU vitamin A; 36 mg vitamin E; 3 mg vitamin C; 15 mg cholesterol

Cowboy Bean Dip

A variation on the usual layered dip, this one with black beans.

15 ounces (420 g) black beans

$^1/_4$ cup (40 g) finely chopped onion

2 tablespoons (28 ml) lime juice

$^1/_4$ teaspoon ground cumin

$^1/_2$ teaspoon finely chopped garlic

$^1/_8$ teaspoon black pepper

8 ounces (225 g) cream cheese, softened

$^1/_4$ cup (25 g) sliced scallions

Drain and rinse the beans. Mix all ingredients except cream cheese and scallions. Cover and refrigerate at least 2 hours. Spread cream cheese on serving plate. Spoon bean mixture evenly over cream cheese. Sprinkle with scallions.

Yield: 12 servings

Per serving: 48 g water; 127 calories (54% from fat, 15% from protein, 31% from carb); 5 g protein; 8 g total fat; 4 g saturated fat; 3 g monounsaturated fat; 0 g polyunsaturated fat; 10 g carbohydrate; 4 g fiber; 0 g sugar; 72 mg phosphorus; 36 mg calcium; 1 mg iron; 139 mg sodium; 164 mg potassium; 318 IU vitamin A; 68 mg vitamin E; 2 mg vitamin C; 21 mg cholesterol

Horseradish Bean Dip

Horseradish adds zip to this dip. Good on toasted pita bread triangles or tortilla chips.

$^1/_4$ cup (60 g) mayonnaise

$^1/_4$ cup (60 ml) low-sodium ketchup

$^1/_4$ cup (60 g) pickle relish

$^1/_2$ cup (80 g) chopped onion

1 tablespoon horseradish

1 tablespoon dry mustard

1 tablespoon (15 ml) Worcestershire sauce

$1^1/_2$ cups (150 g) cooked kidney beans, drained and mashed

Mix mayonnaise and ketchup. Mix in other ingredients, adding kidney beans last. Refrigerate. Serve with crackers.

Yield: 24 servings

Per serving: 15 g water; 39 calories (42% from fat, 12% from protein, 46% from carb); 1 g protein; 2 g total fat; 0 g saturated fat; 0 g monounsaturated fat; 1 g polyunsaturated fat; 5 g carbohydrate; 1 g fiber; 1 g sugar; 19 mg phosphorus; 10 mg calcium; 0 mg iron; 50 mg sodium; 71 mg potassium; 38 IU vitamin A; 2 mg vitamin E; 2 mg vitamin C; 1 mg cholesterol

Red Bean Dip

Great bean-and-cheese dip that not only tastes better than commercial ones, but is healthier too.

2 tablespoons (28 ml) olive oil

$^1/_2$ teaspoon crushed garlic

1 cup (160 g) finely chopped onion

1 jalapeño, finely chopped

1 teaspoon chili powder

2 cups (100 g) cooked kidney beans

$^1/_2$ cup (58 g) shredded Cheddar cheese

Heat oil in a skillet. Add garlic, onion, jalapeño, and chili powder and cook gently 4 minutes. Drain kidney beans, reserving juice. Process beans in a blender or food processor to a puree. Add to onion mixture and stir in 2 tablespoons of reserved bean liquid; mix well. Stir in cheese. Cook gently about 2 minutes, stirring until cheese melts. If mixture becomes too thick, add a little more reserved bean liquid. Spoon into serving dish and serve warm with tortilla chips.

Yield: 12 servings

Per serving: 19 g water; 151 calories (26% from fat, 23% from protein, 52% from carb); 9 g protein; 4 g total fat; 2 g saturated fat; 1 g monounsaturated fat; 1 g polyunsaturated fat; 20 g carbohydrate; 8 g fiber; 1 g sugar; 158 mg phosphorus; 87 mg calcium; 3 mg iron; 44 mg sodium; 463 mg potassium; 126 IU vitamin A; 14 mg vitamin E; 3 mg vitamin C; 6 mg cholesterol

White Bean Dip

A tasty appetizer, good either warm or cold.

1 cup (208 g) dry navy beans

$^{1}/_{2}$ cup (80 g) chopped onion

$^{3}/_{4}$ teaspoon minced garlic

1 tablespoon (15 ml) Dijon mustard

$^{1}/_{4}$ cup (25 g) chopped scallions

2 tablespoons (28 ml) lime juice

1 teaspoon tarragon

Bring beans to a boil for 1 minute and remove from heat to soak for 1 hour. Rinse well. Add onion and garlic and cook beans until tender, about 1 hour. Drain beans and rinse well. In a food processor place mustard, scallions, lime juice, and tarragon. Pulse to combine. Add beans and blend until smooth.

Yield: 8 servings

Per serving: 40 g water; 45 calories (5% from fat, 24% from protein, 72% from carb); 3 g protein; 0 g total fat;

0 g saturated fat; 0 g monounsaturated fat; 0 g polyunsaturated fat; 8 g carbohydrate; 2 g fiber; 1 g sugar; 51 mg phosphorus; 23 mg calcium; 1 mg iron; 169 mg sodium; 128 mg potassium; 38 IU vitamin A; 0 mg vitamin E; 3 mg vitamin C; 0 mg cholesterol

Tip: This is a nice dip with tortilla chips.

Bean Hominy Dip

A seemingly unusual combination that works very well.

16 ounces hominy

16 ounces (455 g) navy beans

4 ounces (115 g) cucumber

$1^{1}/_{2}$ cups (390 g) salsa

4 ounces (115 g) diced green chiles

1 tablespoon (15 ml) lime juice

$^{1}/_{2}$ teaspoon cumin

Puree hominy, beans, and cucumber in food processor until smooth. Put mixture into bowl and add remaining ingredients. Heat and serve with tortilla chips.

Yield: 36 servings

Per serving: 26 g water; 65 calories (4% from fat, 14% from protein, 83% from carb); 2 g protein; 0 g total fat; 0 g saturated fat; 0 g monounsaturated fat; 0 g polyunsaturated fat; 14 g carbohydrate; 2 g fiber; 1 g sugar; 43 mg phosphorus; 13 mg calcium; 1 mg iron; 25 mg sodium; 105 mg potassium; 35 IU vitamin A; 0 mg vitamin E; 0 mg vitamin C; 0 mg cholesterol

Split Pea Spread

An unusual spread made with split peas. Good on toasted wedges of pita bread.

1 cup (196 g) cooked split peas

2 tablespoons (27 g) cottage cheese

2 tablespoons grated Parmesan cheese

2 tablespoons (28 ml) olive oil

$^1/_4$ teaspoon dried basil

$^1/_2$ teaspoon crushed garlic

After cooked split peas have cooled, mash them up. Mix in other ingredients and refrigerate.

Yield: 6 servings

Per serving: 26 g water; 90 calories (51% from fat, 18% from protein, 31% from carb); 4 g protein; 5 g total fat; 1 g saturated fat; 3 g monounsaturated fat; 1 g polyunsaturated fat; 7 g carbohydrate; 3 g fiber; 1 g sugar; 51 mg phosphorus; 30 mg calcium; 0 mg iron; 33 mg sodium; 124 mg potassium; 15 IU vitamin A; 3 mg vitamin E; 0 mg vitamin C; 2 mg cholesterol

Garbanzo Dip

A tasty garbanzo dip topped with crunchy vegetables.

2 cups (450 g) canned garbanzo beans, drained and rinsed

1 cup (230 g) plain fat-free yogurt

2 tablespoons (30 ml) lemon juice

2 tablespoons (30 ml) olive oil

Dash of hot pepper sauce

1 cup (135 g) cucumber, peeled and diced

$^1/_4$ cup (40 g) red onion, chopped

$^1/_4$ cup (30 g) carrots, grated

$^1/_2$ cup (90 g) roma tomatoes, chopped

Blend the garbanzos, yogurt, lemon juice, olive oil, and hot pepper sauce in a blender or food processor until smooth. Transfer the dip to a shallow serving bowl. Mix the remaining ingredients together and spread over the dip.

Yield: 16 servings

Per serving: 63 calories (29% from fat, 15% from protein, 56% from carbohydrate); 2 g protein; 2 g total fat; 0 g saturated fat; 1 g monounsaturated fat; 0 g polyunsaturated fat; 9 g carbohydrate; 2 g fiber; 2 g sugar; 55 mg phosphorus; 43 mg calcium; 0 mg iron; 103 mg sodium; 124 mg potassium; 391 IU vitamin A; 0 mg ATE vitamin E; 3 mg vitamin C; 0 mg cholesterol; 50 g water

Tip: Serve with toasted pita bread or flatbread.

Hummus

A traditional Middle Eastern dip. You should be able to find dried garbanzo beans, or chickpeas, with the other dried beans in most large grocery stores. Tahini, a sesame-seed paste, should also be available in large grocery stores or natural food stores. Feel free to adjust the spices or use different herbs to suit your own taste.

1 cup (240 g) cooked garbanzo beans

$^3/_4$ teaspoon (0.2 g) minced garlic

3 tablespoons (45 ml) lemon juice

$^1/_4$ cup (60 ml) water

$^1/_4$ cup (60 g) tahini

1 teaspoon (2.5 g) cumin

$^1/_2$ teaspoon (1.3 g) paprika

1 tablespoon (15 ml) olive oil

In a food processor combine the cooked garbanzo beans, garlic, lemon juice, and water. Process for 1 minute, or until smooth. If the mixture is too thick, add more water to reach the desired consistency. Add the tahini, cumin, and paprika; stir until well combined. If desired, add more lemon juice, tahini, cumin, or paprika to taste. Spread into a shallow bowl and drizzle with olive oil. Serve chilled.

Yield: 8 servings

Per serving: 98 calories (53% from fat, 11% from protein, 35% from carbohydrate); 3 g protein; 6 g total fat; 1 g saturated fat; 3 g monounsaturated fat; 2 g polyunsaturated fat; 9 g carbohydrate; 2 g fiber; 0 g sugar; 84 mg phosphorus; 45 mg calcium; 1 mg iron; 99 mg sodium; 99 mg potassium; 92 IU vitamin A; 0 mg ATE vitamin E; 4 mg vitamin C; 0 mg cholesterol; 34 g water

Black Bean Spread

A good-for-you dip that tastes good too.

$^1/_2$ cup (125 g) dried black beans

2 teaspoons (10 ml) olive oil

$^1/_4$ cup (40 g) onion, finely chopped

$^1/_2$ teaspoon (1.5 g) minced garlic

4 ounces (115 g) fresh mushrooms, sliced

$^1/_2$ cup (75 g) walnuts

$^1/_4$ teaspoon (0.3 g) dried thyme

$^1/_4$ teaspoon (0.5 g) pepper

Soak the beans in 2 cups (470 ml) of water overnight or combine them with 2 cups (470 ml) of water in a saucepan, boil for 2 minutes, and let stand 1 hour. Cook in soaking water over medium heat for 1 hour, or until very tender, then drain and purée in a food processor. Heat the oil in a skillet over medium heat and sauté the onion for 3 minutes, or until soft. Add the garlic and cook 1 minute. Add the mushrooms, cover, and cook 5 minutes. Remove from heat. Place the walnuts in a blender or food processor and grind to the consistency of cornmeal. Combine the beans, sautéed vegetables, ground walnuts, thyme, and pepper in a blender or food processor until fairly smooth but not creamy. Spoon into a serving dish and chill.

Yield: 16 servings

Per serving: 39 calories (63% from fat, 16% from protein, 21% from carbohydrate); 2 g protein; 3 g total fat; 0 g saturated fat; 1 g monounsaturated fat; 1 g polyunsaturated fat; 2 g carbohydrate; 1 g fiber; 0 g sugar; 35 mg phosphorus; 5 mg calcium; 0 mg iron; 1 mg sodium; 66 mg potassium; 4 IU vitamin A; 0 mg ATE vitamin E; 0 mg vitamin C; 0 mg cholesterol; 13 g water

Tip: Serve with chips or crackers.

Black-Eyed Pea Pâté

Especially good with one of the pita chips recipes, but also great with vegetable dippers or tortilla chips.

8 ounces (225 g) cream cheese, softened

16 ounces (455 g) black-eyed peas, drained

$^1/_2$ cup (80 g) onion, quartered

$^1/_2$ teaspoon minced garlic

$^1/_2$ cup (130 g) salsa

1 teaspoon Tabasco sauce

3 tablespoons (45 ml) Worcestershire sauce

2 packets unflavored gelatin

2 tablespoons (30 ml) cold water

$^1/_4$ cup minced fresh parsley

Put cream cheese, peas, onion, garlic, salsa, Tabasco, and Worcestershire sauce in food processor with knife blade. Process until smooth. Sprinkle gelatin over cold water in small saucepan; let stand 1 minute. Cook over low heat, stirring until dissolved. Add gelatin mixture to pea mixture. Spin again until well blended. Spoon into glass casserole dish. Cover and chill until firm. Unmold and sprinkle with parsley.

Yield: 20 servings

Per serving: 34 g water; 107 calories (34% from fat, 13% from protein, 53% from carb); 4 g protein; 4 g total fat; 3 g saturated fat; 1 g monounsaturated fat; 0 g polyunsaturated fat; 15 g carbohydrate; 2 g fiber; 9 g sugar; 58 mg phosphorus; 18 mg calcium; 1 mg iron; 113 mg sodium; 147 mg potassium; 258 IU vitamin A; 41 mg vitamin E; 6 mg vitamin C; 12 mg cholesterol

Shortcut Black Bean Salsa

Combine canned beans and canned salsa with some extra spices for a quick dip that's more than the sum of its parts.

1 cup (172 g) cooked black beans, drained

12 ounces (340 g) salsa

$^1/_4$ cup chopped fresh cilantro

$^1/_4$ teaspoon cumin

2 tablespoons (28 ml) lime juice

Roughly chop beans in food processor. Do not puree them. Stir in remaining ingredients. Serve immediately or refrigerate overnight. Serve with corn chips or raw vegetables.

Yield: 20 servings

Per serving: 23 g water; 17 calories (4% from fat, 23% from protein, 73% from carb); 1 g protein; 0 g total fat; 0 g saturated fat; 0 g monounsaturated fat; 0 g polyunsaturated fat; 3 g carbohydrate; 1 g fiber; 1 g sugar; 18 mg phosphorus; 8 mg calcium; 0 mg iron; 40 mg sodium; 86 mg potassium; 87 IU vitamin A; 0 mg vitamin E; 1 mg vitamin C; 0 mg cholesterol

Avocado Salsa

Sort of a combination of salsa and guacamole, this dip is sure to please lovers of both. If you like your salsa hotter, add another jalapeño or a few drops of Tabasco sauce.

1 avocado, peeled and diced

$^1/_2$ cup (90 g) chopped tomato

$^1/_2$ cup (80 g) chopped red onion

$^1/_4$ cup (38 g) chopped green bell pepper

1 jalapeño pepper, finely chopped

$^1/_2$ teaspoon minced garlic

2 tablespoons (28 ml) red wine vinegar

1 tablespoon (15 ml) olive oil

Combine the vegetables in a medium bowl. Mash the garlic in a cup or small bowl. Add the vinegar and oil to the garlic. Pour the dressing over the vegetables and toss to combine the ingredients. Serve chilled or at room temperature.

Yield: 4 servings

Per serving: 79 g water; 103 calories (72% from fat, 4% from protein, 23% from carb); 1 g protein; 9 g total fat; 1 g saturated fat; 6 g monounsaturated fat; 1 g polyunsaturated fat; 6 g carbohydrate; 3 g fiber; 2 g sugar; 33 mg phosphorus; 13 mg calcium; 0 mg iron; 5 mg sodium; 273 mg potassium; 268 IU vitamin A; 0 mg vitamin E; 16 mg vitamin C; 0 mg cholesterol

Tomato and Avocado Salsa

Can't make up your mind if you want salsa or guacamole? Then have both together!

5 plum tomatoes

$^1/_4$ cup (40 g) red onion, diced

1 jalapeno, seeded and chopped

1 avocado, diced

2 tablespoons (30 ml) lime juice

1 tablespoon (4 g) cilantro

Halve the tomatoes and remove the seeds, then chop finely. Put into a bowl with other ingredients. Stir to mix.

Yield: 8 servings

Per serving: 34 calories (65% from fat, 6% from protein, 30% from carbohydrate); 1 g protein; 3 g total fat; 0 g saturated fat; 2 g monounsaturated fat; 0 g polyunsaturated fat; 3 g carbohydrate; 1 g fiber; 1 g sugar; 14 mg phosphorus; 5 mg calcium; 0 mg iron; 2 mg sodium; 125 mg potassium; 140 IU vitamin A; 0 mg ATE vitamin E; 5 mg vitamin C; 0 mg cholesterol; 31 g water

Texas Caviar

A traditional southern dip made with black-eyed peas. Serve with corn chips or toasted pita bread.

$^1/_3$ cup (55 g) onion, chopped

$^1/_2$ cup (75 g) green bell pepper, chopped

$^1/_2$ cup (50 g) scallions, chopped

$^1/_4$ cup (36 g) jalapeno peppers, chopped

1 tablespoon (10 g) minced garlic

20 cherry tomatoes, quartered

8 ounces (235 ml) reduced fat Italian dressing

2 cups (450 g) canned black eyed peas, drained

$^1/_2$ teaspoon (1 g) ground coriander

$^1/_4$ cup (15 g) fresh cilantro, chopped

In a large bowl, mix together onion, green bell pepper, scallions, jalapeno peppers, garlic, cherry tomatoes, Italian dressing, black-eyed peas, and coriander. Cover and chill in the refrigerator approximately 2 hours. Toss with fresh cilantro just before serving.

Yield: 16 servings

Per serving: 78 calories (47% from fat, 11% from protein, 42% from carbohydrate); 2 g protein; 4 g total fat; 1 g saturated fat; 1 g monounsaturated fat; 2 g polyunsaturated fat; 9 g carbohydrate; 2 g fiber; 3 g sugar; 32 mg phosphorus; 12 mg calcium; 1 mg iron; 237 ; 165 mg potassium; 258 IU vitamin A; 0 mg ATE vitamin E; 10 mg vitamin C; 0 mg cholesterol; 34 g water

Seven-Layer Dip

Just like you'd find at your favorite Mexican restaurant, except this one you'll feel good about eating.

$1/2$ cup (115 g) refried beans

$1/2$ cup (112 g) guacamole

$1/4$ cup (60 g) fat-free sour cream

1 cup (180 g) chopped tomato

$1/4$ cup (30 g) shredded low fat Cheddar cheese

$1/4$ cup (25 g) chopped scallions

$1/4$ cup (56 g) salsa

In a serving dish, layer the ingredients in the order shown.

Yield: 8 servings

Per serving: 54 calories (36% from fat, 22% from protein, 42% from carbohydrate); 3 g protein; 2 g total fat; 0 g saturated fat; 1 g monounsaturated fat; 0 g polyunsaturated fat; 5 g carbohydrate; 2 g fiber; 1 g sugar; 54 mg phosphorus; 38 mg calcium; 0 mg iron; 126 mg sodium; 177 mg potassium; 260 IU vitamin A; 10 mg ATE vitamin E; 5 mg vitamin C; 5 mg cholesterol; 55 g water

Carrot Cheese Ball

A little different type of appetizer, with carrots providing color and crunch.

$1 1/2$ cups (165 g) shredded carrot

8 ounces (225 g) cream cheese, softened

2 cups (225 g) shredded Cheddar cheese

$1/2$ teaspoon minced garlic

1 teaspoon Worcestershire sauce

$1/2$ teaspoon Tabasco sauce

3 tablespoons chopped fresh parsley

$1/2$ cup (55 g) chopped pecans

Press shredded carrot between paper towels to remove excess moisture; set aside. Combine cream cheese and Cheddar cheese in a medium bowl; stir well. Add carrot, garlic, Worcestershire sauce, and Tabasco sauce; stir well. Cover and chill 1 hour. These ingredients may also be combined in a food processor and mixed. Shape cheese mixture into a ball; roll in parsley and nuts. Wrap in waxed paper and chill at least 1 hour.

Yield: 24 servings

Per serving: 17 g water; 97 calories (78% from Fat, 15% from protein, 6% from carb); 4 g protein; 9 g total fat; 5 g saturated fat; 3 g monounsaturated fat; 1 g polyunsaturated fat; 2 g carbohydrate; 1 g fiber; 1 g sugar; 76 mg phosphorus; 92 mg calcium; 0 mg iron; 105 mg sodium; 62 mg potassium; 1625 IU vitamin A; 62 mg vitamin E; 2 mg vitamin C; 22 mg cholesterol

Chicken Pecan Pâté

The kind of party food that will have everyone guessing about the ingredients. What they will be sure of is that they like it.

2 cups (280 g) chicken, cooked

8 ounces (225 g) cream cheese, cut into chunks and softened

$1/2$ teaspoon minced garlic

1 cup (110 g) finely chopped pecans

6 tablespoons (84 g) mayonnaise

4 teaspoons fresh dill

Combine chicken, cream cheese, and garlic with chopped pecans in food processor or blender and blend just until smooth. Add mayonnaise and dill and blend again. Form into a ball and arrange on a bed of lettuce. Sprinkle with additional dill.

Yield: 24 servings

Per serving: 13 g water; 112 calories (80% from fat, 16% from protein, 4% from carb); 5 g protein; 10 g total fat; 3 g saturated fat; 4 g monounsaturated fat; 3 g polyunsaturated fat; 1 g carbohydrate; 1 g fiber; 0 g sugar; 47 mg phosphorus; 16 mg calcium; 0 mg iron; 58 mg sodium; 65 mg potassium; 156 IU vitamin A; 39 mg vitamin E; 0 mg vitamin C; 22 mg cholesterol

Tip: Serve with whole grain crackers.

Olive Nut Spread

An easy-to-make spread that's great on either crackers or vegetables.

6 ounces (170 g) cream cheese, softened

$^1/_2$ cup (115 g) mayonnaise

$^1/_2$ cup (55 g) chopped pecans

1 cup (100 g) sliced green olives

$^1/_8$ teaspoon black pepper

Combine all ingredients. Refrigerate for a few hours until spreading consistency. Will keep several weeks.

Yield: 16 servings

Per serving: 14 g water; 120 calories (91% from fat, 4% from protein, 5% from carb); 1 g protein; 12 g total fat; 3 g saturated fat; 4 g monounsaturated fat; 4 g polyunsaturated fat; 2 g carbohydrate; 1 g fiber; 0 g sugar; 23 mg phosphorus; 20 mg calcium; 1 mg iron; 144 mg sodium; 30 mg potassium; 199 IU vitamin A; 44 mg vitamin E; 0 mg vitamin C; 14 mg cholesterol

Ranch Cheese Ball

Powdered dressing mix makes ordinary cream cheese special.

8 ounces (225 g) cream cheese

1 packet ranch dressing mix (such as Hidden Valley)

2 cups (220 g) broken pecans

Soften cream cheese, then mix in dressing. Shape into ball. Then roll in pecan pieces. Chill overnight.

Yield: 16 servings

Per serving: 8 g water; 144 calories (88% from fat, 6% from protein, 6% from carb); 2 g protein; 15 g total fat; 4 g saturated fat; 7 g monounsaturated fat; 3 g polyunsaturated fat; 2 g carbohydrate; 1 g fiber; 1 g sugar; 53 mg phosphorus; 21 mg calcium; 1 mg iron; 42 mg sodium; 73 mg potassium; 198 IU vitamin A; 51 mg vitamin E; 0 mg vitamin C; 16 mg cholesterol

Hot Pecan Dip

Dried beef and toasted pecans provide the flavor here.

$^2/_3$ cup (74 g) pecans, toasted

2 tablespoons (28 g) unsalted butter

8 ounces (225 g) cream cheese

$^1/_2$ cup (115 g) sour cream

$^1/_4$ teaspoon garlic powder

$^1/_4$ teaspoon black pepper

$^1/_2$ cup (80 g) grated onion

$^1/_4$ cup (38 g) chopped green bell pepper

3 ounces (85 g) chopped dried beef

Toast pecans in butter. Cream together remaining ingredients. Spread creamed mixture in buttered 9-inch (23-cm) pie plate. Top with toasted pecans and bake 20 minutes in 350°F (180°C, gas mark 4) oven.

Yield: 12 servings

Per serving: 32 g water; 153 calories (81% from fat, 12% from protein, 7% from carb); 5 g protein; 14 g total fat; 7 g saturated fat; 5 g monounsaturated fat; 2 g polyunsaturated fat; 3 g carbohydrate; 1 g fiber; 1 g sugar; 63 mg phosphorus; 33 mg calcium; 1 mg iron; 258 mg sodium; 98 mg potassium; 366 IU vitamin A; 94 mg vitamin E; 3 mg vitamin C; 35 mg cholesterol

Layered Middle Eastern Dip

Serve this Middle Eastern dip with pita bread chips.

$^1/_2$ cup (75 g) tabbouleh

$^3/_4$ cup hummus

1 cup (180 g) chopped tomato

$^1/_2$ cup (80 g) chopped onion

$^3/_4$ cup (113 g) feta cheese

Layer ingredients in glass bowl so each is $^1/_2$ to $^3/_4$ inch (1 to 2 cm) thick: first tabbouleh, then hummus, then tomato-onion mix—squeeze out extra juice before layering in the feta cheese.

Yield: 12 servings

Per serving: 38 g water; 64 calories (47% from fat, 15% from protein, 38% from carb); 2 g protein; 3 g total fat; 2 g saturated fat; 1 g monounsaturated fat; 0 g polyunsaturated fat; 6 g carbohydrate; 2 g fiber; 1 g sugar; 57 mg phosphorus; 65 mg calcium; 0 mg iron; 143 mg sodium; 98 mg potassium; 172 IU vitamin A; 12 mg vitamin E; 5 mg vitamin C; 8 mg cholesterol

Deviled Nut Ball

This tasty spread is kick-started with canned deviled ham.

9 ounces (252 g) deviled ham

12 ounces (340 g) cream cheese, softened

$^1/_2$ cup (80 g) crushed pineapple, drained

3 tablespoons (27 g) minced green bell pepper

1 teaspoon minced onion

$^1/_4$ teaspoon Tabasco sauce

$^1/_2$ cup (55 g) chopped pecans

$^1/_2$ cup (30 g) chopped fresh parsley

In a medium bowl, mix together ham and cream cheese. Stir in pineapple, bell pepper, onion, and Tabasco sauce. Chill 2 to 3 hours. On waxed paper, form mixture into a ball or log and roll in pecans and parsley to coat completely. Serve with crackers.

Yield: 16 servings

Per serving: 32 g water; 137 calories (79% from fat, 10% from protein, 11% from carb); 3 g protein; 12 g total fat; 6 g saturated fat; 5 g monounsaturated fat; 1 g polyunsaturated fat; 4 g carbohydrate; 1 g fiber; 1 g sugar; 53 mg phosphorus; 25 mg calcium; 1 mg iron; 210 mg sodium; 85 mg potassium; 457 IU vitamin A; 76 mg vitamin E; 5 mg vitamin C; 29 mg cholesterol

Tuna-Pecan Ball

Tuna and veggies make this dip just a little different from the ordinary cheese ball.

8 ounces (225 g) cream cheese, softened

$6^1/_2$ ounces (184 g) white albacore tuna, drained and flaked

3 tablespoons (27 g) diced green bell pepper

3 tablespoons (30 g) diced onion

3 tablespoons (24 g) diced celery

5 pimento-stuffed diced olives

2 teaspoons horseradish

$^1/_2$ teaspoon Tabasco sauce

$^1/_2$ teaspoon Worcestershire sauce

$^1/_2$ cup (55 g) chopped pecans

Combine all ingredients except pecans; stir well. Shape into a ball; cover and chill at least 1 hour. Roll in pecans; cover and chill. Serve with assorted crackers.

Yield: 16 servings

Per serving: 21 g water; 90 calories (76% from fat, 18% from protein, 5% from carb); 4 g protein; 8 g total fat; 3 g saturated fat; 3 g monounsaturated fat; 1 g polyunsaturated fat; 1 g carbohydrate; 1 g fiber; 0 g sugar; 51 mg phosphorus; 17 mg calcium; 0 mg iron; 53 mg sodium; 70 mg potassium; 209 IU vitamin A; 52 mg vitamin E; 2 mg vitamin C; 20 mg cholesterol

Salmon Appetizer Ball

Pretty and delicious, this makes a great party food that guests can eat without guilt.

16 ounces (455 g) canned salmon

8 ounces (225 g) fat-free cream cheese, softened

2 teaspoons (6 g) grated onion

1 tablespoon (15 ml) fresh lemon juice

2 teaspoons (10 g) prepared horseradish

$^1/_4$ teaspoon (1.2 ml) liquid smoke

$^1/_2$ cup (60 g) chopped pecans

3 tablespoons (12 g) fresh parsley

Drain and flake salmon. Combine salmon, cream cheese, onion, lemon juice, horseradish, and liquid smoke. Mix thoroughly. Chill for several hours. Combine pecans and parsley on a sheet of waxed paper. Shape salmon mixture into ball and roll in nut mixture. Chill well. Serve with assorted crackers.

Yield: 16 servings

Per serving: 97 calories (60% from fat, 33% from protein, 7% from carbohydrate); 8 g protein; 7 g total fat; 2 g saturated fat; 3 g monounsaturated fat; 1 g polyunsaturated fat; 2 g carbohydrate; 0 g fiber; 0 g sugar; 131 mg phosphorus; 90 mg calcium; 1 mg iron; 66 mg sodium; 130 mg potassium; 175 IU vitamin A; 31 mg ATE vitamin E; 2 mg vitamin C; 19 mg cholesterol; 32 g water

Peanut Butter Dip

This dip is made for apple slices or celery, but don't stop there. You'll be surprised how many things it goes well with.

$^1/_2$ cup (130 g) crunchy peanut butter

$^1/_4$ cup (85 g) honey

$^1/_4$ cup (60 g) sour cream

In small bowl, combine peanut butter, honey, and sour cream; blend well. Serve with fresh vegetables or fruit dippers. Store in refrigerator.

Yield: 8 servings

Per serving: 8 g water; 137 calories (55% from fat, 11% from protein, 34% from carb); 4 g protein; 9 g total fat; 2 g saturated fat; 4 g monounsaturated fat; 2 g polyunsaturated fat; 13 g carbohydrate; 1 g fiber; 10 g sugar; 59 mg phosphorus; 16 mg calcium; 0 mg iron; 82 mg sodium; 135 mg potassium; 28 IU vitamin A; 8 mg vitamin E; 0 mg vitamin C; 3 mg cholesterol

Apple Nut Dip

A great dip for apples, pears, grapes, and other fruit. Also good as a spread for raisin bread or other sweet breakfast breads.

1 cup (230 g) sour cream

8 ounces (225 g) cream cheese, softened

$^1/_4$ teaspoon cinnamon

1 cup (150 g) shredded apple

$^1/_2$ cup (55 g) chopped pecans

2 tablespoons (30 g) brown sugar

Beat sour cream, cream cheese, and cinnamon in medium bowl. Stir in remaining ingredients. Chill. Serve with fruit dippers.

Yield: 16 servings

Per serving: 26 g water; 103 calories (78% from fat, 7% from protein, 15% from carb); 2 g protein; 9 g total fat; 4 g saturated fat; 3 g monounsaturated fat; 1 g polyunsaturated fat; 4 g carbohydrate; 1 g fiber; 3 g sugar; 40 mg phosphorus; 32 mg calcium; 0 mg iron; 49 mg sodium; 63 mg potassium; 252 IU vitamin A; 66 mg vitamin E; 0 mg vitamin C; 21 mg cholesterol

Orange and Nut Spread

A nice sweet fruity dip or spread.

1 orange

1 cup (110 g) broken pecans

$2^1/_2$ cups (365 g) raisins

$^3/_4$ cup (175 g) mayonnaise

Do not peel orange. Quarter and seed orange. In a food processor, process orange and pecans, covered, until finely chopped. Add half of the raisins and all of the mayonnaise. Cover; process until raisins are chopped. Add remaining raisins; cover and process until finely chopped. Transfer to a covered container; chill.

Yield: 28 servings

Per serving: 9 g water; 117 calories (54% from fat, 3% from protein, 43% from carb); 1 g protein; 8 g total fat; 1 g saturated fat; 3 g monounsaturated fat; 3 g

polyunsaturated fat; 13 g carbohydrate; 1 g fiber; 10 g sugar; 28 mg phosphorus; 14 mg calcium; 0 mg iron; 35 mg sodium; 140 mg potassium; 34 IU vitamin A; 5 mg vitamin E; 4 mg vitamin C; 2 mg cholesterol

Tip: To serve, spread on orange slices, celery, or crackers.

Veggie Dippers

Really not a recipe, just a reminder that you don't have to use crackers or other such things for dipping. Most of the recipes for dips and spreads in this book are great with fresh vegetables.

1 cup (116 g) radishes

1 cup (71 g) broccoli florets

1 cup (150 g) red bell pepper, cut in strips

1 cup (150 g) green bell pepper, cut in strips

1 cup (100 g) green beans, steamed until crisp-tender

1 cup (70 g) mushrooms

Assorted raw vegetables for dipping.

Yield: 6 servings

Per serving: 103 g water; 26 calories (7% from fat, 21% from protein, 72% from carb); 2 g protein; 0 g total fat; 0 g saturated fat; 0 g monounsaturated fat; 0 g polyunsaturated fat; 6 g carbohydrate; 2 g fiber; 2 g sugar; 40 mg phosphorus; 22 mg calcium; 1 mg iron; 14 mg sodium; 255 mg potassium; 1352 IU vitamin A; 0 mg vitamin E; 69 mg vitamin C; 0 mg cholesterol

4

Snacks and Nibbles

Ah, snacks. We all love them, even though we know we shouldn't be eating most of them. And how are you going to deal with things like game day or a children's party without them? But they don't *have* to be unhealthy. This chapter contains sixty nine recipes to prove that. They range from traditional appetizers like chicken wings and meatballs though a wide selection of finger food, healthy crispy dippers like crackers and low fat, low sodium versions of tortilla and potato chips to a wide variety of nut and snack mixes. So nibble away and don't feel guilty about it.

Boneless Buffalo Wings

Chicken wings tend to be fairly high in saturated fat, since it isn't easy to avoid eating the skin, where most of it is. But that doesn't mean you have to do without that Buffalo wing taste at your party. Make boneless wings from chicken breasts, cooking them in the oven instead of frying them.

6 boneless, skinless chicken breasts

3 tablespoons (45 ml) hot pepper sauce

2 tablespoons (30 ml) white vinegar

Preheat oven to 350°F (180°C, or gas mark 4). Cut the breasts into strips, about eight per breast. Place in roasting pan sprayed with nonstick vegetable oil spray and roast for 20 minutes, or until done. Mix hot pepper sauce and white vinegar. Place chicken pieces in a large bowl with a tight-sealing cover. Pour vinegar mixture over the pieces and shake to coat. Remove, allowing extra sauce to drain.

Yield: 16 servings

Per serving: 30 calories (11% from fat, 88% from protein, 1% from carbohydrate); 6 g protein; 0 g total fat; 0 g saturated fat; 0 g monounsaturated fat; 0 g polyunsaturated fat; 0 g carbohydrate; 0 g fiber; 0 g sugar; 53 mg phosphorus; 3 mg calcium; 0 mg iron; 34 mg sodium; 73 mg potassium; 49 IU vitamin A; 2 mg ATE vitamin E; 0 mg vitamin C; 15 mg cholesterol; 24 g water

Chicken Wings Nibblers

These can be used as an appetizer or the basis of a meal.

20 chicken wings

2 eggs

2 tablespoons (30 ml) skim milk

1$^1/_2$ cups (190 g) Reduced-Fat Biscuit Mix (see recipe page 38)

$^1/_2$ cup (60 g) sesame seeds

2 teaspoons (5 g) paprika

1$^1/_2$ teaspoons (4.5 g) dry mustard

Preheat oven to 425°F (220°C, or gas mark 7). Separate chicken wings at joints; discard tips. Spray two rectangular 9 × 13-inch (23 × 33-cm) pans with nonstick vegetable oil spray. Beat eggs and milk with fork in bowl. Mix biscuit mix, sesame seeds, paprika, and mustard in a second bowl. Soak chicken in egg mixture and then coat with sesame seed mixture. Arrange close together in baking pans. Bake uncovered for 35 to 40 minutes, or until brown and crisp.

Yield: 10 servings

Per serving: 139 calories (23% from fat, 33% from protein, 44% from carbohydrate); 11 g protein; 4 g total fat; 1 g saturated fat; 1 g monounsaturated fat; 1 g polyunsaturated fat; 15 g carbohydrate; 1 g fiber; 0 g sugar; 171 mg phosphorus; 70 mg calcium; 2 mg iron; 69 mg sodium; 75 mg potassium; 395 IU vitamin A; 2 mg ATE vitamin E; 1 mg vitamin C; 60 mg cholesterol; 41 g water

Taco Chicken Wings

You can use these taco-flavored wings either as appetizers or the main dish. This particular dish seems to be very popular with young people.

12 chicken wings

$^1/_2$ cup (62 g) flour

2 tablespoons (15 g) chili powder

1 teaspoon (2.5 g) cumin

1 teaspoon (1 g) dried oregano

$^1/_2$ teaspoon (1.5 g) onion powder

$^1/_4$ teaspoon (0.8 g) garlic powder

$^1/_8$ teaspoon (0.3 g) cayenne pepper

1 egg

1 cup (28 g) corn chips, crushed

Preheat oven to 350°F (180°C, or gas mark 4). Cut wings into sections, discarding the tips. Combine flour and next 6 ingredients (through cayenne pepper) in a plastic bag. Pour egg into a shallow dish. Spread crushed corn chips in another shallow dish. Shake a few wing sections at a time in the flour mixture, then roll in the egg, then the corn chips. Place in a 9 × 13-inch (23 × 33-cm) pan. Bake for 45 minutes, or until done.

Yield: 6 servings

Per serving: 198 calories (34% from fat, 23% from protein, 43% from carbohydrate); 11 g protein; 8 g total fat; 1 g saturated fat; 2 g monounsaturated fat; 3 g polyunsaturated fat; 22 g carbohydrate; 2 g fiber; 1 g sugar; 117 mg phosphorus; 56 mg calcium; 2 mg iron; 189 mg sodium; 75 mg potassium; 830 IU vitamin A; 6 mg ATE vitamin E; 2 mg vitamin C; 49 mg cholesterol; 36 g water

Steak Bites

These little steak bites will please the toughest one in your party crowd.

$^1/_2$ cup (120 ml) Dick's Reduced Sodium Soy Sauce (see recipe page 25)

6 tablespoons (78 g) sugar

3 tablespoons (45 ml) sesame oil

2 pounds (1 kg) round steak, cubed

$^1/_2$ cup (50 g) chopped scallions

2 tablespoons (30 ml) white wine

Combine soy sauce, sugar, and sesame oil in a shallow dish. Add steak, and refrigerate for 4 hours. Remove steak from marinade, reserving marinade. Place a large skillet over medium-high heat, and cook steak to desired doneness. Pour the reserved marinade into a medium saucepan and place over medium-high heat. Bring to a boil and cook for 5 minutes. Add cooked steak, scallions, and wine to the boiling marinade. Transfer the entire contents of the saucepan to a large bowl, and serve hot.

Yield: 16 servings

Per serving: 141 calories (14% from fat, 20% from protein, 66% from carbohydrate); 16 g protein; 5 g total fat; 1 g saturated fat; 2 g monounsaturated fat; 2 g polyunsaturated fat; 54 g carbohydrate; 0 g fiber; 6 g sugar; 111 mg phosphorus; 10 mg calcium; 1 mg iron; 74 mg sodium; 163 mg potassium; 34 IU vitamin A; 0 mg ATE vitamin E; 1 mg vitamin C; 33 mg cholesterol, 52 g water

Turkey Cocktail Meatballs

These tasty little meatballs can also be used as the basis of a dinner, served over rice with a vegetable. When we've made them for a get-together, they are always one of the first items to disappear.

1 pound (455 g) ground turkey breast

1 egg

³/₄ cup (50 g) saltine crackers, crushed

4 ounces part-skim shredded mozzarella

¹/₄ cup (40 g) chopped onion

¹/₂ teaspoon (0.9 g) ground ginger

6 tablespoons (90 g) Dijon mustard, divided

1¹/₄ cups (295 ml) unsweetened pineapple juice

¹/₄ cup (37 g) chopped green bell pepper

2 tablespoons (30 ml) honey

1 tablespoon (8 g) cornstarch

¹/₄ teaspoon (0.7 g) onion powder

Preheat oven to 350°F (180°C, or gas mark 4). In a bowl, combine turkey, egg, cracker crumbs, mozzarella, onion, ginger, and 3 tablespoons (45 g) mustard. Form into 30 balls, 1 inch (2.5 cm) each. Spray a 9 × 13-inch (23 × 33-cm) baking dish with nonstick vegetable oil spray. Place meatballs in dish. Bake, uncovered, for 20 to 25 minutes, or until cooked through. In a saucepan, combine pineapple juice, green pepper, honey, cornstarch, onion powder, and remaining mustard. Bring to a boil, stirring constantly. Cook and stir until thickened. Brush meatballs with about ¹/₄ cup (60 ml) sauce and return to the oven for 10 minutes. Serve remaining sauce as a dip for meatballs.

Yield: 15 servings

Per serving: 100 calories (23% from fat, 41% from protein, 36% from carbohydrate); 10 g protein; 2 g total fat; 1 g saturated fat; 1 g monounsaturated fat; 0 g polyunsaturated fat; 9 g carbohydrate; 0 g fiber; 5 g sugar; 116 mg phosphorus; 75 mg calcium; 1 mg iron; 181 mg sodium; 67 mg potassium; 66 IU vitamin A; 9 mg ATE vitamin E; 4 mg vitamin C; 64 mg cholesterol; 58 g water

Asian Tuna Bites

Tasty little tuna bites are sure to be a hit with everyone. Serve with the teriyaki sauce in Chapter 2 for dipping.

1 pound tuna steaks, cut in 1" cubes

¹/₄ cup sesame seeds

¹/₄ teaspoon black pepper

Spray tuna with non-stick cooking spray. Sprinkle with sesame seeds and pepper. In a large non-stick skillet brown on all sides until slightly pink in the center. Thread on cocktail toothpicks to serve.

Yield: 10 servings

Per serving: 86 calories (43% from fat, 53% from protein , 4% from carb); 11 g protein ; 4 g total fat; 1 g saturated fat; 1 g monounsaturated fat; 1 g polyunsaturated fat; 1 g carb; 0 g fiber; 0 g sugar; 138 mg phosphorus; 39 mg calcium; 18 mg sodium; 132 mg potassium; 991 IU vitamin A; 297 mg ATE vitamin E; 0 mg vitamin C; 17 mg cholesterol

Quiche Nibblers

Low fat, crustless quiche bites that are sure to be a hit, whether they're just for your family or for guests. No one will ever know that we've taken out the fat, the cholesterol, and the calories.

1 tablespoon (15 ml) olive oil

$1/2$ cup (75 g) red bell pepper, finely chopped

$1/4$ cup (25 g) scallions, finely chopped

3 eggs

2 tablespoons (30 ml) skim milk

2 ounces (55 g) low fat Cheddar cheese, shredded

$1/8$ teaspoon (0.3 g) ground black pepper

Preheat oven to 425°F (220°C, or gas mark 7). Grease 24 mini-muffin cups with nonstick vegetable oil spray. In a small saucepan, heat olive oil over moderate heat. Add red bell pepper and scallions; sauté for 5 minutes, or until soft. Remove the pan from the heat and let the mixture cool slightly. In a medium bowl, combine eggs, milk, cheese, and pepper. Stir in the bell pepper mixture. Spoon about 1 tablespoon of the mixture into each muffin cup. Bake for 8 to 10 minutes, or until the centers are set. Let cool for 1 minute. Using a knife, loosen the quiches around the edges and remove.

Yield: 12 servings

Per serving: 35 calories (52% from fat, 38% from protein, 10% from carbohydrate); 3 g protein; 2 g total fat; 0 g saturated fat; 1 g monounsaturated fat; 0 g polyunsaturated fat; 1 g carbohydrate; 0 g fiber; 0 g sugar; 47 mg phosphorus; 34 mg calcium; 0 mg iron; 59 mg sodium; 29 mg potassium; 287 IU vitamin A; 4 mg ATE vitamin E; 8 mg vitamin C; 1 mg cholesterol; 76 g water

Antipasto on a Skewer

This is handy finger food for your next outdoor meal, much easier to carry around than a plate from a typical antipasto tray.

$1/2$ teaspoon minced garlic

1 teaspoon black pepper

1 teaspoon Italian seasoning

1 teaspoon dry mustard

$1/2$ teaspoon crushed oregano

$1/3$ cup (78 ml) red wine vinegar

1 cup (235 ml) olive oil

8 ounces (225 g) mozzarella cheese, cut in $1/2 \times 1/4 \times$ 2-inch ($1 \times .5 \times 5$-cm) sticks

12 slices salami

24 cherry tomatoes

24 black olives

12 mushrooms

10 ounces (283 g) artichoke hearts, cooked

In a tight-sealing container, combine seasonings and vinegar; shake well. Add oil and shake again for about 30 seconds. Pour marinade in a $13 \times 9 \times 2$-inch ($33 \times 23 \times 5$-cm) baking dish. Wrap each cheese stick in one slice of salami. On each of 12 skewers, thread tomato, olive, mushroom, salami and cheese, artichoke heart, olive, and tomato. Place skewers in marinade. Marinate in refrigerator at least 24 hours, turning several times to coat all sides.

Yield: 12 servings

Per serving: 72 g water; 341 calories (78% from fat, 15% from protein, 7% from carb); 13 g protein; 30 g total fat; 8 g saturated fat; 19 g monounsaturated fat; 3 g polyunsaturated fat; 6 g carbohydrate; 2 g fiber; 1 g sugar; 168 mg phosphorus; 169 mg calcium; 1 mg iron; 742 mg sodium; 317 mg potassium; 403 IU vitamin A; 24 mg vitamin E; 9 mg vitamin C; 38 mg cholesterol

Mexican Pinwheels

These make a great snack or lunch. You can also slice them about $^3/_4$ inch (2 cm) thick and serve as an appetizer.

1 avocado, chopped

3 ounces (85 g) cream cheese, softened

6 whole wheat tortillas, 6 inch (15 cm)

4 ounces (113 g) shredded Monterey Jack cheese

1 ounce (28 g) leaf lettuce

$^1/_2$ cup (17 g) alfalfa sprouts

$^1/_2$ cup (130 g) salsa

Combine avocado and cream cheese; blend dip. Spread each tortilla evenly with avocado mixture to within $^1/_2$ inch (1 cm) of edge. Arrange cheese, lettuce, and sprouts over avocado mixture. Spoon on salsa. Roll up each tortilla; cut in half; secure with toothpicks. Serve immediately or wrap in plastic wrap and refrigerate.

Yield: 6 servings

Per serving: 67 g water; 259 calories (57% from fat, 14% from protein, 30% from carb); 9 g protein; 17 g total fat; 8 g saturated fat; 6 g monounsaturated fat; 1 g polyunsaturated fat; 19 g carbohydrate; 3 g fiber; 1 g sugar; 158 mg phosphorus; 203 mg calcium; 2 mg iron; 388 mg sodium; 269 mg potassium; 787 IU vitamin A; 87 mg vitamin E; 3 mg vitamin C; 32 mg cholesterol

Tortilla Roll-Ups

Tasty little tortilla snacks, with just enough heat to be interesting.

8 whole wheat tortillas

8 ounces (225 g) cream cheese, softened

4 ounces (115 g) black olives, chopped

4 ounces (115 g) diced green chiles

$^1/_4$ teaspoon Tabasco sauce

Cream together cream cheese, olives, chiles, and Tabasco sauce. Spread approximately 2 tablespoons onto a tortilla, roll jelly-roll fashion, roll in plastic wrap, and chill. Before serving cut into $^3/_8$-inch-wide (1-cm) pieces.

Yield: 16 servings

Per serving: 25 g water; 105 calories (59% from fat, 9% from protein, 32% from carb); 2 g protein; 7 g total fat; 3 g saturated fat; 3 g monounsaturated fat; 0 g polyunsaturated fat; 9 g carbohydrate; 2 g fiber; 0 g sugar; 34 mg phosphorus; 37 mg calcium; 1 mg iron; 200 mg sodium; 41 mg potassium; 221 IU vitamin A; 51 mg vitamin E; 0 mg vitamin C; 16 mg cholesterol

Black Bean Tortilla Pinwheels

While intended as an appetizer, you could make a meal of this by not cutting it into slices.

8 ounces (225 g) cream cheese, softened

1 cup (230 g) sour cream

1 cup (115 g) shredded Monterey Jack cheese

$^1/_4$ cup (25 g) pimento-stuffed olives

$^1/_4$ cup (40 g) chopped red onion

$^1/_8$ teaspoon garlic powder

2 cups (344 g) cooked black beans, drained

6 whole wheat tortillas

Combine cream cheese and sour cream; mix until well blended. Stir in Monterey Jack cheese, olives, onion, and garlic powder. Chill 2 hours. Spread thin layer of cream cheese mixture on each tortilla. Puree beans in food processor or blender. Starting in middle of tortilla, spread a layer covering half of tortilla with beans. Roll up tortilla tightly, starting with end that has the beans. Chill. Cut into $^3/_4$-inch (2-cm) slices. Serve with salsa.

Yield: 20 servings

Per serving: 36 g water; 134 calories (56% from fat, 15% from protein, 29% from carb); 5 g protein; 8 g total fat; 5 g saturated fat; 3 g monounsaturated fat; 0 g polyunsaturated fat; 10 g carbohydrate; 2 g fiber; 0 g sugar; 89 mg phosphorus; 89 mg calcium; 1 mg iron; 146 mg sodium; 113 mg potassium; 256 IU vitamin A; 65 mg vitamin E; 0 mg vitamin C; 23 mg cholesterol

New York Goodwich Roll-Ups

I'm not sure where the name comes from, but someone told me that's what this veggie roll-up is called. Whatever you call it, it's tasty and filling.

$^1/_2$ cup (80 g) sliced onion

2 teaspoons (10 ml) olive oil

1 teaspoon (5 ml) barbecue sauce

2 whole wheat tortillas

1 tablespoon mayonnaise

1 cup (71 g) broccoli, cut in florets and steamed

$^1/_2$ cup (50 g) cauliflower, crumbled and steamed

2 slices dill pickle

2 tablespoons grated carrot

2 tablespoons grated red cabbage

2 tablespoons grated yellow squash

$^1/_2$ cup (28 g) shredded lettuce

$^1/_2$ cup (17 g) alfalfa sprouts

2 slices avocado

Sauté onion in oil until it begins to soften. Add barbecue sauce and sauté until tender. In hot dry skillet, heat tortillas, turning from one side to the other until soft but not crisp. Place on large sheet of plastic wrap. Spread tortillas with mayonnaise. Add broccoli in a line down center. Add cauliflower, then pickle, grated vegetables and a line of barbecued onions. Top with lettuce, sprouts, and avocado. Roll, crepe style, around vegetables. Wrap tightly until ready to serve.

Yield: 2 servings

Per serving: 258 g water; 462 calories (62% from fat, 7% from protein, 31% from carb); 8 g protein; 34 g total fat; 5 g saturated fat; 19 g monounsaturated fat; 7 g polyunsaturated fat; 38 g carbohydrate; 14 g fiber; 6 g sugar; 181 mg phosphorus; 106 mg calcium; 3 mg iron; 294 mg sodium; 1076 mg potassium; 2036 IU vitamin A; 6 mg vitamin E; 75 mg vitamin C; 3 mg cholesterol

Skillet Nachos

Great as an appetizer, served right from the skillet. But also good as a meal, wrapped up in a tortilla.

1 pound (455 g) ground beef

1 cup (160 g) chopped onion

2 cups (520 g) salsa

2 cups (344 g) cooked black beans, drained

1 teaspoon chili powder

1 cup (180 g) chopped tomato

1 avocado, seeded and diced

$^1/_2$ cup (50 g) sliced black olives

1 cup (115 g) shredded Cheddar cheese

1 cup (230 g) sour cream

In 12-inch (30-cm) skillet, brown beef with onion; drain. Add salsa, beans, and chili powder; bring to a boil. Reduce heat and simmer uncovered 5 minutes. Stir in tomato, avocado, and olives; remove from heat. Sprinkle with cheese. Spoon sour cream onto center of meat mixture. Serve with tortilla chips and/or flour tortillas.

Yield: 6 servings

Per serving: 276 g water; 486 calories (41% from fat, 30% from protein, 29% from carb); 28 g protein; 17 g total fat; 7 g saturated fat; 7 g monounsaturated fat; 1 g polyunsaturated fat; 27 g carbohydrate; 9 g fiber; 5 g sugar; 392 mg phosphorus; 267 mg calcium; 4 mg iron; 360 mg sodium; 970 mg potassium; 1035 IU vitamin A; 97 mg vitamin E; 9 mg vitamin C; 91 mg cholesterol

Veggie Pizza Bites

Like miniature pieces of pizza, these small wedges are sure to be a hit with nibblers of all ages.

2 teaspoons chopped garlic

1 cup (180 g) sliced tomato

2 tablespoons (28 ml) olive oil

$^1/_8$ teaspoon black pepper

6 ounces (170 g) mozzarella cheese, sliced

2 whole wheat tortillas

2 tablespoons minced fresh basil

$^1/_2$ cup (50 g) grated Parmesan cheese

Preheat the oven to 350°F (180°C, gas mark 4). In a small bowl place the garlic, tomato, olive oil, and pepper. Thoroughly coat the tomatoes. Place the cheese slices over the tortillas. Place the soaked tomatoes on top. Sprinkle on the basil and Parmesan. Place the tortillas on a baking sheet and bake them for 8 minutes or until the cheese is melted. Cut the pizza into wedges.

Yield: 6 servings

Per serving: 43 g water; 201 calories (63% from fat, 21% from protein, 16% from carb); 11 g protein; 14 g total fat; 6 g saturated fat; 6 g monounsaturated fat; 1 g polyunsaturated fat; 8 g carbohydrate; 1 g fiber; 1 g sugar; 184 mg phosphorus; 267 mg calcium; 1 mg iron; 372 mg sodium; 131 mg potassium; 449 IU vitamin A; 59 mg vitamin E; 7 mg vitamin C; 30 mg cholesterol

Pizza Pitas

Pizza snacks are always a hit. And you don't have to tell anyone that these are actually good for them.

1 whole wheat pita

2 tablespoons pizza sauce

$^1/_8$ teaspoon crushed dried oregano

$^1/_2$ cup (75 g) sliced red bell pepper

$^1/_2$ cup (80 g) sliced onion

2 ounces (56 g) shredded mozzarella cheese

Split pita bread round in half, forming 2 thin circles. Spread each circle with half of the sauce. Sprinkle half of the oregano over each. Top each circle with half of the veggies and half of the cheese. Place pita bread halves on a baking sheet. Bake in a 375°F (190°C, gas mark 5) oven for 8 to 10 minutes or until cheese is bubbly and edges of pita bread are crisp. Remove from baking sheet; cool slightly.

Yield: 2 servings

Per serving: 109 g water; 189 calories (26% from fat, 22% from protein, 52% from carb); 11 g protein; 6 g total fat; 3 g saturated fat; 1 g monounsaturated fat; 1 g polyunsaturated fat; 26 g carbohydrate; 4 g fiber; 5 g sugar; 216 mg phosphorus; 241 mg calcium; 1 mg iron; 434 mg sodium; 278 mg potassium; 1434 IU vitamin A; 35 mg vitamin E; 53 mg vitamin C; 18 mg cholesterol

Crostini with Mushrooms

Another appetizer that's fancy enough to serve to company, but still easy to make.

2 cups (140 g) mushrooms, whole

1 tablespoon (15 ml) olive oil

$^1/_4$ teaspoon (0.8 g) crushed garlic

1 tablespoon (4 g) fresh parsley, chopped

12 slices Italian bread, sliced $^1/_4$-inch (0.64 cm) thick

Clean and cut the mushrooms into very thin little pieces. In a large saucepan, heat oil with crushed garlic. Cook over medium heat until the garlic turns light brown, and then add the mushrooms. Cook the mushrooms for 10 minutes, or until the liquid from the mushrooms dries. Turn off the heat and allow to cool. Add parsley and stir. Toast the bread and spread the mushroom mixture on top. Serve at once.

Yield: 6 servings

Per serving: 188 calories (21% from fat, 13% from protein, 66% from carbohydrate); 6 g protein; 4 g total fat; 1 g saturated fat; 2 g monounsaturated fat; 1 g polyunsaturated fat; 31 g carbohydrate; 2 g fiber; 1 g sugar; 82 mg phosphorus; 49 mg calcium; 2 mg iron; 352 mg sodium; 144 mg potassium; 53 IU vitamin A; 0 mg ATE vitamin E; 1 mg vitamin C; 0 mg cholesterol; 44 g water

Tuscan Bruschetta

The simplest form of bruschetta, with just enough garlic to taste and a little olive oil.

4 slices low sodium Italian bread, sliced no more than $^1/_2$-inch (1.3 cm) thick

1 small clove garlic

2 tablespoons (30 ml) extra-virgin olive oil

Toast bread until light brown. Take off the garlic skin and rub garlic firmly across the face of the toast. Drizzle with just enough olive oil to cover the entire surface of the bread.

Yield: 4 servings

Per serving: 143 calories (49% from fat, 8% from protein, 43% from carbohydrate); 3 g protein; 8 g total fat; 1 g saturated fat; 5 g monounsaturated fat; 1 g polyunsaturated fat; 15 g carbohydrate; 1 g fiber; 0 g sugar; 26 mg calcium; 1 mg iron; 16 mg sodium; 39 mg potassium; 0 IU vitamin A; 0 mg vitamin C; 0 mg cholesterol; exchanges = 1 starch–$1^1/_2$ fat; 12 g water

Chicken and Mushroom Quesadillas

If you have an indoor grill like the George Foreman models, it is perfect for making these quesadillas. Otherwise, place them on a baking sheet and bake at 350°F (180°C, or gas mark 4) until crisp.

1 tablespoon (15 ml) olive oil

$2^1/_2$ teaspoons (6.5 g) chili powder

$^1/_2$ teaspoon (1.5 g) minced garlic

1 teaspoon (1 g) dried oregano

8 ounces (225 g) mushrooms, sliced

1 cup (110 g) chicken breast, cooked and shredded

$^2/_3$ cup (110 g) onion, finely chopped

$^1/_2$ cup (30 g) fresh cilantro, chopped

$1^1/_2$ cups (170 g) shredded low fat Monterey Jack cheese

16 5$^1/_2$-inch (13.75-cm) corn tortillas

Heat olive oil in a large skillet over medium-high heat. Add chili powder, garlic, and oregano and sauté for 1 minute. Add mushrooms and sauté for 10 minutes, or until tender. Remove from heat and stir in the chicken, onion, and cilantro. Cool for 10 minutes, then mix in the cheese. Spray olive oil spray on one side of 8 of the tortillas and place them oiled-side down on a baking sheet. Divide chicken mixture among tortillas, spreading to an even thickness. Top with the remaining tortillas and spray the tops with olive oil spray. Grill quesadillas for 3 minutes per side, or until heated through and golden brown. Cut into wedges to serve.

Yield: 12 servings

Per serving: 122 calories (26% from fat, 32% from protein, 43% from carbohydrate); 10 g protein; 4 g total fat; 1 g saturated fat; 2 g monounsaturated fat; 1 g polyunsaturated fat; 13 g carbohydrate; 2 g fiber; 1 g sugar; 206 mg phosphorus; 97 mg calcium; 1 mg iron; 128 mg sodium; 181 mg potassium; 315 IU vitamin A; 11 mg ATE vitamin E; 2 mg vitamin C; 13 mg cholesterol; 57 g water

Tip: Serve with salsa and fat-free sour cream.

Fat-Free Potato Skins

Because they're baked instead of fried, these tasty potato skins contain no fat.

4 potatoes

1¹/₂ teaspoons (3 g) ground coriander

¹/₂ teaspoon (1 g) black pepper

1¹/₂ teaspoons (4 g) chili powder

1¹/₂ teaspoons (3 g) curry powder

Preheat the oven to 400°F (200°C, or gas mark 6). Bake the potatoes for 1 hour. Remove the potatoes from the oven, but keep the oven on. Slice the potatoes in half lengthwise, and let them cool for 10 minutes. Scoop out most of the potato flesh, leaving about ¹/₄ inch (0.6 cm) of flesh against the potato skin (you can save the potato flesh for another use, like mashed potatoes). Cut each potato half crosswise into 3 pieces. Spray with olive oil spray. Combine the spices and sprinkle the mixture over the potatoes. Bake the potato skins for 15 minutes or until they are crispy and brown.

Yield: 24 servings

Per serving: 44 calories (3% from fat, 11% from protein, 87% from carbohydrate); 1 g protein; 0 g total fat; 0 g saturated fat; 0 g monounsaturated fat; 0 g polyunsaturated fat; 10 g carbohydrate; 1 g fiber; 1 g sugar; 39 mg phosphorus; 8 mg calcium; 1 mg iron; 5 mg sodium; 287 mg potassium; 54 IU vitamin A; 0 mg ATE vitamin E; 6 mg vitamin C; 0 mg cholesterol; 50 g water

Potstickers

A fairly traditional recipe for Chinese dumplings.

For Filling:

4 ounces (115 g) napa cabbage, shredded

¹/₂ pound (225 g) ground pork loin

2 tablespoons (12 g) scallions, chopped

¹/₂ tablespoon (7.5 ml) white wine

¹/₂ teaspoon (1.3 g) cornstarch

¹/₂ teaspoon (2.5 ml) sesame oil

Dash white pepper

For Dough:

1 cup (125 g) flour

¹/₂ cup (120 ml) boiling water

1 tablespoon (15 ml) olive oil

To make the filling: In a large bowl, mix the cabbage, pork, scallions, wine, cornstarch, sesame oil, and pepper. Set aside.

To make the dough: In a bowl, mix the flour and boiling water until a soft dough forms. Knead the dough on a lightly floured surface for 5 minutes, or until smooth. Shape into a roll 12 inches (30 cm) long and cut into ¹/₂-inch (1.3-cm) slices.

To assemble, roll 1 slice of dough into a 3-inch (7.5-cm) circle and place 1 tablespoon (13 g) pork mixture in the center of the circle. Lift up the edges of the circle and pinch 5 pleats to create a sealed pouch to encase the mixture. Repeat with the remaining dough and filling. Heat a wok or nonstick skillet until very hot. Add 1 tablespoon (15 ml) olive oil, tilting the wok to coat the sides. Place 12 dumplings in a single layer in the wok and fry 2 minutes, or until the bottoms are golden brown. Add $^1/_2$ cup (120 ml) water. Cover and cook 6 to 7 minutes, or until the water is absorbed. Repeat with the remaining dumplings.

Yield: 24 servings

Per serving: 46 calories (33% from fat, 29% from protein, 37% from carbohydrate); 3 g protein; 2 g total fat; 0 g saturated fat; 1 g monounsaturated fat; 0 g polyunsaturated fat; 4 g carbohydrate; 0 g fiber; 0 g sugar; 28 mg phosphorus; 3 mg calcium; 0 mg iron; 6 mg sodium; 46 mg potassium; 18 IU vitamin A; 0 mg ATE vitamin E; 0 mg vitamin C; 8 mg cholesterol; 17 g water

Chickpea-Stuffed Eggs

A healthier alternative to the usual deviled eggs, these have no cholesterol, but 2 grams of fiber.

7 eggs, hard boiled, peeled

1 cup (164 g) cooked chickpeas, drained

2 tablespoons (30 g) plain fat-free yogurt

1 teaspoon Dijon mustard

$^1/_2$ teaspoon minced garlic

Slice eggs in half and discard yolks. In food processor, combine all other ingredients. Spoon mixture into egg cavities.

Yield: 7 servings

Per serving: 58 g water; 61 calories (7% from fat, 37% from protein, 56% from carb); 6 g protein; 0 g total fat; 0 g saturated fat; 0 g monounsaturated fat; 0 g polyunsaturated fat; 8 g carbohydrate; 2 g fiber; 1 g sugar; 44 mg phosphorus; 23 mg calcium; 1 mg iron; 169 mg

sodium; 126 mg potassium; 9 IU vitamin A; 0 mg vitamin E; 1 mg vitamin C; 0 mg cholesterol

Broccoli Bites

A tasty little snack or a nice side dish.

10 ounces (280 g) frozen broccoli

1 cup (72 g) stuffing mix

$^1/_2$ cup (50 g) grated Parmesan cheese

3 eggs, beaten

4 tablespoons (55 g) unsalted butter, softened

$^1/_4$ teaspoon black pepper

Cook broccoli according to package directions; drain well. In a medium bowl, combine cooked broccoli, stuffing mix, cheese, eggs, butter, and pepper. Shape mixture into small balls, about 1 inch (2.5 cm). Freeze, well covered, for at least 3 hours. Preheat oven to 350°F (180°C, gas mark 4). Place frozen balls on baking sheet coated with nonstick vegetable oil spray. Bake until brown, about 15 minutes.

Yield: 15 servings

Per serving: 27 g water; 63 calories (72% from fat, 20% from protein, 8% from carb); 3 g protein; 5 g total fat; 3 g saturated fat; 2 g monounsaturated fat; 0 g polyunsaturated fat; 1 g carbohydrate; 1 g fiber; 0 g sugar; 56 mg phosphorus; 50 mg calcium; 0 mg iron; 116 mg sodium; 47 mg potassium; 377 IU vitamin A; 45 mg vitamin E; 8 mg vitamin C; 58 mg cholesterol

Eggplant Fingers

Fried eggplant snacks provide a big fiber boost.

1 eggplant

$^1/_2$ cup (120 ml) canola oil

1 cup (235 ml) skim milk

1 cup (120 g) whole wheat flour

1 cup (115 g) whole wheat bread crumbs

Peel eggplant and cut into $^1/_2$-inch (1-cm) strips. Heat oil to 375°F (190°C, gas mark 5). Dip eggplant into milk, then flour, then milk again, then bread crumbs. Deep-fry and drain completely until no trace of oil appears on paper towel.

Yield: 8 servings

Per serving: 83 g water; 254 calories (52% from fat, 9% from protein, 39% from carb); 6 g protein; 15 g total fat; 1 g saturated fat; 8 g monounsaturated fat; 5 g polyunsaturated fat; 26 g carbohydrate; 4 g fiber; 2 g sugar; 123 mg phosphorus; 79 mg calcium; 1 mg iron; 39 mg sodium; 275 mg potassium; 79 IU vitamin A; 19 mg vitamin E; 2 mg vitamin C; 1 mg cholesterol

Spinach Balls

You could serve these as a side dish, but they make a great snack or buffet item, kind of like spinach dip that you can carry around with you.

10 ounces (280 g) frozen spinach, thawed and drained

1 cup (72 g) stuffing mix, crushed

$^1/_2$ cup (50 g) grated Parmesan cheese

3 eggs, beaten

$^1/_4$ cup (55 g) unsalted butter, softened

$^1/_8$ teaspoon nutmeg

Place spinach on paper towels and squeeze until barely moist. Combine spinach and next 5 ingredients in a bowl. Mix well. Shape into $2^1/_2$-inch (6-cm) balls with an ice cream scoop. Place on waxed paper–lined baking sheet. Cover and refrigerate 8 hours. To bake, place spinach balls on a baking sheet coated with nonstick vegetable oil spray and bake at 350°F (180°C, gas mark 4) for 15 minutes until hot. Drain on paper towels.

Yield: 20 servings

Per serving: 20 g water; 70 calories (52% from fat, 18% from protein, 29% from carb); 3 g protein; 4 g total fat; 2 g saturated fat; 1 g monounsaturated fat; 0 g polyunsaturated fat; 5 g carbohydrate; 1 g fiber; 1 g sugar; 50 mg phosphorus; 60 mg calcium; 1 mg iron; 154 mg sodium; 72 mg potassium; 1833 IU vitamin A; 34 mg vitamin E; 0 mg vitamin C; 44 mg cholesterol

Zucchini Sticks

Healthy and crunchy, these baked treats offer taste and nutrition without the fat of deep-frying.

3 medium zucchini

$^1/_2$ cup (56 g) wheat germ

$^1/_2$ cup (55 g) finely chopped almonds

$^1/_4$ cup (25 g) grated Parmesan cheese

2 tablespoons (28 g) unsalted butter, melted

Cut each zucchini lengthwise into fourths, then lengthwise into halves to form sticks. Cut each stick lengthwise into halves (each zucchini makes 16 sticks). Mix wheat germ, almonds, and cheese in plastic bag. Roll about 8 zucchini sticks at a time in butter until evenly coated. Lift with fork. Shake sticks in wheat germ. Lay on an ungreased baking sheet. Cook in 350°F (180°C, gas mark 4) oven until crisp and tender, about 15 minutes.

Yield: 6 servings

Per serving: 61 g water; 168 calories (62% from fat, 17% from protein, 21% from carb); 8 g protein; 12 g total fat; 4 g saturated fat; 5 g monounsaturated fat; 2 g polyunsaturated fat; 9 g carbohydrate; 3 g fiber; 2 g sugar; 221 mg phosphorus; 87 mg calcium; 2 mg iron; 74 mg sodium; 341 mg potassium; 271 IU vitamin A; 37 mg vitamin E; 11 mg vitamin C; 14 mg cholesterol

Stuffed Artichokes

Walnuts give this appetizer both crunch and extra fiber.

10 ounces (280 g) frozen spinach

1/4 cup (30 g) chopped walnuts

1 cup (235 ml) fat-free evaporated milk

1/2 teaspoon crushed garlic

1 can artichoke bottoms, drained and rinsed

2 tablespoons (30 ml) lemon juice

1/4 cup (25 g) grated Parmesan cheese

Cook and drain spinach. Process spinach in blender with chopped walnuts, evaporated milk, and crushed garlic until coarsely chopped. Arrange artichoke bottoms in baking dish coated with nonstick vegetable oil spray. Drizzle with lemon juice. Stuff with spinach mixture and top with Parmesan cheese.

Bake in oven at 350°F (180°C, gas mark 4) for 20 to 25 minutes.

Yield: 4 servings

Per serving: 181 g water; 301 calories (44% from fat, 32% from protein, 25% from carb); 25 g protein; 15 g total fat; 7 g saturated fat; 4 g monounsaturated fat; 3 g polyunsaturated fat; 19 g carbohydrate; 6 g fiber; 9 g sugar; 493 mg phosphorus; 701 mg calcium; 2 mg iron; 710 mg sodium; 680 mg potassium; 9058 IU vitamin A; 116 mg vitamin E; 9 mg vitamin C; 33 mg cholesterol

Marinated Veggies

This version of marinated vegetables is also good on a salad, but if you cut them a bit smaller, it makes a great relish for sandwiches, similar to New Orleans's muffaletta.

1/2 teaspoon minced garlic

1/2 cup (120 ml) vinegar

1/2 cup (120 ml) olive oil

1 teaspoon oregano

1/2 cup (35 g) chopped mushrooms

1/4 cup (25 g) chopped black olives

1/4 cup (25 g) chopped green olives

1/2 cup (82 g) cooked chickpeas

1/2 cup (80 g) chopped onion

1/2 cup (150 g) chopped artichoke hearts

Combine first 4 ingredients. Add any or all of the remaining ingredients, cutting raw vegetables into bite-size chunks and draining liquids from those in cans. Marinate up to 24 hours.

Yield: 24 servings

Per serving: 18 g water; 53 calories (81% from fat, 3% from protein, 15% from carb); 0 g protein; 5 g total fat; 1 g saturated fat; 4 g monounsaturated fat; 1 g polyunsaturated fat; 2 g carbohydrate; 1 g fiber; 0 g sugar; 10 mg phosphorus; 7 mg calcium; 0 mg iron; 42 mg sodium; 32 mg potassium; 21 IU vitamin A; 0 mg vitamin E; 1 mg vitamin C; 0 mg cholesterol

Veggie Antipasto

An easy antipasto platter full of fresh veggies.

Herb Marinade

$^2/_3$ cup (157 ml) red wine vinegar

$^1/_3$ cup (78 ml) olive oil

3 diced scallions

1 teaspoon basil

1 teaspoon oregano

$^1/_2$ teaspoon black pepper, fresh ground

$^1/_2$ teaspoon minced garlic

Vegetables

8 ounces (225 g) mushrooms, sliced

6 ounces (170 g) artichoke hearts, halved

1 cup (130 g) sliced carrot

1 cup (150 g) sliced red bell pepper

1 cup (100 g) sliced celery

8 ounces (225 g) cherry tomatoes

2 tablespoons fresh cilantro

4 ounces (115 g) olives

16 ounces (455 g) chickpeas

Mix all marinade ingredients in saucepan and boil for 2 or 3 minutes. Cool for 10 minutes and pour over vegetables in a large bowl that has a tight-fitting cover. Refrigerate covered for at least 24 hours. Invert bowl several times during the 24-hour period to make sure that all vegetables absorb flavor from the marinade.

Yield: 8 servings

Per serving: 158 g water; 203 calories (50% from fat, 10% from protein, 40% from carb); 5 g protein; 12 g total fat; 2 g saturated fat; 8 g monounsaturated fat; 2 g polyunsaturated fat; 21 g carbohydrate; 6 g fiber; 2 g sugar; 105 mg phosphorus; 55 mg calcium; 2 mg iron; 330 mg sodium; 445 mg potassium; 3658 IU vitamin A; 0 mg vitamin E; 35 mg vitamin C; 0 mg cholesterol

Tip: Vary by using your favorite vegetables in place of or in addition to those listed.

Vegetable Wrap

This makes a great lunch. It's easy and quick to put together, tastes great, and packs a lot of nutrition into not many calories.

1 cup (119 g) sliced cucumber

1 cup (113 g) sliced zucchini

$^1/_2$ cup (65 g) sliced carrot

4 ounces (115 g) mushrooms, chopped

$^1/_4$ cup (25 g) chopped scallions

$^1/_2$ teaspoon minced garlic

3 ounces (85 g) cream cheese

4 whole wheat tortillas

$^1/_4$ cup (65 g) salsa

Combine all veggies. Spread cream cheese on tortilla. Spread veggies and salsa over cream cheese. Roll up.

Yield: 4 servings

Per serving: 135 g water; 197 calories (44% from fat, 12% from protein, 44% from carb); 6 g protein; 10 g total fat; 5 g saturated fat; 3 g monounsaturated fat; 1 g polyunsaturated fat; 22 g carbohydrate; 3 g fiber; 3 g sugar; 115 mg phosphorus; 80 mg calcium; 2 mg iron; 309 mg sodium; 399 mg potassium; 3175 IU vitamin A; 76 mg vitamin E; 9 mg vitamin C; 23 mg cholesterol

Spinach Roll-Ups

Sort of like spinach salad to take with you. Colorful roll-ups with spinach and bacon flavor.

10 ounces (280 g) frozen spinach

$^1/_2$ cup (115 g) sour cream

$^1/_2$ cup (115 g) mayonnaise

2 tablespoons bacon bits

3 whole wheat tortillas

Cook spinach and drain well. Mix sour cream, mayonnaise, and bacon bits. Mix in cooked spinach. Equally divide on top of tortillas. Spread mixture evenly over each tortilla. Roll up each tortilla. Store overnight in refrigerator. Slice into 1-inch (2.5-cm) slices.

Yield: 15 servings

Per serving: 26 g water; 92 calories (71% from fat, 8% from protein, 21% from carb); 2 g protein; 7 g total fat; 2 g saturated fat; 2 g monounsaturated fat; 3 g

polyunsaturated fat; 5 g carbohydrate; 1 g fiber; 0 g sugar; 27 mg phosphorus; 48 mg calcium; 1 mg iron; 124 mg sodium; 80 mg potassium; 2330 IU vitamin A; 14 mg vitamin E; 1 mg vitamin C; 6 mg cholesterol

Vegetable Quesadillas

If you have an indoor grill like the George Foreman models, it is perfect for making these quesadillas. If not, place them on a baking sheet in a 350°F (180°C, gas mark 4) oven until crisp. Serve them with salsa and sour cream.

$^1/_4$ cup (55 g) unsalted butter

$2^1/_2$ teaspoons chili powder

1 teaspoon minced garlic

1 teaspoon oregano

8 ounces (225 g) mushrooms, sliced

1 cup (150 g) sliced green bell pepper

$^2/_3$ cup (110 g) finely chopped onion

$^1/_2$ cup chopped fresh cilantro

$1^1/_2$ cups (175 g) shredded Monterey Jack cheese

2 tablespoons (28 ml) olive oil

16 corn tortillas, $5^1/_2$ inch (14 cm)

Melt the butter in a large skillet over medium-high heat. Add chili powder, garlic, and oregano and sauté about 1 minute. Add mushrooms and sauté until tender, about 10 minutes. Remove from heat and mix in the bell pepper, onion, and cilantro. Cool for 10 minutes, then mix in the cheese. Lightly brush oil on one side of 8 of the tortillas and place them oil side down on a baking sheet. Divide vegetable mixture among tortillas, spreading to even thickness. Top with the remaining 8 tortillas and brush tops with oil. Grill quesadillas until heated through and golden brown, about 3 minutes per side. Cut into wedges (4 to 6) to serve.

Yield: 12 servings

Per serving: 62 g water; 205 calories (52% from fat, 13% from protein, 35% from carb); 7 g protein; 12 g total fat; 6 g saturated fat; 4 g monounsaturated fat; 1 g polyunsaturated fat; 19 g carbohydrate; 3 g fiber; 1 g sugar; 207 mg phosphorus; 193 mg calcium; 1 mg iron; 101 mg sodium; 184 mg potassium; 569 IU vitamin A; 63 mg vitamin E; 12 mg vitamin C; 25 mg cholesterol

Vegetable Pita Pockets

I just love it when things that are good for you also taste great. This is one of those things.

1 cup (71 g) sliced broccoli

1 cup (100 g) sliced cauliflower

1 cup (130 g) sliced carrot

$^1/_2$ cup (80 g) sliced onion

1 tablespoon unsalted butter

1 cup (180 g) chopped tomato

$^1/_4$ teaspoon oregano leaves

$^1/_4$ teaspoon basil leaves

1 cup (110 g) shredded Swiss cheese

4 whole wheat pitas

Sauté broccoli, cauliflower, carrot, and onion in butter for 3 to 4 minutes until crisp and tender. Toss sautéed vegetables with tomato, oregano, basil, and cheese. Cut pita bread in half to form two half-circle pockets. Divide vegetable mixture evenly in all the pita halves.

Yield: 4 servings

Per serving: 163 g water; 364 calories (33% from fat, 19% from protein, 48% from carb); 18 g protein; 14 g total fat; 8 g saturated fat; 3 g monounsaturated fat; 1 g polyunsaturated fat; 46 g carbohydrate; 8 g fiber; 4 g sugar; 367 mg phosphorus; 361 mg calcium; 3 mg iron; 384 mg sodium; 478 mg potassium; 6123 IU vitamin A; 93 mg vitamin E; 47 mg vitamin C; 38 mg cholesterol

Veggie Bars

This makes both a pretty and a tasty appetizer. It's light enough that people won't get filled up on it, so it's also a good choice before a meal. We've used it to satisfy the family munchies while roast beef is cooking for New Year's dinner.

1 package crescent rolls

$^1/_4$ cup (60 g) sour cream

1 tablespoon (15 ml) ranch dressing

8 ounces (225 g) cream cheese

$^1/_2$ cup (75 g) finely chopped green bell pepper

$^1/_2$ cup (80 g) finely chopped onion

$^1/_2$ cup (36 g) finely chopped broccoli

$^1/_2$ cup (65 g) finely chopped carrot

$^1/_2$ cup (50 g) finely chopped cauliflower

$^1/_4$ cup (25 g) finely chopped black olives

$^1/_2$ cup (35 g) finely chopped mushrooms

$^1/_2$ cup (58 g) shredded Cheddar cheese

Carefully unroll crescent rolls and place dough in 8 × 13-inch (20 × 33-cm) pan. Gently press and shape to cover bottom. Bake at 350°F (180°C, gas mark 4) for 8 minutes. Let cool. Mix sour cream, dressing, and cream cheese. Spread on cooled crust. Sprinkle remaining ingredients on top, cover with plastic wrap, and press vegetables down into cream. Chill for 3 to 4 hours. Cut into bars and serve.

Yield: 16 servings

Per serving: 35 g water; 90 calories (73% from fat, 12% from protein, 15% from carb); 3 g protein; 7 g total fat; 4 g saturated fat; 2 g monounsaturated fat; 0 g polyunsaturated fat; 3 g carbohydrate; 1 g fiber; 1 g sugar; 51 mg phosphorus; 55 mg calcium; 0 mg iron; 108 mg sodium; 78 mg potassium; 965 IU vitamin A; 65 mg vitamin E; 9 mg vitamin C; 22 mg cholesterol

Pecan-Stuffed Mushrooms

This appetizer always disappears fast. Something about the crunch of pecans just makes these different from other mushrooms.

12 large mushrooms

2 tablespoons (20 g) chopped onion

2 tablespoons (28 g) unsalted butter

$^1/_2$ cup (55 g) chopped pecans

$^1/_2$ cup (60 g) whole wheat bread crumbs

1 teaspoon lemon juice

Wash mushrooms gently in cool water or wipe with damp cloth. Remove and chop stems. Sauté onion in butter; add chopped stems, pecans, bread crumbs, and lemon juice. Mix well. Mound mushroom caps

with stuffing. Broil 4 minutes about 4 inches (10 cm) from heat or cook in microwave oven on 100 percent power 2 to 3 minutes until heated through.

Yield: 12 servings

Per serving: 14 g water; 70 calories (68% from fat, 8% from protein, 24% from carb); 1 g protein; 5 g total fat; 2 g saturated fat; 2 g monounsaturated fat; 1 g polyunsaturated fat; 4 g carbohydrate; 1 g fiber; 1 g sugar; 31 mg phosphorus; 13 mg calcium; 0 mg iron; 7 mg sodium; 68 mg potassium; 62 IU vitamin A; 16 mg vitamin E; 1 mg vitamin C; 5 mg cholesterol

Pineapple Kabobs

Sweet grilled pineapple wedges. Try this with pork chops.

$^1/_4$ cup (85 g) honey

2 tablespoons (28 g) unsalted butter

1 teaspoon cinnamon

1 pineapple

Combine honey, butter, and cinnamon. Pare and cut fresh pineapple into long wedges. Grill over medium heat 15 minutes, basting with sauce. Turn frequently.

Yield: 4 servings

Per serving: 15 g water; 123 calories (40% from fat, 1% from protein, 60% from carb); 0 g protein; 6 g total fat; 4 g saturated fat; 1 g monounsaturated fat; 0 g polyunsaturated fat; 20 g carbohydrate; 1 g fiber; 19 g sugar; 4 mg phosphorus; 12 mg calcium; 0 mg iron; 2 mg sodium; 28 mg potassium; 183 IU vitamin A; 48 mg vitamin E; 1 mg vitamin C; 15 mg cholesterol

Banana Bites

A quick way to add crunch and flavor to bananas.

3 cups (450 g) sliced banana

6 ounces (213 g) orange juice concentrate

2 cups (164 g) granola

Cut bananas into bite-size pieces. Pour orange juice concentrate into mixing bowl. Spread granola on baking sheet. Dip banana bits into the orange juice. Roll in granola.

Yield: 6 servings

Per serving: 103 g water; 251 calories (6% from fat, 6% from protein, 88% from carb); 4 g protein; 2 g total fat; 0 g saturated fat; 1 g monounsaturated fat; 0 g polyunsaturated fat; 59 g carbohydrate; 5 g fiber; 34 g sugar; 116 mg phosphorus; 25 mg calcium; 1 mg iron; 105 mg sodium; 671 mg potassium; 179 IU vitamin A; 0 mg vitamin E; 49 mg vitamin C; 0 mg cholesterol

Date Chews

Sweet little treats to nibble on.

1 cup (145 g) cut-up dates

3 teaspoons flour

1 cup (110 g) finely chopped pecans

$^1/_2$ cup (100 g) sugar

2 eggs

1 teaspoon vanilla extract

Combine dates with flour and stir to coat. Stir all ingredients enough to blend. Place 1 teaspoon each

in mini muffin pans that have been sprayed with nonstick vegetable oil spray. Bake at 375°F (190°C, gas mark 5) for 12 to 15 minutes.

Yield: 32 servings

Per serving: 4 g water; 58 calories (42% from fat, 6% from protein, 52% from carb); 1 g protein; 3 g total fat; 0 g saturated fat; 2 g monounsaturated fat; 1 g polyunsaturated fat; 8 g carbohydrate; 1 g fiber; 7 g sugar; 20 mg phosphorus; 7 mg calcium; 0 mg iron; 5 mg sodium; 56 mg potassium; 20 IU vitamin A; 5 mg vitamin E; 0 mg vitamin C; 15 mg cholesterol

Apricot Chews

Treats that are perfect when you just want a little something sweet.

2 ounces (57 g) cream cheese, softened

1 tablespoon confectioners' sugar

$^1/_4$ teaspoon vanilla extract

8 ounces (225 g) dried apricots

1 tablespoon wheat germ

3 tablespoons (27 g) slivered almonds

Blend cream cheese, confectioners' sugar, and vanilla until softened. Place small amount of mixture between two halves of apricots. Sprinkle wheat germ and almonds on top. Chill for 15 minutes.

Yield: 15 servings

Per serving: 15 g water; 35 calories (57% from fat, 10% from protein, 33% from carb); 1 g protein; 2 g total fat; 1 g saturated fat; 1 g monounsaturated fat; 0 g polyunsaturated fat; 3 g carbohydrate; 1 g fiber; 2 g sugar;

21 mg phosphorus; 10 mg calcium; 0 mg iron; 12 mg sodium; 47 mg potassium; 307 IU vitamin A; 14 mg vitamin E; 1 mg vitamin C; 4 mg cholesterol

Cheese Crisps

These little snacks taste great either warm from the oven or cold. There usually aren't any left to eat cold, however, when we make them.

1 cup (120 g) grated Cheddar cheese

$1/4$ cup (55 g) unsalted butter

$1/2$ cup (60 g) whole wheat flour

In large bowl, combine the cheese and butter. Add the flour and mix thoroughly. Roll into small balls. Place the balls on an baking sheet sprayed with nonstick vegetable oil spray and flatten. Bake at 400°F (200°C, gas mark 6) for 5 to 8 minutes. Do not let the edges get browned.

Yield: 12 servings

Per serving: 5 g water; 95 calories (70% from fat, 14% from protein, 16% from carb); 3 g protein; 8 g total fat; 5 g saturated fat; 2 g monounsaturated fat; 0 g polyunsaturated fat; 4 g carbohydrate; 1 g fiber; 0 g sugar; 75 mg phosphorus; 82 mg calcium; 0 mg iron; 69 mg sodium; 32 mg potassium; 229 IU vitamin A; 60 mg vitamin E; 0 mg vitamin C; 22 mg cholesterol

Wheat Germ Crackers

Tasty little crackers, these are good without anything, but also make a healthy dipper for any of the dips and spreads in Chapter 3.

3 cups (240 g) quick-cooking oats

2 cups (240 g) whole wheat pastry flour

1 cup (112 g) wheat germ

3 tablespoons (39 g) sugar

1 cup (235 ml) water

$3/4$ cup (175 ml) canola oil

Mix dry ingredients together. Add water and oil; stir until all is wet. Roll out thin on upside-down baking sheet. Score and prick with fork. Bake at 325°F (170°C, gas mark 3) for 30 minutes or more, until brown. This is enough for 2 baking sheets, approximately 10 × 15 inches (25 × 37 cm) or 11 × 16 inches (27 × 40 cm).

Yield: 60 servings

Per serving: 5 g water; 63 calories (46% from fat, 11% from protein, 44% from carb); 2 g protein; 3 g total fat; 0 g saturated fat; 2 g monounsaturated fat; 1 g polyunsaturated fat; 7 g carbohydrate; 1 g fiber; 1 g sugar; 55 mg phosphorus; 4 mg calcium; 0 mg iron; 1 mg sodium; 48 mg potassium; 2 IU vitamin A; 0 mg vitamin E; 0 mg vitamin C; 0 mg cholesterol

Pita Chips

Simple and easy. Make your own low-fat, high-fiber chips for snacking or dipping in about 5 minutes.

2 whole wheat pitas

Cut pita into triangles, then separate. Place on foil-covered baking sheet. Spray with nonstick vegetable oil spray; season if desired. Bake in 375°F (190°C, gas mark 5) oven until crisp, about 5 minutes. Remove and cool.

Yield: 4 servings

Per serving: 10 g water; 85 calories (8% from fat, 14% from protein, 78% from carb); 3 g protein; 1 g total fat; 0 g saturated fat; 0 g monounsaturated fat; 0 g polyunsaturated fat; 18 g carbohydrate; 2 g fiber; 0 g sugar; 58 mg phosphorus; 5 mg calcium; 1 mg iron; 170 mg sodium; 54 mg potassium; 0 IU vitamin A; 0 mg vitamin E; 0 mg vitamin C; 0 mg cholesterol

Parmesan-Garlic Pita Toasts

Use these flavorful pita crisps for any of the spreads or dips in the book. Or just nibble on them for a healthier-than-usual snack option.

2 whole wheat pitas, cut into 8 triangles each

3 tablespoons (42 g) unsalted butter

1 teaspoon minced garlic

$^1/_2$ teaspoon black pepper, fresh ground

$^1/_4$ cup (25 g) grated Parmesan cheese

Melt butter; cook garlic in butter over low heat, stirring occasionally, for 5 minutes. Brush mixture lightly on rough side of pita triangles. Arrange butter side up in 1 layer on baking sheet. Sprinkle pepper and Parmesan cheese on top. Bake in oven

preheated to 350°F (180°C, gas mark 4) for 12 to 15 minutes, until crisp and light brown. Cool on racks and store in airtight container in dry place.

Yield: 8 servings

Per serving: 7 g water; 95 calories (51% from fat, 12% from protein, 37% from carb); 3 g protein; 6 g total fat; 3 g saturated fat; 1 g monounsaturated fat; 0 g polyunsaturated fat; 9 g carbohydrate; 1 g fiber; 0 g sugar; 54 mg phosphorus; 40 mg calcium; 1 mg iron; 134 mg sodium; 35 mg potassium; 147 IU vitamin A; 39 mg vitamin E; 0 mg vitamin C; 14 mg cholesterol

Spicy Pita Dippers

Pepper and cumin give these pita triangles a southwestern flavor that goes particularly well with bean dips.

$^1/_2$ cup (112 g) unsalted butter, melted

2 teaspoons lemon pepper

2 teaspoons ground cumin

6 whole wheat pitas, cut into triangles

To make dippers, preheat the broiler. Combine the melted butter, lemon pepper, and cumin in a bowl. Dip the pita pieces quickly in the mixture, then place on a baking sheet. Broil 2 to 4 minutes, until crisp. Cool on a rack.

Yield: 12 servings

Per serving: 12 g water; 155 calories (48% from fat, 8% from protein, 44% from carb); 3 g protein; 9 g total fat; 5 g saturated fat; 2 g monounsaturated fat; 1 g polyunsaturated fat; 18 g carbohydrate; 2 g fiber; 0 g sugar; 62 mg phosphorus; 12 mg calcium; 1 mg iron; 172 mg sodium; 67 mg potassium; 242 IU vitamin A; 63 mg vitamin E; 0 mg vitamin C; 20 mg cholesterol

Pecan Cheese Wafers

Savory little pecan and cheese crackers are great to snack on or as dippers.

$^1/_2$ cup (112 g) unsalted butter, softened

2 cups (225 g) shredded Cheddar cheese

1 cup (110 g) finely chopped pecans

1 cup (120 g) whole wheat pastry flour

$^1/_4$ teaspoon cayenne pepper

Cream butter and cheese. Add pecans, flour, and cayenne. Mix well. Form into 2 rolls, 1 inch (2.5 cm) in diameter. Wrap in plastic and refrigerate several hours or overnight. (Can also be frozen.) Slice rolls into thin rounds and place on baking sheet coated with nonstick vegetable oil spray. Bake at 350°F (180°C, gas mark 4) for 15 minutes or until edges brown lightly. Remove to rack to cool.

Yield: 40 servings

Per serving: 3 g water; 76 calories (75% from fat, 12% from protein, 13% from carb); 2 g protein; 7 g total fat; 3 g saturated fat; 2 g monounsaturated fat; 1 g polyunsaturated fat; 3 g carbohydrate; 1 g fiber; 0 g sugar; 52 mg phosphorus; 51 mg calcium; 0 mg iron; 41 mg sodium; 31 mg potassium; 143 IU vitamin A; 36 mg vitamin E; 0 mg vitamin C; 13 mg cholesterol

Macadamia Cheese Crisps

Savory little crackers with the added bonus of macadamia nuts. You'll find it hard to limit yourself to the recommended serving size.

$^1/_2$ cup (112 g) unsalted butter

$^1/_4$ pound (115 g) grated Swiss cheese

1 egg

1$^1/_2$ cups (180 g) whole wheat pastry flour

$^1/_3$ cup (45 g) chopped macadamia nuts

Preheat oven to 400°F (200°C, gas mark 6). Blend butter, cheese, and egg. Gradually work in flour and nuts. Mold into roll 1$^1/_2$ inches (4 cm) in diameter. Wrap in waxed paper and chill until firm. Slice dough into $^1/_4$-inch (0.5-cm) slices. Place on lightly buttered baking sheet and bake for 10 to 15 minutes or until lightly browned.

Yield: 18 servings

Per serving: 6 g water; 126 calories (64% from fat, 12% from protein, 24% from carb); 4 g protein; 9 g total fat; 5 g saturated fat; 3 g monounsaturated fat; 0 g polyunsaturated fat; 8 g carbohydrate; 1 g fiber; 0 g sugar; 84 mg phosphorus; 69 mg calcium; 1 mg iron; 7 mg sodium; 62 mg potassium; 229 IU vitamin A; 61 mg vitamin E; 0 mg vitamin C; 31 mg cholesterol

Fat-Free Potato Chips

These potato chips are very easy to make in the microwave. Also, they are healthier for you since they are not cooked in any oils. They can be made plain or with your choice of herbs and spices. They need to be sliced fairly thin to get crisp, but not paper thin. The original recipe called for a covered microwave bacon rack, but I found that putting them between two plates worked great. You may need to spray the plates with a little nonstick vegetable oil spray before the first batch to keep them from sticking.

4 medium potatoes

Your choice of spices or herbs

If the potatoes are old, peel them before slicing. If the potatoes are new or have good skins, do not peel, just scrub well. Slice potatoes $^1/_{16}$ inch (1.5 mm) in thickness, slicing across the potato. Sprinkle with your choice of spices or herbs, if desired. If you have a microwave bacon tray, place the sliced potatoes flat on the tray in a single layer. Cover with a microwavable, round, heavy plastic cover. If you do not have a bacon tray, place potatoes between two microwave-safe plates. Microwave on high (full power) for 7 to 8 minutes. Cooking time could vary slightly, depending on the wattage of your microwave. You do not have to turn the sliced potatoes over. Plates will be hot by the time potatoes are done. Continue to microwave the remainder of sliced potatoes as directed above.

Yield: 8 servings

Per serving: 129 calories (2% from fat, 10% from protein, 88% from carbohydrate); 3 g protein; 0 g total fat; 0 g saturated fat; 0 g monounsaturated fat; 0 g polyunsaturated fat; 29 g carbohydrate; 3 g fiber; 2 g sugar; 113 mg phosphorus; 18 mg calcium; 1 mg iron; 11 mg sodium; 839 mg potassium; 13 IU vitamin A; 0 mg ATE vitamin E; 16 mg vitamin C; 0 mg cholesterol; 149 g water

Low Fat Tortilla Chips

Just like you used to get at your favorite Mexican restaurant. I like these sprinkled with a little salt-free taco seasoning.

1 corn tortilla

Nonstick vegetable oil spray

Preheat oven to 350°F (180°C, or gas mark 4). Cut tortilla into 6 wedges. Place tortilla pieces on a baking sheet. Spray with nonstick vegetable oil spray. Turn tortillas over and spray the other side. Bake for 10 minutes, or until crispy and browned on the edges.

Yield: 1 serving

Per serving: 58 calories (10% from fat, 10% from protein, 80% from carbohydrate); 1 g protein; 1 g total fat; 0 g saturated fat; 0 g monounsaturated fat; 0 g polyunsaturated fat; 12 g carbohydrate; 1 g fiber; 0 g sugar; 82 mg phosphorus; 46 mg calcium; 0 mg iron; 3 mg sodium; 40 mg potassium; 0 IU vitamin A; 0 mg ATE vitamin E; 0 mg vitamin C; 0 mg cholesterol; 11 g water

Sweet Potato Chips

High-fiber, fat-free snack. And they taste great.

3 sweet potatoes

$^1/_2$ teaspoon cumin

$^1/_2$ teaspoon chili powder

Scrub sweet potatoes. Slice, in rounds, very thin. Spray baking sheet with nonstick vegetable oil spray. Lay rounds on sheet and spray the tops. Place in preheated 350°F (180°C, gas mark 4) oven and bake until crisp, about 10 minutes. Sprinkle with spices.

Yield: 6 servings

Per serving: 61 g water; 59 calories (3% from fat, 7% from protein, 90% from carb); 1 g protein; 0 g total fat; 0 g saturated fat; 0 g monounsaturated fat; 0 g polyunsaturated fat; 14 g carbohydrate; 2 g fiber; 4 g sugar; 26 mg phosphorus; 23 mg calcium; 1 mg iron; 23 mg sodium; 181 mg potassium; 11948 IU vitamin A; 0 mg vitamin E; 10 mg vitamin C; 0 mg cholesterol

Tip: Vary the spices to suit your mood.

Roasted Chickpeas

A healthy, tasty snack, high in fiber and very low in fat. Vary the seasonings according to your taste.

4 cups (656 g) cooked chickpeas

$^1/_4$ teaspoon cayenne pepper

1 teaspoon garlic powder

1 teaspoon cumin

1 teaspoon paprika

Preheat oven to 400°F (200°C, gas mark 6). In a mesh strainer, gently rinse beans. Drain on paper towels and gently roll them dry. Line a baking sheet with aluminum foil and spread chickpeas evenly across sheet. Bake chickpeas, checking at 10-minute intervals. When chickpeas are dried and crunchy, about 30 to 40 minutes, remove from oven and spray with an olive oil cooking spray. Place spices in a plastic bowl with a tight-fitting lid or resealable plastic bag. Add chickpeas and shake to coat. For best results, store in an airtight container in the refrigerator.

Yield: 12 servings

Per serving: 33 g water; 92 calories (14% from fat, 21% from protein, 65% from carb); 5 g protein; 1 g total fat;

0 g saturated fat; 0 g monounsaturated fat; 1 g polyunsaturated fat; 15 g carbohydrate; 4 g fiber; 3 g sugar; 94 mg phosphorus; 29 mg calcium; 2 mg iron; 4 mg sodium; 170 mg potassium; 133 IU vitamin A; 0 mg vitamin E; 1 mg vitamin C; 0 mg cholesterol

Whole Wheat Honey Mustard Pretzels

This was one of those extended work-in-progress recipes as I tried different combinations to get the taste I wanted. The breakthrough was finding the large hard pretzels in a honey wheat with sesame seeds variety from Harry's Premium Snacks at a gourmet food store not too far away. They are great tasting alone, but they also made a great base for this recipe.

$^1/_4$ cup (55 g) unsalted butter

2 tablespoons (40 g) honey

$^1/_4$ cup (60 ml) honey mustard

$^1/_2$ teaspoon onion powder

$^1/_4$ teaspoon Tabasco sauce

8 ounces (225 g) whole wheat pretzels, broken up

Melt butter in microwave. Stir in honey, honey mustard, and spices. Pour over pretzels and stir to coat evenly. Bake at 300°F (150°C, gas mark 2) for 30 minutes, stirring every 10 minutes. Cool on waxed paper. Store in an airtight container.

Yield: 10 servings

Per serving: 8 g water; 137 calories (32% from fat, 7% from protein, 60% from carb); 3 g protein; 5 g total fat; 3 g saturated fat; 1 g monounsaturated fat; 0 g polyunsaturated fat; 22 g carbohydrate; 2 g fiber; 4 g

sugar; 32 mg phosphorus; 9 mg calcium; 1 mg iron; 83 mg sodium; 110 mg potassium; 236 IU vitamin A; 38 mg vitamin E; 1 mg vitamin C; 12 mg cholesterol

Ranch-Style Pretzels

Flavorful pretzel snacks with the taste of ranch dressing.

12 ounces (340 g) whole wheat pretzels, broken

1 packet Hidden Valley Ranch or other ranch dressing mix

$^1/_4$ cup (235 ml) olive oil

1 teaspoon lemon pepper

1 teaspoon dill weed

1 teaspoon garlic powder

Mix all ingredients in large bowl and toss to coat. Spread on baking sheet. Don't preheat oven. Bake at 300°F (150°C, gas mark 2) for 20 minutes, 10 minutes on one side, then turn and bake another 10 minutes.

Yield: 24 servings

Per serving: 1 g water; 72 calories (31% from fat, 8% from protein, 61% from carb); 2 g protein; 3 g total fat; 0 g saturated fat; 2 g monounsaturated fat; 0 g polyunsaturated fat; 12 g carbohydrate; 1 g fiber; 0 g sugar; 19 mg phosphorus; 5 mg calcium; 0 mg iron; 29 mg sodium; 65 mg potassium; 3 IU vitamin A; 0 mg vitamin E; 0 mg vitamin C; 0 mg cholesterol

Spicy Snack Mix

Marti, a subscriber to my email newsletter, sent me this recipe for a snack mix. It makes a nice alternative to Chex mix.

1 egg white

2 teaspoons (10 ml) water

3 tablespoons (39 g) sugar

$^3/_4$ teaspoon (1.7 g) cinnamon

$^1/_8$ teaspoon (0.3 g) nutmeg

$^1/_8$ teaspoon (0.2 g) ground ginger

5 cups (250 g) spoon-sized shredded wheat squares

$1^1/_2$ cups (220 g) unsalted dry roasted peanuts

Preheat oven to 250°F (120°C, or gas mark $^1/_2$). Combine egg white and water; stir in sugar, cinnamon, nutmeg, and ginger. Beat until frothy. Mix cereal and nuts in a 9 × 13-inch (23 × 33-cm) baking pan. Add egg white mixture; toss to coat. Bake for 15 minutes. Cool 5 minutes. Remove from pan; cool completely. Store in tightly covered container.

Yield: 14 servings

Per serving: 169 calories (40% from fat, 12% from protein, 48% from carbohydrate); 5 g protein; 8 g total fat; 1 g saturated fat; 4 g monounsaturated fat; 2 g polyunsaturated fat; 22 g carbohydrate; 3 g fiber; 8 g sugar; 108 mg phosphorus; 13 mg calcium; 1 mg iron; 8 mg sodium; 169 mg potassium; 0 IU vitamin A; 0 mg ATE vitamin E; 0 mg vitamin C; 0 mg cholesterol; 4 g water

Cajun Party Mix

A little spicier than some party mixes, this one will definitely let you know that you are eating it.

12 ounces (340 g) almonds

6 cups (180 g) Crispix or other hexagonal multigrain cereal

1 cup (45 g) goldfish-shaped or other small crackers

$^1/_4$ cup (55 g) unsalted butter

1 tablespoon (15 ml) Worcestershire sauce

$^1/_2$ teaspoon paprika

$^1/_2$ teaspoon thyme

$^1/_4$ teaspoon black pepper

$^1/_4$ teaspoon Tabasco sauce

Preheat oven to 250°F (120°C, gas mark $^1/_2$). In a large shallow roasting pan, combine almonds, cereal, and goldfish crackers. Melt butter and stir in seasonings. Pour over mixture and toss to coat. Bake 1 hour, stirring every 20 minutes. Spread on paper towel to cool. Store in airtight container.

Yield: 36 servings

Per serving: 1 g water; 86 calories (61% from fat, 11% from protein, 28% from carb); 2 g protein; 6 g total fat; 1 g saturated fat; 3 g monounsaturated fat; 1 g polyunsaturated fat; 6 g carbohydrate; 1 g fiber; 1 g sugar; 51 mg phosphorus; 22 mg calcium; 2 mg iron; 45 mg sodium; 76 mg potassium; 212 IU vitamin A; 55 mg vitamin E; 2 mg vitamin C; 3 mg cholesterol

Curried Snack Mix

A savory version of the old favorite Chex mix, with curry powder dominating.

2 cups (60 g) round toasted oat cereal, such as Cheerios

2 cups (60 g) square wheat cereal, such as Wheat Chex

2 cups (50 g) square rice cereal, such as Rice Chex

2 cups (90 g) pretzel sticks

$1^1/_2$ cups bite-size shredded wheat cereal

$1^1/_2$ teaspoons onion powder

1 teaspoon garlic powder

$^1/_2$ tablespoon curry powder

1 teaspoon ground celery seeds

$1^1/_2$ tablespoons (22 ml) Worcestershire sauce

1 teaspoon Tabasco sauce

Combine first 5 ingredients in large roasting pan. Spray thoroughly with nonstick vegetable oil spray. Combine remaining ingredients. Pour over cereal mixture, tossing to coat. Bake at 250°F (120°C, gas mark $^1/_2$) for 2 hours, stirring and spraying with butter-flavored nonstick cooking spray every 15 minutes. Cool and store in an airtight container.

Yield: 25 servings

Per serving: 1 g water; 48 calories (6% from fat, 10% from protein, 83% from carb); 1 g protein; 0 g total fat; 0 g saturated fat; 0 g monounsaturated fat; 0 g polyunsaturated fat; 11 g carbohydrate; 1 g fiber; 1 g sugar; 39 mg phosphorus; 27 mg calcium; 4 mg iron; 79 mg sodium; 68 mg potassium; 117 IU vitamin A; 34 mg vitamin E; 3 mg vitamin C; 0 mg cholesterol

Barbecued Nuts

Not your usual nut. The flavor and spiciness can be varied depending on what kind of barbecue sauce you use.

4 cups (580 g) mixed nuts

1 cup (250 g) barbecue sauce

2 tablespoons grated Parmesan cheese

Heat oven to 300°F (150°C, gas mark 2). In medium bowl, combine mixed nuts and barbecue sauce; stir until evenly coated. Spread on ungreased baking sheet; sprinkle with Parmesan cheese. Bake at 350°F (180°C, gas mark 4) for 20 to 25 minutes, or until nuts are dry. Transfer to waxed paper. Cool completely. Store in tightly covered container.

Yield: 16 servings

Per serving: 10 g water; 254 calories (68% from fat, 10% from protein, 23% from carb); 6 g protein; 20 g total fat; 3 g saturated fat; 11 g monounsaturated fat; 5 g polyunsaturated fat; 15 g carbohydrate; 3 g fiber; 7 g sugar; 170 mg phosphorus; 47 mg calcium; 1 mg iron; 312 mg sodium; 207 mg potassium; 6 IU vitamin A; 1 mg vitamin E; 0 mg vitamin C; 1 mg cholesterol

Hot Spiced Nuts

These make a great snack during the game (whatever game happens to be on). Make sure you have plenty of drinks available. Nuts contain the good kind of fat, so you can feel good about this snack.

1 egg white

1 cup (145 g) unsalted peanuts

1 cup (150 g) unsalted cashews

1 cup (100 g) unsalted pecans

1 teaspoon (2 g) curry powder

1 teaspoon (2.3 g) cinnamon

1 teaspoon (2.5 g) cumin

$1/4$ teaspoon (0.5 g) cayenne pepper

3 tablespoons (35 g) brown sugar

Preheat oven to 250°F (120°C, or gas mark $1/2$). Beat egg white until foamy. Add peanuts, cashews, and pecans, tossing to coat. Combine remaining ingredients in a medium bowl; toss with nuts to coat. Spread nuts on a greased baking sheet in a single layer. Bake for 1 hour, stirring once. Cool slightly and break apart. Cool completely and store in an airtight container for up to two weeks.

Yield: 15 servings

Per serving: 129 calories (69% from fat, 9% from protein, 23% from carbohydrate); 3 g protein; 10 g total fat; 1 g saturated fat; 6 g monounsaturated fat; 3 g polyunsaturated fat; 8 g carbohydrate; 1 g fiber; 4 g sugar; 76 mg phosphorus; 18 mg calcium; 1 mg iron; 38 mg sodium; 108 mg potassium; 20 IU vitamin A; 0 mg ATE vitamin E; 0 mg vitamin C; 0 mg cholesterol; 4 g water

Spicy Pecans

Tabasco adds a little heat to these pecans.

2 tablespoons (28 g) unsalted butter

$1/2$ teaspoon salt-free seasoning blend (such as Mrs. Dash)

$1/8$ teaspoon Tabasco sauce

1 pound (455 g) pecan halves

3 tablespoons (45 ml) Worcestershire sauce

Put butter, seasoning, and Tabasco sauce in 12 × 8 × 2-inch (30 × 20 × 5-cm) baking dish. Place in 300°F (150°C, gas mark 2) oven until butter melts. Add pecans, stirring until all are butter-coated. Bake for about 15 minutes, stirring occasionally. Sprinkle with Worcestershire sauce and stir again. Continue baking another 10 minutes until crisp.

Yield: 12 servings

Per serving: 3 g water; 281 calories (87% from fat, 5% from protein, 8% from carb); 4 g protein; 29 g total fat; 4 g saturated fat; 16 g monounsaturated fat; 8 g polyunsaturated fat; 6 g carbohydrate; 4 g fiber; 2 g sugar; 109 mg phosphorus; 27 mg calcium; 1 mg iron; 37 mg sodium; 186 mg potassium; 85 IU vitamin A; 16 mg vitamin E; 7 mg vitamin C; 5 mg cholesterol

Spicy Nut Mix

Unlike the cinnamon-sugar nuts in this chapter, these are chili spiced, providing a savory snack.

1¹/₄ cups (175 g) cashews

³/₄ cup (109 g) soy nuts

1 cup (145 g) sunflower seeds

2 tablespoons (28 ml) canola oil

1¹/₂ teaspoons chili powder

¹/₈ teaspoon garlic powder

1 teaspoon Worcestershire sauce

Combine nuts and seeds in large bowl. Place oil, spices, and Worcestershire sauce in covered container. Cover and shake. Sprinkle over nuts and seeds. Toss to coat. Spread in baking pan. Bake 20 minutes at 300°F (150°C, gas mark 2). Cool and store in covered containers in refrigerator.

Yield: 16 servings

Per serving: 0 g water; 161 calories (66% from fat, 15% from protein, 19% from carb); 6 g protein; 12 g total fat; 2 g saturated fat; 5 g monounsaturated fat; 5 g polyunsaturated fat; 8 g carbohydrate; 2 g fiber; 1 g sugar; 198 mg phosphorus; 22 mg calcium; 1 mg iron; 8 mg

sodium; 246 mg potassium; 71 IU vitamin A; 0 mg vitamin E; 1 mg vitamin C; 0 mg cholesterol

Party Nut Mix

A sweet and spicy variation on the traditional cereal mix, this one is mostly nuts.

8 ounces (225 g) dry-roasted peanuts

8 ounces (225 g) dry-roasted cashews

6 ounces (170 g) almonds

2 cups (60 g) square wheat cereal, such as Wheat Chex

¹/₄ cup (55 g) unsalted butter, melted

1¹/₂ tablespoons (22 ml) Dick's Reduced Sodium Soy Sauce (see recipe page 25)

1¹/₂ tablespoons (22 ml) Worcestershire sauce

¹/₄ teaspoon Tabasco sauce

1 cup (145 g) raisins

Combine first 4 ingredients in a large bowl; stir well. Combine butter, soy sauce, Worcestershire sauce, and Tabasco; mix well and pour over nut mixture, tossing to coat. Spread half of mixture in a 15 × 10 × 1-inch (37 × 25 × 2.5-cm) jelly-roll pan. Bake at 325°F (170°C, gas mark 3) for 15 minutes; cool and place in a large bowl. Repeat with remaining mixture. Add raisins and stir well. Store in an airtight container.

Yield: 28 servings

Per serving: 3 g water; 174 calories (61% from fat, 11% from protein, 28% from carb); 5 g protein; 13 g total fat; 3 g saturated fat; 7 g monounsaturated fat; 3 g polyunsaturated fat; 13 g carbohydrate; 2 g fiber; 5 g

sugar; 118 mg phosphorus; 27 mg calcium; 2 mg iron; 44 mg sodium; 209 mg potassium; 60 IU vitamin A; 14 mg vitamin E; 3 mg vitamin C; 4 mg cholesterol

Sweet Spiced Nuts

I've been trying for several years to come up with a recipe that is similar to the cinnamon nuts they sell at Nissan Pavilion in Virginia. This isn't it. The ones there have a hard sugar and spice coating and are made in a machine that spins them around, similar to a cotton candy machine. These have a flavor I like, though, so I'm including them here.

1 egg white

1 teaspoon (5 ml) water

2 cups (300 g) unsalted cashews

2 cups (300 g) unsalted almonds

$^1/_2$ cup (100 g) sugar

$^1/_2$ teaspoon (1.2 g) cinnamon

$^1/_8$ teaspoon (0.2 g) ground ginger

$^1/_8$ teaspoon (0.3 g) nutmeg

Preheat oven to 250°F (120°C, or gas mark $^1/_2$). Beat the egg white and water until frothy, but not stiff. Add the cashews and almonds, and stir to coat. Combine the remaining ingredients and pour over the nuts. Stir until the sugar is dissolved. Place on a greased baking sheet and bake for 1 hour, stirring occasionally. Cool on waxed paper. Store in an airtight container.

Yield: 16 servings

Per serving: 229 calories (63% from fat, 11% from protein, 26% from carbohydrate); 7 g protein; 17 g total fat; 2 g saturated fat; 11 g monounsaturated fat; 4 g polyunsaturated fat; 16 g carbohydrate; 2 g fiber; 8 g sugar; 171 mg phosphorus; 48 mg calcium; 2 mg iron; 11 mg sodium; 225 mg potassium; 2 IU vitamin A; 0 mg ATE vitamin E; 0 mg vitamin C; 0 mg cholesterol; 3 g water

S'more Snack Mix

This is a great idea. Everyone likes s'mores, so why not a snack mix that gives you that flavor whenever you want it? And all you have to do is mix it up.

2 cups (80 g) honey grahams cereal , such as Golden Grahams

1 cup (50 g) miniature marshmallows

1 cup (145 g) peanuts

$^1/_2$ cup (87.5 g) chocolate chips

$^1/_2$ cup (75 g) raisins

Combine all ingredients and mix thoroughly.

Yield: 20 servings

Per serving: 3 g water; 68 calories (29% from fat, 6% from protein, 65% from carb); 1 g protein; 2 g total fat; 1 g saturated fat; 1 g monounsaturated fat; 0 g polyunsaturated fat; 11 g carbohydrate; 1 g fiber; 8 g sugar; 24 mg phosphorus; 12 mg calcium; 1 mg iron; 51 mg sodium; 58 mg potassium; 86 IU vitamin A; 26 mg vitamin E; 1 mg vitamin C; 1 mg cholesterol

Sugared Pecans

Sweet and just slightly spicy nuts. I came up with the recipe while on a search to duplicate the spiced nuts sold at places like the Maryland Renaissance Festival. They aren't quite the same, but they're closer than the baked ones.

$^3/_4$ cup (150 g) sugar

2 teaspoons cinnamon

$^1/_4$ cup (60 ml) water

2 cups (220 g) pecans

Mix sugar and cinnamon in pan. Pour in water. Put in nuts. Bring to boil over medium heat; turn heat down and simmer, barely bubbling, 20 minutes or until syrup dries. Place nuts on waxed paper. Cool.

Yield: 12 servings

Per serving: 6 g water; 176 calories (63% from fat, 4% from protein, 33% from carb); 2 g protein; 13 g total fat; 1 g saturated fat; 7 g monounsaturated fat; 4 g polyunsaturated fat; 15 g carbohydrate; 2 g fiber; 13 g sugar; 51 mg phosphorus; 18 mg calcium; 1 mg iron; 0 mg sodium; 77 mg potassium; 11 IU vitamin A; 0 mg vitamin E; 0 mg vitamin C; 0 mg cholesterol

Honey Nutty Snack

Kind of a healthier version of peanut brittle, this starts with honey-nut cereal for taste as well as nutrition.

1 cup (225 g) packed brown sugar

$^1/_2$ cup (112 g) unsalted butter, softened

$^1/_4$ cup (60 ml) light corn syrup

$^1/_2$ teaspoon baking soda

6 cups (180 g) honey-nut–flavored round toasted oat cereal, such as Honey Nut Cheerios

1 cup (145 g) peanuts

1 cup (145 g) raisins

Heat oven to 250°F (120°C, gas mark $^1/_2$). Coat 2 rectangular pans, 13 × 9 × 2 (33 × 23 × 5-cm) inches, or 1 jelly-roll pan, 15$^1/_2$ × 10$^1/_2$ × 1 inch (37 × 25 × 2.5-cm), with nonstick vegetable oil spray. Heat brown sugar, butter, and corn syrup in 2-quart (2-L) saucepan over medium heat, stirring constantly, until bubbly around edges. Cook uncovered, stirring occasionally, 2 minutes longer. Remove from heat; stir in baking soda until foamy and light colored. Pour over cereal, peanuts, and raisins in 4-quart (4-L) bowl coated with nonstick vegetable oil spray; stir until mixture is coated. Spread evenly in pans. Bake 15 minutes; stir. Let stand just until cool, about 10 minutes. Loosen mixture with metal spatula. Let stand until firm, about 30 minutes. Break into bite-size pieces.

Yield: 24 servings

Per serving: 4 g water; 144 calories (30% from fat, 4% from protein, 66% from carb); 2 g protein; 5 g total fat; 3 g saturated fat; 1 g monounsaturated fat; 0 g polyunsaturated fat; 25 g carbohydrate; 1 g fiber; 17 g sugar; 49 mg phosphorus; 48 mg calcium; 2 mg iron; 90 mg sodium; 127 mg potassium; 285 IU vitamin A; 82 mg vitamin E; 2 mg vitamin C; 10 mg cholesterol

Pecan Crunch Snack

Easy-to-make snack mix, full of nuts and crunchy cereal.

1 cup (225 g) unsalted butter

1 cup (225 g) brown sugar

8 cups mini shredded wheat cereal

1 pound (455 g) pecans

Melt butter and brown sugar; boil 2 minutes. Place cereal and nuts in two 9 × 13-inch (23 × 33-cm)

cake pans. Pour butter-sugar mixture over cereal-nuts mixture. Bake at 375°F (190°C, gas mark 5) for 8 minutes. Stir occasionally. Store in covered container.

Yield: 20 servings

Per serving: 3 g water; 280 calories (78% from fat, 3% from protein, 19% from carb); 2 g protein; 26 g total fat; 7 g saturated fat; 12 g monounsaturated fat; 5 g polyunsaturated fat; 14 g carbohydrate; 2 g fiber; 11 g sugar; 68 mg phosphorus; 28 mg calcium; 1 mg iron; 6 mg sodium; 134 mg potassium; 296 IU vitamin A; 76 mg vitamin E; 0 mg vitamin C; 24 mg cholesterol

Fruit and Nut Popcorn

Sweetly spiced popcorn-and-fruit mixture. Perfect with a glass of apple cider.

2 quarts (64 g) popped popcorn

1 cup (86 g) chopped dried apples

1 cup (130 g) chopped dried apricots

1 cup (145 g) raisins

1 cup (120 g) coarsely chopped walnuts

$1/4$ teaspoon confectioners' sugar

$1 1/2$ teaspoons cinnamon

$1/2$ teaspoon nutmeg

In a large bowl, combine hot popcorn, fruits, and nuts. Combine sugar, cinnamon, and nutmeg. Sprinkle over popcorn mixture to coat. Store in an airtight container. Will keep for up to 3 days.

Yield: 12 servings

Per serving: 28 g water; 164 calories (48% from fat, 8% from protein, 44% from carb); 4 g protein; 9 g total fat; 1 g saturated fat; 2 g monounsaturated fat; 5 g polyunsaturated fat; 19 g carbohydrate; 2 g fiber; 11 g sugar; 87 mg phosphorus; 20 mg calcium; 1 mg iron; 80 mg sodium; 214 mg potassium; 364 IU vitamin A; 0 mg vitamin E; 2 mg vitamin C; 0 mg cholesterol

Cinnamon Apple Popcorn

A nice sweet treat to nibble while you are watching television.

1 cup (86 g) chopped dried apples

5 cups (40 g) popped popcorn

1 cup (55 g) halved pecans

4 tablespoons (55 g) unsalted butter, melted

1 teaspoon cinnamon

$1/4$ teaspoon nutmeg

2 tablespoons (30 g) brown sugar

$1/4$ teaspoon vanilla extract

Preheat oven to 250°F (120°C, gas mark $1/2$). Place apples in a large shallow baking pan. Bake 20 minutes. Remove pan from oven and stir in popcorn and pecans. In a small bowl, combine remaining ingredients. Drizzle butter mixture over popcorn mixture, stirring well. Bake for 30 minutes, stirring every 10 minutes. Pour onto waxed paper to cool. Store in airtight container.

Yield: 14 servings

Per serving: 8 g water; 118 calories (77% from fat, 3% from protein, 19% from carb); 1 g protein; 11 g total

fat; 3 g saturated fat; 4 g monounsaturated fat; 3 g polyunsaturated fat; 6 g carbohydrate; 1 g fiber; 3 g sugar; 32 mg phosphorus; 11 mg calcium; 0 mg iron; 43 mg sodium; 55 mg potassium; 115 IU vitamin A; 27 mg vitamin E; 0 mg vitamin C; 9 mg cholesterol

Caramel Corn

This is an easier version than most for caramel corn, not requiring candy thermometers and all that. But the taste is just as good.

$^1/_2$ cup (112 g) unsalted butter

1 cup (225 g) brown sugar

$^1/_4$ cup (60 ml) corn syrup

$^1/_2$ teaspoon baking soda

4 quarts (128 g) popped popcorn

2 cups (290 g) peanuts

Cook butter, brown sugar, and syrup 1$^1/_2$ minutes; stir and cook an additional 2 to 3 minutes until at a rolling boil. Take off heat and add soda. Stir well. Pour mixture over popped corn and nuts in grocery bag and shake. Microwave 1 minute, shake; 1 minute, shake; 30 seconds, shake; 30 seconds, shake. Pour into pan, cool, and eat.

Yield: 18 servings

Per serving: 5 g water; 184 calories (52% from fat, 4% from protein, 45% from carb); 2 g protein; 11 g total fat; 4 g saturated fat; 3 g monounsaturated fat; 3 g polyunsaturated fat; 21 g carbohydrate; 1 g fiber; 13 g sugar; 38 mg phosphorus; 17 mg calcium; 0 mg iron; 164 mg sodium; 74 mg potassium; 173 IU vitamin A; 42 mg vitamin E; 0 mg vitamin C; 14 mg cholesterol

Rocky Road Popcorn Bars

Easy microwave recipe for tasty popcorn-and-peanut bars.

$^1/_4$ cup (55 g) unsalted butter

2 tablespoons (28 g) shortening

12 ounces (340 g) chocolate chips

5 cups (250 g) miniature marshmallows

$^3/_4$ cup (109 g) peanuts

6 cups (48 g) popped popcorn

Spray a 9 × 12 × 2-inch (23 × 30 × 5-cm) microwave-safe dish with nonstick vegetable oil spray. Set aside. Measure and mix butter, shortening, and chocolate chips in bowl. Microwave uncovered on high (100%) until chips are softened and mixture becomes smooth when stirred—about 2$^1/_2$ minutes. Stir in marshmallows. Microwave uncovered until they are almost melted—15 to 20 seconds. Stir in peanuts and popcorn until evenly covered with mixture. When cool, press in pan with spoon. Refrigerate until firm—about 1 hour. Cut into squares.

Yield: 10 servings

Per serving: 8 g water; 378 calories (49% from fat, 4% from protein, 46% from carb); 4 g protein; 21 g total fat; 9 g saturated fat; 8 g monounsaturated fat; 3 g polyunsaturated fat; 45 g carbohydrate; 2 g fiber; 32 g sugar; 97 mg phosphorus; 69 mg calcium; 1 mg iron; 153 mg sodium; 150 mg potassium; 211 IU vitamin A; 54 mg vitamin E; 0 mg vitamin C; 20 mg cholesterol

5

Breakfasts

I'm a great believer in the idea that breakfast is the most important meal of the day. I need something in the morning to get me going and keep me going until lunch. So there are a lot of breakfast recipes here. Even though traditional breakfast meat tends to be high in fat and sodium, we have some options for you like a low fat turkey sausage with only 35 mg of sodium per serving. Along with lots of egg dishes we have a great selection of whole grain pancakes and waffles, fruit breakfasts, cookies and bars and smoothies. And if you get tired of these you can move on to the muffins in Chapter 20.

Turkey Breakfast Sausage

I've been back at the chemistry table—I mean, kitchen counter—trying various recipes for sausage again. This is my favorite so far. It contains about 5% of the sodium, 10% of the fat, and one-third of the calories of the average store-bought sausage.

1 pound (455 g) ground turkey

$^1/_4$ teaspoon (0.5 g) black pepper

$^1/_4$ teaspoon (0.5 g) white pepper

$^3/_4$ teaspoon (0.6 g) dried sage

$^1/_4$ teaspoon (0.4 g) ground mace

$^1/_2$ teaspoon (1.5 g) garlic powder

$^1/_4$ teaspoon (0.8 g) onion powder

$^1/_4$ teaspoon (0.5 g) ground allspice

1 teaspoon (5 ml) olive oil

Combine all ingredients, mixing well. Fry, grill, or preheat oven to 325°F (170°C, or gas mark 3) and cook on a greased baking sheet to desired doneness.

Yield: 8 servings

Per serving: 69 calories (20% from fat, 77% from protein, 2% from carbohydrate); 13 g protein; 1 g total fat; 0 g saturated fat; 1 g monounsaturated fat; 0 g polyunsaturated fat; 0 g carbohydrate; 0 g fiber; 0 g sugar; 106 mg phosphorus; 9 mg calcium; 1 mg iron; 35 mg sodium; 153 mg potassium; 5 IU vitamin A; 0 mg ATE vitamin E; 0 mg vitamin C; 41 mg cholesterol; 43 g water

Snowy Day Breakfast Casserole

My wife came up with this one winter when we were snowed in. It has since become a standard in our house, just the sort of thing you need to sit in front of the fire with.

2 slices low sodium bacon

3 potatoes, shredded

$^1/_2$ cup (80 g) onion, chopped

$^1/_4$ cup (37 g) green bell pepper, chopped

4 eggs

$^1/_4$ cup (30 g) low fat Cheddar cheese, shredded

Preheat oven to 350°F (180°C, or gas mark 4). Fry bacon in a large skillet. Remove bacon to a paper towel—covered plate to drain. Add potatoes, onion, and green pepper to skillet and sauté until potatoes are crispy and onion soft. Stir in crumbled bacon. Transfer to greased 8-inch (20-cm) square baking dish. Pour eggs over. Sprinkle with cheese. Bake until eggs are set, about 20 minutes.

Yield: 4 servings

Per serving: 292 calories (14% from fat, 22% from protein, 63% from carbohydrate); 17 g protein; 5 g total fat; 1 g saturated fat; 1 g monounsaturated fat; 1 g polyunsaturated fat; 47 g carbohydrate; 5 g fiber; 4 g sugar; 314 mg phosphorus; 101 mg calcium; 4 mg iron; 221 mg sodium; 1310 mg potassium; 299 IU vitamin A; 5 mg ATE vitamin E; 33 mg vitamin C; 207 mg cholesterol; 308 g water

Breakfast Skillet

This was originally a Sunday-morning breakfast in late summer. At that time of year, I usually have extra peppers from the garden, and this recipe used up a few of them.

1 tablespoon (15 ml) olive oil

$^1/_4$ cup (40 g) onion, finely chopped

$^1/_4$ cup (38 g) red bell pepper, finely chopped

$^1/_2$ cup (105 g) frozen hash brown potatoes, thawed

3 eggs, beaten

Heat oil in a large skillet over medium heat. Sauté onion and red bell pepper until tender. Add hash browns and cook until potatoes are softened and beginning to brown, stirring occasionally. Pour eggs over vegetables and continue to cook for 5 minutes, or until set, stirring occasionally.

Yield: 2 servings

Per serving: 195 calories (47% from fat, 26% from protein, 26% from carbohydrate); 13 g protein; 10 g total fat; 2 g saturated fat; 6 g monounsaturated fat; 2 g polyunsaturated fat; 13 g carbohydrate; 1 g fiber; 2 g sugar; 149 mg phosphorus; 61 mg calcium; 3 mg iron; 180 mg sodium; 129 mg potassium; 922 IU vitamin A; 0 mg ATE vitamin E; 30 mg vitamin C; 300 mg cholesterol; 154 g water

Vegetable Omelet

This can be either a breakfast or the main part of an evening meal.

1 tablespoon (15 ml) olive oil

2 ounces (55 g) mushrooms, sliced

$^1/_4$ cup (40 g) onion, diced

$^1/_4$ cup (37 g) green bell peppers, diced

$^1/_4$ cup (28 g) zucchini, sliced

$^1/_2$ cup (90 g) tomato, diced

4 eggs

2 tablespoons (30 g) fat-free sour cream

2 tablespoons (30 ml) water

2 ounces (55 g) Swiss cheese, shredded

Add olive oil to a large skillet and sauté mushrooms, onion, green bell pepper, zucchini, and tomato until soft, adding tomato last. Whisk together eggs, sour cream, and water until fluffy. Coat an omelet pan or skillet with nonstick vegetable spray and place over medium-high heat. Pour egg mixture into pan. Lift the edges as it cooks to allow uncooked egg to run underneath. When eggs are nearly set, cover half the eggs with the cheese and sautéed vegetables and fold the other half over. Continue cooking until eggs are completely set.

Yield: 2 servings

Per serving: 263 calories (46% from fat, 41% from protein, 13% from carbohydrate); 25 g protein; 13 g total fat; 3 g saturated fat; 6 g monounsaturated fat; 3 g polyunsaturated fat; 8 g carbohydrate; 2 g fiber; 4 g sugar; 386 mg phosphorus; 369 mg calcium; 3 mg iron; 309 mg sodium; 246 mg potassium; 962 IU vitamin A; 6 mg ATE vitamin E; 25 mg vitamin C; 395 mg cholesterol; 259 g water

Cinnamon Apple Omelet

A little different version of an omelet. I remember years ago there were often recipes for omelets with jelly or other sweet fillings, but you don't see them much any more. This one makes me think they are still a good idea.

1 tablespoon unsalted butter, divided

1 apple, peeled and sliced thin

$^1/_2$ teaspoon cinnamon

1 tablespoon (15 g) brown sugar

3 eggs

1 tablespoon cream

1 tablespoon sour cream

Melt 2 teaspoons butter in egg pan. Add apple, cinnamon, and brown sugar. Sauté until tender. Set aside. Whip eggs and cream until fluffy; set aside. Clean egg pan. Melt remaining butter, pour in egg mixture. Cook as you would for an omelet. When eggs are ready to flip, turn them, then add to the center of the eggs the sour cream and on top of that the apple mixture. Fold it onto a plate.

Yield: 2 servings

Per serving: 129 g water; 252 calories (57% from fat, 17% from protein, 25% from carb); 11 g protein; 16 g total fat; 8 g saturated fat; 5 g monounsaturated fat; 1 g polyunsaturated fat; 16 g carbohydrate; 1 g fiber; 14 g sugar; 181 mg phosphorus; 73 mg calcium; 2 mg iron; 126 mg sodium; 211 mg potassium; 695 IU vitamin A; 187 mg vitamin E; 3 mg vitamin C; 379 mg cholesterol

Spinach Quiche

This versatile dish can work for breakfast, lunch, or dinner.

8 slices low-sodium bacon

1 cup (160 g) chopped onion

4 eggs, beaten

1 cup (235 ml) light cream

1 cup (235 ml) skim milk

1 tablespoon flour

$^1/_8$ teaspoon nutmeg

12 ounces (340 g) frozen spinach, thawed and chopped

4 ounces (115 g) mushrooms, sliced

1 cup (115 g) shredded Monterey Jack cheese

1 cup (115 g) shredded Cheddar cheese

1 prepared piecrust

Cook together bacon and onion. Crumble bacon. Mix all ingredients together. Pour into piecrust in quiche-baking dish. Bake at 325°F (170°C, gas mark 3) for 50 minutes. Let stand 10 minutes before serving.

Yield: 8 servings

Per serving: 141 g water; 296 calories (65% from fat, 25% from protein, 11% from carb); 19 g protein; 22 g total fat; 12 g saturated fat; 7 g monounsaturated fat; 1 g polyunsaturated fat; 8 g carbohydrate; 2 g fiber; 2 g sugar; 338 mg phosphorus; 382 mg calcium; 2 mg iron; 379 mg sodium; 387 mg potassium; 5775 IU vitamin A; 174 mg vitamin E; 3 mg vitamin C; 177 mg cholesterol

Spinach Pie

A great breakfast idea, but also a great side dish to go with chicken, turkey, or beef.

10 ounces (280 g) frozen spinach

6 eggs, stirred

2 cups (450 g) cottage cheese

1/4 cup (55 g) unsalted butter, melted

6 tablespoons (48 g) flour

10 ounces (283 g) Cheddar cheese, cut into cubes

Preheat oven to 350°F (180°C, gas mark 4). Cook spinach according to package directions; drain thoroughly and squeeze dry. Mix all ingredients together in a 9 × 13-inch (23 × 33-cm) pan. Bake for 1 hour.

Yield: 6 servings

Per serving: 143 g water; 423 calories (62% from fat, 28% from protein, 10% from carb); 30 g protein; 29 g total fat; 17 g saturated fat; 9 g monounsaturated fat; 2 g polyunsaturated fat; 10 g carbohydrate; 2 g fiber; 2 g sugar; 433 mg phosphorus; 462 mg calcium; 3 mg iron; 425 mg sodium; 290 mg potassium; 6696 IU vitamin A; 268 mg vitamin E; 1 mg vitamin C; 310 mg cholesterol

Black Bean and Spinach Breakfast Burrito

Almost as quick as fast food, this will get your day off to a good start with something a little different, and provide 12 grams of fiber while doing it.

1 egg

1 egg white

1 cup (30 g) fresh spinach

1/4 cup (45 g) diced tomato

1/4 cup (43 g) cooked black beans, drained

1 tablespoon grated Cheddar cheese

1 tablespoon (16 g) salsa

1 whole wheat tortilla

Preheat the oven to 350°F (180°C, gas mark 4). Mix the egg and egg white and scramble them quickly in a small frying pan. Fold in the next five ingredients. Place this mixture in the middle of the tortilla. Wrap the two sides over tightly and place the roll, seam side down, on a baking sheet coated with nonstick vegetable oil spray. Bake at 350°F (180°C, gas mark 4) for about 6 minutes until the tortilla is crisp and the filling is heated through.

Yield: 1 serving

Per serving: 320 g water; 363 calories (32% from fat, 28% from protein, 41% from carb); 26 g protein; 13 g total fat; 5 g saturated fat; 5 g monounsaturated fat; 2 g polyunsaturated fat; 39 g carbohydrate; 12 g fiber; 4 g sugar; 349 mg phosphorus; 438 mg calcium; 7 mg iron; 616 mg sodium; 1040 mg potassium; 23694 IU vitamin A; 110 mg vitamin E; 9 mg vitamin C; 219 mg cholesterol

Breakfast Burrito

This breakfast burrito is filled with good things. It also is perfect for grabbing on your way out the door.

2 ounces (55 g) chorizo, finely chopped

1/4 cup (40 g) chopped onion

1/4 cup (38 g) chopped red bell pepper

1 whole wheat tortilla

1 egg, beaten

2 tablespoons (30 g) sour cream

2 ounces (55 g) Monterey Jack cheese, shredded or crumbled

Preheat oven to 400°F (200°C, gas mark 6). In a small pan, cook the chorizo, onion, and bell pepper over medium heat until cooked through. Drain excess fat. Place the tortilla on a baking sheet covered with a very damp, clean dish towel. Let the tortilla cook for about 3 minutes. Whisk together the egg and sour cream. Pour the egg mixture into the pan over the chorizo and cook over medium heat; stir while cooking to scramble the eggs. Take the tortilla out of the oven and place eggs down the center; then top with shredded cheese. Fold up the burrito and let it sit for about 1 minute to let the burrito mold itself closed.

Yield: 1 serving

Per serving: 187 g water; 710 calories (64% from fat, 22% from protein, 14% from carb); 39 g protein; 51 g total fat; 24 g saturated fat; 20 g monounsaturated fat; 4 g polyunsaturated fat; 25 g carbohydrate; 2 g fiber; 5 g sugar; 531 mg phosphorus; 539 mg calcium; 4 mg iron; 1289 mg sodium; 569 mg potassium; 1988 IU vitamin A; 217 mg vitamin E; 51 mg vitamin C; 349 mg cholesterol

Breakfast Quesadilla

These are easy to make if you have a portable contact grill like the George Foreman models. If not, you can also grill them in a dry skillet, turning once.

4 eggs

1/4 cup (56 g) salsa

1/4 cup (30 g) low fat Cheddar cheese, shredded

8 corn tortillas

Scramble eggs, stirring in salsa and cheese when it is almost set. Lightly spray one side of the tortillas in nonstick olive oil spray and place 4 of them oiled-side down on a baking sheet. Divide egg mixture among tortillas, spreading to even thickness. Top with the remaining tortillas, oiled-side up. Grill quesadillas for 3 minutes per side, or until heated through and golden brown. Cut into quarters to serve.

Yield: 4 servings

Per serving: 152 calories (22% from fat, 31% from protein, 47% from carbohydrate); 12 g protein; 4 g total fat; 1 g saturated fat; 1 g monounsaturated fat; 2 g polyunsaturated fat; 18 g carbohydrate; 3 g fiber; 1 g sugar; 237 mg phosphorus; 102 mg calcium; 2 mg iron; 275 mg sodium; 130 mg potassium; 291 IU vitamin A; 5 mg ATE vitamin E; 0 mg vitamin C; 202 mg cholesterol; 89 g water

Breakfast Enchiladas

A make-ahead breakfast, you can assemble this the night before and then just bake it in the morning. This and the large number of servings make it a great choice when you have company staying overnight.

12 ounces (340 g) ham, finely chopped

1/2 cup (50 g) chopped scallions

2 cups (300 g) chopped green bell pepper

1 cup (160 g) chopped onion

2¹/₂ cups (300 g) grated Cheddar cheese

8 whole wheat tortillas

4 eggs

2 cups (475 ml) skim milk

1 tablespoon flour

¹/₄ teaspoon garlic powder

1 teaspoon Tabasco sauce

Preheat oven to 350°F (180°C, gas mark 4). Mix together ham, scallions, bell pepper, onion, and cheese. Put 5 tablespoons of mixture on each tortilla and roll up. Place seam side down in 12 × 7 × 2-inch (30 × 18 × 5-cm) pan coated with nonstick vegetable oil spray. In separate bowl, beat together eggs and milk, flour, garlic, and Tabasco. Pour over enchiladas. Place in refrigerator overnight. Cover with foil and bake for 30 minutes, uncovering for the last 10 minutes.

Yield: 8 servings

Per serving: 188 g water; 418 calories (49% from fat, 27% from protein, 24% from carb); 28 g protein; 23 g total fat; 11 g saturated fat; 8 g monounsaturated fat; 2 g polyunsaturated fat; 25 g carbohydrate; 2 g fiber; 3 g sugar; 482 mg phosphorus; 455 mg calcium; 3 mg iron; 984 mg sodium; 500 mg potassium; 885 IU vitamin A; 183 mg vitamin E; 33 mg vitamin C; 180 mg cholesterol

Tip: Serve with dollop of sour cream, salsa, and avocado slices.

California Breakfast Sandwich

A sort of Mexican version of eggs Benedict, this is a great weekend breakfast.

6 eggs

³/₄ cup (120 g) chopped onion

1 tablespoon unsalted butter

2 ounces (55 g) mushrooms, sliced

1 avocado, sliced

¹/₂ cup (90 g) chopped tomato

¹/₂ cup (60 g) grated Cheddar cheese

6 whole wheat English muffins

Mix eggs with wire whisk. In large skillet, brown onion with butter until clear and limp. Add mushrooms, avocado, and tomato. Stir. Add beaten eggs. Cook until almost set; add grated cheese. Spoon onto toasted English muffins.

Yield: 6 servings

Per serving: 126 g water; 319 calories (43% from fat, 19% from protein, 37% from carb); 16 g protein; 16 g total fat; 6 g saturated fat; 6 g monounsaturated fat; 2 g polyunsaturated fat; 31 g carbohydrate; 5 g fiber; 3 g sugar; 254 mg phosphorus; 220 mg calcium; 3 mg iron; 368 mg sodium; 396 mg potassium; 581 IU vitamin A; 122 mg vitamin E; 5 mg vitamin C; 254 mg cholesterol

Tip: Serve with salsa and sour cream.

Breakfast Wraps

For those days when you want a little something different for breakfast. This is similar to the breakfast burritos served at several fast food restaurants, but with a lot less fat.

1 medium potato

$^1/_2$ pound (225 g) Turkey Breakfast Sausage (see recipe page 89)

$^1/_2$ cup (80 g) onion, chopped

1 teaspoon (2.6 g) chili powder

$^1/_4$ teaspoon (0.5 g) cayenne pepper

2 eggs, beaten

6 flour tortillas

$^1/_2$ cup (58 g) low fat Cheddar cheese, shredded

Boil or microwave potato until tender. Peel and cut into cubes. Brown sausage in a frying pan. Add chopped onion, chili powder, and cayenne pepper and cook for 10 minutes. Drain and discard any fat. Add potato and eggs. Stir until eggs are set. Divide mixture evenly among warmed tortillas, top with shredded cheese, and roll up tortillas to enclose mixture.

Yield: 6 servings

Per serving: 269 calories (36% from fat, 22% from protein, 42% from carbohydrate); 15 g protein; 11 g total fat; 4 g saturated fat; 3 g monounsaturated fat; 2 g polyunsaturated fat; 28 g carbohydrate; 2 g fiber; 2 g sugar; 211 mg phosphorus; 116 mg calcium; 2 mg iron; 524 mg sodium; 190 mg potassium; 254 IU vitamin A; 7 mg ATE vitamin E; 16 mg vitamin C; 95 mg cholesterol; 108 g water

Frittata

A frittata is an Italian-style omelet, with the filling mixed in with the eggs. It's cooked without turning and then the top set under the broiler. This version does not have any of the meat and potatoes that they often have, providing you with a filling weekend breakfast low in sodium, fat, and carbohydrates.

$^1/_4$ cup (60 ml) olive oil

2 baking potatoes, peeled and thinly sliced

1 cup (160 g) thinly sliced onion

2 cups (226 g) thinly sliced zucchini

1 cup (150 g) red bell pepper, cut in $^1/_2$-inch (1-cm) cubes

1 cup (150 g) green bell pepper, cut in $^1/_2$-inch (1-cm) cubes

12 eggs

2 tablespoons chopped fresh parsley

Preheat oven to 450°F (230°C, gas mark 8). Pour oil into 12-inch (30-cm) square or round baking dish. Heat oil in oven for 5 minutes, then remove. Place potatoes and onion over bottom of dish and bake until potatoes are just tender, 20 minutes. Arrange zucchini slices over potatoes and onion, then sprinkle peppers over all. Beat eggs. Add chopped parsley to eggs. Pour eggs over vegetables. Bake until eggs are set and sides are "puffy," about 25 minutes. Top should be golden brown. Serve hot or at room temperature.

Yield: 6 servings

Per serving: 293 g water; 364 calories (50% from fat, 19% from protein, 31% from carb); 18 g protein; 20 g total fat; 5 g saturated fat; 11 g monounsaturated fat; 3 g polyunsaturated fat; 29 g carbohydrate; 5 g fiber; 5 g sugar; 320 mg phosphorus; 92 mg calcium; 4 mg iron; 172 mg sodium; 918 mg potassium; 1606 IU vitamin A; 156 mg vitamin E; 87 mg vitamin C; 474 mg cholesterol

Sausage Frittata

We like this for breakfast on those rare occasions when the entire family is around, but it also makes a good dinner with a salad and a slice of freshly baked bread.

4 eggs

$^1/_4$ cup (60 ml) skim milk

8 ounces (225 g) Turkey Breakfast Sausage (see recipe page 89)

$^1/_2$ cup (75 g) green bell pepper, chopped

4 ounces (115 g) low fat Cheddar cheese, shredded

Preheat broiler. Combine eggs and milk in medium bowl; whisk until well blended. Set aside. Place a 12-inch (30-cm) broiler-proof nonstick skillet over medium-high heat until hot. Add sausage; cook and stir for 4 minutes or until no longer pink, breaking up sausage with spoon. Drain sausage on paper towels; set aside. Add pepper to same skillet; cook and stir for 2 minutes, or until crisp-tender. Return sausage to skillet. Add egg mixture; stir until blended. Cover; cook over medium-low heat for 10 minutes, or until eggs are almost set. Sprinkle cheese over frittata. Broil for 2 minutes, or until cheese is melted and eggs are set. Cut into wedges.

Yield: 4 servings

Per serving: 245 calories (54% from fat, 40% from protein, 6% from carbohydrate); 24 g protein; 14 g total fat; 6 g saturated fat; 4 g monounsaturated fat; 3 g polyunsaturated fat; 4 g carbohydrate; 0 g fiber; 1 g sugar; 339 mg phosphorus; 193 mg calcium; 2 mg iron; 626 mg sodium; 198 mg potassium; 385 IU vitamin A; 6 mg ATE vitamin E; 32 mg vitamin C; 241 mg cholesterol; 137 g water

Vegetable Frittata

$^1/_2$ cup (75 g) red bell pepper, diced

$^1/_2$ cup (80 g) onion, chopped

1 cup (70 g) broccoli florets

8 ounces (225 g) mushrooms, sliced

1 cup (113 g) zucchini, sliced

6 eggs

1 tablespoon (0.4 g) dried parsley

$^1/_4$ teaspoon (0.5 g) black pepper

2 ounces (55 g) Swiss cheese, shredded

Spray a large oven-proof skillet with nonstick vegetable oil spray. Stir-fry the red bell pepper, onions, and broccoli until crisp-tender. Add the mushrooms and zucchini and stir-fry for 1 to 2 minutes more. Stir together the eggs, parsley, and pepper, and pour over vegetable mixture, spreading to cover. Cover and cook over medium heat for 10 to 12 minutes, or until eggs are nearly set. Sprinkle cheese over the top. Place under the broiler until eggs are set and cheese is melted.

Yield: 4 servings

Per serving: 140 calories (26% from fat, 51% from protein, 22% from carbohydrate); 18 g protein; 4 g total fat; 1 g saturated fat; 1 g monounsaturated fat; 2 g polyunsaturated fat; 8 g carbohydrate; 2 g fiber; 4 g sugar; 283 mg phosphorus; 209 mg calcium; 3 mg iron; 216 mg sodium; 321 mg potassium; 1618 IU vitamin A; 6 mg ATE vitamin E; 50 mg vitamin C; 306 mg cholesterol; 220 g water

Pasta Frittata

This makes a wonderful meatless meal. It's kind of like macaroni and cheese, only a little fancier.

2 tablespoons (30 ml) olive oil

1 cup (150 g) red bell pepper, diced

1 cup (160 g) onion, chopped

2 cups (100 g) cooked pasta

$^1/_4$ cup (25 g) grated Parmesan

4 eggs

Heat a 10-inch (25-cm) nonstick skillet that is broiler safe. When the pan is hot, add the oil, then sauté red bell pepper and onion for 2 to 3 minutes, stirring frequently. Add the pasta to the pan, mixing well. When ingredients are thoroughly combined, press down on pasta with spatula to flatten it against the bottom of the pan. Let it cook a few minutes more. Whisk grated Parmesan into the eggs. Pour egg mixture over the top of the pasta, making sure the eggs spread evenly. Gently lift the edges of the pasta to let egg flow underneath and completely coat the pasta. Let the eggs cook for 6 to 9 minutes. Slide the pan into a preheated broiler and finish cooking until eggs are set.

Yield: 4 servings

Per serving: 360 calories (29% from fat, 20% from protein, 51% from carbohydrate); 18 g protein; 12 g total fat; 3 g saturated fat; 6 g monounsaturated fat; 2 g polyunsaturated fat; 46 g carbohydrate; 3 g fiber; 5 g sugar; 242 mg phosphorus; 125 mg calcium; 2 mg iron; 213 mg sodium; 169 mg potassium; 1421 IU vitamin A; 7 mg ATE vitamin E; 51 mg vitamin C; 206 mg cholesterol; 128 g water

Easy Breakfast Strata

This is another great fix-ahead breakfast. We usually have some variation of this on special holidays when there is a lot to do in the morning, but we want a special family breakfast.

1 pound (455 g) sausage

8 eggs

10 slices whole wheat bread, cubed

3 cups (710 g) skim milk

2 cups (225 g) shredded Cheddar cheese

10 ounces (280 g) frozen chopped broccoli, thawed

2 tablespoons (28 g) unsalted butter, melted

2 tablespoons (16 g) flour

1 tablespoon dry mustard

2 teaspoons basil

In large skillet, brown sausage, drain. In large bowl, beat eggs. Add remaining ingredients and mix well. Spoon into 13 × 9-inch (33 × 23-cm) baking pan coated with nonstick vegetable oil spray. Cover and refrigerate 8 hours or overnight. Preheat oven to 350°F (180°C, gas mark 4). Bake 60 to 70 minutes or until knife inserted near center comes out clean.

Yield: 8 servings

Per serving: 181 g water; 379 calories (49% from fat, 25% from protein, 26% from carb); 24 g protein; 21 g total fat; 11 g saturated fat; 6 g monounsaturated fat; 2 g polyunsaturated fat; 24 g carbohydrate; 2 g fiber; 3 g sugar; 449 mg phosphorus; 462 mg calcium; 3 mg iron; 593 mg sodium; 396 mg potassium; 1293 IU vitamin A; 243 mg vitamin E; 15 mg vitamin C; 281 mg cholesterol

Breakfast Potatoes

Sometimes called O'Brien potatoes, this is a traditional breakfast kind of dish, but it works just as well as a side dish at dinner.

4 potatoes

1 cup (160 g) onion, chopped

$^1/_4$ cup (37 g) green bell peppers, chopped

1 tablespoon (14 g) unsalted butter

$^1/_2$ teaspoon (1 g) freshly ground black pepper

Boil or microwave potatoes until almost cooked through. Drain. Coarsely chop potatoes and combine with onion and green bell pepper. Melt butter in a heavy skillet. Add potato mixture. Sprinkle black pepper over the top. Fry until browned, turning frequently.

Yield: 6 servings

Per serving: 201 calories (10% from fat, 10% from protein, 81% from carbohydrate); 5 g protein; 2 g total fat; 1 g saturated fat; 1 g monounsaturated fat; 0 g polyunsaturated fat; 42 g carbohydrate; 5 g fiber; 4 g sugar; 161 mg phosphorus; 34 mg calcium; 2 mg iron; 37 mg sodium; 1174 mg potassium; 141 IU vitamin A; 23 mg ATE vitamin E; 28 mg vitamin C; 5 mg cholesterol; 229 g water

Latkes

You don't need to be Jewish to enjoy these. In fact, we have them often with pork chops.

4 potatoes

1 tablespoon finely chopped onion

1 egg

$^1/_2$ cup (60 g) bread crumbs

2 tablespoons (28 ml) canola oil

Peel and grate potatoes. Squeeze in a kitchen towel to remove excess moisture. Mix all ingredients together. Heat oil in heavy skillet. Drop batter onto hot skillet in $^1/_4$-cup measures and flatten with fork into pancakes. Cook until browned. Turn over and finish cooking.

Yield: 4 servings

Per serving: 11 g water; 139 calories (61% from fat, 10% from protein, 29% from carb); 3 g protein; 9 g total fat; 1 g saturated fat; 5 g monounsaturated fat; 3 g polyunsaturated fat; 10 g carbohydrate; 1 g fiber; 1 g sugar; 47 mg phosphorus; 32 mg calcium; 1 mg iron; 42 mg sodium; 47 mg potassium; 84 IU vitamin A; 22 mg vitamin E; 0 mg vitamin C; 53 mg cholesterol

Tip: Serve with butter, sour cream, or applesauce.

Zucchini Pancakes

These make a great side dish with almost any kind of meat, but I have to admit to having them for breakfast a time or two also. Maybe that's just because I get desperate when the garden is really producing zucchini.

4 cups (452 g) shredded zucchini

4 eggs

$^1/_2$ cup (62 g) flour

$^1/_8$ teaspoon black pepper

$^1/_4$ teaspoon garlic powder

$^1/_4$ cup chopped fresh parsley

3 tablespoons (45 ml) canola oil

Wash zucchini and trim the ends. Grate or grind into a bowl. Squeeze dry. In a bowl, combine the zucchini and all the other ingredients except the oil. Heat the oil in a heavy skillet over medium heat. Drop zucchini mixture by heaping tablespoons into hot oil. Flatten them a little, fry until golden brown on bottom. Turn and brown second side. Drain on paper towels. (If mixture is thin, add more flour.)

Yield: 6 servings

Per serving: 110 g water; 168 calories (58% from fat, 16% from protein, 26% from carb); 7 g protein; 11 g total fat; 2 g saturated fat; 6 g monounsaturated fat; 3 g polyunsaturated fat; 11 g carbohydrate; 1 g fiber; 2 g sugar; 116 mg phosphorus; 37 mg calcium; 2 mg iron; 62 mg sodium; 293 mg potassium; 560 IU vitamin A; 52 mg vitamin E; 17 mg vitamin C; 158 mg cholesterol

Whole Wheat Buttermilk Pancakes

A great tasty, old-fashioned pancake. Reminds me of the kind of breakfasts my grandmother made.

1 cup (120 g) whole wheat pastry flour

$1/2$ teaspoon baking soda

$1/4$ teaspoon cinnamon

$1 1/4$ cups (295 ml) buttermilk

2 eggs

3 tablespoons (45 ml) canola oil

Blend dry ingredients. Blend wet ingredients except oil. Mix the two mixtures together. Will be slightly lumpy. Heat oil in cast-iron skillet. Pour one-quarter of the batter into pan. When pancake bubbles, turn, cook 1 to 2 minutes.

Yield: 4 servings

Per serving: 93 g water; 266 calories (48% from fat, 15% from protein, 38% from carb); 10 g protein; 15 g total fat; 2 g saturated fat; 8 g monounsaturated fat; 4 g polyunsaturated fat; 26 g carbohydrate; 4 g fiber; 4 g sugar; 226 mg phosphorus; 116 mg calcium; 2 mg iron; 121 mg sodium; 275 mg potassium; 159 IU vitamin A; 44 mg vitamin E; 1 mg vitamin C; 122 mg cholesterol

Cornmeal Pancakes

Another of those old-fashioned breakfast meals. Do you suppose that I keep saying that because people ate healthier food in the good old days?

1 cup (235 ml) boiling water

$3/4$ cup (105 g) cornmeal

$1 1/4$ cups (295 ml) buttermilk

2 eggs

1 cup (120 g) whole wheat pastry flour

1 tablespoon baking powder

$1/4$ teaspoon baking soda

$1/4$ cup (60 ml) canola oil

Pour water over cornmeal, stir until thick. Add buttermilk; beat in eggs. Mix flour, baking powder, and baking soda. Add to cornmeal mixture. Stir in canola oil. Bake on hot griddle.

Yield: 7 servings

Per serving: 89 g water; 233 calories (40% from fat, 12% from protein, 48% from carb); 7 g protein; 11 g total fat; 1 g saturated fat; 6 g monounsaturated fat; 3 g polyunsaturated fat; 29 g carbohydrate; 3 g fiber; 3 g

sugar; 190 mg phosphorus; 182 mg calcium; 2 mg iron; 280 mg sodium; 184 mg potassium; 127 IU vitamin A; 25 mg vitamin E; 0 mg vitamin C; 69 mg cholesterol

Multigrain Pancakes

These are great pancakes, thicker and full of much more flavor than regular ones. Try them with the apple topping in Chapter 23.

$1^1/_2$ cups (180 g) whole wheat pastry flour

$^1/_4$ cup (35 g) cornmeal

$^1/_4$ cup (20 g) rolled oats

2 tablespoons oat bran

2 tablespoons wheat germ

2 tablespoons (18 g) toasted wheat cereal, such as Wheatena

1 teaspoon baking soda

$^1/_2$ teaspoon baking powder

1 teaspoon vanilla extract

$1^1/_2$ cups (355 g) skim milk

2 egg whites

Mix all dry ingredients. Add milk and vanilla to make batter. Thicker batter makes thicker pancakes. Set aside to rest for a half an hour. Beat egg whites until stiff peaks form. Gently fold into batter after it has rested. Spoon onto moderate griddle and cook until bubbles break. Turn and cook until done. Bake more slowly than with regular pancakes because of the heavy batter.

Yield: 6 servings

Per serving: 70 g water; 195 calories (6% from fat, 20% from protein, 74% from carb); 10 g protein; 1 g total

fat; 0 g saturated fat; 0 g monounsaturated fat; 1 g polyunsaturated fat; 37 g carbohydrate; 5 g fiber; 1 g sugar; 249 mg phosphorus; 127 mg calcium; 2 mg iron; 101 mg sodium; 316 mg potassium; 154 IU vitamin A; 40 mg vitamin E; 1 mg vitamin C; 1 mg cholesterol

Oat Bran Pancakes

Why should breakfast be boring or unhealthy? Try these pancakes and you will not be bored.

1 cup (100 g) oat bran

$^1/_2$ cup (60 g) flour

2 teaspoons (9 g) sugar

2 teaspoons (9.2 g) baking powder

1 cup (235 ml) skim milk

1 tablespoon (15 ml) canola oil

1 egg white

Heat griddle over medium-high heat. Spray lightly with nonstick vegetable oil spray. Stir first 4 ingredients together. Combine remaining ingredients, add to the oat bran mixture, and mix well. Spoon batter onto griddle and cook until bubbles form on the tops. Turn over and cook until done.

Yield: 4 servings

Per serving: 171 calories (24% from fat, 15% from protein, 61% from carbohydrate); 6 g protein; 5 g total fat; 1 g saturated fat; 2 g monounsaturated fat; 1 g polyunsaturated fat; 27 g carbohydrate; 2 g fiber; 4 g sugar; 205 mg phosphorus; 251 mg calcium; 5 mg iron; 336 mg sodium; 105 mg potassium; 263 IU vitamin A; 71 mg ATE vitamin E; 2 mg vitamin C; 1 mg cholesterol; 64 g water

Cinnamon–Oat Bran Pancakes

These are the kind of pancakes you want on a snowy day, warm and flavorful. The good news is they are also a lot better for you than regular, boring pancakes.

$^3/_4$ cup (75 g) oat bran

$^3/_4$ cup (90 g) whole wheat pastry flour

1 tablespoon sugar

$^1/_2$ teaspoon baking powder

$^1/_2$ teaspoon cinnamon

$^1/_4$ teaspoon baking soda

$1^1/_4$ cups (295 ml) buttermilk

1 tablespoon (15 ml) canola oil

$^1/_2$ cup (55 g) finely chopped pecans

In medium mixing bowl, combine dry ingredients. Set bowl aside. In a small mixing bowl, combine buttermilk and oil. Add to dry ingredients, stirring until just combined. Stir in pecans. Cook on hot griddle. Use $^1/_4$ cup batter for each pancake.

Yield: 4 servings

Per serving: 72 g water; 277 calories (46% from fat, 11% from protein, 43% from carb); 8 g protein; 15 g total fat; 2 g saturated fat; 8 g monounsaturated fat; 4 g polyunsaturated fat; 32 g carbohydrate; 5 g fiber; 9 g sugar; 241 mg phosphorus; 160 mg calcium; 4 mg iron; 174 mg sodium; 302 mg potassium; 113 IU vitamin A; 30 mg vitamin E; 2 mg vitamin C; 3 mg cholesterol

Oatmeal Pancakes

A nice change for Sunday morning breakfast.

$1^1/_4$ cups (285 ml) skim milk

1 cup (80 g) quick-cooking oats

2 eggs

$^1/_2$ cup (60 g) whole wheat flour

1 tablespoon (15 g) brown sugar

1 teaspoon (2.3 g) cinnamon

1 tablespoon (13.8 g) baking powder

Combine milk and oats in a bowl and let stand 5 minutes. Add eggs and mix well. Add remaining ingredients and stir until just blended. Cook on a hot griddle, turning when bubbles form on the tops of the pancakes and burst. Flip pancakes and finish cooking on the other side.

Yield: 6 servings

Per serving: 135 calories (12% from fat, 23% from protein, 65% from carbohydrate); 8 g protein; 2 g total fat; 0 g saturated fat; 1 g monounsaturated fat; 1 g polyunsaturated fat; 22 g carbohydrate; 3 g fiber; 3 g sugar; 232 mg phosphorus; 237 mg calcium; 2 mg iron; 313 mg sodium; 160 mg potassium; 181 IU vitamin A; 31 mg ATE vitamin E; 1 mg vitamin C; 71 mg cholesterol; 66 g water

Banana Pancakes

During a search for a breakfast that would use up some overripe bananas, I came up with this recipe. They are very good and sweet enough that you don't really need to add anything (although a little powdered sugar sprinkled over them is good).

1 cup (125 g) flour

1 tablespoon (13 g) sugar

1 tablespoon (14 g) baking powder

$^1/_2$ cup (120 ml) skim milk

1 egg

1 tablespoon (15 ml) canola oil

1 cup (225 g) banana, chopped

Stir together flour, sugar, and baking powder. Combine the milk, egg, and oil. Stir in banana. Add milk mixture all at once to flour mixture. Stir until blended but still slightly lumpy. Pour about $^1/_4$ cup (60 ml) of batter onto a hot griddle sprayed with nonstick vegetable oil spray. Cook until browned on bottom (when bubbles form and then break on the top). Turn and cook on the other side until done. Repeat with remaining batter.

Yield: 4 servings

Per serving: 235 calories (17% from fat, 12% from protein, 71% from carbohydrate); 7 g protein; 5 g total fat; 1 g saturated fat; 2 g monounsaturated fat; 1 g polyunsaturated fat; 43 g carbohydrate; 2 g fiber; 10 g sugar; 175 mg phosphorus; 263 mg calcium; 2 mg iron; 413 mg sodium; 243 mg potassium; 155 IU vitamin A; 19 mg ATE vitamin E; 5 mg vitamin C; 51 mg cholesterol; 86 g water

Tip: The griddle is hot enough when a drop of water sizzles and breaks up immediately.

Apple Pancakes

This makes a great breakfast for a weekend (or maybe when you are snowed in). Kind of like apple fritters, only the syrup flavor gets baked right into the pancakes.

4 cups (440 g) sliced apple

$^1/_2$ cup (120 ml) maple syrup

2 tablespoons (28 g) unsalted butter

$1^1/_2$ cups (192 g) biscuit baking mix

1 cup (235 ml) skim milk

2 eggs

$^1/_2$ teaspoon cinnamon

$^1/_4$ teaspoon nutmeg

Combine apples in skillet with syrup and butter. Cook until tender but firm, about 25 minutes. Meanwhile combine rest of ingredients and mix until smooth. Remove apples from skillet with slotted spoon and add to batter. Fold gently until apples are covered. Lift batter-covered apples onto hot griddle coated with nonstick vegetable oil spray. Grill until edges are cooked. Turn pancakes once. Serve with remaining syrup in which apples were cooked.

Yield: 6 servings

Per serving: 126 g water; 306 calories (30% from fat, 8% from protein, 62% from carb); 7 g protein; 10 g total fat; 4 g saturated fat; 4 g monounsaturated fat; 1 g polyunsaturated fat; 48 g carbohydrate; 2 g fiber; 27 g sugar; 258 mg phosphorus; 145 mg calcium; 2 mg iron; 417 mg sodium; 269 mg potassium; 323 IU vitamin A; 83 mg vitamin E; 4 mg vitamin C; 91 mg cholesterol

High-Protein Blueberry Pancakes

When you are looking for a great-tasting breakfast, but want something that also is good for you, you should give these pancakes a try.

4 eggs

1 cup (225 g) cottage cheese

$^1/_4$ cup (28 g) wheat germ

$^1/_4$ cup (20 g) quick-cooking oats

2 tablespoons (28 ml) canola oil

1 cup (145 g) blueberries

Place all the ingredients except blueberries in a blender and mix thoroughly. Stir in blueberries. Drop by tablespoons onto a hot frying pan or griddle coated with nonstick vegetable oil spray.

Yield: 4 servings

Per serving: 103 g water; 240 calories (51% from fat, 27% from protein, 22% from carb); 16 g protein; 14 g total fat; 3 g saturated fat; 7 g monounsaturated fat; 3 g polyunsaturated fat; 13 g carbohydrate; 2 g fiber; 5 g sugar; 254 mg phosphorus; 49 mg calcium; 2 mg iron; 84 mg sodium; 200 mg potassium; 311 IU vitamin A; 81 mg vitamin E; 4 mg vitamin C; 239 mg cholesterol

Oven-Baked Pancake

Mix it up, stick it in the oven, and enjoy it. A great weekend breakfast choice.

3 eggs

$^1/_2$ cup (60 g) whole wheat pastry flour

$^1/_2$ cup (120 ml) skim milk

$^1/_4$ cup (55 g) unsalted butter, divided

2 tablespoons (26 g) sugar

2 tablespoons (18 g) slivered almonds, toasted

2 tablespoons (30 ml) lemon juice

Beat eggs with an electric mixer at medium speed until well blended. Gradually add flour, beating until smooth. Add milk and 2 tablespoons (28 g) melted butter; beat until batter is smooth. Pour batter into a 10-inch (25-cm) skillet coated with nonstick vegetable oil spray. Bake at 400°F (200°C, gas mark 6) for 15 minutes or until pancake is puffed and golden brown. Sprinkle with sugar and toasted almonds. Combine remaining butter and lemon juice; heat until butter melts. Serve over hot pancake.

Yield: 3 servings

Per serving: 94 g water; 370 calories (58% from fat, 13% from protein, 29% from carb); 13 g protein; 24 g total fat; 12 g saturated fat; 8 g monounsaturated fat; 2 g polyunsaturated fat; 28 g carbohydrate; 3 g fiber; 9 g sugar; 255 mg phosphorus; 116 mg calcium; 2 mg iron; 106 mg sodium; 291 mg potassium; 832 IU vitamin A; 230 mg vitamin E; 5 mg vitamin C; 278 mg cholesterol

Baked Pancake

This is a German-style pancake, baked in one large pan in the oven, then cut into serving-size pieces.

1$^1/_2$ cups (180 g) whole wheat pastry flour

1$^1/_2$ cups (35 ml) skim milk

4 eggs, slightly beaten

$^1/_4$ cup (55 g) unsalted butter

1 cup (170 g) sliced strawberries

Gradually add flour and milk to eggs. Melt butter in 9 × 13-inch (23 × 33-cm) pan. Pour batter over melted butter. Bake at 400°F (200°C, gas mark 6) for about 30 minutes. Serve with fresh sliced strawberries.

Per serving: 167 g water; 378 calories (42% from fat, 17% from protein, 41% from carb); 17 g protein; 18 g total fat; 9 g saturated fat; 5 g monounsaturated fat; 2 g polyunsaturated fat; 41 g carbohydrate; 6 g fiber; 7 g sugar; 368 mg phosphorus; 169 mg calcium; 3 mg iron; 201 mg sodium; 462 mg potassium; 823 IU vitamin A; 229 mg vitamin E; 22 mg vitamin C; 269 mg cholesterol

Wheat Waffles

You can certainly have these for breakfast, but we also like them for dinner, topped with something like chicken à la king.

2 cups (240 g) whole wheat pastry flour

4 teaspoons (18 g) baking powder

2 tablespoons (40 g) honey

1³/₄ cups (410 ml) skim milk

4 tablespoons (60 ml) canola oil

2 eggs

Mix dry ingredients together. Stir in remaining ingredients. For lighter waffles, separate eggs. Beat egg whites and carefully fold in. Pour into a waffle iron coated with nonstick vegetable oil spray.

Yield: 8 servings

Per serving: 63 g water; 223 calories (35% from fat, 14% from protein, 51% from carb); 8 g protein; 9 g total fat; 1 g saturated fat; 5 g monounsaturated fat; 3 g polyunsaturated fat; 30 g carbohydrate; 4 g fiber; 5 g sugar; 241 mg phosphorus; 230 mg calcium; 2 mg iron; 297 mg sodium; 241 mg potassium; 180 IU vitamin A; 52 mg vitamin E; 1 mg vitamin C; 60 mg cholesterol

Oatmeal Waffles

Great waffles, and easy to make. These don't require the separated eggs and beaten whites that most waffle recipes call for. This and the whole grains make them a little crisper than some waffles, but the taste is wonderful.

1¹/₂ cups (180 g) whole wheat pastry flour

1 cup (80 g) quick-cooking oats

1 tablespoon baking powder

1 teaspoon cinnamon

2 tablespoons (30 g) brown sugar

3 tablespoons (42 g) unsalted butter

1¹/₂ cups (355 ml) skim milk

2 eggs, slightly beaten

In large bowl, mix all dry ingredients together and set aside. Melt butter and add milk and eggs. Mix well and then add to flour mixture. Stir until well blended. Pour into a waffle iron coated with nonstick vegetable oil spray.

Yield: 5 servings

Per serving: 91 g water; 326 calories (29% from fat, 15% from protein, 56% from carb); 13 g protein; 11 g total fat; 5 g saturated fat; 3 g monounsaturated fat; 1 g polyunsaturated fat; 47 g carbohydrate; 6 g fiber; 10 g sugar; 382 mg phosphorus; 299 mg calcium; 3 mg iron; 360 mg sodium; 371 mg potassium; 476 IU vitamin A; 133 mg vitamin E; 0 mg vitamin C; 115 mg cholesterol

Oat Bran Waffles

If you have a waffle iron, you might want give these a try. They make a crunchy waffle that's great for a dinner meal when topped with something like chicken à la king.

$^1/_2$ cup (60 g) flour

$^1/_2$ cup (40 g) quick-cooking oats

$^1/_2$ cup (50 g) oat bran

1 teaspoon (4.6 g) baking powder

1 egg

$^3/_4$ cup (180 ml) skim milk

1 tablespoon (15 ml) honey

2 tablespoons (28 g) unsalted butter, melted

Mix together first 4 ingredients. Combine egg, milk, honey, and butter. Add to dry ingredients, mixing until just blended. Cook according to waffle iron instructions.

Yield: 3 servings

Per serving: 288 calories (30% from fat, 14% from protein, 56% from carbohydrate); 10 g protein; 6 g total fat; 4 g saturated fat; 2 g monounsaturated fat; 1 g polyunsaturated fat; 40 g carbohydrate; 3 g fiber; 7 g sugar; 255 mg phosphorus; 216 mg calcium; 4 mg iron; 265 mg sodium; 190 mg potassium; 610 IU vitamin A; 132 mg ATE vitamin E; 2 mg vitamin C; 80 mg cholesterol; 79 g water

French Toast

French toast is one of those breakfasts that we don't seem to have very often, but wonder why not every time we do.

2 eggs

$^3/_4$ cup (180 ml) skim milk

2 teaspoons (10 ml) vanilla extract

$^1/_2$ teaspoon (1.2 g) cinnamon

8 slices day-old whole wheat bread

Combine eggs, milk, vanilla, and cinnamon in a wide bowl or dish. Dip bread in egg mixture, ensuring both sides are soaked. Coat a griddle or nonstick skillet with nonstick vegetable oil spray and place over medium-high heat. Place bread slices in skillet or griddle and cook for 3 minutes on each side, or until both sides of bread are golden brown.

Yield: 4 servings

Per serving: 185 calories (15% from fat, 25% from protein, 60% from carbohydrate); 11 g protein; 3 g total fat; 1 g saturated fat; 1 g monounsaturated fat; 1 g polyunsaturated fat; 27 g carbohydrate; 2 g fiber; 3 g sugar; 167 mg phosphorus; 157 mg calcium; 3 mg iron; 344 mg sodium; 184 mg potassium; 207 IU vitamin A; 28 mg ATE vitamin E; 1 mg vitamin C; 51 mg cholesterol; 86 g water

Tip: Top with confectioner's sugar and fresh fruit.

Praline French Toast

Like a taste of old New Orleans, this breakfast treat will definitely be on your list to make again.

8 eggs

$1^1/_2$ cups (355 ml) skim milk

$^1/_2$ cup (115 g) brown sugar, divided

2 teaspoons vanilla extract

8 slices whole wheat bread

$1/4$ cup (55 g) unsalted butter

$1/4$ cup (60 ml) maple syrup

$1/2$ cup (55 g) chopped pecans

Thoroughly blend eggs, milk, 1 tablespoon brown sugar, and vanilla. Pour half of egg mixture into 9 × 13-inch (23 × 33-cm) baking dish. Place bread slices in mixture. Pour remaining egg mixture over bread. Cover and refrigerate several hours or overnight. Preheat oven to 350°F (180°C, gas mark 4). Remove bread from baking dish and set aside. Place butter in 9 × 13-inch (23 × 33-cm) baking dish and put in oven until butter melts. Stir in remaining brown sugar and syrup. Sprinkle with pecans. Carefully place reserved bread slices on pecans. Pour any remaining egg mixture over bread. Bake uncovered until puffed and lightly brown, 30 to 35 minutes. Invert slices to serve.

Yield: 8 servings

Per serving: 98 g water; 345 calories (45% from fat, 14% from protein, 41% from carb); 12 g protein; 17 g total fat; 6 g saturated fat; 7 g monounsaturated fat; 3 g polyunsaturated fat; 36 g carbohydrate; 2 g fiber; 22 g sugar; 221 mg phosphorus; 156 mg calcium; 2 mg iron; 243 mg sodium; 304 mg potassium; 547 IU vitamin A; 154 mg vitamin E; 1 mg vitamin C; 253 mg cholesterol

Breakfast Citrus Cups

Quick and easy. But the citrus and grape combination and the addition of the almonds make it a little more than just grapefruit and oranges.

4 grapefruits

2 cups (300 g) seedless green grapes

2 oranges, sectioned

$1/4$ cup (27 g) slivered almonds, toasted

Cut grapefruits in half. Remove sections and membrane, leaving shells intact. Combine grapefruit sections, grapes, and oranges; mix lightly. Chill. Add nuts to fruit mixture just before serving. Spoon fruit mixture onto grapefruit shells.

Yield: 8 servings

Per serving: 210 g water; 116 calories (18% from fat, 8% from protein, 74% from carb); 3 g protein; 3 g total fat; 0 g saturated fat; 1 g monounsaturated fat; 1 g polyunsaturated fat; 24 g carbohydrate; 4 g fiber; 20 g sugar; 44 mg phosphorus; 51 mg calcium; 0 mg iron; 2 mg sodium; 389 mg potassium; 1666 IU vitamin A; 0 mg vitamin E; 82 mg vitamin C; 0 mg cholesterol

Fruit with Orange Cream Dip

A nice dip with fruit for a party or company, but it wouldn't be a bad idea to have it for family also, since it's got so many good things for you.

1 cup (230 g) sour cream

2 tablespoons (30 g) firmly packed brown sugar

1 tablespoon (15 ml) orange juice

1 teaspoon orange peel

1 cup (165 g) pineapple chunks

1 cup (195 g) orange sections

1 cup (177 g) sliced kiwifruit

1 cup (145 g) strawberries

In medium-size serving bowl, stir together all ingredients except fruit. Cover; refrigerate at least 2 hours. Serve with skewered fresh fruit for dipping.

Yield: 6 servings

Per serving: 120 g water; 112 calories (39% from fat, 6% from protein, 55% from carb); 2 g protein; 5 g total fat; 3 g saturated fat; 1 g monounsaturated fat; 0 g polyunsaturated fat; 16 g carbohydrate; 2 g fiber; 11 g sugar; 57 mg phosphorus; 67 mg calcium; 0 mg iron; 20 mg sodium; 256 mg potassium; 198 IU vitamin A; 40 mg vitamin E; 47 mg vitamin C; 16 mg cholesterol

Fruit Sauce

A simple, uncooked fruit sauce. For a real treat, try this over multigrain pancakes.

1 cup (235 ml) apple juice

4 apples, peeled and cored

2 cups (300 g) sliced banana

1 pear, peeled and cored

1 teaspoon cinnamon

1 teaspoon nutmeg

Put apple juice and fruits in blender. Blend until smooth. Then add spices and mix.

Yield: 6 servings

Per serving: 183 g water; 138 calories (4% from fat, 3% from protein, 93% from carb); 1 g protein; 1 g total fat; 0 g saturated fat; 0 g monounsaturated fat; 0 g polyunsaturated fat; 35 g carbohydrate; 4 g fiber; 24 g sugar; 32 mg phosphorus; 17 mg calcium; 1 mg iron; 4 mg sodium; 423 mg potassium; 82 IU vitamin A; 0 mg vitamin E; 11 mg vitamin C; 0 mg cholesterol

Breakfast Bars

These contain a little more nutrition than commercial granola bars and are equally good for a breakfast on the run.

1 cup (80 g) quick-cooking oats

$^1/_2$ cup (60 g) whole wheat flour

$^1/_2$ cup (58 g) crunchy wheat-barley cereal, such as Grape-Nuts

$^1/_2$ teaspoon cinnamon

1 egg

$^1/_4$ cup (60 g) applesauce

$^1/_4$ cup (85 g) honey

3 tablespoons (45 g) brown sugar

2 tablespoons (28 ml) canola oil

$^1/_4$ cup (36 g) sunflower seeds, unsalted

$^1/_4$ cup (30 g) chopped walnuts

7 ounces (198 g) dried fruit

Preheat oven to 325°F (170°C, gas mark 3). Line a 9-inch (23-cm) square baking pan with aluminum foil. Spray the foil with nonstick vegetable oil spray. In a large bowl, stir together the oats, flour, cereal, and cinnamon. Add the egg, applesauce, honey, brown sugar, and oil. Mix well. Stir in the sunflower seeds, walnuts, and dried fruit. Spread mixture evenly in the prepared pan. Bake 30 minutes, or until firm and lightly browned around the edges. Let cool. Use the foil to lift from the pan. Cut into bars and store in the refrigerator.

Yield: 12 servings

Per serving: 16 g water; 222 calories (26% from fat, 9% from protein, 65% from carb); 6 g protein; 7 g total fat; 1 g saturated fat; 2 g monounsaturated fat; 3 g polyunsaturated fat; 38 g carbohydrate; 4 g fiber; 10 g sugar; 164 mg phosphorus; 27 mg calcium; 3 mg iron;

43 mg sodium; 284 mg potassium; 492 IU vitamin A; 6 mg vitamin E; 1 mg vitamin C; 20 mg cholesterol

sodium; 99 mg potassium; 25 IU vitamin A; 5 mg vitamin E; 1 mg vitamin C; 15 mg cholesterol

Banana Cereal Cookies

Bananas and oatmeal are a great combination. And these cookies are great either for breakfast or as a snack.

1$^1/_4$ cups (281 g) shortening

2 cups (400 g) sugar

3 eggs

3 cups (360 g) whole wheat pastry flour

$^1/_2$ teaspoon nutmeg

1$^1/_4$ teaspoons cinnamon

3$^1/_2$ cups (280 g) quick-cooking oats

1 teaspoon baking soda

2 cups (450 g) mashed banana

1 cup (110 g) chopped pecans

Cream shortening and sugar. Add eggs; cream well. Sift flour, baking soda, nutmeg, and cinnamon together. Add oats to shortening mixture. Add flour mixture alternately with mashed banana. Add chopped pecans. Drop on baking sheet coated with nonstick vegetable oil spray. Bake at 375°F (190°C, gas mark 5) for 12 to 15 minutes.

Yield: 48 servings

Per serving: 11 g water; 157 calories (43% from fat, 7% from protein, 50% from carb); 3 g protein; 8 g total fat; 2 g saturated fat; 4 g monounsaturated fat; 2 g polyunsaturated fat; 20 g carbohydrate; 2 g fiber; 10 g sugar; 69 mg phosphorus; 10 mg calcium; 1 mg iron; 6 mg

Apple Pecan Breakfast Cookies

Personally, I like the idea of cookies for breakfast. It makes me feel like I'm getting away with something, especially when they taste as good as these do.

$^1/_2$ cup (112 g) unsalted butter

1 cup (225 g) firmly packed brown sugar

2 eggs

1 tablespoon (15 ml) skim milk

1 teaspoon vanilla extract

1$^1/_4$ cups (150 g) whole wheat pastry flour

$^1/_2$ teaspoon baking soda

2 cups (164 g) granola

$^1/_2$ cup (43 g) dried apples

$^1/_2$ cup (55 g) chopped pecans

Preheat oven to 350°F (180°C, gas mark 4). Coat baking sheets with nonstick vegetable oil spray. Cream together butter and brown sugar in a large bowl. Add eggs, milk, and vanilla. Beat well. In a medium bowl, combine flour and baking soda. Mix well and add to sugar mixture. Stir in granola, apples, and pecans. Drop by teaspoons onto prepared baking sheets. Bake 10 to 12 minutes until edges are browned.

Per serving: 6 g water; 94 calories (40% from fat, 6% from protein, 54% from carb); 2 g protein; 4 g total fat; 2 g saturated fat; 2 g monounsaturated fat; 1 g

polyunsaturated fat; 13 g carbohydrate; 1 g fiber; 8 g sugar; 40 mg phosphorus; 12 mg calcium; 0 mg iron; 25 mg sodium; 64 mg potassium; 97 IU vitamin A; 26 mg vitamin E; 0 mg vitamin C; 20 mg cholesterol

Yield: 36 servings

Cereal Breakfast Cookies

These are tasty little things and keep well. This recipe makes a lot, but they freeze well and you can save time by making a big batch—then just take out a bagful whenever you need more.

1 cup (235 ml) canola oil

1 cup (225 g) brown sugar

1 cup (200 g) sugar

1 teaspoon vanilla extract

2 eggs

4 cups (480 g) whole wheat pastry flour

1 teaspoon baking powder

1 teaspoon baking soda

1 cup (80 g) rolled oats

1 cup (40 g) bran flakes cereal

1 cup (110 g) chopped pecans

Mix together oil, sugars, vanilla, and eggs. Add the flour, baking powder, baking soda, oats, bran flakes, and pecans. Mix well. Batter will be sticky. Flour your hands and roll into 1-inch (2.5-cm) balls (go easy on the flour on your hands, or your cookies will come out dry). Bake on ungreased baking sheet at 350°F (180°C, gas mark 4) for 8 to 9 minutes. Do not overbake—cookies should be chewy in the middle.

Yield: 80 servings

Per serving: 2 g water; 81 calories (44% from fat, 6% from protein, 50% from carb); 1 g protein; 4 g total fat; 0 g saturated fat; 2 g monounsaturated fat; 1 g polyunsaturated fat; 10 g carbohydrate; 1 g fiber; 5 g sugar; 34 mg phosphorus; 10 mg calcium; 0 mg iron; 9 mg sodium; 45 mg potassium; 8 IU vitamin A; 2 mg vitamin E; 0 mg vitamin C; 6 mg cholesterol

Breakfast Carrot Cookies

Another quick grab-and-go breakfast option.

1 cup (110 g) grated carrot

$1/2$ cup (115 g) plain fat-free yogurt

$1/4$ cup (60 g) brown sugar

2 tablespoons (28 ml) canola oil

1 teaspoon vanilla extract

$1^1/2$ cups (220 g) chopped dates

$1^1/2$ cups (180 g) whole wheat pastry flour

$1/4$ cup (29 g) crunchy wheat-barley cereal, such as Grape-Nuts

$1/2$ teaspoon baking soda

Preheat oven to 350°F (180°C, gas mark 4). Spray baking sheets with nonstick vegetable oil spray or line with parchment paper or silicone sheet. In medium mixing bowl, stir carrot, yogurt, sugar, oil, vanilla, and dates. Let stand 15 minutes. Stir in remaining dry ingredients until well blended. Drop tablespoons of mixture onto baking sheets, spacing $1^1/2$ inches (4 cm) apart. Reduce to teaspoon drops for mini-size cookies. Bake 15 minutes or until cookie top springs back when lightly touched. Cool.

Yield: 30 servings

Per serving: 10 g water; 69 calories (14% from fat, 8% from protein, 78% from carb); 1 g protein; 1 g total fat; 0 g saturated fat; 1 g monounsaturated fat; 0 g polyunsaturated fat; 14 g carbohydrate; 2 g fiber; 8 g sugar; 36 mg phosphorus; 16 mg calcium; 1 mg iron; 13 mg sodium; 115 mg potassium; 733 IU vitamin A; 1 mg vitamin E; 0 mg vitamin C; 0 mg cholesterol

Tip: You can substitute raisins or other dried fruit for the dates.

Breakfast Cookies

These are good for breakfast on the run. They are fairly soft, but they're portable and fat-free.

3 cups (675 g) mashed banana

$^1/_3$ cup (82 g) applesauce

2 cups (160 g) quick-cooking oats

$^1/_4$ cup (60 ml) skim milk

$^1/_2$ cup (75 g) dried cranberries

1 teaspoon (5 ml) vanilla

1 teaspoon (2.3 g) cinnamon

1 tablespoon (13 g) sugar

$^1/_2$ cup (50 g) pecans, chopped

Preheat oven to 350°F (180°C, or gas mark 4). Mix all ingredients in a bowl until well combined. Let this mixture stand for at least 5 minutes. Heap the dough by teaspoonfuls onto a greased baking sheet. Bake for 15 to 20 minutes and let cool.

Yield: 20 servings

Per serving: 127 calories (22% from fat, 10% from protein, 68% from carbohydrate); 3 g protein; 3 g total fat; 0 g saturated fat; 1 g monounsaturated fat; 1 g polyunsaturated fat; 23 g carbohydrate; 3 g fiber; 8 g sugar; 101 mg phosphorus; 18 mg calcium; 1 mg iron; 3 mg sodium; 209 mg potassium; 30 IU vitamin A; 2 mg ATE vitamin E; 3 mg vitamin C; 0 mg cholesterol; 33 g water

Tip: You can leave out the nuts if you prefer and substitute other dried fruit like raisins or dried apples for the cranberries.

Crunchy Breakfast Topping

Sprinkle over oatmeal, toast, fresh fruit, yogurt, pancakes, waffles, or French toast.

$^1/_4$ cup (55 g) unsalted butter

1$^1/_4$ cups (140 g) wheat germ

$^1/_2$ cup (115 g) packed brown sugar

$^1/_2$ cup (47 g) ground almonds

1 tablespoon grated orange peel

$^1/_2$ teaspoon cinnamon

Melt butter in a 9 × 13-inch (23 × 33-cm) baking pan in oven about 4 minutes. Add remaining ingredients and mix well. Bake 10 to 12 minutes or until deep golden brown. Stir. Cool and store in the refrigerator for up to 3 months.

Yield: 12 servings

Per serving: 2 g water; 149 calories (47% from fat, 12% from protein, 41% from carb); 5 g protein; 8 g total fat; 3 g saturated fat; 3 g monounsaturated fat; 2 g polyunsaturated fat; 16 g carbohydrate; 3 g fiber; 10 g sugar; 167 mg phosphorus; 29 mg calcium; 2 mg iron; 6 mg sodium; 187 mg potassium; 133 IU vitamin A; 32 mg vitamin E; 1 mg vitamin C; 10 mg cholesterol

Toasty Nut Granola

Great as a snack or breakfast cereal.

6 cups (480 g) rolled oats

1 cup (110 g) chopped pecans

³/₄ cup (84 g) wheat germ

¹/₂ cup (115 g) firmly packed brown sugar

¹/₂ cup (40 g) shredded coconut

¹/₂ cup (72 g) sesame seeds

¹/₂ cup (120 ml) canola oil

¹/₂ cup (170 g) honey

1¹/₂ teaspoons vanilla extract

Toast oats in a 9 × 13-inch (23 × 33-cm) pan at 350°F (180°C, gas mark 4) for 10 minutes. Combine remaining ingredients in a large bowl and add toasted oats. Bake on 2 baking sheets at 350°F (180°C, gas mark 4) for 20 to 25 minutes. Stir when cool and store in refrigerator.

Yield: 28 servings

Per serving: 4 g water; 194 calories (44% from fat, 9% from protein, 47% from carb); 5 g protein; 10 g total fat; 2 g saturated fat; 4 g monounsaturated fat; 4 g polyunsaturated fat; 24 g carbohydrate; 3 g fiber; 9 g sugar; 146 mg phosphorus; 42 mg calcium; 2 mg iron;

3 mg sodium; 139 mg potassium; 6 IU vitamin A; 0 mg vitamin E; 0 mg vitamin C; 0 mg cholesterol

Granola

Some healthy cereals are available, if you are careful about reading the ingredient labels. But it would be hard to find one healthier or tastier than this homemade granola.

6 cups (480 g) rolled oats

6 cups rolled wheat

2 cups (290 g) sunflower seeds

4 ounces (113 g) sesame seeds

2 cups (190 g) peanuts

3 cups (255 g) coconut

1 cup (112 g) wheat germ

1¹/₂ cups (355 ml) canola oil

1 cup (340 g) honey

¹/₂ cup (170 g) molasses

1 tablespoon (15 ml) vanilla extract

1 cup (145 g) raisins

Mix all dry ingredients except raisins together in large bowl. Put aside. Heat the oil, honey, molasses, and vanilla together and mix with dry ingredients. Spread mixture on baking sheets. Bake at 350°F (180°C, gas mark 4) for 30 to 40 minutes or until light brown. Stir frequently to brown evenly. Remove from oven and add raisins or any other dried fruit.

Yield: 30 servings

Per serving: 10 g water; 391 calories (49% from fat, 8% from protein, 43% from carb); 8 g protein; 22 g total fat; 4 g saturated fat; 9 g monounsaturated fat; 8 g

polyunsaturated fat; 44 g carbohydrate; 5 g fiber; 18 g sugar; 290 mg phosphorus; 75 mg calcium; 5 mg iron; 75 mg sodium; 372 mg potassium; 205 IU vitamin A; 60 mg vitamin E; 1 mg vitamin C; 0 mg cholesterol

Tip: Experiment with walnuts, cashews, dried fruits, crushed rye, barley, cornmeal, wheat bran, flax seed, soy grits, cinnamon, ginger, etc. Also you might try adding 1 cup peanut butter or corn syrup to moist ingredients. In general keep the ratio of dry ingredients to wet ingredients 21 to 3.

Cashew Granola

Cashews are my favorite nuts, and this granola is a real treat, just full of good things.

8 cups (640 g) rolled oats

1 cup (80 g) shredded coconut

1$^1/_2$ cups (168 g) wheat germ

$^2/_3$ cup (93 g) chopped cashews

1 cup (144 g) sesame seeds

1 cup (145 g) sunflower seeds

$^1/_2$ teaspoon vanilla extract

1$^1/_4$ cups (295 ml) canola oil

1 cup (340 g) honey

Combine first 6 ingredients in large bowl; mix well. Blend vanilla, oil, and honey in small bowl. Add to oats mixture; mix quickly until evenly coated. Spread on 3 ungreased baking sheets. Bake at 350°F (180°C, gas mark 4) for 10 minutes. Turn mixture over with spatula. Bake for 10 minutes longer. Reduce heat to 250°F (120°C, gas mark $^1/_2$). Bake until brown. Cool. Store in airtight container.

Yield: 32 servings

Per serving: 6 g water; 358 calories (45% from fat, 11% from protein, 44% from carb); 10 g protein; 18 g total fat; 3 g saturated fat; 8 g monounsaturated fat; 6 g polyunsaturated fat; 41 g carbohydrate; 6 g fiber; 9 g sugar; 356 mg phosphorus; 72 mg calcium; 3 mg iron; 3 mg sodium; 302 mg potassium; 6 IU vitamin A; 0 mg vitamin E; 0 mg vitamin C; 0 mg cholesterol

Date Granola

Great as a cereal, a snack, or a topping for oatmeal, ice cream, or whatever pleases you.

6 cups (480 g) rolled oats

1 cup (80 g) shredded coconut, unsweetened

1 cup (112 g) wheat germ

1 cup (145 g) sunflower seeds

$^1/_2$ cup (72 g) sesame seeds

$^2/_3$ cup (45 g) powdered milk

1 cup (340 g) honey

1 cup (110 g) slivered almonds

1 cup (145 g) chopped dates, lightly floured

In a large bowl, combine oats, coconut, wheat germ, sunflower seeds, sesame seeds, and powdered milk. Warm the honey until it pours easily. Add honey to dry ingredients, stirring until well mixed. Pour mixture into a large shallow baking pan that has been generously brushed with oil. Spread mixture evenly in the pan. Bake at 325°F (170°C, gas mark 3)for 1 hour, stirring every 15 minutes. When lightly browned, remove from oven and add almonds and dates. Allow to cool completely before storing in airtight container.

Yield: 24 servings

Per serving: 7 g water; 265 calories (32% from fat, 12% from protein, 56% from carb); 8 g protein; 10 g total

fat; 2 g saturated fat; 4 g monounsaturated fat; 4 g polyunsaturated fat; 39 g carbohydrate; 5 g fiber; 20 g sugar; 286 mg phosphorus; 88 mg calcium; 2 mg iron; 23 mg sodium; 319 mg potassium; 51 IU vitamin A; 13 mg vitamin E; 1 mg vitamin C; 0 mg cholesterol

Apple-Coconut Granola

Apple juice adds a whole different flavor to this granola mix.

8 cups (640 g) rolled oats

1 pound (455 g) coconut

1$^1/_2$ cups (150 g) wheat bran

1 tablespoon cinnamon

$^2/_3$ cup (230 g) honey

$^2/_3$ cup (160 ml) canola oil

6 ounces (170 g) apple juice concentrate

Mix all the ingredients together well. Place in shallow pan. Bake at 225°F for 2$^1/_2$ hours; stir every 30 minutes.

Yield: 24 servings

Per serving: 13 g water; 291 calories (42% from fat, 7% from protein, 51% from carb); 6 g protein; 14 g total fat; 6 g saturated fat; 4 g monounsaturated fat; 3 g polyunsaturated fat; 39 g carbohydrate; 5 g fiber; 11 g sugar; 186 mg phosphorus; 25 mg calcium; 2 mg iron; 7 mg sodium; 237 mg potassium; 1 IU vitamin A; 0 mg vitamin E; 6 mg vitamin C; 0 mg cholesterol

Baked Breakfast Cereal

Baking softens the apple and raisins and allows the flavors to blend more with the oatmeal.

2 cups (467 g) cooked rolled oats

1$^1/_2$ cups (225 g) diced apple

1 cup (110 g) chopped pecans

$^1/_2$ cup (75 g) raisins

$^1/_4$ cup (85 g) molasses

2 tablespoons (40 g) honey

1 teaspoon cinnamon

Combine all ingredients in a vegetable casserole dish coated with nonstick vegetable oil spray and bake in a 400°F (200°C, gas mark 6) oven for 20 minutes.

Yield: 6 servings

Per serving: 31 g water; 244 calories (45% from fat, 3% from protein, 51% from carb); 2 g protein; 13 g total fat; 1 g saturated fat; 7 g monounsaturated fat; 4 g polyunsaturated fat; 34 g carbohydrate; 3 g fiber; 25 g sugar; 72 mg phosphorus; 55 mg calcium; 2 mg iron; 7 mg sodium; 414 mg potassium; 22 IU vitamin A; 0 mg vitamin E; 2 mg vitamin C; 0 mg cholesterol

Tip: Serve warm with milk.

Baked Oatmeal

Okay, it seems like a strange idea, but this really works. What you end up with is not at all the same as just microwaving your oatmeal. Try it and see if it's not worth the effort.

$^1/_2$ cup (125 g) applesauce

$^3/_4$ cup (170 g) brown sugar

2 eggs

1 cup (235 ml) skim milk

3 cups (240 g) quick-cooking oats

2 teaspoons baking powder

$^1/_2$ teaspoon cinnamon

$^2/_3$ cup (80 g) chopped walnuts

Combine applesauce, sugar, eggs, and milk; mix well. Mix remaining ingredients together and then combine with first mixture. Bake in a 9 × 13-inch (23 × 33-cm) pan coated with nonstick vegetable oil spray for 30 minutes at 350°F (180°C, gas mark 4). Serve with hot milk.

Yield: 6 servings

Per serving: 72 g water; 406 calories (27% from fat, 13% from protein, 60% from carb); 14 g protein; 13 g total fat; 2 g saturated fat; 4 g monounsaturated fat; 6 g polyunsaturated fat; 63 g carbohydrate; 5 g fiber; 31 g sugar; 386 mg phosphorus; 215 mg calcium; 3 mg iron; 226 mg sodium; 423 mg potassium; 183 IU vitamin A; 51 mg vitamin E; 1 mg vitamin C; 80 mg cholesterol

Pumpkin Oatmeal

Oatmeal is one of the few foods that has been approved to claim it reduces cholesterol, so that makes it our friend. But it can get boring after a while. Adding pumpkin spices it up with a little fall flavor.

2 cups (160 g) quick-cooking oats

3 cups (710 ml) skim milk

$^1/_2$ cup (160 g) canned pumpkin

$^1/_4$ teaspoon (0.5 g) pumpkin pie spice

$^1/_8$ teaspoon (0.3 g) cinnamon

$^1/_4$ cup (40 g) raisins

Place oats in a microwave-safe bowl and stir in milk. Microwave on high for 2 to 3 minutes. Remove from microwave and stir in pumpkin, pumpkin pie spice, and cinnamon. Heat for 40 to 60 seconds, or until heated through. Stir in raisins.

Yield: 4 servings

Per serving: 273 calories (10% from fat, 21% from protein, 69% from carbohydrate); 14 g protein; 3 g total fat; 1 g saturated fat; 1 g monounsaturated fat; 1 g polyunsaturated fat; 48 g carbohydrate; 5 g fiber; 8 g sugar; 420 mg phosphorus; 300 mg calcium; 2 mg iron; 113 mg sodium; 619 mg potassium; 5141 IU vitamin A; 113 mg ATE vitamin E; 4 mg vitamin C; 4 mg cholesterol; 198 g water

Cranberry Orange Oat Bran Cereal

If you are looking for a little different taste for breakfast, this could be it. This works with regular oatmeal just as well too. Dried fruits are a favorite of mine. They make great snacks when you want something sweet.

$^1/_2$ cup (120 ml) water

$^1/_2$ cup (120 ml) orange juice

$^1/_3$ cup (33 g) oat bran

$^1/_4$ cup (38 g) dried cranberries

Combine ingredients in a microwave-safe bowl and cook according to oat bran package microwave directions.

Yield: 1 serving

Per serving: 205 calories (6% from fat, 5% from protein, 89% from carbohydrate); 3 g protein; 2 g total fat; 0 g saturated fat; 0 g monounsaturated fat; 1 g polyunsaturated fat; 49 g carbohydrate; 3 g fiber; 22 g sugar; 95 mg phosphorus; 48 mg calcium; 5 mg iron; 61 mg sodium; 316 mg potassium; 244 IU vitamin A; 44 mg ATE vitamin E; 43 mg vitamin C; 0 mg cholesterol; 234 g water

Apple Oat Bran Cereal

How about a nice easy-to-fix hot breakfast? An added benefit is that oat bran has been shown to reduce cholesterol.

$^1/_2$ cup (50 g) oat bran

$^1/_2$ cup (120 ml) apple juice

$^3/_4$ cup (180 ml) water

$^1/_4$ cup (35 g) raisins

$^1/_2$ teaspoon (1.2 g) cinnamon

Combine ingredients in a microwave-safe bowl. Microwave on high power for $2^1/_2$ to 3 minutes. Serve with skim milk and honey.

Yield: 1 serving

Per serving: 182 calories (2% from fat, 3% from protein, 95% from carbohydrate); 1 g protein; 0 g total fat; 0 g saturated fat; 0 g monounsaturated fat; 0 g

polyunsaturated fat; 47 g carbohydrate; 2 g fiber; 38 g sugar; 51 mg phosphorus; 47 mg calcium; 2 mg iron; 19 mg sodium; 467 mg potassium; 3 IU vitamin A; 0 mg ATE vitamin E; 2 mg vitamin C; 0 mg cholesterol; 289 g water

Couscous Cereal with Fruit

I get bored sometimes. This is a somewhat different take on hot breakfast cereal.

$^3/_4$ cup (180 ml) water

$^1/_2$ cup (88 g) couscous

2 tablespoons (20 g) raisins

2 tablespoons (19 g) dried cranberries

1 tablespoon (15 ml) honey

$^1/_2$ teaspoon (1.2 g) cinnamon

Bring water to a boil. Add the couscous and stir, then cover and remove from heat. Let stand for 5 minutes. Stir in the remaining ingredients.

Yield: 2 servings

Per serving: 250 calories (2% from fat, 9% from protein, 89% from carbohydrate); 6 g protein; 0 g total fat; 0 g saturated fat; 0 g monounsaturated fat; 0 g polyunsaturated fat; 57 g carbohydrate; 3 g fiber; 20 g sugar; 85 mg phosphorus; 27 mg calcium; 1 mg iron; 9 mg sodium; 161 mg potassium; 2 IU vitamin A; 0 mg ATE vitamin E; 0 mg vitamin C; 0 mg cholesterol; 97 g water

Breakfast Couscous

We usually think of couscous as a dinner item, perhaps with curry or some other savory topping. But this sweeter version makes a great breakfast.

$^1/_4$ cup (55 g) unsalted butter, divided

$^1/_4$ teaspoon cinnamon

$^1/_4$ teaspoon cardamom

$2^1/_4$ cups (535 ml) orange juice

$^1/_2$ cup (75 g) currants

$1^1/_2$ cups (263 g) whole wheat couscous

$^1/_4$ cup (35 g) chopped cashews

Melt 2 tablespoons butter, add spices, and cook 2 minutes. Add juice and currants. Bring to a boil. Mix in couscous and add remaining butter. Cover. Remove from heat and let stand 5 minutes. Fluff with fork and put in bowl. Add cashews. Serve.

Yield: 4 servings

Per serving: 144 g water; 466 calories (31% from fat, 9% from protein, 59% from carb); 11 g protein; 16 g total fat; 8 g saturated fat; 5 g monounsaturated fat; 1 g polyunsaturated fat; 69 g carbohydrate; 4 g fiber; 0 g sugar; 180 mg phosphorus; 47 mg calcium; 2 mg iron; 11 mg sodium; 473 mg potassium; 496 IU vitamin A; 95 mg vitamin E; 71 mg vitamin C; 31 mg cholesterol

Banana-Peach-Blueberry Smoothie

Smoothies make a quick and easy breakfast, and they are packed with nutrition. The fiber and protein will help to keep you from being hungry as the morning goes on.

2 cups (490 g) peach low-fat yogurt

1 cup (145 g) blueberries

2 cups (300 g) sliced banana

Mix all ingredients in a blender and serve.

Yield: 2 servings

Per serving: 415 g water; 485 calories (7% from fat, 10% from protein, 83% from carb); 13 g protein; 4 g total fat; 2 g saturated fat; 1 g monounsaturated fat; 0 g polyunsaturated fat; 108 g carbohydrate; 8 g fiber; 81 g sugar; 325 mg phosphorus; 354 mg calcium; 1 mg iron; 133 mg sodium; 1296 mg potassium; 282 IU vitamin A; 27 mg vitamin E; 28 mg vitamin C; 12 mg cholesterol

Chocolate-Raspberry Smoothie

How could anyone not like the taste of chocolate and raspberries for breakfast?

1 cup (235 ml) skim milk

$^1/_2$ cup (141 g) chocolate syrup

3 cups (750 g) frozen raspberries

Pour the milk and chocolate syrup into a blender. Slowly add the raspberries, 1 cup at a time, and blend for 15 to 30 seconds after adding each cup. Do not overmix, as this will thin the drink down. Serve immediately.

Yield: 2 servings

Per serving: 268 g water; 146 calories (9% from fat, 18% from protein, 73% from carb); 7 g protein; 2 g total fat;

0 g saturated fat; 0 g monounsaturated fat; 1 g polyunsaturated fat; 29 g carbohydrate; 12 g fiber; 8 g sugar; 191 mg phosphorus; 222 mg calcium; 1 mg iron; 74 mg sodium; 502 mg potassium; 311 IU vitamin A; 75 mg vitamin E; 50 mg vitamin C; 2 mg cholesterol

Tip: Substitute other frozen fruit for the raspberries (strawberry, banana, etc.).

Raspberry-Banana Smoothie

Another great-tasting smoothie. The raspberries give this one a special boost in fiber.

2 cups (250 g) fresh raspberries

2 cups (300 g) sliced banana

2 cups (475 ml) skim milk

$1/4$ cup (60 g) low-fat vanilla yogurt

1 tablespoon (20 g) honey

Combine all ingredients in a blender or food processor and process until smooth.

Yield: 2 servings

Per serving: 496 g water; 397 calories (5% from fat, 13% from protein, 83% from carb); 14 g protein; 2 g total fat; 1 g saturated fat; 0 g monounsaturated fat; 1 g polyunsaturated fat; 88 g carbohydrate; 14 g fiber; 42 g sugar; 361 mg phosphorus; 394 mg calcium; 2 mg iron; 149 mg sodium; 1444 mg potassium; 684 IU vitamin A; 150 mg vitamin E; 55 mg vitamin C; 5 mg cholesterol

Bananaberry Breakfast Shake

So why not a shake for breakfast? Besides, it's really just a smoothie.

1 cup (145 g) strawberries

1 cup (150 g) sliced banana

$1^1/_2$ cups (355 ml) skim milk

1 cup (230 g) vanilla yogurt

1 tablespoon (20 g) honey

Place all ingredients in a blender. Process until well blended.

Yield: 2 servings

Per serving: 417 g water; 336 calories (7% from fat, 17% from protein, 76% from carb); 15 g protein; 3 g total fat; 1 g saturated fat; 1 g monounsaturated fat; 0 g polyunsaturated fat; 67 g carbohydrate; 4 g fiber; 43 g sugar; 415 mg phosphorus; 492 mg calcium; 1 mg iron; 192 mg sodium; 1129 mg potassium; 508 IU vitamin A; 127 mg vitamin E; 58 mg vitamin C; 10 mg cholesterol

Tip: Great with toast or muffins.

Oat Bran–Berry Smoothie

Adding oat bran to a smoothie is probably not something you'd thought about doing. But it really works, adding flavor, texture, and lots of good nutrition.

1 cup (235 ml) cranberry juice

1 cup (255 g) strawberries, frozen

8 ounces (225 g) vanilla yogurt

²/₃ cup (66 g) oat bran

1 cup ice cubes

Place all ingredients except ice in blender. Cover. Blend on high about 2 minutes or until smooth. Gradually add ice, blending on high until smooth. Serve immediately.

Yield: 2 servings

Per serving: 267 g water; 246 calories (9% from fat, 13% from protein, 79% from carb); 8 g protein; 2 g total fat; 1 g saturated fat; 1 g monounsaturated fat; 0 g polyunsaturated fat; 50 g carbohydrate; 3 g fiber; 22 g sugar; 251 mg phosphorus; 241 mg calcium; 5 mg iron; 135 mg sodium; 449 mg potassium; 217 IU vitamin A; 58 mg vitamin E; 60 mg vitamin C; 6 mg cholesterol

Cranberry Orange Smoothie

If you have a little cranberry sauce left (as I always seem to after the holidays), this is a tasty way to use it.

¹/₂ cup (135 g) cranberry sauce

¹/₂ cup (120 ml) orange juice

1 cup (230 g) plain nonfat yogurt

1 cup (225 g) banana, sliced

¹/₂ cup (120 ml) skim milk

Combine all ingredients in a blender and process until smooth.

Yield: 2 servings

Per serving: 326 calories (3% from fat, 13% from protein, 84% from carbohydrate); 11 g protein; 1 g total fat; 0 g saturated fat; 0 g monounsaturated fat; 0 g polyunsaturated fat; 72 g carbohydrate; 4 g fiber; 49 g sugar; 297 mg phosphorus; 346 mg calcium; 1 mg iron; 152 mg sodium; 963 mg potassium; 283 IU vitamin A; 40 mg ATE vitamin E; 33 mg vitamin C; 4 mg cholesterol; 341 g water

Banana Melon Smoothies

I like smoothies for a quick breakfast, but I find that I'm often hungry before noon. Adding some extra protein with the tofu seems to help fill me up longer.

6 ounces (170 g) soft tofu

1 banana

1 cup (155 g) cantaloupe

¹/₂ cup (120 ml) skim milk

¹/₂ cup (120 ml) apple juice

Place all ingredients in a blender and process until smooth.

Yield: 2 servings

Per serving: 230 calories (11% from fat, 14% from protein, 75% from carbohydrate); 9 g protein; 3 g total fat; 1 g saturated fat; 1 g monounsaturated fat; 1 g polyunsaturated fat; 46 g carbohydrate; 4 g fiber; 28 g sugar; 164 mg phosphorus; 131 mg calcium; 1 mg iron; 60 mg sodium; 979 mg potassium; 3190 IU vitamin A; 38 mg ATE vitamin E; 43 mg vitamin C; 1 mg cholesterol; 347 g water

Bananaberry Smoothies

I developed this as a way to store and use later those last couple of bananas that always seem to be near the end of their useful life just when you don't have a use for them. Peel bananas, cut in halves or thirds, and freeze in a resealable plastic bag to use them in smoothies later. Using frozen bananas also gives you a nice, thick smoothie that isn't diluted by ice.

$^1/_2$ cup (120 ml) orange juice

$1^1/_2$ cups (340 g) frozen bananas

$^1/_2$ cup (55 g) frozen strawberries

Pour juice into blender. Add frozen bananas and berries and blend until smooth.

Yield: 2 servings

Per serving: 190 calories (4% from fat, 5% from protein, 91% from carbohydrate); 3 g protein; 1 g total fat; 0 g saturated fat; 0 g monounsaturated fat; 0 g polyunsaturated fat; 48 g carbohydrate; 5 g fiber; 22 g sugar; 53 mg phosphorus; 21 mg calcium; 1 mg iron; 3 mg sodium; 781 mg potassium; 161 IU vitamin A; 0 mg ATE vitamin E; 58 mg vitamin C; 0 mg cholesterol; 216 g water

Tip: Vary the flavor by using different ingredients. For the liquid, you can use apple juice or other fruit juice. For the fruit, you can use any kind of fresh or frozen berries, peaches, nectarines, grapes, or cherries. Just be sure to remove any pits before blending.

Peach Smoothies

The yogurt in this smoothie adds calcium, protein, and other nutrients, making it even more healthful than some of the fruit-only ones.

1 cup (235 ml) orange juice

1 cup (225 g) banana

1 cup (230 g) low fat vanilla yogurt

$^3/_4$ cup (150 g) peaches, sliced and frozen

Place all ingredients in a blender and process until thick and smooth.

Yield: 1 serving

Per serving: 563 calories (7% from fat, 12% from protein, 81% from carbohydrate); 18 g protein; 5 g total fat; 2 g saturated fat; 1 g monounsaturated fat; 1 g polyunsaturated fat; 121 g carbohydrate; 8 g fiber; 71 g sugar; 431 mg phosphorus; 462 mg calcium; 1 mg iron; 166 mg sodium; 2034 mg potassium; 820 IU vitamin A; 29 mg ATE vitamin E; 111 mg vitamin C; 12 mg cholesterol; 685 g water

Strawberry Smoothie

Another breakfast treat. Feel free to add a banana, if you like.

$1^1/_4$ cups (140 g) strawberries

$1^1/_2$ cups (355 ml) skim milk

1 tablespoon (13 g) sugar

1 teaspoon (5 ml) lemon juice

Put all ingredients in a blender and process until smooth.

Yield: 2 servings

Per serving: 131 calories (5% from fat, 24% from protein, 71% from carbohydrate); 8 g protein; 1 g total fat; 0 g saturated fat; 0 g monounsaturated fat; 0 g polyunsaturated fat; 24 g carbohydrate; 2 g fiber; 11 g sugar; 230 mg phosphorus; 279 mg calcium; 1 mg iron; 110 mg sodium; 484 mg potassium; 386 IU vitamin A; 113 mg ATE vitamin E; 59 mg vitamin C; 4 mg cholesterol; 254 g water

Yogurt Parfait

This makes a nice change of pace for breakfast. Even though the total fat may seem high, it's almost all from the walnuts, which provide healthy fat.

1 cup (110 g) strawberries

2 tablespoons (26 g) sugar

8 ounces (225 g) plain fat-free yogurt

$^1/_2$ cup (50 g) granola

$^1/_4$ cup (31 g) chopped walnuts

Chop the strawberries and toss with the sugar. Layer in parfait glasses in this order: fruit, yogurt, granola, and nuts. Repeat layers.

Yield: 2 servings

Per serving: 313 calories (29% from fat, 15% from protein, 55% from carbohydrate); 12 g protein; 11 g total fat; 1 g saturated fat; 3 g monounsaturated fat; 6 g polyunsaturated fat; 45 g carbohydrate; 4 g fiber; 32 g sugar; 333 mg phosphorus; 255 mg calcium; 1 mg iron; 166 mg sodium; 545 mg potassium; 23 IU vitamin A; 2 mg ATE vitamin E; 46 mg vitamin C; 2 mg cholesterol; 168 g water

6

Main Dishes:
Poultry

Poultry is a great healthy meat choice. It tends to be significantly lower in saturated fat then red meats. There are poultry dishes here that range from down home Sunday dinner comfort food like roast or fried chicken to a variety of dishes with flavors from around the world. A number of them use boneless skinless chicken breasts to lower the fat content even more. But you won't miss the fat with the great taste.

Grilled Roaster

If you cook a large chicken on the weekend, you can have a great meal and lots of leftovers to use during the week. This one has a smoky flavor, but not so much as to overpower other ingredients.

1 large roasting chicken, 5 to 6 pounds (2.3 to 2.7 kg)

2 tablespoons (30 ml) olive oil

1 teaspoon (2.5 g) paprika

1 teaspoon (3 g) onion powder

$^1/_2$ teaspoon (1 g) black pepper

$^1/_2$ teaspoon (0.5 g) dried thyme

$^1/_4$ teaspoon (0.8 g) garlic powder

1 teaspoon (5 ml) liquid smoke

Split chicken in half along the backbone and breastbone. Mix together remaining ingredients and rub into both sides of chicken halves. Grill over indirect heat, turning occasionally, for $1^1/_2$ to 2 hours, or until done. Place over low heat the last 15 minutes to brown skin.

Yield: 12 servings

Per serving: 289 calories (69% from fat, 30% from protein, 1% from carbohydrate); 22 g protein; 22 g total fat; 6 g saturated fat; 9 g monounsaturated fat; 4 g polyunsaturated fat; 1 g carbohydrate; 0 g fiber; 0 g sugar; 2 mg phosphorus; 15 mg calcium; 2 mg iron; 0 mg sodium; 255 mg potassium; 209 IU vitamin A; 0 mg ATE vitamin E; 3 mg vitamin C; 113 mg cholesterol; 0 g water

Rotisserie-Flavored Chicken Breasts

This recipe gives you a flavor reminiscent of carryout rotisserie chicken, but with lower-fat chicken breasts as the basis.

$^1/_4$ cup (60 ml) honey

1 teaspoon (2.5 g) paprika

1 teaspoon (3 g) onion powder

$^1/_2$ teaspoon (1 g) black pepper

$^1/_2$ teaspoon (0.5 g) dried thyme

$^1/_4$ teaspoon (0.8 g) garlic powder

4 boneless chicken breasts

Preheat oven to 325°F (170°C, or gas mark 3). Mix honey, paprika, onion powder, black pepper, thyme, and garlic powder. Rub onto chicken. Roast for 45 minutes, or until done, basting occasionally with pan juices.

Yield: 4 servings

Per serving: 148 calories (6% from fat, 44% from protein, 50% from carbohydrate); 17 g protein; 1 g total fat; 0 g saturated fat; 0 g monounsaturated fat; 0 g polyunsaturated fat; 19 g carbohydrate; 0 g fiber; 18 g sugar; 145 mg phosphorus; 16 mg calcium; 1 mg iron; 48 mg sodium; 217 mg potassium; 324 IU vitamin A; 4 mg ATE vitamin E; 2 mg vitamin C; 41 mg cholesterol; 57 g water

Grilled Marinated Chicken Breasts

These thin grilled chicken breasts make great sandwiches. They are also good sliced on top of a salad or stirred into a pasta salad.

$^1/_4$ cup (60 ml) olive oil

$^1/_4$ cup (60 ml) red wine vinegar

$^1/_4$ teaspoon (0.8 g) minced garlic

1 teaspoon (3 g) onion powder

$1^1/_2$ teaspoons (1 g) Italian seasoning

$^1/_2$ teaspoon (0.5 g) dried thyme

2 boneless chicken breasts

Combine all ingredients except chicken in a resealable plastic bag and mix well. Slice breasts in half crosswise, making two thin fillets from each. Add the chicken to the bag, seal, and marinate for at least 2 hours, turning occasionally. Remove chicken from marinade and grill over medium heat until done, turning once.

Yield: 4 servings

Per serving: 165 calories (77% from fat, 20% from protein, 2% from carbohydrate); 8 g protein; 14 g total fat; 2 g saturated fat; 10 g monounsaturated fat; 2 g polyunsaturated fat; 1 g carbohydrate; 0 g fiber; 0 g sugar; 74 mg phosphorus; 16 mg calcium; 1 mg iron; 25 mg sodium; 110 mg potassium; 38 IU vitamin A; 2 mg ATE vitamin E; 1 mg vitamin C; 21 mg cholesterol; 41 g water

Grilled Chicken and Vegetables

Chicken and vegetables grilled with a lemon and herb marinade.

$1^1/_2$ teaspoons basil

$1^1/_2$ teaspoon garlic powder

$^1/_4$ teaspoon black pepper

1 teaspoon lemon peel, gated

1 tablespoon lemon juice

1 tablespoon olive oil

4 boneless skinless chicken breasts

1 small eggplant, sliced

1 zucchini, sliced lengthwise

1 red bell peppers, sliced crosswise

Combine first six ingredients. Heat grill to medium heat. Brush chicken and vegetables with herb mixture. Grill chicken until no longer pink in the center, about 5–10 minutes per side. Grill vegetables until crisp tender, about 5 minutes per side.

Yield: 4 servings

Total Recipe: 543 calories (30% from fat, 52% from protein, 19% from carb); 71 g protein; 18 g total fat; 3 g saturated fat; 11 g monounsaturated fat; 3 g polyunsaturated fat; 26 g carb; 9 g fiber; 13 g sugar; 711 mg phosphorus; 109 mg calcium; 210 mg sodium; 1826 mg potassium; 5220 IU vitamin A; 17 mg ATE vitamin E; 331 mg vitamin C; 165 mg cholesterol

Italian Chicken Kabobs

Sort of like pizza on a stick, these tasty kabobs are sure to please young and old alike.

1 pound boneless skinless chicken breast, cut in 1″ cubes

1 cup green bell peppers, cut in 1″ pieces

1 cup red bell peppers, cut in 1″ pieces

8 ounces mushrooms

$^1/_4$ cup reduced fat Italian dressing (recipe in Chapter 2)

1 teaspoon Italian seasoning

$^1/_4$ cup parmesan cheese, grated

Heat grill to medium. Thread chicken and vegetables on skewers. Brush with dressing and sprinkle with Italian seasoning. Grill until chicken is no longer pink in center, about 10 minutes. Remove from skewers and sprinkle with cheese.

Yield: 4 servings

Per serving: 193 calories (21% from fat, 65% from protein , 14% from carb); 31 g protein ; 5 g total fat; 2 g saturated fat; 1 g monounsaturated fat; 1 g polyunsaturated fat; 7 g carb; 2 g fiber; 4 g sugar; 335 mg phosphorus; 95 mg calcium; 178 mg sodium; 636 mg potassium; 1373 IU vitamin A; 14 mg ATE vitamin E; 104 mg vitamin C; 72 mg cholesterol

Tip: Serve with spaghetti sauce for dipping.

Lemon Thyme Chicken

Lemon and honey add a sort of sweet and sour flavor to these grilled chicken breasts.

$^1/_4$ cup honey

1 tablespoon lemon peel, grated

1 tablespoon lemon juice

$^1/_2$ teaspoon thyme

$^1/_4$ teaspoon black pepper

4 boneless skinless chicken breasts

Heat grill to medium heat. Combine honey, lemon peel, lemon juice, thyme, and pepper. Grill chicken until no longer pink in the center, about 15–20 minutes. Brush with sauce during the last 10 minutes.

Yield: 4 servings

Per serving: 145 calories (6% from fat, 45% from protein , 50% from carb); 17 g protein ; 1 g total fat; 0 g saturated fat; 0 g monounsaturated fat; 0 g polyunsaturated fat; 18 g carb; 0 g fiber; 18 g sugar; 141 mg phosphorus; 14 mg calcium; 47 mg sodium; 202 mg potassium; 21 IU vitamin A; 4 mg ATE vitamin E; 5 mg vitamin C; 41 mg cholesterol

Oven-Fried Chicken

Fried chicken doesn't have to be as unhealthy as it usually is. Get rid of the skin and "fry" the chicken in the oven, and it's a perfectly acceptable food. Not to mention that it tastes good.

¹/₄ cup (55 g) unsalted butter, melted

¹/₄ teaspoon (0.5 g) black pepper

3 pounds (1.4 kg) chicken, cut into pieces, skin removed

1 cup (56 g) corn flake crumbs

Preheat oven to 350°F (180°C, or gas mark 4). Combine butter and pepper. Roll chicken in butter mixture , then corn flake crumbs. Place in an ungreased baking pan and bake about 1 hour, or until done.

Yield: 8 servings

Per serving: 267 calories (38% from fat, 57% from protein, 5% from carbohydrate); 37 g protein; 12 g total fat; 7 g saturated fat; 3 g monounsaturated fat; 1 g polyunsaturated fat; 3 g carbohydrate; 0 g fiber; 0 g sugar; 297 mg phosphorus; 22 mg calcium; 3 mg iron; 159 mg sodium; 395 mg potassium; 423 IU vitamin A; 104 mg ATE vitamin E; 6 mg vitamin C; 129 mg cholesterol; 130 g water

Potato-Coated Oven-Fried Chicken

This is my favorite recipe for oven-fried chicken.

1 egg

2 tablespoons (30 ml) water

¹/₄ cup (25 g) Parmesan cheese, grated

3 pounds (1.4 kg) chicken, cut into pieces, skin removed

1 cup (60 g) instant mashed potato flakes

Preheat oven to 375°F (190°C, or gas mark 5). Combine egg, water, and cheese. Dip chicken in egg mixture, then roll in potato flakes. Place in ungreased baking pan. Bake for 1 hour, or until done.

Yield: 8 servings

Per serving: 249 calories (24% from fat, 65% from protein, 10% from carbohydrate); 39 g protein; 6 g total fat; 2 g saturated fat; 2 g monounsaturated fat; 1 g polyunsaturated fat; 6 g carbohydrate; 0 g fiber; 0 g sugar; 338 mg phosphorus; 61 mg calcium; 2 mg iron; 201 mg sodium; 402 mg potassium; 131 IU vitamin A; 31 mg ATE vitamin E; 10 mg vitamin C; 152 mg cholesterol; 140 g water

Baked Chicken Nuggets

You can greatly reduce the amount of fat in chicken nuggets by baking them instead of frying them. The flavor is just as good, and they are a lot better for you.

¹/₂ cup (14 g) crushed corn flakes

2 tablespoons (15 g) nonfat dry milk

1 tablespoon (0.4 g) dried parsley

1 tablespoon (7 g) paprika

1 teaspoon (3 g) onion powder

¹/₄ teaspoon (0.8 g) garlic powder

¹/₂ teaspoon (0.4 g) poultry seasoning

1 pound (455 g) boneless chicken breasts, cut in strips

1 egg, beaten

Preheat oven to 350°F (180°C, or gas mark 4). Mix together crushed corn flakes and next 6 ingredients (through poultry seasoning) in a resealable plastic bag. Dip chicken pieces in egg, then place in bag. Shake to coat evenly. Place on baking sheet coated with nonstick vegetable oil spray. Bake for 20 minutes, or until chicken is done and coating is crispy.

Yield: 4 servings

Per serving: 167 calories (12% from fat, 73% from protein, 14% from carbohydrate); 29 g protein; 2 g total fat; 1 g saturated fat; 1 g monounsaturated fat; 1 g polyunsaturated fat; 6 g carbohydrate; 1 g fiber; 2 g sugar; 274 mg phosphorus; 61 mg calcium; 2 mg iron; 116 mg sodium; 342 mg potassium; 1088 IU vitamin A; 22 mg ATE vitamin E; 3 mg vitamin C; 136 mg cholesterol; 98 g water

Honey Mustard Fruit Sauced Chicken

What can I say? I was looking for something a little different, and this just came to me. It is a true original. I actually used tropical fruit cocktail, but the regular kind should work just as well.

6 boneless chicken breasts

1 cup (240 g) fruit cocktail, in juice

2 tablespoons (30 ml) red wine vinegar

2 tablespoons (30 ml) honey

2 tablespoons (30 ml) honey mustard

Preheat oven to 350°F (180°C, or gas mark 4). Place chicken breasts in a roasting pan. Purée fruit cocktail, vinegar, honey, and mustard in a blender. Pour over chicken. Bake for 50 to 60 minutes, or until done.

Yield: 6 servings

Per serving: 122 calories (8% from fat, 56% from protein, 36% from carbohydrate); 17 g protein; 1 g total fat; 0 g saturated fat; 0 g monounsaturated fat; 0 g polyunsaturated fat; 11 g carbohydrate; 1 g fiber; 10 g sugar; 151 mg phosphorus; 15 mg calcium; 1 mg iron; 105 mg sodium; 231 mg potassium; 139 IU vitamin A; 4 mg ATE vitamin E; 2 mg vitamin C; 41 mg cholesterol; 98 g water

Maple Glazed Chicken

Maple sweetness and mustard tanginess is a winning combination for these grilled chicken breasts.

$^3/_4$ cup maple syrup

$^1/_4$ cup Dijon mustard

2 tablespoons chives

4 boneless skinless chicken breasts

$^1/_4$ teaspoon salt free seasoning blend such as Mrs. Dash

$^1/_4$ teaspoon black pepper

Heat grill to medium. Combine syrup, mustard, and chives. Sprinkle chicken with seasoning blend and pepper. Grill until no longer pink in center, about 15–20 minutes, brushing with sauce occasionally. Heat remaining sauce to boiling and boil for one minute. Serve with chicken.

Yield: 4 servings

Per serving: 247 calories (5% from fat, 27% from protein, 67% from carb); 17 g protein ; 1 g total fat; 0 g saturated fat; 1 g monounsaturated fat; 0 g polyunsaturated fat; 42 g carb; 1 g fiber; 36 g sugar; 155 mg phosphorus; 62 mg calcium; 227 mg sodium; 333 mg potassium; 104 IU vitamin A; 4 mg ATE vitamin E; 2 mg vitamin C; 41 mg cholesterol

Chicken and Snow Peas

The stir-frying and ingredients give this an Asian feel, although it doesn't use the typical seasonings. It's good over rice, and I would think it would go well with pasta too.

2 tablespoons (30 ml) olive oil, divided

1 pound (455 g) boneless chicken breasts, sliced

1 egg, beaten

$^{1}/_{3}$ cup (43 g) cornstarch

$1^{1}/_{2}$ cups (240 g) onions, sliced

$^{1}/_{2}$ cup (75 g) green bell pepper, sliced

6 ounces (170 g) snow peas

$^{1}/_{4}$ cup (60 ml) honey

2 tablespoons (16 g) almonds, slivered

Heat 1 tablespoon (15 ml) of the oil in a wok. Dip half the chicken in the egg and dust with cornstarch. Stir-fry for 4 to 5 minutes, or until just cooked. Remove cooked chicken from pan and repeat with remaining chicken. Remove chicken from pan; add the rest of the oil to the wok. Stir-fry the onion until it begins to soften. Add the green bell pepper and snow peas and stir-fry for 4 minutes, or until crisp-tender. Add the honey and toss the vegetables in it until well coated. Add the chicken and toss until coated and heated through. Sprinkle the almonds over the top.

Yield: 4 servings

Per serving: 375 calories (27% from fat, 33% from protein, 40% from carbohydrate); 31 g protein; 11 g total fat; 2 g saturated fat; 7 g monounsaturated fat; 2 g polyunsaturated fat; 38 g carbohydrate; 3 g fiber; 22 g sugar; 309 mg phosphorus; 66 mg calcium; 3 mg iron; 109 mg sodium; 489 mg potassium; 613 IU vitamin A; 7 mg ATE vitamin E; 46 mg vitamin C; 136 mg cholesterol; 211 g water

Chicken Polynesian

A kind of variation on sweet-and-sour chicken, made different by the citrus fruit sections in the sauce.

2 chicken breasts, halved

4 chicken thighs

1 grapefruit

3 oranges

$^{1}/_{2}$ cup (120 ml) light corn syrup

$^{1}/_{4}$ cup (60 ml) mustard

$^{1}/_{4}$ cup (60 ml) cider vinegar

$^{1}/_{4}$ teaspoon Tabasco sauce

$^{1}/_{8}$ teaspoon ginger

2 teaspoons cornstarch

1 tablespoon (15 ml) water

9 ounces (255 g) crushed pineapple

$^{1}/_{3}$ cup (36 g) slivered toasted almonds

Place chicken skin side down in shallow baking dish. Section grapefruit, holding over bowl to catch juice. Measure juice. Section oranges, adding enough orange juice to grapefruit juice to make $^{1}/_{2}$ cup (120 ml). In saucepan, blend corn syrup, mustard, vinegar, Tabasco, ginger, and fruit juices. Add cornstarch mixed with water; bring to boil. Boil 5 minutes, stirring constantly. Brush chicken with this mixture. Bake at 350°F (180°C, gas mark 4) for 1 hour, basting with sauce occasionally and turning once. Add crushed pineapple, orange and grapefruit sections, and almonds to remaining sauce. Heat; pour over chicken for last 5 minutes of baking time.

Yield: 8 servings

Per serving: 159 g water; 223 calories (22% from fat, 19% from protein, 59% from carb); 11 g protein; 6 g total fat; 1 g saturated fat; 3 g monounsaturated fat; 1 g polyunsaturated fat; 34 g carbohydrate; 3 g fiber; 19 g sugar; 97 mg phosphorus; 62 mg calcium; 1 mg iron; 39 mg sodium; 341 mg potassium; 573 IU vitamin A; 4 mg vitamin E; 54 mg vitamin C; 26 mg cholesterol

Tip: Serve over brown rice.

Lemon Rosemary Chicken

This technique has become my new favorite way of grilling chicken. It allows it to cook relatively quickly, stay juicy, and not get too blackened. Plus, you usually have some left over for sandwiches or salads the next day. Whole chickens can be very low in saturated fat as long as you don't eat the skin.

1 whole chicken, 3 to 4 pounds (1.4 to 1.8 kg)

$^1/_2$ cup (120 ml) lemon juice

1 teaspoon (1.2 g) dried rosemary

Split chicken in half, cutting along backbone and breast bone. Place in resealable plastic bag with lemon juice and rosemary. Marinate at least two hours, turning frequently. Preheat grill, making one side hot and the other low heat. Cook over the low side, turning several times, for about 1 hour or until done. Discard the skin.

Yield: 8 servings

Per serving: 33 calories (20% from fat, 64% from protein, 16% from carbohydrate); 5 g protein; 1 g total fat; 0 g saturated fat; 0 g monounsaturated fat; 0 g polyunsaturated fat; 1 g carbohydrate; 0 g fiber; 0 g sugar; 44 mg phosphorus; 4 mg calcium; 0 mg iron; 19 mg sodium; 76 mg potassium; 18 IU vitamin A; 4 mg ATE vitamin E; 8 mg vitamin C; 17 mg cholesterol; 32 g water

Pulled Chicken

Here's a good use for leftover smoked or grilled chicken. Try it with Onion Rolls in Chapter 21 and a scoop of coleslaw on it and you won't even miss the expensive sandwiches at your favorite barbecue restaurant.

8 ounces (225 g) no-salt-added tomato sauce

$^1/_4$ cup (60 ml) vinegar

$^1/_4$ cup (60 ml) molasses

$^1/_2$ teaspoon (1.5 g) onion powder

$^1/_2$ teaspoon (1.3 g) chili powder

$^1/_2$ teaspoon (1.5 g) dry mustard

$^1/_4$ teaspoon (0.5 g) cayenne pepper

$^1/_4$ teaspoon (0.8 g) garlic powder

2 cups (220 g) smoked chicken, shredded

Mix the first 8 ingredients (through garlic powder). Add chicken and stir to combine or place chicken on rolls and spoon sauce over chicken.

Yield: 6 servings

Per serving: 146 calories (23% from fat, 39% from protein, 38% from carbohydrate); 14 g protein; 4 g total fat; 1 g saturated fat; 1 g monounsaturated fat; 1 g polyunsaturated fat; 14 g carbohydrate; 1 g fiber; 8 g sugar; 116 mg phosphorus; 45 mg calcium; 3 mg iron; 227 mg sodium; 475 mg potassium; 490 IU vitamin A; 7 mg ATE vitamin E; 3 mg vitamin C; 42 mg cholesterol; 76 g water

Moroccan Chicken

Sweet spices contrast with olives and tomatoes in this chicken dish that invokes the flavors of North Africa.

1 tablespoon olive oil

4 boneless skinless chicken breasts

14 ounces no salt added tomatoes

$^1/_4$ cup ripe olives

2 cups zucchini, sliced

1 cup red bell peppers, sliced

$1^1/_2$ teaspoon cumin

$^1/_2$ teaspoon cinnamon

1 teaspoon lemon peel, grated

Heat oil over medium heat in a large non-stick skillet. Add chicken and cook until browned on each side, about 5 minutes. Combine remaining ingredients and pour over chicken. Cover and simmer until chicken is no longer pink in the center, about 20 minutes.

Yield: 4 servings

Per serving: 160 calories (31% from fat, 45% from protein , 24% from carb); 19 g protein ; 6 g total fat; 1 g

saturated fat; 4 g monounsaturated fat; 1 g polyunsaturated fat; 10 g carb; 3 g fiber; 6 g sugar; 195 mg phosphorus; 68 mg calcium; 138 mg sodium; 664 mg potassium; 1479 IU vitamin A; 4 mg ATE vitamin E; 97 mg vitamin C; 41 mg cholesterol

Indian-Flavored Chicken

This is similar to the recipe for country captain soup, a curried chicken dish that supposedly came to England from India originally. The curry powder I use most often is a Blue Mountain brand from Jamaica that I get at a local Hispanic market. It's milder than most Asian curries, so if you can't find something similar, you may want to reduce the amount.

6 chicken thighs

2 cups (480 g) no-salt-added canned tomatoes

1 cup (160 g) chopped onion

$^1/_2$ teaspoon garlic powder

1 cup (130 g) frozen peas

$1^1/_2$ tablespoons curry powder

Place chicken in a 9 x 13-inch (23 x 33-cm) baking dish. Mix other ingredients together and pour over chicken. Bake at 350°F (180°C, gas mark 4) until chicken is done, about 45 minutes

Yield: 6 servings

Per serving: 152 g water; 100 calories (18% from fat, 41% from protein, 41% from carb); 11 g protein; 2 g total fat; 0 g saturated fat; 1 g monounsaturated fat; 1 g polyunsaturated fat; 11 g carbohydrate; 3 g fiber; 4 g sugar; 119 mg phosphorus; 49 mg calcium; 2 mg iron; 67 mg sodium; 340 mg potassium; 696 IU vitamin A; 8 mg vitamin E; 12 mg vitamin C; 34 mg cholesterol

Indian Chicken

A slightly tangy, not overly hot chicken flavored like the classic Tandoori chicken. If you like hotter food, you can add more cayenne pepper.

1 cup (230 g) plain fat-free yogurt

$^1/_2$ teaspoon (0.9 g) cardamom

$^1/_2$ teaspoon (1.3 g) ground cumin

$^1/_2$ teaspoon (1.1 g) turmeric

$^1/_8$ teaspoon (0.3 g) cayenne pepper

1 teaspoon (0.6 g) bay leaf, crushed

$^1/_2$ teaspoon (1.5 g) garlic powder

$^3/_4$ teaspoon (1.4 g) ground ginger

$^1/_4$ cup (40 g) onion, minced

$^1/_4$ cup (60 ml) lime juice

$^1/_4$ teaspoon (0.5 g) black pepper

1 teaspoon (2.3 g) cinnamon

1 teaspoon (2 g) ground coriander

8 boneless chicken breasts

Combine yogurt and remaining ingredients except chicken, mixing well. Prick chicken with a fork. In a resealable plastic bag or glass pan large enough to hold chicken, cover chicken with yogurt marinade, making sure all surfaces of chicken are coated. Cover and refrigerate at least 3 hours, or overnight. Turn at least once while marinating. Grill over medium heat until done or preheat oven to 375°F (190°C, or gas mark 5) and place chicken in a greased roasting pan with marinade and cook for 45 minutes to 1 hour, or until chicken is tender.

Yield: 8 servings

Per serving: 103 calories (9% from fat, 73% from protein, 17% from carbohydrate); 18 g protein; 1 g total fat; 0 g saturated fat; 0 g monounsaturated fat; 0 g polyunsaturated fat; 4 g carbohydrate; 0 g fiber; 3 g sugar; 193 mg phosphorus; 79 mg calcium; 1 mg iron; 71 mg sodium; 293 mg potassium; 44 IU vitamin A; 5 mg ATE vitamin E; 4 mg vitamin C; 42 mg cholesterol; 91 g water

Slow-Cooker Chicken Curry

I'm fond of curries. They make a particularly nice slow-cooker meal because they fill the house with such a great aroma for you to come home to. This one calls for a number of spices that are typical of curry powder.

5 medium potatoes, diced

1 cup (150 g) coarsely chopped green bell pepper

1 cup (160 g) coarsely chopped onion

1 pound (455 g) boneless chicken breasts, cubed

2 cups (480 g) no-salt-added canned tomatoes

1 tablespoon coriander

1 $^1/_2$ tablespoons paprika

1 tablespoon ginger

$^1/_4$ teaspoon red pepper flakes

$^1/_2$ teaspoon turmeric

$^1/_4$ teaspoon cinnamon

$^1/_8$ teaspoon cloves

1 cup (235 ml) low-sodium chicken broth

2 tablespoons (28 ml) cold water

4 tablespoons (32 g) cornstarch

Place potatoes, bell pepper, and onion in slow cooker. Place chicken on top. Mix together tomatoes, spices, and chicken broth. Pour over chicken. Cook on low 8 to 10 hours or on high 5 to 6 hours. Remove meat and vegetables. Turn heat to high. Stir cornstarch into water. Add to cooker. Cook until sauce is slightly thickened, about 15 to 20 minutes. Stir meat and vegetables into thickened sauce.

Yield: 5 servings

Per serving: 440 g water; 351 calories (4% from fat, 12% from protein, 84% from carb); 11 g protein; 2 g total fat; 0 g saturated fat; 0 g monounsaturated fat; 1 g polyunsaturated fat; 76 g carbohydrate; 8 g fiber; 7 g sugar; 202 mg phosphorus; 78 mg calcium; 3 mg iron; 54 mg sodium; 1407 mg potassium; 1352 IU vitamin A; 1 mg vitamin E; 61 mg vitamin C; 9 mg cholesterol

Tip: If you have a favorite curry powder on the shelf, you could substitute a couple of tablespoons of that for the other spices.

Chicken and Chickpea Curry

Low fat chicken and chickpeas give this a super boost of protein and other vegetables provide additional nutrients. And the combination provides plenty of volume without the need for rice or other starch.

1 cup plain low-fat yogurt

3 teaspoons curry powder

3 teaspoons turmeric

1 tablespoon canola oil

12 ounces boneless skinless chicken breast, chopped

1 tablespoon lemon juice

1 tablespoon fresh coriander, chopped

$^1/_2$ teaspoon garlic, minced

$^1/_2$ cup onion, chopped

$^1/_2$ cup green pepper, chopped

1 cup cooked chickpeas

Heat the canola oil in a large pan and add the onion, coriander, green peppers, garlic, and chick peas. Fry lightly. Add the curry powder and turmeric to the onion mix. Add a little bit of water if fluid is needed. Remove from pan. Put chicken in pan and fry until cooked. Sprinkle with lemon juice. Add onion and curry mix to chicken and simmer for about 20 minutes. Add yogurt, heat through, and remove from stove.

Yield: 3 servings

Per serving: 120 g water; 341 calories (24% from fat, 43% from protein, 33% from carb); 36 g protein; 9 g total fat; 2 g saturated fat; 4 g monounsaturated fat; 2 g polyunsaturated fat; 28 g carbohydrate; 6 g fiber; 10 g sugar; 461 mg phosphorus; 221 mg calcium; 0 mg iron; 140 mg sodium; 846 mg potassium; 228 IU vitamin A; 18 mg vitamin E; 31 mg vitamin C; 71 mg cholesterol

Chicken Zucchini Pie

An easy and tasty one-dish meal based on the concept of the Bisquick impossible pies, which make their own crust.

1 cup (110 g) cooked chicken breast, cubed

1 cup (113 g) zucchini, cubed

1 cup (180 g) tomatoes, chopped

1 cup (160 g) onion, chopped

$^1/_4$ cup (20 g) Parmesan cheese, shredded

1 cup (235 ml) skim milk

$^1/_2$ cup (60 g) Reduced Fat Biscuit Mix (see recipe page 38)

2 eggs

$^1/_4$ teaspoon (0.5 g) black pepper

Preheat oven to 400°F (200°C, or gas mark 6) and coat a 9-inch (23-cm) pie plate with nonstick vegetable oil spray. Mix chicken, zucchini, tomatoes, onion, and cheese and spoon evenly into prepared pie plate. Beat remaining ingredients in a blender or with a wire whisk until smooth. Pour evenly over chicken mixture. Bake for 35 minutes, or until a knife inserted in center comes out clean. Let stand 5 minutes before cutting.

Yield: 6 servings

Per serving: 156 calories (23% from fat, 38% from protein, 39% from carbohydrate); 15 g protein; 4 g total fat; 1 g saturated fat; 1 g monounsaturated fat; 1 g polyunsaturated fat; 15 g carbohydrate; 1 g fiber; 2 g sugar; 231 mg phosphorus; 160 mg calcium; 2 mg iron; 157 mg sodium; 333 mg potassium; 423 IU vitamin A; 41 mg ATE vitamin E; 12 mg vitamin C; 95 mg cholesterol; 138 g water

Chicken and Sausage Pie

An old-fashioned country-style dish, with both chicken and sausage and a crispy cornmeal crust.

2 potatoes, cut in $^1/_2$-inch (1-cm) pieces

$^1/_2$ pound (225 g) breakfast sausage

$^1/_2$ pound (225 g) boneless skinless chicken breasts

1 cup (160 g) diced onion

$^1/_2$ teaspoon garlic powder

$^1/_2$ cup (60 g) diced celery

$^1/_2$ cup (65 g) diced carrot

2 tablespoons (16 g) flour

$^1/_4$ cup (60 ml) white wine

1$^1/_2$ cups (355 ml) low-sodium chicken broth

1 teaspoon thyme

1 teaspoon poultry seasoning

Cornmeal Crust

$^3/_4$ cup (90 g) flour

$^1/_2$ cup (70 g) cornmeal

$^1/_4$ cup (55 g) unsalted butter

2 tablespoons (28 ml) cold water

Boil potatoes until just soft. Drain. Crumble the sausage and place in a large, deep pan. Add the chicken. Cook over medium heat. Add onion, garlic powder, celery, and carrot, and cook about 5 minutes or until vegetables are tender. Stir together flour, wine, and broth. Add to pan and bring to a boil. Turn heat to low, add thyme, poultry seasoning, and potatoes and cook until thickened and bubbly. Pour into 8 x 8-inch (20 x 20-cm) baking dish and set aside. To make the crust, mix flour and cornmeal in a large bowl. Cut in butter until texture resembles coarse meal. Sprinkle water over dough and knead with hands, adding only enough to make the dough form a ball. Refrigerate dough 30 minutes to 24 hours. Roll dough on a floured surface to $^1/_4$-inch (0.5-cm) thickness. Place dough over top of filling. Bake pie at 375°F (190°C, gas mark 5) for 30 minutes or until crust is lightly browned and filling is bubbly.

Yield: 6 servings

Per serving: 204 g water; 344 calories (31% from fat, 11% from protein, 58% from carb); 9 g protein; 12 g total fat; 6 g saturated fat; 4 g monounsaturated fat; 1 g polyunsaturated fat; 50 g carbohydrate; 4 g fiber; 3 g sugar; 136 mg phosphorus; 38 mg calcium; 2 mg iron; 114 mg sodium; 568 mg potassium; 2113 IU vitamin A; 64 mg vitamin E; 11 mg vitamin C; 31 mg cholesterol

Zucchini Moussaka

A variation of the typical Greek dish using ground turkey and zucchini, rather than the more common lamb and eggplant.

6 cups (675 g) zucchini, sliced lengthwise

$1/2$ pound (225 g) ground turkey

1 cup (160 g) onion, chopped

2 teaspoons (6 g) garlic, minced

$1/2$ teaspoon (1.2 g) cinnamon

$1/2$ teaspoon (0.5 g) dried oregano

1 cup (235 ml) low sodium chicken broth

$2/3$ cup (130 g) rice

8 ounces (235 ml) no-salt-added tomato sauce

2 tablespoons (30 ml) olive oil

$1/4$ cup (30 g) flour

$1 1/2$ cups (355 ml) skim milk

2 eggs, beaten

$1/4$ teaspoon (0.6 g) nutmeg

Preheat oven to 350°F (180°C, or gas mark 4). Lightly grease a shallow 2-quart (1.9-L) baking dish. Bring 3 cups (705 ml) water to boil in a large nonstick skillet. Add zucchini, cover, reduce heat, and simmer 10 minutes or until crisp-tender. Remove to paper towels to drain. Wipe out skillet. Add turkey, onion, and garlic Cook until turkey is no longer pink. Stir in cinnamon and oregano, then broth and rice. Cover and simmer 10 minutes, stirring two or three times. Stir in tomato sauce. Remove from heat. Heat oil in a 2-quart (1.9-L) saucepan. Whisk in flour and cook, stirring 1 to 2 minutes without letting mixture brown. Gradually whisk in milk. Cook, whisking constantly, 4 to 5 minutes until thickened and smooth. Whisk one-third of the hot mixture into the eggs, then whisk egg mixture into remaining sauce. Remove from heat; stir in nutmeg.

To assemble: Cover the bottom of prepared baking dish with half the zucchini slices. Spoon the turkey mixture over the slices, then cover with remaining zucchini. Pour the milk mixture over everything. Bake for 20 to 25 minutes, or until hot and bubbly and top is lightly golden.

Yield: 4 servings

Per serving: 327 calories (27% from fat, 32% from protein, 41% from carbohydrate); 26 g protein; 10 g total fat; 2 g saturated fat; 6 g monounsaturated fat; 2 g polyunsaturated fat; 34 g carbohydrate; 4 g fiber; 8 g sugar; 390 mg phosphorus; 217 mg calcium; 4 mg iron; 190 mg sodium; 1159 mg potassium; 879 IU vitamin A; 56 mg ATE vitamin E; 44 mg vitamin C; 144 mg cholesterol; 491 g water

Chicken and Spaghetti Bake

This comes more or less directly from my daughter's theory of cooking, namely, if you can't think of anything else for dinner, make something Italian. Works for me!

8 ounces (225 g) spaghetti

2 eggs, beaten

1 cup (225 g) fat-free cottage cheese

1 pound (455 g) boneless chicken breast, sliced

$^1/_2$ cup (80 g) onion, chopped

$^1/_2$ cup (75 g) green bell pepper, chopped

2 cups (360 g) canned no-salt-added tomatoes

6 ounces (170 g) no-salt-added tomato paste

1 teaspoon (4 g) sugar

1 teaspoon (1 g) dried oregano

$^1/_2$ teaspoon (1.5 g) garlic powder

$^1/_2$ cup (60 g) mozzarella, shredded

Preheat oven to 350°F (180°C, or gas mark 4). Cook spaghetti according to package directions. Drain. Mix in eggs. Form into a "crust" in a greased 10-inch (25-cm) pie pan. Top with cottage cheese. In a large skillet cook chicken, onion, and green bell pepper until meat is done and vegetables are tender. Add remaining ingredients except mozzarella and heat through. Spread over spaghetti and cottage cheese. Bake for 20 minutes. Sprinkle with mozzarella about 5 minutes before the end of baking.

Yield: 6 servings

Per serving: 218 calories (9% from fat, 50% from protein, 41% from carbohydrate); 27 g protein; 2 g total fat; 1 g saturated fat; 1 g monounsaturated fat; 1 g polyunsaturated fat; 22 g carbohydrate; 4 g fiber; 8 g sugar; 274 mg phosphorus; 70 mg calcium; 3 mg iron; 128 mg sodium; 666 mg potassium; 704 IU vitamin A; 7 mg ATE vitamin E; 26 mg vitamin C; 116 mg cholesterol; 239 g water

Pasta with Chicken and Vegetables

This is a good way to use up a few fresh vegetables. These were what we had available, but you can vary them to match what you have. It makes a simple one-dish meal that's perfect for a warm evening with just a little homemade bread.

8 ounces (225 g) linguine or spaghetti

2 tablespoons (30 ml) olive oil

1 cup (113 g) zucchini, cut in strips

$^1/_2$ cup (35 g) mushrooms, sliced

$^1/_2$ teaspoon (0.3 g) dried basil

$^1/_2$ teaspoon (1.5 g) minced garlic

1 cup (235 ml) skim milk

2 cups (220 g) chicken breast, cooked and cubed

1 cup (180 g) roma tomatoes, sliced

2 tablespoons (10 g) Parmesan cheese, grated

$^1/_8$ teaspoon (0.3 g) black pepper

Cook linguini or spaghetti according to package directions. Meanwhile, heat the oil in a skillet. Add zucchini, mushrooms, basil, and garlic. Cook and stir for 20 to 30 minutes, or until zucchini is crisp-tender. Drain pasta and return to saucepan. Stir in milk, chicken, and zucchini mixture and heat through. Add tomatoes, cheese, and pepper. Toss and serve.

Yield: 6 servings

Per serving: 297 calories (26% from fat, 31% from protein, 42% from carbohydrate); 23 g protein; 9 g total fat; 2 g saturated fat; 5 g monounsaturated fat; 1 g polyunsaturated fat; 31 g carbohydrate; 2 g fiber; 2 g sugar; 278 mg phosphorus; 110 mg calcium; 1 mg iron; 102 mg sodium; 424 mg potassium; 379 IU vitamin A; 37 mg ATE vitamin E; 7 mg vitamin C; 74 mg cholesterol; 119 g water

Pasta with Chicken, Asparagus, and Tomatoes

A simple Balsamic vinegar and oil dressing add just the right touch to this tasty, quick to fix main dish.

8 ounces whole wheat pasta, such as rotini

1 pound boneless skinless chicken breast, cut in $1/4$ inch strips

$1/2$ teaspoon black pepper, freshly ground

1 cup asparagus, cut in 1 inch slices

1 cup cherry tomatoes, cut in half

$1/2$ teaspoon garlic, minced

$1/2$ teaspoon basil

2 tablespoons balsamic vinegar

1 tablespoon olive oil

Cook pasta according to package directions, omitting salt. Heat a non-stick skillet over medium heat. Add chicken and asparagus and cook until chicken is no longer pink, about 5 minutes. Add tomatoes and garlic and cook one minute longer. Remove from heat, stir in pasta and remaining ingredients.

Yield: 4 servings

Per serving: 256 calories (19% from fat, 47% from protein , 34% from carb); 31 g protein ; 5 g total fat; 1 g saturated fat; 3 g monounsaturated fat; 1 g polyunsaturated fat; 22 g carb; 4 g fiber; 2 g sugar; 293 mg phosphorus; 41 mg calcium; 77 mg sodium; 628 mg potassium; 934 IU vitamin A; 7 mg ATE vitamin E; 23 mg vitamin C; 66 mg cholesterol

Chicken with Pasta and Mozzarella

Fresh cherry tomatoes and mozzarella make this chicken and pasta dish special.

1 pound boneless skinless chicken breast, cut in strips

$1/4$ cup olive oil, divided

$1^1/2$ teaspoons Italian seasoning

8 ounces whole wheat pasta

2 cups cherry tomatoes, cut in half

8 ounces fresh mozzarella, cut in $1/2$ inch cubes

$1/4$ cup parmesan, grated

$1/4$ cup fresh parsley

Heat 2 tablespoons oil in a large skillet over medium heat. Add chicken and cook until no longer pink. Meanwhile cook pasta according to package directions, omitting salt. Drain and toss with remaining oil. And chicken and other ingredients and toss to combine.

Yield: 4 servings

Per serving: 524 calories (46% from fat, 37% from protein , 17% from carb); 48 g protein ; 27 g total fat; 10 g saturated fat; 14 g monounsaturated fat; 2 g polyunsaturated fat; 22 g carb; 3 g fiber; 1 g sugar; 618 mg phosphorus; 521 mg calcium; 183 mg sodium; 629 mg potassium; 1322 IU vitamin A; 90 mg ATE vitamin E; 26 mg vitamin C; 102 mg cholesterol

Chicken and Bean Skillet

This is a great, quick dinner for those nights when you don't have something planned and everyone is hungry. Simple and fast, but loaded with flavor and nutrition.

1 cup (160 g) chopped onion

$^1/_3$ cup (50 g) chopped red bell pepper

$^3/_4$ teaspoon crushed garlic

2 teaspoons (10 ml) olive oil

$^1/_2$ pound (225 g) boneless chicken breast, cut in 1-inch (2.5-cm) cubes

$^3/_4$ teaspoon cumin

$^1/_2$ teaspoon cinnamon

10 ounces (280 g) navy beans, drained

10 ounces (280 g) kidney beans, drained

2 cups (510 g) no-salt-added stewed tomatoes, undrained

Sauté onion, pepper, and garlic in oil in medium saucepan 2 to 3 minutes. Add chicken, cumin, and cinnamon; cook over medium-high heat until chicken is lightly browned, about 3 to 4 minutes. Add beans and tomatoes; heat to boiling. Reduce heat and simmer, uncovered, until slightly thickened, 5 to 8 minutes. Season to taste with salt and pepper.

Yield: 4 servings

Per serving: 299 g water; 325 calories (10% from fat, 33% from protein, 57% from carb); 27 g protein; 4 g total fat; 1 g saturated fat; 2 g monounsaturated fat; 1 g polyunsaturated fat; 47 g carbohydrate; 16 g fiber; 8 g sugar; 353 mg phosphorus; 163 mg calcium; 6 mg iron; 53 mg sodium; 1076 mg potassium; 631 IU vitamin A; 3 mg vitamin E; 31 mg vitamin C; 33 mg cholesterol

Tip: This dish is delicious served over cooked rice, couscous, or pasta.

Chicken and Black Beans

A Mexican-flavored skillet meal featuring marinated chicken and black beans.

$^1/_2$ cup (120 ml) Italian dressing

$^1/_2$ teaspoon crushed garlic

$^1/_4$ teaspoon red pepper flakes

12 ounces (340 g) boneless chicken breast, cut in 1-inch (2.5-cm) cubes

2 teaspoons (10 ml) olive oil

1 cup (150 g) chopped green bell pepper

$^3/_4$ cup (120 g) chopped onion

$^3/_4$ teaspoon oregano

$^1/_4$ teaspoon black pepper, fresh ground

$^1/_4$ teaspoon cumin

2 cups (344 g) cooked black beans, drained and rinsed

2 cups (480 g) no-salt-added canned tomatoes

$^1/_4$ cup chopped fresh cilantro

Combine dressing, garlic, and red pepper. Place chicken in large glass bowl, pour dressing over chicken, cover, and refrigerate 30 to 60 minutes (or overnight). Remove chicken from marinade, drain well, and discard marinade. Heat oil in large skillet over medium-high heat until hot. Add chicken, cook 5 to 7 minutes, stirring until chicken is slightly brown, spooning off any excess liquid. Add bell pepper, onion, oregano, pepper, and cumin. Cook, stirring 4 to 5 minutes or until vegetables are tender. Add black beans and tomatoes. Cook 2 to 3 minutes more, or until thoroughly heated. Garnish with cilantro; serve immediately.

Yield: 4 servings

Per serving: 314 g water; 355 calories (31% from fat, 32% from protein, 37% from carb); 29 g protein; 12 g total fat; 2 g saturated fat; 4 g monounsaturated fat; 5 g polyunsaturated fat; 33 g carbohydrate; 10 g fiber; 7 g sugar; 332 mg phosphorus; 90 mg calcium; 4 mg iron; 562 mg sodium; 896 mg potassium; 550 IU vitamin A; 5 mg vitamin E; 46 mg vitamin C; 49 mg cholesterol

Tip: Serve over rice.

Chicken with Asparagus

My wife came home with some asparagus recently, and this recipe came up while searching our recipe file. It had been a long time since we made it, but it turned out very well. It's definitely something we will keep in mind for the future.

4 boneless chicken breasts

1 tablespoon (4 g) cilantro, chopped

2 tablespoons (30 ml) olive oil

$^1/_2$ pound (225 g) asparagus, cut in 3-inch (7.5-cm) lengths

$1^1/_2$ cups (355 ml) low sodium chicken broth

1 tablespoon (8 g) cornstarch

1 tablespoon (15 ml) lemon juice

$^1/_2$ teaspoon (1 g) black pepper

Slice the chicken breasts into strips about $^1/_4$-inch (62-mm) thick. Sprinkle with cilantro and toss to coat. Heat the oil in a large frying pan and fry the chicken quickly in small batches, 1 to 2 minutes per side. Remove from pan when no longer pink. Add asparagus and chicken broth to pan and bring to a boil. Cook for 4 to 5 minutes, or until asparagus is tender. Mix the cornstarch with a little water and stir into the broth. Cook until thickened. Add the chicken. Stir in the lemon juice and pepper. Cook until chicken is heated through.

Yield: 4 servings

Per serving: 170 calories (49% from fat, 43% from protein, 8% from carbohydrate); 18 g protein; 9 g total fat; 2 g saturated fat; 6 g monounsaturated fat; 1 g polyunsaturated fat; 3 g carbohydrate; 0 g fiber; 0 g sugar; 148 mg phosphorus; 14 mg calcium; 1 mg iron; 66 mg sodium; 225 mg potassium; 67 IU vitamin A; 3 mg ATE vitamin E; 2 mg vitamin C; 44 mg cholesterol; 126 g water

Stir-Fried Chicken and Brown Rice

Asian-style chicken stir-fry.

2 tablespoons (28 ml) olive oil, divided

8 ounces (225 g) boneless chicken breast sliced into strips

$^1/_2$ cup (75 g) chopped red bell pepper

$^1/_2$ cup (50 g) chopped scallions

3 cups (660 g) cooked, cooled brown rice

2 tablespoons (28 ml) Dick's Reduced Sodium Soy Sauce (see recipe page 25)

1 tablespoon (15 ml) rice wine vinegar

1 cup (130 g) frozen peas, thawed

Heat large nonstick skillet over medium heat. Add 1 tablespoon oil. Add chicken, bell pepper, and scallions. Cook 5 minutes until chicken is cooked through. Remove to plate. Heat remaining oil in skillet. Add rice and cook 1 minute. Stir in soy sauce, vinegar, and peas; cook 1 minute. Stir in chicken and vegetable mixture.

Yield: 4 servings

Per serving: 213 g water; 349 calories (26% from fat, 25% from protein, 49% from carb); 21 g protein; 10 g total fat; 2 g saturated fat; 6 g monounsaturated fat; 2 g polyunsaturated fat; 43 g carbohydrate; 6 g fiber; 3 g sugar; 313 mg phosphorus; 49 mg calcium; 2 mg iron; 77 mg sodium; 425 mg potassium; 1560 IU vitamin A; 3 mg vitamin E; 31 mg vitamin C; 33 mg cholesterol

Chicken-Pasta Stir-Fry

An Asian-flavored use for leftover chicken, quick and easy to make.

2 tablespoons (28 ml) olive oil

1 cup (160 g) coarsely chopped onion

1 cup (150 g) coarsely chopped bell pepper

2 cups (142 g) broccoli florets

1 teaspoon minced garlic

2 cups (280 g) cubed cooked chicken

8 ounces (225 g) whole wheat pasta, cooked

1/4 cup (60 ml) Dick's Reduced Sodium Soy Sauce (see recipe page 25)

3 tablespoons (45 ml) rice wine

1 1/2 tablespoons (19 g) sugar

1 1/2 tablespoons (25 ml) Worcestershire sauce

1/2 teaspoon ginger

Heat oil in wok or skillet. Sauté garlic and vegetables in hot oil until just tender. Stir in chicken and pasta. Mix together remaining ingredients and stir in until meat, pasta, and vegetables are well coated.

Yield: 4 servings

Per serving: 128 g water; 343 calories (20% from fat, 13% from protein, 67% from carb); 11 g protein; 8 g total fat; 1 g saturated fat; 2 g monounsaturated fat; 4 g polyunsaturated fat; 59 g carbohydrate; 6 g fiber; 8 g sugar; 219 mg phosphorus; 57 mg calcium; 3 mg iron; 172 mg sodium; 470 mg potassium; 2238 IU vitamin A; 0 mg vitamin E; 94 mg vitamin C; 0 mg cholesterol

Chicken Pot Pie

A chicken and dumplings variation that is topped with mashed potatoes. This makes a large amount and is good for a family meal or leftovers for lunch.

2 pounds (905 g) boneless chicken breasts

2 cups (470 ml) low sodium chicken broth

1 cup (160 g) onion, coarsely chopped

1 cup (130 g) carrot, sliced

1 1/3 cups (170 g) frozen peas, thawed

2/3 cup (84 g) flour

1 cup (235 g) water

1 tablespoon (0.4 g) dried parsley

1 teaspoon (1 g) dried thyme

6 potatoes, peeled and diced

1 cup (235 ml) skim milk

Preheat broiler. Place chicken and broth in a slow cooker or Dutch oven and cook until chicken is done. Remove chicken from broth, chop coarsely. Strain any fat from broth and add enough water to make 5 cups (1.2 L). Return broth to Dutch oven. Add onions, carrots, and peas and cook for 15 minutes, or until carrots are tender. Add flour to water in a jar with a tight-fitting lid. Shake until dissolved. Add to broth and cook until thickened. Stir in chicken, parsley, and thyme. While chicken mixture is cooking boil potatoes until done. Mash with milk. Drop mashed potatoes by spoonful onto top of chicken mixture. Broil until potatoes start to brown.

Yield: 8 servings

Per serving: 411 calories (5% from fat, 35% from protein, 59% from carbohydrate); 36 g protein; 2 g total fat; 1 g saturated fat; 1 g monounsaturated fat; 1 g polyunsaturated fat; 61 g carbohydrate; 7 g fiber; 5 g sugar; 486 mg phosphorus; 109 mg calcium; 4 mg iron; 209 mg sodium; 1791 mg potassium; 3265 IU vitamin A; 26 mg ATE vitamin E; 30 mg vitamin C; 66 mg cholesterol; 474 g water

Reduced Fat Chicken and Dumplings

This is classic comfort food any time of year, but especially as the weather gets colder. You can also make the dumplings using 2 cups (250 g) of Reduced Fat Biscuit Mix (see recipe page 38) rather than the flour, baking powder, and butter called for here.

For Chicken:

1 $^1/_2$ cups (165 g) chicken breast, cooked and cubed

3 cups (710 ml) low sodium chicken broth

3 cups (710 ml) water

1 $^1/_2$ cups (195 g) carrot, sliced

6 potatoes, peeled and cubed

1 cup (160 g) onion, chopped

For Dumplings:

2 cups (250 g) flour

1 tablespoon (14 g) baking powder

2 tablespoons (28 g) butter

$^2/_3$ cup (160 g) skim milk

To make the chicken: Place chicken, broth, water, carrots, potatoes, and onion in a large pan. Bring to a boil.

To make the dumplings: Stir together the flour and baking powder. Cut in butter until mixture resembles coarse crumbs. Stir in milk until dough holds together in a ball. Drop dumplings on top of boiling chicken mixture by spoonfuls. Reduce heat and simmer uncovered for 10 minutes. Cover and simmer 10 minutes more.

Yield: 6 servings

Per serving: 556 calories (11% from fat, 19% from protein, 71% from carbohydrate); 26 g protein; 7 g total fat; 6 g saturated fat; 1 g monounsaturated fat; 0 g polyunsaturated fat; 100 g carbohydrate; 9 g fiber; 7 g sugar; 488 mg phosphorus; 251 mg calcium; 6 mg iron; 413 mg sodium; 2113 mg potassium; 5668 IU vitamin A; 65 mg ATE vitamin E; 36 mg vitamin C; 30 mg cholesterol; 637 g water

Reduced Fat Chicken Salad

This makes great sandwiches, and the food processor makes it easy. A few seconds will give you perfectly ground and mixed salad. I often cook a whole chicken in the slow cooker and then use the meat for this and other recipes.

1 cup (110 g) chicken, cooked

1/4 cup (25 g) celery, chopped

2 tablespoons (28 g) low fat mayonnaise

2 tablespoons (30 g) fat-free sour cream

1/2 teaspoon (1.5 g) onion powder

Place chicken and celery in food processor and process until finely ground. Add remaining ingredients and process until well mixed.

Yield: 4 servings

Per serving: 104 calories (49% from fat, 45% from protein, 6% from carbohydrate); 10 g protein; 5 g total fat; 1 g saturated fat; 1 g monounsaturated fat; 1 g polyunsaturated fat; 1 g carbohydrate; 0 g fiber; 1 g sugar; 82 mg phosphorus; 17 mg calcium; 0 mg iron; 98 mg sodium; 118 mg potassium; 89 IU vitamin A; 13 mg ATE vitamin E; 0 mg vitamin C; 37 mg cholesterol; 39 g water

Smoked Turkey

If you have a smoker, this makes a sweet and juicy meal for a crowd, with a slightly southwestern flavor. Remember to discard the skin. It has most of the saturated fat, and it tends to get rubbery in the smoker anyway, so you're less tempted to cheat.

10-pound (4.5 kg) turkey

1 apple, quartered

1 onion, quartered

1 cup (100 g) celery, sliced

1/4 cup (60 ml) honey

1/4 cup (60 ml) lime juice

1/2 teaspoon (1.3 g) paprika

1 tablespoon (7 g) cumin

1/2 teaspoon (0.9 g) cayenne pepper

1/2 teaspoon (1.5 g) garlic powder

Place apple, onion, and celery inside turkey cavity. Combine remaining ingredients. Loosen the skin of the breast, legs, and thighs. Rub the honey spice mixture under the skin, spreading it as far as possible. Smoke for 8 to 10 hours, or until done.

Yield: 20 servings

Per serving: 271 calories (13% from fat, 79% from protein, 9% from carbohydrate); 51 g protein; 4 g total fat; 1 g saturated fat; 1 g monounsaturated fat; 1 g polyunsaturated fat; 6 g carbohydrate; 0 g fiber; 5 g sugar; 424 mg phosphorus; 35 mg calcium; 4 mg iron; 144 mg sodium; 634 mg potassium; 79 IU vitamin A; 0 mg ATE vitamin E; 2 mg vitamin C; 166 mg cholesterol; 191 g water

Turkey Cutlets Scaloppini

I don't usually pay the price they want for turkey cutlets, but I do occasionally buy a turkey breast and slice it into "cutlets," freezing most for later use and making soup of the carcass once most of the meat has been removed.

1 1/4 pounds (570 g) turkey cutlets

1 1/2 teaspoons (3 g) lemon pepper

1 tablespoon (7 g) paprika

3 tablespoons (45 ml) lemon juice

3/8 cups (90 ml) water

1 tablespoon (15 ml) olive oil

Coat a skillet with nonstick vegetable oil spray. Flatten cutlets to about 1/4-inch (0.6 cm) thickness. Place in skillet. Sprinkle with lemon pepper and paprika. Cook 3 to 4 minutes, turn over, and cook 4 to 5 minutes more or until done. Remove turkey from skillet. Add lemon juice, water, and oil. Heat until hot, stirring up any browned bits stuck on the bottom of the skillet. Serve sauce over cutlets.

Yield: 4 servings

Per serving: 257 calories (29% from fat, 67% from protein, 4% from carbohydrate); 42 g protein; 8 g total fat; 2 g saturated fat; 4 g monounsaturated fat; 2 g polyunsaturated fat; 2 g carbohydrate; 1 g fiber; 0 g sugar; 314 mg phosphorus; 29 mg calcium; 3 mg iron; 77 mg sodium; 460 mg potassium; 914 IU vitamin A; 0 mg ATE vitamin E; 7 mg vitamin C; 128 mg cholesterol; 129 g water

Turkey and Zucchini Meatloaf

The glaze gives this a nice sweet-tart taste. The turkey keeps it low in fat. The zucchini keeps it moist. What more could you ask?

1 1/4 pounds (570 g) ground turkey

1 cup (125 g) zucchini, grated

1/2 cup (60 g) low sodium bread crumbs

1 egg

1 tablespoon (0.4 g) dried parsley

1/2 teaspoon (1 g) black pepper

1/2 teaspoon (1.5 g) garlic powder

1 teaspoon (3 g) onion powder

1/4 cup (80 g) peach preserves

2 teaspoons (10 g) Dijon mustard

Preheat oven to 350°F (180°C, or gas mark 4). Combine first 8 ingredients (through onion powder) in a large bowl and mix well. Shape mixture into a loaf on a baking sheet. Bake for 45 minutes. Stir preserves and mustard together. Spread on top of loaf. Return to the oven and bake for 20 minutes, or until the internal temperature is 165°F (74°C).

Yield: 8 servings

Per serving: 144 calories (12% from fat, 51% from protein, 37% from carbohydrate); 18 g protein; 2 g total fat; 1 g saturated fat; 0 g monounsaturated fat; 1 g polyunsaturated fat; 13 g carbohydrate; 1 g fiber; 6 g sugar; 162 mg phosphorus; 32 mg calcium; 2 mg iron; 126 mg sodium; 242 mg potassium; 100 IU vitamin A; 0 mg ATE vitamin E; 4 mg vitamin C; 82 mg cholesterol; 80 g water

Turkey and Wild Rice Bake

An easy and tasty casserole that uses leftover turkey.

6 ounces (170 g) wild and white rice mix

2 1/3 cups (544 ml) water

$^1/_2$ cup (35 g) sliced mushrooms

14 ounces (400 g) artichoke hearts, quartered

2 ounces (55 g) pimento, drained and chopped

2 cups (350 g) cubed cooked turkey

1 cup (110 g) shredded Swiss cheese

Preheat oven to 350°F (180°C, gas mark 4). In 2-quart (2-L) casserole dish, combine rice and water. Stir in mushrooms, artichoke hearts, pimento, and turkey. Cover and bake about 1$^1/_4$ hours or until liquid is absorbed. Top with cheese and bake uncovered for 5 to 10 minutes or until cheese is melted and golden brown.

Yield: 4 servings

Per serving: 315 g water; 366 calories (11% from fat, 43% from protein, 46% from carb); 40 g protein; 5 g total fat; 2 g saturated fat; 1 g monounsaturated fat; 1 g polyunsaturated fat; 43 g carbohydrate; 8 g fiber; 3 g sugar; 599 mg phosphorus; 366 mg calcium; 3 mg iron; 195 mg sodium; 716 mg potassium; 597 IU vitamin A; 13 mg vitamin E; 17 mg vitamin C; 80 mg cholesterol

Tip: Chicken is just as good if you don't have turkey but are longing for this dish.

Turkey and Rice Loaf

Make use of leftover rice in this tasty turkey meatloaf.

1 egg white

2 tablespoons skim milk

1 pound ground turkey

1 cup cooked rice

$^1/_2$ cup carrot, shredded

$^1/_4$ cup onion, minced

$^1/_2$ teaspoon garlic, minced

$^1/_2$ teaspoon dry mustard

$^1/_4$ teaspoon black pepper

Preheat oven to 350°F. In a large bowl beat together the egg white and milk. Add the remaining ingredients and combine. Shape the mixture into a 9 × 4-inch loaf pan. Bake for one hour or until loaf registers 165°F in the center using an instant read thermometer. Let stand covered for 10 minutes. Turn out and slice.

Yield: 4 servings

Per serving: 201 calories (9% from fat, 61% from protein, 30% from carb); 29 g protein ; 2 g total fat; 1 g saturated fat; 0 g monounsaturated fat; 1 g polyunsaturated fat; 14 g carb; 1 g fiber; 1 g sugar; 267 mg phosphorus; 38 mg calcium; 102 mg sodium; 457 mg potassium; 1942 IU vitamin A; 5 mg ATE vitamin E; 2 mg vitamin C; 68 mg cholesterol

Turkey Vegetable Sauté

Turkey and vegetable sauce with just a hint of Mexican flavor. I particularly like this one over whole wheat spaghetti, but it's also good over brown rice.

1 pound (455 g) ground turkey

1 cup (160 g) onion, cut in rings

1 cup (130 g) sliced carrot

$^1/_2$ cup (50 g) sliced celery

$^1/_2$ cup (75 g) chunked green bell pepper

4 ounces (115 g) mushrooms, sliced

$^1/_2$ teaspoon cumin

$^1/_2$ teaspoon garlic salt

1 cup (180 g) chopped tomato

15 black olives, halved

3 slices low-sodium bacon, cooked and broken into pieces (optional)

Brown turkey. Add onion, carrot, celery, bell pepper, and mushrooms; add cumin and garlic salt and cook over medium heat until vegetables are crisp-tender. Add tomatoes, olives, and bacon and heat through.

Yield: 6 servings

Per serving: 161 g water; 197 calories (32% from fat, 52% from protein, 17% from carb); 25 g protein; 7 g total fat; 2 g saturated fat; 2 g monounsaturated fat; 1 g polyunsaturated fat; 8 g carbohydrate; 2 g fiber; 3 g sugar; 226 mg phosphorus; 50 mg calcium; 2 mg iron; 217 mg sodium; 521 mg potassium; 3873 IU vitamin A; 0 mg vitamin E; 20 mg vitamin C; 62 mg cholesterol

Turkey Skillet Pie

This is a great dish to make with leftover holiday turkey and stuffing.

1 tablespoon (15 ml) olive oil

$^1/_3$ cup (35 g) celery, chopped

2 tablespoons (20 g) onion, finely chopped

$^2/_3$ cup (160 ml) fat-free evaporated milk

2 cups (400 g) prepared stuffing

3 cups (525 g) cooked turkey, chopped

1 cup (110 g) low fat Swiss cheese, shredded

Heat olive oil in a small skillet; cook celery and onion until soft. In a large bowl, combine milk, stuffing, and onion mixture. Stir in turkey. Pour into a large skillet and sprinkle with cheese. Cook until heated through, about 10 minutes.

Yield: 6 servings

Per serving: 305 calories (33% from fat, 42% from protein, 25% from carbohydrate); 31 g protein; 11 g total fat; 3 g saturated fat; 5 g monounsaturated fat; 3 g polyunsaturated fat; 19 g carbohydrate; 2 g fiber; 5 g sugar; 359 mg phosphorus; 325 mg calcium; 2 mg iron; 501 mg sodium; 364 mg potassium; 370 IU vitamin A; 113 mg ATE vitamin E; 1 mg vitamin C; 77 mg cholesterol; 133 g water

Turkey-Stuffed Zucchini

This is perfect for those times when you don't get back to check the garden as often as you should and find a couple of zucchini that would make great softball bats. Discard the seeds and any center part of the squash that has gotten hard or stringy, and put the rest of what you scoop out into the filling.

3 large zucchini

$1^1/_4$ pounds (570 g) ground turkey

1 cup (160 g) onion, chopped

2 cloves garlic, crushed

2 cups (360 g) canned no-salt-added tomatoes

$1^1/_2$ cups (250 g) cooked rice, or small pasta

1 teaspoon (0.7 g) dried basil

12 ounces (340 g) Swiss cheese, sliced

Preheat broiler. Cut the zucchini in half lengthwise. Scrape out the center, leaving a thickness of about $^{1}/_{2}$ inch (1.2 cm). Discard the seeds and chop the remainder of the flesh; set aside. In a large skillet, cook the turkey, onion, and garlic until turkey is done. Stir in tomatoes, rice, basil, and chopped zucchini flesh. Cook the zucchini halves in boiling water until it begins to soften. Drain and place in baking pan. Divide the filling between the zucchini halves. Place a slice of cheese on top of each. Place under broiler until cheese is melted and bubbly.

Yield: 6 servings

Per serving: 309 calories (15% from fat, 54% from protein, 32% from carbohydrate); 42 g protein; 5 g total fat; 2 g saturated fat; 1 g monounsaturated fat; 1 g polyunsaturated fat; 24 g carbohydrate; 4 g fiber; 7 g sugar; 633 mg phosphorus; 625 mg calcium; 4 mg iron; 236 mg sodium; 1012 mg potassium; 563 IU vitamin A; 22 mg ATE vitamin E; 41 mg vitamin C; 89 mg cholesterol; 408 g water

Shepherd's Pie with Cornbread Crust

A meal in a pan. The cornbread on the bottom adds some substance to this while adding minimal fat and sodium.

1 pound (455 g) ground turkey

1 cup (160 g) chopped onion

12 ounces (340 g) mixed vegetables

3 cups (675 g) mashed potatoes

4 ounces (113 g) shredded Cheddar cheese

Cornbread Crust

1 cup (120 g) whole wheat pastry flour

$^{1}/_{2}$ cup (70 g) cornmeal

1 tablespoon sugar

2 teaspoons baking powder

1 cup (235 ml) skim milk

1 egg

2 tablespoons (28 ml) canola oil

Sauté turkey and onion. Drain. Cook vegetables until almost done. Drain. To make crust, stir together flour, cornmeal, sugar, and baking powder. Combine milk, egg, and oil. Stir into dry ingredients until just mixed. Spread cornbread in the bottom of a 9 x 13-inch (23 x 33-cm) baking dish sprayed with nonstick vegetable oil spray. On top of cornbread, layer meat mixture, veggies, and potatoes. Sprinkle with cheese. Bake at 425°F (220°C, gas mark 7) for 20 minutes.

Yield: 8 servings

Per serving: 131 g water; 417 calories (27% from fat, 27% from protein, 46% from carb); 28 g protein; 13 g total fat; 5 g saturated fat; 3 g monounsaturated fat; 3 g polyunsaturated fat; 48 g carbohydrate; 6 g fiber; 5 g sugar; 390 mg phosphorus; 258 mg calcium; 3 mg iron; 320 mg sodium; 672 mg potassium; 2091 IU vitamin A; 66 mg vitamin E; 21 mg vitamin C; 85 mg cholesterol

Chicken and Sun-Dried Tomato Pasta

Easy and delicious pasta with chicken. Serve with crusty bread and salad for a quick dinner.

12 ounces (340 g) bow tie, fusilli, or other shape
pasta

$1/_2$ teaspoon (2.5 ml) olive oil

$1/_2$ teaspoon (1.5 g) minced garlic

2 boneless chicken breasts, cut into bite-sized pieces

$1/_4$ cup (28 g) oil-packed sun-dried tomatoes,
chopped

$1/_4$ cup (65 g) prepared pesto

Cook pasta according to package directions. Drain.
Heat oil in a large skillet over medium heat. Sauté
garlic until tender, then stir in chicken. Cook until
chicken is golden and cooked through. In a large
bowl, combine pasta, chicken, sun-dried tomatoes,
and pesto. Toss to coat evenly.

Yield: 4 servings

Per serving: 462 calories (25% from fat, 20% from
protein, 55% from carbohydrate); 23 g protein; 13 g total
fat; 3 g saturated fat; 7 g monounsaturated fat; 2 g
polyunsaturated fat; 63 g carbohydrate; 3 g fiber; 2 g
sugar; 285 mg phosphorus; 139 mg calcium; 3 mg iron;
162 mg sodium; 458 mg potassium; 303 IU vitamin A;
17 mg ATE vitamin E; 9 mg vitamin C; 96 mg cholesterol;
38 g water

7

Main Dishes:
Beef

A S noted in the Introduction, beef has gotten a reputation for being bad for you. And it can be. The key to heart healthy beef lies in the selection of the cut used and the preparation. Most of the dishes here use low fat cuts like round steak or extra lean ground beef. The preparation is careful to keep it tender and flavorful without adding fat or sodium. We still eat beef more often than is recommended, but recipes like these make it tasty as well as good for you. Many contain the nutrition and fiber boost of whole grains and legumes.

Big Juicy Burgers

Extra lean ground beef doesn't have to be dry. If you prefer your burger medium or medium rare, you can have great grilled burgers that are still juicy without the fat content. If you prefer a more well done burger, you might try this recipe, where low fat beef broth provides the extra moistness.

1 cup (235 ml) low sodium beef broth

2 slices white bread, torn into pieces

1 1/2 pounds (680 g) extra-lean ground beef (93% lean)

1 egg

1/2 teaspoon (1 g) black pepper

Microwave broth in a glass bowl for 30 seconds. Add bread pieces and combine with your hands. Combine broth mixture and remaining ingredients. Shape into 5 patties. Grill patties over medium-high heat 6 to 8 minutes on each side or to desired doneness.

Yield: 5 servings

Per serving: 328 calories (43% from fat, 56% from protein, 0% from carbohydrate); 27 g protein; 9 g total fat; 4 g saturated fat; 4 g monounsaturated fat; 0 g polyunsaturated fat; 0 g carbohydrate; 0 g fiber; 0 g sugar; 206 mg phosphorus; 17 mg calcium; 3 mg iron; 129 mg sodium; 336 mg potassium; 23 IU vitamin A; 0 mg ATE vitamin E; 0 mg vitamin C; 134 mg cholesterol; 138 g water

Barbecued Beef

This is a quick sandwich meal that will cook while you are out. Small children and teenagers seem to like this too, so it's great for a party or family get-together.

1 1/2 pounds (680 g) extra-lean ground beef (93% lean)

1 onion, chopped

1 cup (240 g) low sodium ketchup

1 green bell pepper, chopped

2 tablespoons (30 g) brown sugar

1/2 teaspoon (1.5 g) garlic powder

2 tablespoons (30 g) prepared mustard

3 tablespoons (45 ml) vinegar

1 tablespoon (15 ml) Worcestershire sauce

1 teaspoon (2.6 g) chili powder

In a skillet, brown beef and onion. Drain. Stir together remaining ingredients in slow cooker. Stir in meat and onion mixture. Cook on low for 6 to 8 hours or on high for 3 to 4 hours.

Yield: 8 servings

Per serving: 249 calories (32% from fat, 40% from protein, 28% from carbohydrate); 17 g protein; 6 g total fat; 2 g saturated fat; 2 g monounsaturated fat; 0 g polyunsaturated fat; 12 g carbohydrate; 0 g fiber; 10 g sugar; 135 mg phosphorus; 18 mg calcium; 2 mg iron; 85 mg sodium; 402 mg potassium; 377 IU vitamin A; 0 mg ATE vitamin E; 8 mg vitamin C; 59 mg cholesterol; 80 g water

London Broil

London broil is traditionally made with flank steak. But now you'll find top round steak labeled as London broil. That is what we'll use here. Cooking under the broiler to medium-rare and slicing thin against the grain give you a tender piece of meat from a lean cut.

$^1/_4$ cup (60 ml) olive oil

1 teaspoon (5 ml) cider vinegar

$^1/_4$ teaspoon (0.8 g) minced garlic

$^1/_4$ teaspoon (0.5 g) freshly ground black pepper

$1^1/_2$ pounds (680 g) beef round steak

Score steak on both sides. Combine oil, vinegar, garlic, and pepper in a resealable plastic bag. Add steak and marinate for several hours, turning occasionally. Preheat broiler. Remove steak from marinade and broil 3 inches (7.5 cm) from heat for 4 to 5 minutes. Turn and broil 4 to 5 minutes longer, or until medium-rare. Carve in thin slices against the grain.

Yield: 5 servings

Per serving: 367 calories (45% from fat, 55% from protein, 0% from carbohydrate); 49 g protein; 18 g total fat; 4 g saturated fat; 11 g monounsaturated fat; 1 g polyunsaturated fat; 0 g carbohydrate; 0 g fiber; 0 g sugar; 308 mg phosphorus; 6 mg calcium; 5 mg iron; 62 mg sodium; 457 mg potassium; 0 IU vitamin A; 0 mg ATE vitamin E; 0 mg vitamin C; 122 mg cholesterol; 81 g water

Tip: We often grill this recipe, rather than broiling.

Oven Swiss Steak

This is an easy recipe for Swiss steak. It's good served with noodles or rice to soak up the sauce.

$1^1/_2$ pounds (690 g) beef round steak

$^1/_4$ cup (30 g) flour

2 tablespoons (30 ml) olive oil

2 cups (360 g) canned no-salt-added tomatoes

$^1/_2$ cup (50 g) celery, finely chopped

$^1/_2$ cup (65 g) carrot, finely chopped

1 tablespoon (15 ml) Worcestershire sauce

Preheat oven to 350°F (180°C, or gas mark 4). Cut meat into serving-sized pieces. Dredge in flour. Heat oil in a heavy skillet. Brown meat on both sides in oil. Transfer meat to a glass baking dish. Blend any remaining flour into pan drippings. Stir in remaining ingredients. Cook and stir until thickened and bubbly. Pour over meat. Bake, covered, for $1^1/_2$ hours, or until tender.

Yield: 6 servings

Per serving: 306 calories (31% from fat, 57% from protein, 12% from carbohydrate); 42 g protein; 10 g total fat; 3 g saturated fat; 6 g monounsaturated fat; 1 g polyunsaturated fat; 9 g carbohydrate; 1 g fiber; 3 g sugar; 286 mg phosphorus; 37 mg calcium; 5 mg iron; 100 mg sodium; 611 mg potassium; 1927 IU vitamin A; 0 mg ATE vitamin E; 13 mg vitamin C; 102 mg cholesterol; 161 g water

Beef Kabobs

The marinade helps to give these kabobs a nice flavor as well as making the leaner cut of meat more tender. You could also cook these in the oven if you don't want to grill them.

$^1/_4$ cup (60 ml) olive oil

$^1/_3$ cup (80 ml) Dick's Reduced Sodium Soy Sauce (see recipe page 25)

$^1/_4$ cup (60 ml) lemon juice

2 tablespoons (30 ml) Worcestershire sauce

$^1/_2$ teaspoon (1.5 g) minced garlic

1 teaspoon (2 g) coarsely ground black pepper

1 pound (455 g) beef round steak, cut in 1-inch (2.5-cm) cubes

2 cups (140 g) mushrooms

Mix together all ingredients except beef and mushrooms. Add beef cubes. Cover and refrigerate overnight, turning meat occasionally. Thread meat and mushrooms on skewers. Grill over hot fire to desired doneness, turning often.

Yield: 4 servings

Per serving: 380 calories (20% from fat, 19% from protein, 61% from carbohydrate); 42 g protein; 19 g total fat; 4 g saturated fat; 12 g monounsaturated fat; 4 g polyunsaturated fat; 135 g carbohydrate; 1 g fiber; 4 g sugar; 313 mg phosphorus; 20 mg calcium; 5 mg iron; 266 mg sodium; 628 mg potassium; 21 IU vitamin A; 0 mg ATE vitamin E; 21 mg vitamin C; 102 mg cholesterol; 142 g water

Meatloaf

This meatloaf, with variations as our diet has changed, has been a family favorite for years. It's a simple loaf with only a few ingredients, which my kids seemed to appreciate. The sauce is the real star here, a sweet and sour barbecue-y marvel that is worlds away from plain tomato sauce or, heaven forbid, tomato soup. It gives the whole house a wonderful aroma while it cooks. I always make at least a double recipe. It makes great sandwiches. You can also use ground turkey and make a lower fat version.

$1^1/_2$ pounds (680 g) extra-lean ground beef (93% lean)

1 cup (115 g) bread crumbs

1 onion, finely chopped

1 egg

$^1/_4$ teaspoon (0.5 g) black pepper

8 ounces (225 g) no-salt-added tomato sauce, divided

$^1/_2$ cup (120 ml) water

2 teaspoons (10 ml) Worcestershire sauce

3 tablespoons (45 ml) vinegar

2 tablespoons (30 g) mustard

3 tablespoons (45 g) brown sugar

Preheat oven to 350°F (180°C, or gas mark 4). Mix together beef, bread crumbs, onion, egg, pepper, and half the tomato sauce. Form into one large loaf or two small ones; mix remaining tomato sauce and remaining ingredients together; pour over loaves. Bake for 1 to $1^1/_2$ hours.

Yield: 6 servings

Per serving: 393 calories (29% from fat, 37% from protein, 33% from carbohydrate); 26 g protein; 9 g total fat; 3 g saturated fat; 3 g monounsaturated fat; 1 g polyunsaturated fat; 23 g carbohydrate; 1 g fiber; 9 g sugar; 218 mg phosphorus; 62 mg calcium; 4 mg iron; 249 mg sodium; 485 mg potassium; 175 IU vitamin A; 0 mg ATE vitamin E; 8 mg vitamin C; 118 mg cholesterol; 142 g water

Tex-Mex Meat Loaf

We love meat loaf and we love food with a Mexican flavor, so it's no surprise that this turned out to be a big hit around our house.

1 1/2 pounds (675 g) ground beef

2 cups (200 g) cooked kidney beans, rinsed and drained

1 1/2 cups (390 g) salsa, divided

1 cup (160 g) chopped onion

1/2 teaspoon minced garlic

1/2 cup (60 g) bread crumbs

2 eggs

1 1/2 teaspoons ground cumin

2 tablespoons (30 g) brown sugar

Combine beef, beans, 1 cup (260 g) salsa, onion, garlic, bread crumbs, eggs, and cumin. Mix well. Press into a loaf shape on a broiler pan or roasting pan. Bake 1 hour at 350°F (180°C, gas mark 4). Carefully pour off any drippings. Combine remaining salsa and brown sugar; mix well. Spread over top of meat loaf. Continue baking 15 minutes; remove and let stand 10 minutes.

Yield: 6 servings

Per serving: 176 g water; 579 calories (20% from fat, 34% from protein, 46% from carb); 41 g protein; 10 g total

fat; 4 g saturated fat; 4 g monounsaturated fat; 1 g polyunsaturated fat; 55 g carbohydrate; 17 g fiber; 10 g sugar; 492 mg phosphorus; 155 mg calcium; 9 mg iron; 223 mg sodium; 1484 mg potassium; 287 IU vitamin A; 26 mg vitamin E; 6 mg vitamin C; 157 mg cholesterol

Reduced-Fat Meatballs

This meatball recipe has been in the family for years, long before we were concerned with heart-healthy cooking. It's been modified a number of times as our diets changed, first to reduce the sodium, and later to make it lower in fat. The meatballs are good by themselves, but they're better if allowed to simmer in the sauce in a slow cooker for a few hours.

1 1/2 pounds (680 g) extra-lean ground beef (93% lean)

3 eggs

1/2 cup Parmesan cheese, shredded

1/2 teaspoon (1.5 g) garlic powder

1 tablespoon (0.4 g) dried parsley

1/2 tablespoon (1.5 g) dried oregano

4 slices bread, crumbled

2 cups (320 g) onion, chopped

6 ounces (170 g) no-salt-added tomato paste

1 1/2 cups (355 ml) water

1/2 cup (120 ml) red wine vinegar

3 tablespoons (45 g) brown sugar

Preheat oven to 375°F (190°C, or gas mark 5). Combine beef, eggs, cheese, garlic powder, parsley, oregano, and bread. Form into 1-inch (2.5-cm) balls.

Bake for 30 to 40 minutes, turning once. Pour a few tablespoons (45 ml) of meat drippings into a skillet; sauté onion. Combine onions, tomato paste, water, vinegar, and brown sugar and place in slow cooker. Add meatballs. Stir to mix and cook on low for several hours.

Yield: 6 servings

Per serving: 457 calories (31% from fat, 37% from protein, 32% from carbohydrate); 32 g protein; 12 g total fat; 5 g saturated fat; 4 g monounsaturated fat; 1 g polyunsaturated fat; 28 g carbohydrate; 4 g fiber; 15 g sugar; 340 mg phosphorus; 173 mg calcium; 5 mg iron; 398 mg sodium; 787 mg potassium; 653 IU vitamin A; 10 mg ATE vitamin E; 11 mg vitamin C; 186 mg cholesterol; 254 g water

German Meatballs

These German-flavored meatballs would traditionally be served over spaetzle, but they are also good with noodles, rice, or mashed potatoes.

1 egg

$^1/_4$ cup (60 ml) skim milk

$^1/_4$ cup (29 g) bread crumbs

$^1/_4$ teaspoon (0.2 g) poultry seasoning

1 pound (455 g) extra-lean ground beef (93% lean)

2 cups (470 ml) low sodium beef broth

$^1/_2$ cup (35 g) mushrooms, sliced

$^1/_2$ cup (80 g) onion, chopped

1 cup (230 g) fat free sour cream

1 tablespoon (8 g) flour

1 teaspoon (2.1 g) caraway seed

Combine egg and milk. Stir in bread crumbs and poultry seasoning. Add beef and mix well. Form into 24 meatballs, each about 1$^1/_2$ inches (3.8-cm). Brown meatballs in skillet. Drain. Add broth, mushrooms, and onion to the skillet. Cover and simmer for 30 minutes. Stir together sour cream, flour, and caraway seed. Add to skillet. Cook and stir until thickened.

Yield: 6 servings

Per serving: 281 calories (32% from fat, 47% from protein, 21% from carbohydrate); 19 g protein; 6 g total fat; 2 g saturated fat; 2 g monounsaturated fat; 1 g polyunsaturated fat; 8 g carbohydrate; 1 g fiber; 1 g sugar; 199 mg phosphorus; 87 mg calcium; 2 mg iron; 172 mg sodium; 317 mg potassium; 212 IU vitamin A; 47 mg ATE vitamin E; 2 mg vitamin C; 105 mg cholesterol; 194 g water

Stuffed Banana Peppers

Another recipe that uses some excess peppers. The original recipe I used to develop this one called for frying, but I decided to make them in the oven instead to reduce the amount of fat, since the meat and cheese already have a significant amount.

12 banana peppers, hot or sweet

1 pound (455 g) extra-lean ground beef (93% lean)

$^1/_2$ cup (80 g) onion, finely chopped

$^1/_2$ cup (55 g) Swiss cheese, shredded

1 egg

$^1/_4$ teaspoon (0.5 g) black pepper

$^1/_4$ cup (30 g) flour

Preheat oven to 350°F (180°C, or gas mark 4). Wash and clean peppers, then cut off the top and a small part of the bottom of peppers. In a large skillet, sauté ground beef and onions until meat is browned. Stir in cheese. Stuff mixture into peppers. Whisk egg and black pepper in a bowl. Dip peppers in egg mixture. Roll in flour, dip in egg again, and roll in flour again. Place in 9 x 13-inch (23 x 33-cm) baking dish and coat surface with nonstick vegetable oil spray until flour is moistened. Bake for 20 minutes, or until cheese is melted and coating begins to brown.

Yield: 4 servings

Per serving: 372 calories (32% from fat, 47% from protein, 21% from carbohydrate); 30 g protein; 9 g total fat; 4 g saturated fat; 4 g monounsaturated fat; 1 g polyunsaturated fat; 14 g carbohydrate; 4 g fiber; 3 g sugar; 325 mg phosphorus; 195 mg calcium; 3 mg iron; 159 mg sodium; 585 mg potassium; 419 IU vitamin A; 7 mg ATE vitamin E; 83 mg vitamin C; 134 mg cholesterol; 204 g water

Beef Barley Skillet

A tasty and healthy family meal that cooks in one pan.

$^3/_4$ pound (338 g) ground beef

$^1/_2$ cup (80 g) chopped onion

$^1/_4$ cup (38 g) chopped green bell pepper

$^1/_4$ cup (25 g) chopped celery

$^1/_4$ teaspoon black pepper

$^1/_2$ teaspoon marjoram

1 teaspoon sugar

1 teaspoon Worcestershire sauce

2 cups (480 g) no-salt-added canned tomatoes, broken up

$1^1/_2$ cups (355 ml) water

$^3/_4$ cup (150 g) pearl barley

Sauté meat, onion, green pepper, and celery in nonstick fry pan. Drain off excess fat; stir in remaining ingredients. Bring to a boil. Reduce heat to simmer; cover and cook about 1 hour.

Yield: 3 servings

Per serving: 389 g water; 477 calories (21% from fat, 31% from protein, 48% from carb); 29 g protein; 9 g total fat; 3 g saturated fat; 3 g monounsaturated fat; 1 g polyunsaturated fat; 45 g carbohydrate; 10 g fiber; 7 g sugar; 326 mg phosphorus; 90 mg calcium; 6 mg iron; 129 mg sodium; 932 mg potassium; 292 IU vitamin A; 0 mg vitamin E; 30 mg vitamin C; 78 mg cholesterol

Brisket of Beef with Beans

Kind of like baked beans with the addition of the beef. The cooking liquid gives the beef a nice flavor, and the beans go well with it.

1 pound (455 g) navy beans

2 pound (900 g) beef brisket

2 slices bacon

$^1/_2$ teaspoon black pepper, freshly ground

2 cups (475 ml) water

$^1/_4$ cup (60 ml) maple syrup

$^1/_2$ cup (115 g) packed brown sugar

$^1/_2$ teaspoon dry mustard

Soak beans in water overnight. Drain the beans. Brown the fat side of the brisket in a Dutch oven or heavy skillet over medium-high heat. Add the bacon and brown the other side. Add the pepper, water, and beans. Reduce heat to medium and cook, covered, for 2 hours or until the beef and beans are tender, stirring occasionally to prevent sticking. Remove the beef and keep warm. Add the maple syrup, brown sugar, and mustard to the beans. Mix thoroughly, and simmer over medium heat for another 10 minutes. Slice the brisket thinly and serve with the beans.

Yield: 6 servings

Per serving: 221 g water; 644 calories (49% from fat, 22% from protein, 29% from carb); 35 g protein; 35 g total fat; 14 g saturated fat; 15 g monounsaturated fat; 2 g polyunsaturated fat; 47 g carbohydrate; 8 g fiber; 26 g sugar; 379 mg phosphorus; 103 mg calcium; 5 mg iron; 165 mg sodium; 829 mg potassium; 2 IU vitamin A; 0 mg vitamin E; 0 mg vitamin C; 125 mg cholesterol

Tip: The beef also makes great sandwiches.

Ground Beef Stroganoff

Fiber up your stroganoff by using whole wheat noodles.

$^1/_2$ pound (225 g) ground beef, extra lean

$^1/_2$ cup (35 g) sliced mushrooms

1 packet onion soup mix

1 tablespoon whole wheat flour

$1^3/_4$ cups (414 ml) water

8 ounces (225 g) whole wheat noodles, cooked and drained

8 tablespoons (120 g) plain fat-free yogurt

Brown beef and drain. Add mushrooms. Whisk dry soup mix and flour into water and heat. Stir until thickened. Combine thickened onion soup and cooked beef. Serve over whole wheat noodles. Garnish with a dollop of yogurt.

Yield: 4 servings

Per serving: 178 g water; 360 calories (26% from fat, 23% from protein, 51% from carb); 21 g protein; 11 g total fat; 4 g saturated fat; 4 g monounsaturated fat; 1 g polyunsaturated fat; 48 g carbohydrate; 2 g fiber; 3 g sugar; 288 mg phosphorus; 95 mg calcium; 3 mg iron; 222 mg sodium; 397 mg potassium; 2 IU vitamin A; 1 mg vitamin E; 1 mg vitamin C; 40 mg cholesterol

Beef Stroganoff

Serve this creamy beef dish over noodles. Lima beans always seem to go well as an accompaniment to me.

1 pound (455 g) beef round steak

2 tablespoons (30 ml) olive oil

$1^1/_2$ cups (105 g) mushrooms, sliced

$^1/_2$ cup (120 ml) dry sherry

$^1/_4$ cup (60 ml) low sodium beef broth

1 cup (230 g) fat-free sour cream

Cut beef into $^1/_4$-inch (63-mm) strips. Heat oil in skillet. Cook beef quickly, 2 to 4 minutes. Remove beef from skillet. Add mushrooms to skillet and cook for 2 to 3 minutes. Remove mushrooms. Add sherry and broth to skillet and cook until liquid is reduced to about $^1/_3$ cup (80 ml). Stir in sour cream. Stir in beef and mushrooms. Heat through, but do not boil.

Yield: 4 servings

Per serving: 419 calories (36% from fat, 55% from protein, 9% from carbohydrate); 44 g protein; 13 g total fat; 3 g saturated fat; 7 g monounsaturated fat; 1 g polyunsaturated fat; 7 g carbohydrate; 0 g fiber; 1 g sugar; 341 mg phosphorus; 72 mg calcium; 4 mg iron; 89 mg sodium; 576 mg potassium; 225 IU vitamin A; 61 mg ATE vitamin E; 1 mg vitamin C; 126 mg cholesterol; 175 g water

Cholent

Cholent is a European delicacy that enabled Jews to prepare a warm Sabbath meal without violating the prohibition against cooking, since the dish is prepared on Friday and slow cooks until Sabbath lunch. If you are not preparing it in the traditional manner, it will be done in 10 to 12 hours, but the longer cooking time makes the meat even more tender and the flavors more developed.

1 cup (250 g) dried kidney beans

1 cup (208 g) dried navy beans

1 cup (225 g) dried split peas

3 pound (1 1/4 kg) beef brisket, cut into large chunks

1 1/2 cups (240 g) sliced onion

1 cup (200 g) pearl barley

4 potatoes, peeled and sliced

1/2 cup (120 ml) water

1/4 teaspoon black pepper

Boil all beans in a separate pot for 5 minutes, then drain and rinse beans. Arrange in a slow cooker layers of meat, onion, beans, barley, and potatoes. Add pepper, then water. Cover tightly. Set slow cooker on lowest setting; it will be done within 24 hours.

Yield: 10 servings

Per serving: 253 g water; 710 calories (40% from fat, 22% from protein, 38% from carb); 40 g protein; 31 g total fat; 12 g saturated fat; 13 g monounsaturated fat; 2 g polyunsaturated fat; 68 g carbohydrate; 16 g fiber; 4 g sugar; 551 mg phosphorus; 107 mg calcium; 7 mg iron; 101 mg sodium; 1749 mg potassium; 16 IU vitamin A; 0 mg vitamin E; 16 mg vitamin C; 110 mg cholesterol

Cornbread-Topped Bean Casserole

A meal in a pan. Preparation is made easier by using canned pork and beans, but the flavor definitely says homemade.

1 pound (455 g) ground beef

1/2 cup (80 g) chopped onion

2 cups (506 g) pork and beans

4 ounces (115 g) chopped green chiles, drained

2 tablespoons taco seasoning mix

1/4 cup (60 ml) water

1 1/4 cups (175 g) cornmeal

1/4 cup (31 g) flour

1 tablespoon baking powder

1 tablespoon sugar

1 cup (115 g) shredded Cheddar cheese

1 cup (235 ml) skim milk

1 egg

3 tablespoons (45 ml) canola oil

Brown ground beef and onion; drain. Stir in pork and beans, chiles, seasoning mix, and water. Spread in

8-inch (20-cm) glass baking dish. Heat oven to 350°F (180°C, gas mark 4). Combine dry ingredients. Add cheese, tossing to coat. Add remaining ingredients, stirring just until dry ingredients are moistened. Spread topping evenly over ground beef mixture. Bake 30 to 35 minutes or until wooden pick comes out clean. Let stand 5 minutes before cutting to serve.

Yield: 9 servings

Per serving: 136 g water; 402 calories (37% from fat, 22% from protein, 41% from carb); 20 g protein; 15 g total fat; 5 g saturated fat; 6 g monounsaturated fat; 2 g polyunsaturated fat; 36 g carbohydrate; 4 g fiber; 5 g sugar; 317 mg phosphorus; 281 mg calcium; 4 mg iron; 669 mg sodium; 445 mg potassium; 440 IU vitamin A; 64 mg vitamin E; 7 mg vitamin C; 78 mg cholesterol

Three Bean Casserole

If you like baked beans, but you are one of those people who want meat with their meal, this one-dish bean and beef dinner should be just the thing for you.

15 ounces (420 g) kidney beans, rinsed and drained

15 ounces (420 g) chickpeas, rinsed and drained

15 ounces (420 g) lima beans, rinsed and drained

1 pound (455 g) ground beef, extra lean

1 cup (160 g) chopped onion

$^1/_2$ teaspoon minced garlic

$^1/_4$ cup (60 g) brown sugar

$^1/_2$ teaspoon black pepper

2 tablespoons (28 ml) mustard

$^1/_2$ cup (120 ml) low-sodium ketchup

1 teaspoon cumin

$^1/_4$ cup (60 ml) water

1 tablespoon (15 ml) cider vinegar

In $2^1/_2$-quart (2.5-L) casserole dish combine beans; set aside. In skillet cook beef, onion, and garlic. Remove from heat and drain. Add remaining ingredients. Mix well. Stir beef mix into beans. Bake 350°F (180°C, gas mark 4) for 45 minutes.

Yield: 6 servings

Per serving: 246 g water; 495 calories (26% from fat, 24% from protein, 50% from carb); 30 g protein; 14 g total fat; 5 g saturated fat; 6 g monounsaturated fat; 1 g polyunsaturated fat; 63 g carbohydrate; 15 g fiber; 15 g sugar; 366 mg phosphorus; 120 mg calcium; 7 mg iron; 295 mg sodium; 1092 mg potassium; 333 IU vitamin A; 0 mg vitamin E; 13 mg vitamin C; 52 mg cholesterol

Western Casserole

A simple beef-and-noodle casserole, updated to give you more fiber without sacrificing taste.

1 pound (455 g) beef stew meat, cut in cubes

$^1/_4$ cup (30 g) whole wheat flour

$^1/_4$ cup (60 ml) olive oil

6 ounces (170 g) no-salt-added tomato paste

$^1/_2$ cup (120 ml) dry red wine

1 cup (235 ml) water

1 teaspoon thyme

1 teaspoon oregano

1 cup (70 g) sliced mushrooms

1 cup (180 g) chopped tomato

4 ounces (115 g) whole wheat noodles, cooked and drained

1 cup (115 g) shredded Cheddar cheese

Coat meat with flour; brown in oil. Add all ingredients except noodles and cheese. Cover and simmer for 1 hour. Add noodles and cheese. Simmer 5 minutes more and serve.

Yield: 4 servings

Per serving: 264 g water; 607 calories (47% from fat, 27% from protein, 26% from carb); 41 g protein; 31 g total fat; 11 g saturated fat; 15 g monounsaturated fat; 2 g polyunsaturated fat; 39 g carbohydrate; 3 g fiber; 6 g sugar; 563 mg phosphorus; 299 mg calcium; 6 mg iron; 341 mg sodium; 1114 mg potassium; 1239 IU vitamin A; 85 mg vitamin E; 20 mg vitamin C; 96 mg cholesterol

Sauerbraten

Round roasts are not the tenderest cut of beef. But marinating followed by slow, moist cooking makes this one a treat to eat, not to mention the great flavor. Serve with egg noodles.

For Marinade:

2$\frac{1}{2}$ cups (590 ml) water

1$\frac{1}{2}$ cups (355 ml) red wine vinegar

1 tablespoon (13 g) sugar

$\frac{1}{4}$ teaspoon (0.5 g) ground ginger

12 whole cloves

6 bay leaves

2 cups (320 g) onion, sliced

For Meat

4 pounds (1.8 kg) beef round roast

2 tablespoons (30 ml) olive oil

$\frac{1}{2}$ cup (65 g) carrot, finely chopped

$\frac{1}{2}$ cup (50 g) celery, finely chopped

$\frac{1}{2}$ cup (80 g) onion, finely chopped

1 cup (100 g) gingersnaps, crushed

$\frac{2}{3}$ cup (160 ml) water

In a large bowl combine the marinade ingredients. Add roast. Cover and refrigerate for 1$\frac{1}{2}$ to 2 days, turning occasionally. Remove meat and wipe dry. Strain and reserve marinade liquid.

In a Dutch oven, brown meat in oil on all sides. Add reserved marinade, carrots, celery, and onion. Cover and simmer until meat is tender, 2 to 2$\frac{1}{2}$ hours. Remove meat to platter and slice thinly. Reserve 2 cups of cooking liquid in pot. Add gingersnaps and water. Cook and stir until thickened. Serve sauce with meat.

Yield: 10 servings

Per serving: 323 calories (30% from fat, 54% from protein, 16% from carbohydrate); 41 g protein; 10 g total fat; 3 g saturated fat; 5 g monounsaturated fat; 1 g polyunsaturated fat; 12 g carbohydrate; 1 g fiber; 5 g sugar; 419 mg phosphorus; 62 mg calcium; 4 mg iron; 183 mg sodium; 792 mg potassium; 1100 IU vitamin A; 0 mg ATE vitamin E; 4 mg vitamin C; 91 mg cholesterol; 288 g water

Beef Paprikash

The origin of this meal is Hungarian. It's the kind of slow-cooker meal that greets you with a wonderful aroma when you return home from work. Stick a loaf of bread in the bread machine on timed bake and you have an instant dinner.

2 pounds (900 g) round steak, cubed

6 potatoes, cut in $^3/_4$-inch (2-cm) pieces

1 cup frozen pearl onions

$^1/_4$ cup (31 g) flour

1 tablespoon paprika

$^1/_2$ teaspoon black pepper

$^1/_4$ teaspoon caraway seed

2 cups (475 ml) low-sodium beef broth

1 cup (130 g) no-salt-added frozen peas

$^1/_2$ cup (115 g) sour cream

Add beef, potatoes, onions, flour, and spices to slow cooker. Pour beef broth over. Cover and cook on low 7 to 8 hours. Stir in peas and sour cream. Cover and cook on low about 15 minutes longer, until peas are tender.

Yield: 6 servings

Per serving: 472 g water; 590 calories (15% from fat, 36% from protein, 49% from carb); 52 g protein; 10 g total fat; 4 g saturated fat; 4 g monounsaturated fat; 1 g polyunsaturated fat; 72 g carbohydrate; 8 g fiber; 5 g sugar; 463 mg phosphorus; 76 mg calcium; 6 mg iron; 148 mg sodium; 1513 mg potassium; 1252 IU vitamin A; 20 mg vitamin E; 28 mg vitamin C; 96 mg cholesterol

Pot Roast with Root Vegetables

This is a simple fall pot roast, featuring root vegetables and not containing a lot of added ingredients. Cooking it in a covered roasting pan will ensure that the meat is very tender.

2 pound (900 g) beef bottom round roast

4 potatoes, quartered

4 turnips, peeled and cut into quarters

6 carrots, sliced

1 onion, peeled and quartered

1 parsnip, peeled and sliced

2 cups (475 ml) low-sodium beef broth

2 cups (480 g) no-salt-added canned tomatoes

Place all ingredients in large roasting pan. Cover and roast at 350°F (180°C, gas mark 4) until vegetables are done and meat is tender, about 2 hours.

Yield: 8 servings

Per serving: 383 g water; 527 calories (38% from fat, 31% from protein, 31% from carb); 40 g protein; 22 g total fat; 9 g saturated fat; 9 g monounsaturated fat; 1 g polyunsaturated fat; 41 g carbohydrate; 6 g fiber; 6 g sugar; 370 mg phosphorus; 72 mg calcium; 5 mg iron; 209 mg sodium; 1492 mg potassium; 4280 IU vitamin A; 0 mg vitamin E; 35 mg vitamin C; 108 mg cholesterol

Country Beef Stew

A hearty stew of beef and beans, perfect for a winter day.

2 tablespoons (28 ml) olive oil

2 pound (900 g) boneless beef chuck, cut into 1-inch (2.5-cm) cubes

2 cups (480 g) canned no-salt-added tomatoes

1 cup (160 g) coarsely chopped onion

$1^1/_2$ cups (355 ml) water

1 tablespoon (15 ml) Worcestershire sauce

$^3/_4$ teaspoon tarragon

$^1/_2$ teaspoon black pepper

$^1/_2$ teaspoon garlic powder

2 cups (260 g) sliced carrot

5 cups (885 g) cooked great northern beans, drained

In large kettle or Dutch oven, heat oil until hot. Add half of the beef and brown on all sides. Remove with slotted spoon and repeat with remaining beef. Return meat to kettle. Add tomatoes, onion, water, Worcestershire sauce, tarragon, black pepper, and garlic powder. Bring to a boil. Reduce heat and simmer, covered, until meat is almost tender, about 1 hour. Add carrot. Simmer, covered, until carrot and meat are tender, about 20 minutes. Stir in beans and cook until beans are heated through, about 5 minutes.

Yield: 8 servings

Per serving: 321 g water; 587 calories (40% from fat, 31% from protein, 29% from carb); 46 g protein; 26 g total fat; 9 g saturated fat; 10 g monounsaturated fat; 3 g polyunsaturated fat; 42 g carbohydrate; 10 g fiber; 4 g sugar; 452 mg phosphorus; 141 mg calcium; 6 mg iron; 110 mg sodium; 1102 mg potassium; 5455 IU vitamin A; 0 mg vitamin E; 15 mg vitamin C; 108 mg cholesterol

Beef and Barley Stew

A hearty stew that makes a meal in a bowl (although I prefer it with a slice of fresh hot bread).

$1^1/_2$ pounds (675 g) beef round steak

$^1/_4$ cup (31 g) flour

2 tablespoons (28 ml) olive oil

1 cup (160 g) chopped onion

$^1/_2$ teaspoon crushed garlic

3 cups (710 ml) low-sodium beef broth

2 cups (260 g) sliced carrot

$^1/_4$ cup (50 g) pearl barley

1 tablespoon (15 ml) Dick's Reduced Sodium Soy Sauce (see recipe page 25)

$^1/_2$ teaspoon oregano

$^1/_2$ cup (50 g) chopped celery

$^1/_2$ teaspoon black pepper

Trim fat from meat and cut into bite-size cubes. Dust beef with flour. Using a heavy pot, brown beef in hot oil, browning all sides. Remove meat and set aside. Add onion and garlic to drippings and cook until onion is transparent. Return the meat to pot. Add broth, barley, soy sauce, and oregano. Cover and simmer for 45 minutes. Add carrot and celery and simmer until meat is tender, about 40 minutes. Add water as needed. Season with pepper.

Yield: 6 servings

Per serving: 257 g water; 352 calories (28% from fat, 52% from protein, 20% from carb); 45 g protein; 11 g total fat; 3 g saturated fat; 6 g monounsaturated fat; 1 g polyunsaturated fat; 17 g carbohydrate; 3 g fiber; 3 g sugar; 327 mg phosphorus; 42 mg calcium; 5 mg iron; 210 mg sodium; 693 mg potassium; 7222 IU vitamin A; 0 mg vitamin E; 5 mg vitamin C; 102 mg cholesterol

Irish Stew

This has become our traditional meal for St. Patrick's Day.

2 pounds (900 g) beef stew meat

$^1/_2$ teaspoon minced garlic

$^1/_4$ teaspoon black pepper, fresh ground

1 cup (160 g) halved and sliced onion

12 ounces (355 ml) dark beer

2 cups (475 ml) low-sodium beef broth

3 tablespoons (48 g) no-salt-added tomato paste

2 cups (260 g) sliced carrot

4 potatoes, cut into quarters

2 turnips, cut into quarters

1 teaspoon rosemary

2 bay leaves

$^1/_4$ cup (32 g) cornstarch

$^1/_2$ cup (120 ml) water

Combine all ingredients except the cornstarch and water in a slow cooker and cook on low for 8 hours. Combine the cornstarch and water in a bowl and stir into the stew. Turn to high, cover the slow cooker, and allow the stew to cook an additional 30 minutes, until thickened slightly.

Yield: 8 servings

Per serving: 420 g water; 461 calories (24% from fat, 38% from protein, 38% from carb); 43 g protein; 12 g total fat; 4 g saturated fat; 5 g monounsaturated fat; 1 g polyunsaturated fat; 43 g carbohydrate; 6 g fiber; 7 g sugar; 387 mg phosphorus; 64 mg calcium; 5 mg iron; 156 mg sodium; 1464 mg potassium; 5489 IU vitamin A; 0 mg vitamin E; 30 mg vitamin C; 127 mg cholesterol

Tip: You could also use lamb in place of the beef if desired.

Eggplant Stew

This recipe is a nice variation on the beef stew theme, with different vegetables and spices than you probably usually use.

1$^1/_2$ pounds (675 g) beef stew meat, cubed

2 tablespoons (28 ml) olive oil

2 cups (480 g) no-salt-added canned tomatoes

1 cup (160 g) chopped onion

2 tablespoons (32 g) no-salt-added tomato paste

$^1/_2$ teaspoon oregano

$^1/_2$ teaspoon basil

$^1/_2$ teaspoon cumin

$^1/_4$ teaspoon red pepper flakes

$^1/_2$ teaspoon garlic powder

1 cup (235 ml) water

1 potato, peeled and cubed

1 cup (235 ml) white wine

1 eggplant, peeled and cubed

1 cup (70 g) sliced mushrooms

In a Dutch oven, brown half the beef at a time in the oil. Drain and return all meat to the pan. Add tomatoes, onion, tomato paste, and spices. Stir in water. Bring to a boil. Reduce heat and simmer, covered, for 45 minutes. Add potato and wine. Cover and simmer 10 minutes more. Stir in eggplant and mushrooms. Cover and simmer until meat and veggies are tender, 15 to 20 minutes.

Yield: 6 servings

Per serving: 356 g water; 504 calories (50% from fat, 30% from protein, 19% from carb); 36 g protein; 27 g total fat; 9 g saturated fat; 13 g monounsaturated fat; 1 g polyunsaturated fat; 23 g carbohydrate; 5 g fiber; 7 g

sugar; 283 mg phosphorus; 71 mg calcium; 4 mg iron; 78 mg sodium; 921 mg potassium; 217 IU vitamin A; 0 mg vitamin E; 17 mg vitamin C; 108 mg cholesterol

Peasant Soup

A quick soup using leftover roast beef. A round roast, trimmed of fat, is a good choice. This is a warming meal on a cold evening, needing just bread to make it complete.

1 pound (455 g) leftover roast beef, chopped

2 cups (470 ml) low sodium beef broth

1 cup (180 g) canned no-salt-added tomatoes

1 pound (455 g) frozen mixed vegetables, thawed

1 cup (70 g) cabbage, shredded

$^1/_2$ cup (75 g) turnips, cubed

Combine all ingredients in a large Dutch oven. Simmer until vegetables are tender, around 45 minutes.

Yield: 6 servings

Per serving: 198 calories (24% from fat, 50% from protein, 26% from carbohydrate); 25 g protein; 5 g total fat; 2 g saturated fat; 2 g monounsaturated fat; 0 g polyunsaturated fat; 13 g carbohydrate; 4 g fiber; 4 g sugar; 197 mg phosphorus; 51 mg calcium; 3 mg iron; 503 mg sodium; 467 mg potassium; 3295 IU vitamin A; 0 mg ATE vitamin E; 13 mg vitamin C; 67 mg cholesterol; 254 g water

Beef and Mushroom Stew

This is a simple and hearty slow-cooker stew, but one with a lot of flavor. It goes well with just a simple multigrain bread to make a complete meal.

1$^1/_2$ pounds (680 g) beef round steak, cut into $^1/_2$-inch (1.3-cm) cubes

1 can (14 ounces, or 395 g) low sodium beef broth

$^1/_2$ cup (120 ml) red wine

$^1/_4$ teaspoon (0.5 g) freshly ground black pepper

5 medium potatoes, cubed

1$^1/_3$ cups (195 g) carrot, sliced

1 cup (70 g) mushrooms, sliced

1 bay leaf

$^1/_4$ teaspoon (0.3 g) dried rosemary

2 cups (360 g) canned no-salt-added tomatoes

3 tablespoons (24 g) flour

$^1/_4$ cup (60 ml) water

Combine first 9 ingredients (through rosemary) and place in slow cooker. Cover and cook on low for 8 to 10 hours. About 45 minutes to 1 hour before done, turn heat to high. Add tomatoes. Stir flour and water together to make a paste and stir into stew. Cook until slightly thickened.

Yield: 6 servings

Per serving: 507 calories (12% from fat, 40% from protein, 48% from carbohydrate); 50 g protein; 7 g total fat; 2 g saturated fat; 2 g monounsaturated fat; 1 g polyunsaturated fat; 59 g carbohydrate; 7 g fiber; 7 g sugar; 501 mg phosphorus; 79 mg calcium; 7 mg iron; 158 mg sodium; 2140 mg potassium; 4898 IU vitamin A; 0 mg ATE vitamin E; 36 mg vitamin C; 102 mg cholesterol; 549 g water

Fall Stew

Apple cider gives this stew its unique flavor.

3 tablespoons (24 g) flour

$^1/_4$ teaspoon (0.5 g) black pepper

$^1/_4$ teaspoon (0.3 g) dried thyme

2 pounds (905 g) beef round steak, cut in 1-inch (2.5-cm) cubes

3 tablespoons (45 ml) olive oil

2 cups (470 ml) apple cider

2 tablespoons (30 ml) cider vinegar

3 medium potatoes, peeled and quartered

$1^1/_2$ cups (195 g) carrot, sliced

1 cup (160 g) onion, quartered

$^1/_2$ cup (50 g) celery, sliced

Combine flour, pepper, and thyme. Dredge meat in flour mixture. Heat oil in Dutch oven. Brown half the meat at a time in the oil. Return all meat to the pan. Stir in cider and vinegar. Cook and stir until mixture boils. Reduce heat, cover and simmer $1^1/_4$ hours, or until the meat is tender. Stir in potatoes, carrot, onion, and celery. Cover and cook until vegetables are done, about 30 minutes more.

Yield: 8 servings

Per serving: 430 calories (24% from fat, 42% from protein, 34% from carbohydrate); 44 g protein; 11 g total fat; 3 g saturated fat; 6 g monounsaturated fat; 1 g polyunsaturated fat; 36 g carbohydrate; 3 g fiber; 10 g sugar; 361 mg phosphorus; 36 mg calcium; 5 mg iron; 89 mg sodium; 1193 mg potassium; 4077 IU vitamin A; 0 mg ATE vitamin E; 18 mg vitamin C; 102 mg cholesterol; 256 g water

Cabbage Beef Soup

This is one of those throw-together meals that turned out to be a keeper. It's quick and easy and has a lot of flavor.

$^1/_2$ pound (225 g) extra-lean ground beef (93% lean)

$^1/_2$ cup (80 g) onion, chopped

1 cup (70 g) cabbage, shredded

1 cup (180 g) canned no-salt-added tomatoes

2 cups (450 g) Mexican beans

1 cup (235 ml) water

Brown beef and onion in a large saucepan. Drain. Add cabbage and continue cooking until cabbage is soft, about 5 minutes. Add tomatoes, beans, and water. Bring to a boil and simmer 10 minutes to blend the flavors.

Yield: 5 servings

Per serving: 213 calories (16% from fat, 37% from protein, 47% from carbohydrate); 16 g protein; 3 g total fat; 1 g saturated fat; 1 g monounsaturated fat; 0 g polyunsaturated fat; 20 g carbohydrate; 8 g fiber; 2 g sugar; 179 mg phosphorus; 77 mg calcium; 4 mg iron; 44 mg sodium; 570 mg potassium; 76 IU vitamin A; 0 mg ATE vitamin E; 13 mg vitamin C; 31 mg cholesterol; 199 g water

Tip: For variety, replace the cabbage with packaged coleslaw or broccoli slaw mix.

Beef and Black Bean Stew

Not quite a chili, but with a definite southwestern flavor, this one is always a big hit at our house.

2 pounds (905 g) extra-lean ground beef (93% lean)

$^1/_2$ teaspoon (1.5 g) minced garlic

1 cup (160 g) onion, chopped

2 cups (360 g) canned no-salt-added tomatoes

1 cup (225 g) salsa

1 teaspoon (2.5 g) ground cumin

$1/_2$ teaspoon (1 g) freshly ground black pepper

1 cup (170 g) frozen corn, thawed

2 cups (450 g) black beans, drained and rinsed

1 tablespoon (4 g) chopped fresh cilantro

In a large skillet, brown ground beef with garlic and onion. Drain and transfer to a slow cooker. Add tomatoes, salsa, cumin, pepper, corn, and black beans. Cook on low 6 to 8 hours or on high for 3 to 4 hours. Add cilantro during the last hour of cooking.

Yield: 8 servings

Per serving: 369 calories (28% from fat, 41% from protein, 32% from carbohydrate); 27 g protein; 8 g total fat; 3 g saturated fat; 3 g monounsaturated fat; 1 g polyunsaturated fat; 21 g carbohydrate; 6 g fiber; 4 g sugar; 268 mg phosphorus; 55 mg calcium; 4 mg iron; 282 mg sodium; 779 mg potassium; 238 IU vitamin A; 0 mg ATE vitamin E; 9 mg vitamin C; 78 mg cholesterol; 220 g water

Tip: To make a meal, top with grated cheese, guacamole, or sour cream, and serve with tortilla chips or cornbread.

Scottish Oxtail Soup

Oxtails may be difficult to find, although you might get some from an old-fashioned butcher or meat market. Here, in the metropolitan Washington, DC, area, I can occasionally get oxtails from the meat department at some of the Giant Food supermarkets.

1 bay leaf

2 tablespoons (4.8 g) fresh thyme

$1/_4$ cup (15 g) fresh parsley

$1/_2$ cup (50 g) celery, chopped, plus one 4-inch (10-cm) piece celery stalk

2 scallions

4 cups (946 ml) low sodium beef broth

1 pound (455 g) oxtail, cut into pieces, fat removed

$1/_2$ cup (80 g) onion, chopped

$1/_2$ cup (65 g) carrot, chopped

4 ounces (115 g) no-salt-added tomato sauce

1 tablespoon (8 g) flour

3 tablespoons (45 ml) port wine

Make a spice bag by placing bay leaf, thyme, parsley (including stalks), one 4-inch (10-cm) piece celery stalk with leaves, and scallions in the center of a square of double thickness cheesecloth. Fold up the sides of the cheesecloth and tie off the top very tightly. Pour the beef broth into a saucepan and add the oxtail and onion, carrot, tomato sauce, and remaining celery, as well as the spice bag. Bring to a boil, and then transfer to a slow cooker and cook on high for $1/_2$- 2 hours (or longer if necessary) until the meat is tender. Strain the stock, cut all the meat from the bones and then return the stock and meat to the saucepan. Bring to a boil. Mix the flour and port together and add to the soup. Simmer for 5 minutes before serving.

Yield: 6 servings

Per serving: 148 calories (23% from fat, 56% from protein, 21% from carbohydrate); 19 g protein; 3 g total fat; 1 g saturated fat; 2 g monounsaturated fat; 0 g polyunsaturated fat; 7 g carbohydrate; 2 g fiber; 3 g sugar; 198 mg phosphorus; 63 mg calcium; 4 mg iron; 161 mg sodium; 566 mg potassium; 2187 IU vitamin A; 0 mg ATE vitamin E; 9 mg vitamin C; 29 mg cholesterol; 269 g water

8

Main Dishes:
Pork

Like beef, pork doesn't have to be as bad for you as it is often portrayed. Most of these recipes use lean cuts of pork from the loin, either as chops or roasts. This lets you get the great taste of pork done up in a variety of ways, from Southern to Indian, without worrying about eating heart healthy.

Skillet Pork Chops

This is a great skillet meal. Not exactly typical Hamburger Helper fare, but the kind of thing that you would want to serve on the patio after a summer day of working in the yard.

6 pork loin chops

1 tablespoon (15 ml) olive oil

1 cup (160 g) onion, chopped

$1/2$ teaspoon (1.5 g) minced garlic

$1/2$ cup (120 ml) low sodium chicken broth

$1/2$ cup (120 ml) barbecue sauce

4 cups (900 g) no-salt-added canned pinto beans, drained

2 jalapeno peppers, chopped

In a large skillet, sear pork chops in oil for 5 minutes, or until brown. Remove pork chops and place on a plate. Add onion and garlic to skillet; cook 10 minutes. Stir in broth, barbecue sauce, beans, and jalapenos. Heat mixture to a boil. Return pork to skillet. Reduce heat; cover and simmer 50 to 60 minutes, stirring sauce and turning chops occasionally until meat is fork-tender.

Yield: 6 servings

Per serving: 370 calories (18% from fat, 35% from protein, 47% from carbohydrate); 33 g protein; 7 g total fat; 2 g saturated fat; 4 g monounsaturated fat; 1 g polyunsaturated fat; 43 g carbohydrate; 11 g fiber; 9 g sugar; 403 mg phosphorus; 73 mg calcium; 3 mg iron; 261 mg sodium; 938 mg potassium; 45 IU vitamin A; 2 mg ATE vitamin E; 6 mg vitamin C; 64 mg cholesterol; 206 g water

Grilled Pork Chops

A quick and easy grill recipe for a summer evening. You could make a little extra of the marinade and put it on zucchini slices to grill as a side dish.

2 tablespoons (30 ml) honey

$1/4$ cup (60 ml) Worcestershire sauce

$1/4$ teaspoon (0.5 g) black pepper

$1/4$ teaspoon (0.8 g) garlic powder

4 boneless pork loin chops

In a shallow glass dish or bowl, mix together honey, Worcestershire sauce, pepper, and garlic powder. Add pork chops and toss to coat. Cover and refrigerate for no more than 4 hours. Lightly oil grill and preheat to medium. Remove pork chops from marinade. Grill 20 to 30 minutes, or until cooked through, turning often.

Yield: 4 servings

Per serving: 174 calories (22% from fat, 50% from protein, 27% from carbohydrate); 22 g protein; 4 g total fat; 1 g saturated fat; 2 g monounsaturated fat; 0 g polyunsaturated fat; 12 g carbohydrate; 0 g fiber; 9 g sugar; 238 mg phosphorus; 14 mg calcium; 2 mg iron; 199 mg sodium; 503 mg potassium; 24 IU vitamin A; 2 mg ATE vitamin E; 28 mg vitamin C; 64 mg cholesterol; 80 g water

Barbecue Pork Chops

A nice sweet-and-sour sort of barbecue sauce gives these chops great flavor.

4 pork loin chops, 1 inch (2.5 cm) thick

1 cup (160 g) onion, finely chopped

2 tablespoons (30 ml) vinegar

1 tablespoon (15 ml) canola oil

$1/2$ teaspoon (1.5 g) dry mustard

1 tablespoon (15 ml) Worcestershire sauce

1 teaspoon (2 g) black pepper

1 tablespoon (13 g) sugar

$1/2$ teaspoon (1.3 g) paprika

Score the edges of the chops to prevent curling. Place into a large baking pan; set aside. Combine remaining ingredients and mix well. Pour over the chops to coat well. Cover and chill for 2 to 4 hours. Grill chops to desired doneness, basting often.

Yield: 4 servings

Per serving: 196 calories (37% from fat, 46% from protein, 17% from carbohydrate); 22 g protein; 8 g total fat; 2 g saturated fat; 4 g monounsaturated fat; 2 g polyunsaturated fat; 8 g carbohydrate; 1 g fiber; 5 g sugar; 238 mg phosphorus; 26 mg calcium; 1 mg iron; 91 mg sodium; 482 mg potassium; 166 IU vitamin A; 2 mg ATE vitamin E; 11 mg vitamin C; 64 mg cholesterol; 118 g water

Southern Pork Chops

Slow-cooked stuffed pork chops. Great with greens and cornbread.

4 pork loin chops, 1 inch (2.5 cm) thick

2 cups (215 g) cornbread stuffing mix

2 tablespoons (30 ml) low sodium chicken broth

$1/3$ cup (80 ml) orange juice

1 tablespoon (8 g) pecans, finely chopped

$1/4$ cup (60 ml) light corn syrup

$1/2$ teaspoon (0.9 g) grated orange peel

With a sharp knife, cut a horizontal slit in side of each chop forming a pocket for stuffing. Combine stuffing with remaining ingredients. Fill pockets with stuffing mixture. Place chops on a metal rack in a slow cooker. Cover and cook on low for 6 to 8 hours. Uncover; turn to high and brush with sauce again. Cook on high for 15 to 20 minutes.

Yield: 4 servings

Per serving: 322 calories (19% from fat, 31% from protein, 50% from carbohydrate); 25 g protein; 7 g total fat; 2 g saturated fat; 3 g monounsaturated fat; 1 g polyunsaturated fat; 41 g carbohydrate; 4 g fiber; 7 g sugar; 262 mg phosphorus; 42 mg calcium; 2 mg iron; 431 mg sodium; 485 mg potassium; 70 IU vitamin A; 2 mg ATE vitamin E; 9 mg vitamin C; 64 mg cholesterol; 106 g water

Stuffed Pork Chops

These make an elegant meal. If possible, get the meat cutter at the store to cut the slit in the chops. The idea is to open it up inside, but not cut the whole way around the chop, so it's easier to close back up.

6 pork loin chops, cut 1$^{1}/_{2}$ inches (3.8 cm) thick

1 tablespoon (15 ml) olive oil

$^{1}/_{4}$ cup (37 g) green bell peppers, chopped

$^{1}/_{4}$ cup (40 g) onion, chopped

1 egg

1$^{1}/_{2}$ cups (120 g) bread cubes

$^{1}/_{4}$ teaspoon (0.6 g) cumin

Make a slit in each chop to allow for stuffing. Heat oil in a small skillet over medium heat. Cook green bell pepper and onion until soft. Combine egg, bread, and cumin in a bowl. Pour pepper and onion mixture over bread mixture and toss to combine. Spoon an equal amount of the stuffing into the pocket of each chop. Secure with a wooden toothpick or skewer. Grill over medium heat about 20 minutes. Turn and grill 15 minutes more, or until done.

Yield: 6 servings

Per serving: 193 calories (36% from fat, 50% from protein, 14% from carbohydrate); 24 g protein; 7 g total fat; 2 g saturated fat; 4 g monounsaturated fat; 1 g polyunsaturated fat; 7 g carbohydrate; 1 g fiber; 1 g sugar; 245 mg phosphorus; 27 mg calcium; 2 mg iron; 123 mg sodium; 340 mg potassium; 69 IU vitamin A; 2 mg ATE vitamin E; 6 mg vitamin C; 99 mg cholesterol; 95 g water

Tip: If you have some raisin bread on hand, it's great in this recipe.

Pineapple-Stuffed Pork Chops

Feel like you need a trip to the islands? Let these pineapple-stuffed chops ferry you away.

4 pork loin chops, 1 inch (2.5-cm) thick

8 ounces (225 g) pineapple slices canned in juice, undrained

$^{1}/_{4}$ cup (60 g) low sodium ketchup

1 tablespoon (6 g) scallions, chopped

$^{1}/_{2}$ teaspoon (1.5 g) dry mustard

Cut a pocket in each chop to make room for pineapple. Drain pineapple, reserving liquid. Cut two pineapple slices in half; cut up remaining pineapple and set aside. Place a half pineapple slice in the pocket of each chop. Heat grill to medium and grill about 20 minutes, turning once. Meanwhile, in a small saucepan combine ketchup, scallions, mustard, and the reserved pineapple juice and pieces. Heat to boiling, reduce heat and simmer 10 minutes. Grill chops 5 minutes more, brushing with sauce and turning several times.

Yield: 4 servings

Per serving: 189 calories (21% from fat, 46% from protein, 33% from carbohydrate); 22 g protein; 4 g total fat; 1 g saturated fat; 2 g monounsaturated fat; 0 g polyunsaturated fat; 15 g carbohydrate; 1 g fiber; 13 g sugar; 230 mg phosphorus; 25 mg calcium; 1 mg iron; 55 mg sodium; 495 mg potassium; 171 IU vitamin A; 2 mg ATE vitamin E; 8 mg vitamin C; 64 mg cholesterol; 131 g water

Hawaiian Kabobs

Serve these with rice for an island treat.

$^1/_2$ cup (120 ml) Dick's Reduced Sodium Soy Sauce (see recipe page 25)

2 tablespoons (30 ml) olive oil

1 tablespoon (15 g) brown sugar

$^1/_2$ teaspoon (1.5 g) minced garlic

1 teaspoon (3 g) dry mustard

1 teaspoon (1.8 g) ground ginger

2 pounds (905 g) pork tenderloin, cut in 1-inch (2.5-cm) cubes

2 cups (300 g) green bell peppers, cut in 1-inch (2.5-cm) pieces

20 cherry tomatoes

6 ounces (170 g) pineapple chunks

In a large bowl combine soy sauce, oil, brown sugar, garlic, mustard, and ginger. Add pork cubes; cover and refrigerate overnight. Drain meat, reserving marinade. Thread meat, green bell pepper, tomatoes, and pineapple on skewers. Grill over medium-hot fire for 15 minutes, or until pork is done. Baste with marinade with cooking.

Yield: 6 servings

Per serving: 279 calories (11% from fat, 17% from protein, 72% from carbohydrate); 33 g protein; 10 g total fat; 2 g saturated fat; 6 g monounsaturated fat; 4 g polyunsaturated fat; 140 g carbohydrate; 2 g fiber; 8 g sugar; 370 mg phosphorus; 34 mg calcium; 2 mg iron; 217 mg sodium; 867 mg potassium; 566 IU vitamin A; 3 mg ATE vitamin E; 54 mg vitamin C; 98 mg cholesterol; 213 g water

Pork Chop and Bean Skillet

This makes a good dinner with fried potatoes.

6 center-cut pork chops

1 tablespoon (15 ml) olive oil

1 cup (160 g) chopped onion

$^1/_2$ teaspoon minced garlic

$^1/_2$ cup (120 ml) low-sodium chicken broth

$^1/_2$ cup (125 g) barbecue sauce

2 jalapeño peppers, chopped

4 cups (684 g) no-salt-added pinto beans, drained

In a large skillet, sear pork chops in oil until brown, about 5 minutes. Remove pork chops and place on plate. Add onion and garlic to skillet; cook 10 minutes. Stir in broth, barbecue sauce, jalapeños, and beans. Heat mixture to a boil. Return pork to skillet. Reduce heat. Cover and simmer 50 to 60 minutes, stirring sauce and turning chops occasionally until meat is fork-tender.

Yield: 6 servings

Per serving: 171 g water; 401 calories (23% from fat, 33% from protein, 43% from carb); 34 g protein; 10 g total fat; 3 g saturated fat; 5 g monounsaturated fat; 1 g polyunsaturated fat; 43 g carbohydrate; 11 g fiber; 9 g sugar; 370 mg phosphorus; 76 mg calcium; 3 mg iron; 269 mg sodium; 874 mg potassium; 43 IU vitamin A; 1 mg vitamin E; 6 mg vitamin C; 63 mg cholesterol

Tip: You can either use canned no-salt-added beans or cook your own dried ones.

Apple and Pork Chop Skillet

A newsletter subscriber originally sent in this recipe. It's just spicy enough to satisfy even those people who aren't on a diet.

1 tablespoon (15 ml) olive oil

$^1/_2$ cup (80 g) onion, chopped

3 pork loin chops

2 tablespoons (13 g) fresh ginger, peeled and thinly sliced

1 apple, peeled and thinly sliced

$^1/_2$ cup (120 ml) water

Heat oil in a nonstick skillet over medium heat. Sauté the chopped onion for 2 to 4 minutes, or until lightly browned. Push the onion pieces to one side of the skillet and place the chops in the center of the skillet. Brown the chops on each side. Spoon the onion pieces on top of each chop, dividing evenly. Layer each chop with sliced ginger and apple. Add the water to the skillet and cover tightly. Cook over low heat for 30 to 40 minutes depending on the thickness of the pork chops.

Yield: 3 servings

Per serving: 213 calories (39% from fat, 42% from protein, 20% from carbohydrate); 22 g protein; 9 g total fat; 2 g saturated fat; 5 g monounsaturated fat; 1 g polyunsaturated fat; 10 g carbohydrate; 1 g fiber; 6 g sugar; 238 mg phosphorus; 27 mg calcium; 1 mg iron; 55 mg sodium; 500 mg potassium; 29 IU vitamin A; 2 mg ATE vitamin E; 5 mg vitamin C; 64 mg cholesterol; 175 g water

Pork and Chickpea Stir-Fry

Another quick, tasty, nutritious dinner.

$^1/_2$ pound (225 g) boneless pork loin chops, cut into $1^1/_2$-inch-thick (4-cm) strips

$^1/_4$ cup (25 g) sliced scallions, with tops

$^1/_2$ teaspoon crushed garlic

2 teaspoons (10 ml) olive oil

$1^1/_2$ cups (106 g) broccoli florets

10 ounces (280 g) chickpeas, drained and rinsed

$^1/_4$ cup (60 ml) low-sodium beef broth

$^1/_4$ cup (60 ml) Dick's Reduced Sodium Soy Sauce (see recipe page 25)

2 teaspoons cornstarch

1 cup (220 g) cooked brown rice

Stir-fry pork, scallions, and garlic in oil in wok or large skillet over high heat until pork is browned, 3 to 5 minutes. Add broccoli and stir-fry 2 to 3 minutes. Add chickpeas and cook, covered, over medium heat until broccoli is crisp-tender, 3 to 4 minutes. Combine broth, soy sauce, and cornstarch. Stir into mixture. Cook and stir until thickened. Serve over rice.

Yield: 4 servings

Per serving: 176 g water; 287 calories (22% from fat, 30% from protein, 49% from carb); 21 g protein; 7 g total fat; 1 g saturated fat; 3 g monounsaturated fat; 2 g polyunsaturated fat; 35 g carbohydrate; 7 g fiber; 4 g sugar; 323 mg phosphorus; 69 mg calcium; 3 mg iron; 185 mg sodium; 579 mg potassium; 884 IU vitamin A; 1 mg vitamin E; 28 mg vitamin C; 36 mg cholesterol

Pork and Apple Curry

Curry flavor creates a new kind of pork dish.

2 tablespoons (30 ml) olive oil

4 pork loin chops

$^1/_2$ cup (80 g) onion, thinly sliced

$^1/_4$ teaspoon (0.8 g) minced garlic

1 apple, peeled and sliced

$^1/_2$ cup (75 g) red bell pepper, cut in strips

$^1/_2$ cup (120 ml) low sodium chicken broth

1 teaspoon (2 g) cornstarch

1 teaspoon (2 g) curry powder

$^1/_2$ teaspoon (1.3 g) ground cumin

$^1/_2$ teaspoon (1.2 g) cinnamon

$^1/_4$ teaspoon (0.5 g) freshly ground black pepper

In a heavy frying pan, heat oil over medium-high heat. Cook pork chops until browned on both sides and almost cooked through; remove from pan and set aside. Over medium heat, cook the onion, garlic, apple, and red bell pepper strips for 2 minutes or until softened. Blend chicken broth with cornstarch; add to pan along with curry powder, cumin, and cinnamon; cook for 1 or 2 minutes, or until slightly reduced and thickened. Return pork chops to frying pan. Cook for 1 or 2 minutes or until heated through. Serve pork chops with sauce and sprinkle with pepper.

Yield: 4 servings

Per serving: 228 calories (45% from fat, 39% from protein, 15% from carbohydrate); 23 g protein; 11 g total fat; 3 g saturated fat; 7 g monounsaturated fat; 1 g polyunsaturated fat; 9 g carbohydrate; 2 g fiber; 5 g sugar; 247 mg phosphorus; 31 mg calcium; 2 mg iron; 63 mg sodium; 513 mg potassium; 612 IU vitamin A; 2 mg ATE vitamin E; 28 mg vitamin C; 64 mg cholesterol; 166 g water

Tip: Serve with quick-cooking couscous flavored with chopped scallions and raisins.

Glazed Pork Roast

I actually grill this when it's warm enough. If you want to do that, it's best to grill using indirect heat. Place a pan of water under the roast and mound the charcoal around it. Close the grill to hold in the heat and smoke. This makes excellent sandwiches when sliced thinly and served cold.

$^1/_4$ cup (60 ml) honey

1 tablespoon (9 g) dry mustard

$^1/_4$ cup (60 ml) white wine vinegar

1 teaspoon (2.6 g) chili powder

2 pounds (905 g) pork tenderloin

Preheat oven to 350°F (180°C, or gas mark 4). Mix together the first 4 ingredients. Trim excess fat from pork roast. Brush with honey glaze. Roast for 1 to $1^1/_2$ hours, or until done, brushing with additional glaze occasionally.

Yield: 8 servings

Per serving: 173 calories (22% from fat, 57% from protein, 21% from carbohydrate); 24 g protein; 4 g total fat; 1 g saturated fat; 2 g monounsaturated fat; 0 g polyunsaturated fat; 9 g carbohydrate; 0 g fiber; 9 g sugar; 258 mg phosphorus; 9 mg calcium; 2 mg iron; 61 mg sodium; 436 mg potassium; 101 IU vitamin A; 2 mg ATE vitamin E; 1 mg vitamin C; 74 mg cholesterol; 94 g water

Stuffed Pork Roast

This pork loin is filled with a traditional cornbread stuffing. If you put a drip pan under the roast during the indirect cooking phase and add some water to it, you will end up with the makings of a delicious gravy. Remember not to let the drip pan dry out.

2 tablespoons (30 ml) olive oil

$^1/_2$ cup (160 g) onion, chopped

1 teaspoon (3 g) minced garlic

1 tablespoon (2 g) dried sage, chopped

4 cups (600 g) Lower Fat Cornbread, cubed (see recipe page 445)

1 egg

1 cup (235 ml) low sodium chicken broth

2 pounds (905 g) pork loin roast

In a skillet, heat oil over medium-high heat. Add onions and garlic and cook until tender. Add sage and cook for about 30 seconds. Remove from heat and add cornbread, onion mixture, and egg. Stir, adding the chicken broth slowly until it becomes spreadable (it should look like stuffing). Butterfly the pork loin. Spread stuffing over the pork loin and roll up. Secure with kitchen twine at 1-inch (2.5-cm) intervals. Preheat grill and prepare for indirect grilling. Place pork loin on grill over direct heat. Turn every two minutes until the surface of the pork loin is seared. Move to indirect portion of grill and continue cooking for about 30 minutes or until the meat reaches an internal temperature of 155°F (68°C). Remove from grill and let rest for 5 minutes. Slice and serve.

Yield: 8 servings

Per serving: 371 calories (31% from fat, 38% from protein, 31% from carbohydrate); 28 g protein; 10 g total fat; 3 g saturated fat; 6 g monounsaturated fat; 2 g polyunsaturated fat; 24 g carbohydrate; 3 g fiber; 4 g sugar; 303 mg phosphorus; 53 mg calcium; 2 mg iron; 222 mg sodium; 452 mg potassium; 391 IU vitamin A; 75 mg ATE vitamin E; 3 mg vitamin C; 102 mg cholesterol; 193 g water

Pork Loin Roast

This pork roast has a Latin flavor. The sauce is good over rice or noodles.

3 pounds (1.4 kg) pork loin roast

1 tablespoon (7.5 g) chili powder

$^1/_2$ cup (120 ml) lime juice

1 teaspoon (2.5 g) cumin

1 teaspoon (1 g) dried oregano

$^1/_2$ teaspoon (1 g) black pepper

$^1/_2$ teaspoon (1.5 g) minced garlic

6 ounces (170 g) orange juice concentrate, thawed, divided

$^1/_4$ cup (60 ml) dry white wine

$^1/_2$ cup (115 g) fat free sour cream

Place pork roast in a shallow glass dish. Mix chili powder, lime juice, cumin, oregano, pepper, garlic, and $^1/_4$ cup (60 ml) of orange juice concentrate and brush mixture onto the pork roast. Cover and refrigerate at least 8 hours. Preheat oven to 325°F (170°C, or gas mark 3). Place pork on a rack in a shallow roasting pan. Roast uncovered for $1^1/_2$ to 2 hours, or until thermometer registers 170°F (77°C). Remove pork and rack from the pan. Strain the drippings from the pan and set aside. Add enough water to remaining orange juice concentrate to measure $^3/_4$ cup (180 ml); stir juice and wine into the drippings, then stir in the sour cream. Serve with the pork roast.

Yield: 9 servings

Per serving: 255 calories (26% from fat, 57% from protein, 17% from carbohydrate); 33 g protein; 7 g total fat; 2 g saturated fat; 3 g monounsaturated fat; 1 g polyunsaturated fat; 10 g carbohydrate; 1 g fiber; 7 g sugar; 361 mg phosphorus; 49 mg calcium; 2 mg iron; 93 mg sodium; 748 mg potassium; 397 IU vitamin A; 16 mg ATE vitamin E; 32 mg vitamin C; 100 mg cholesterol; 151 g water

Pork Loin Roast with Asian Vegetables

Serve this Asian-style pork roast with rice for a complete meal.

1 teaspoon (1.8 g) ground ginger

2 tablespoons (30 ml) olive oil

2 pounds (905 g) pork loin roast

$1^1/_4$ cups (295 ml) water, divided

1 cup (160 g) onion, coarsely chopped

$^1/_4$ cup (60 ml) Dick's Reduced Sodium Soy Sauce (see recipe page 25)

$^1/_4$ cup (60 ml) red wine vinegar

2 tablespoons (30 g) brown sugar

$^1/_2$ teaspoon (1.5 g) garlic powder

$^1/_4$ teaspoon (0.5 g) black pepper

4 cups (250 g) snow pea pods

2 cups (360 g) canned no-salt-added tomatoes, undrained

8 ounces (225 g) water chestnuts

1 cup mushrooms (70 g), sliced

2 tablespoons (16 g) cornstarch

In a large Dutch oven, sauté ginger in oil for 30 seconds. Add pork roast and brown meat on all sides. Add 1 cup (235 ml) water, onion, soy sauce, vinegar, brown sugar, garlic powder, and pepper. Cover and simmer for $1^1/_2$ hours, or until tender. Add pea pods, tomatoes and liquid, water chestnuts, and mushrooms. Cover and simmer for 3 to 5 minutes, or until crisp-tender. Remove vegetables and meat. Skim any fat from pan juices. Blend the remaining $^1/_4$ cup (60 ml) water with the cornstarch and stir into the pot. Cook and stir until bubbly. Serve sauce with vegetables and meat.

Yield: 8 servings

Per serving: 273 calories (16% from fat, 23% from protein, 60% from carbohydrate); 27 g protein; 8 g total fat; 2 g saturated fat; 5 g monounsaturated fat; 2 g polyunsaturated fat; 70 g carbohydrate; 3 g fiber; 10 g sugar; 325 mg phosphorus; 72 mg calcium; 3 mg iron; 128 mg sodium; 893 mg potassium; 615 IU vitamin A; 2 mg ATE vitamin E; 39 mg vitamin C; 71 mg cholesterol; 285 g water

Apple Cranberry Stuffed Pork Roast

When I said I was going to make this, my wife wondered about going to the trouble of butterflying the roast, but the results were worth what turned out to be not a lot of effort. This is the kind of meal you could serve to anyone without worrying that it seems like a special "diet" food.

$^2/_3$ cup (160 ml) apple cider

$^1/_4$ cup (60 ml) cider vinegar

$^1/_2$ cup (115 g) light brown sugar, packed

1 tablespoon (0.9 g) dried shallots

1 cup (86 g) dried apples

$^1/_2$ cup (75 g) dried cranberries

1 teaspoon (1.8 g) ground ginger

$^1/_2$ teaspoon (1.9 g) mustard seed

$^1/_2$ teaspoon (0.8 g) ground allspice

$^1/_8$ teaspoon (0.3 g) cayenne pepper

2 pounds (905 g) boneless pork loin roast

Combine all ingredients except pork in medium saucepan and bring to a simmer over medium-high heat. Cover; reduce heat to low, and cook until apples are very soft, about 20 minutes. Strain through a fine-mesh sieve, using a rubber spatula to press against the apple mixture in the sieve to extract as much liquid as possible; reserve the liquid. Return liquid to saucepan and simmer over medium-high heat until reduced to $^1/_2$ cup (120 ml), about 5 minutes. Remove from heat, set aside, and reserve for use as a glaze.

Preheat oven to 350°F (180°C, or gas mark 4) or prepare your grill for indirect heat. Lay the roast down, fat side up. Insert a knife into the roast $^1/_2$ inch (1.3 cm) horizontally from the bottom of the roast, along the long side of the roast. Make a long cut along the bottom of the roast, stopping $^1/_2$ inch (1.3 cm) before the edge of the roast. You might find it easier to handle by starting at a corner of the roast. Open up the roast and continue to cut through the thicker half of the roast, again keeping $^1/_2$ inch (1.3 cm) from the bottom. Repeat until the roast is an even $^1/_2$-inch (1.3-cm) thickness all over when laid out. Spread out the filling on the roast, leaving a $^1/_2$-inch (1.3-cm) border from the edges. Starting with the short side of the roast, roll it up very tightly. Secure with kitchen twine at 1-inch (2.5-cm) intervals. If baking, place the roast on a rack in a roasting pan and cook on the middle rack of the oven. If you are grilling using indirect heat, preheat the grill and wipe the grates with olive oil. Place roast, fat side up, on the side of the grill that has no coals underneath. Cover the grill with the lid. Cook for 45 to 60 minutes (if you are grilling, turn roast halfway through the cooking). Brush the roast with half of the glaze and cook for 5 minutes longer. Remove the roast from the oven or grill. Place it on a cutting board. Cover with foil to rest and keep warm for 15 minutes before slicing. Slice into $^1/_2$-inch (1.3-cm) pieces, removing the cooking twine as you cut the roast. Serve with remaining glaze.

Yield: 8 servings

Per serving: 269 calories (26% from fat, 38% from protein, 37% from carbohydrate); 25 g protein; 8 g total fat; 3 g saturated fat; 3 g monounsaturated fat; 1 g polyunsaturated fat; 24 g carbohydrate; 1 g fiber; 22 g sugar; 245 mg phosphorus; 24 mg calcium; 1 mg iron; 58 mg sodium; 581 mg potassium; 41 IU vitamin A; 2 mg ATE vitamin E; 1 mg vitamin C; 62 mg cholesterol; 121 g water

Winter Pork Stew

One of those meals that just takes too long to fix when you get home from work, transformed into an easy slow-cooker creation.

4 sweet potatoes, peeled and sliced

2 pounds (905 g) pork loin roast

$1/2$ cup (115 g) brown sugar

$1/4$ teaspoon (0.5 g) cayenne pepper

$1/4$ teaspoon (0.5 g) black pepper

$1/4$ teaspoon (0.8 g) garlic powder

$1/2$ teaspoon (1.5 g) onion powder

Place sweet potatoes in the bottom of a slow cooker. Place pork on top. Combine remaining ingredients and sprinkle over pork and potatoes. Cover and cook on low 8 to 10 hours. Remove pork and slice. Serve juices over pork and potatoes.

Yield: 8 servings

Per serving: 256 calories (18% from fat, 40% from protein, 43% from carbohydrate); 25 g protein; 5 g total fat; 2 g saturated fat; 2 g monounsaturated fat; 1 g polyunsaturated fat; 27 g carbohydrate; 2 g fiber; 18 g sugar; 276 mg phosphorus; 48 mg calcium; 2 mg iron; 84 mg sodium; 645 mg potassium; 11915 IU vitamin A; 2 mg ATE vitamin E; 11 mg vitamin C; 71 mg cholesterol; 144 g water

Pineapple Boats

This would make a great luncheon dish, but it also works as a full dinner, perfect for those hot summer evenings when you don't feel like cooking.

2 pineapples

4 kiwifruits

1 cup (150 g) seedless green grapes

2 cups (300 g) sliced banana

$1/4$ cup (60 g) packed brown sugar

1 teaspoon poppyseeds

$1/2$ pound (225 g) ham, thinly sliced

$1/4$ pound (115 g) Swiss cheese

Slice pineapple lengthwise in half, crown to stem. Leave leafy crown on. Remove tough core. Loosen fruit by cutting to rind; cut in bite-size pieces. Place in large bowl. Peel kiwifruit and bananas and slice into wedges. Cut grapes in half and add all other fruit to pineapple. Toss with brown sugar and poppyseeds. Line pineapple shells with ham. Spoon in fruit mixture. Dice Swiss cheese and tuck among fruit.

Yield: 4 servings

Per serving: 248 g water; 441 calories (27% from fat, 20% from protein, 53% from carb); 23 g protein; 14 g total fat; 7 g saturated fat; 4 g monounsaturated fat; 1 g polyunsaturated fat; 61 g carbohydrate; 6 g fiber; 42 g sugar; 366 mg phosphorus; 342 mg calcium; 2 mg iron; 620 mg sodium; 1039 mg potassium; 415 IU vitamin A; 60 mg vitamin E; 97 mg vitamin C; 49 mg cholesterol

Stir-Fried Pork and Cabbage

Not a traditional Asian stir-fry, but it still has an interesting flavor combination and is good served over rice.

1 pound (455 g) pork loin chops, sliced thinly

1 tablespoon (15 ml) olive oil

1 cup (150 g) apple, sliced thinly

3 tablespoons (45 ml) honey

4 cups (280 g) cabbage, shredded

Slice pork. Heat oil in wok or skillet, add pork and stir-fry until no longer pink, about 5 minutes. Add apples and honey, stir-fry 1 minute. Add cabbage and stir-fry for 30 to 45 seconds, or until heated through, but still crispy.

Yield: 4 servings

Per serving: 259 calories (28% from fat, 38% from protein, 33% from carbohydrate); 25 g protein; 8 g total fat; 2 g saturated fat; 5 g monounsaturated fat; 1 g polyunsaturated fat; 22 g carbohydrate; 3 g fiber; 19 g sugar; 274 mg phosphorus; 53 mg calcium; 2 mg iron; 75 mg sodium; 604 mg potassium; 106 IU vitamin A; 2 mg ATE vitamin E; 35 mg vitamin C; 71 mg cholesterol; 192 g water

9

Main Dishes:
Fish and Seafood

Fish is one thing we should all eat more of. Not only is it low in fat, but cold water varieties like salmon and tuna also contain significant quantities of omerga-3 fatty acids, which have been shown to reduce cholesterol and promote heart health. You wouldn't go wrong eating fish two or three times a week. And with the variety of recipes here you could. They use a number of different kinds of fish and different preparations like grilling, baking, oven frying, and casseroles, so you have lots of fish options to choose from.

Tuna Steaks

If you get them on sale, tuna steaks are a good bargain, as well as containing lots of omega-3 fatty acids. The key to cooking them is not to overcook them and dry them out. It's fine for them to be medium or even medium-rare. Soaking them in a simple marinade also helps to keep them moist and flavorful.

2 tablespoons (30 ml) olive oil

2 tablespoons (30 ml) lemon juice

6 ounces (170 g) tuna steaks

$^1/_2$ teaspoon (1 g) freshly ground black pepper

Combine the olive oil and lemon juice. Marinate the steaks in the mixture for at least 30 minutes, turning occasionally. Heat a skillet over high heat. Add the steaks and cook 2 minutes. Sprinkle with pepper, turn over, and cook 2 minutes longer.

Yield: 2 servings

Per serving: 247 calories (65% from fat, 32% from protein, 3% from carbohydrate); 20 g protein; 18 g total fat; 3 g saturated fat; 11 g monounsaturated fat; 3 g polyunsaturated fat; 2 g carbohydrate; 0 g fiber; 0 g sugar; 218 mg phosphorus; 10 mg calcium; 1 mg iron; 34 mg sodium; 240 mg potassium; 1861 IU vitamin A; 557 mg ATE vitamin E; 7 mg vitamin C; 32 mg cholesterol; 72 g water

Grilled Tuna Steaks

Tuna steaks tend to get tough if you cook them too long, so take them off the grill while they are still pink in the center to keep them juicy.

$^1/_2$ cup (120 ml) balsamic vinegar

2 tablespoons (26 g) sugar

1 tablespoon (2.1 g) Italian seasoning

$^1/_2$ teaspoon (1.5 g) garlic powder

1 tablespoon (15 ml) olive oil

1 pound (455 g) tuna steaks

1 tablespoon (15 ml) lemon juice

Combine all ingredients except tuna and lemon juice and pour in a 9 × 9-inch (23 × 23-cm) glass baking dish. Add tuna and marinate 15 minutes, turning frequently. Heat grill to high. Place fish on grill and grill until medium doneness, about 3 minutes per side. Place on serving plates and drizzle lemon juice over.

Yield: 4 servings

Per serving: 228 calories (37% from fat, 49% from protein, 14% from carbohydrate); 27 g protein; 9 g total fat; 2 g saturated fat; 4 g monounsaturated fat; 2 g polyunsaturated fat; 8 g carbohydrate; 0 g fiber; 7 g sugar; 294 mg phosphorus; 24 mg calcium; 2 mg iron; 46 mg sodium; 329 mg potassium; 2528 IU vitamin A; 743 mg ATE vitamin E; 2 mg vitamin C; 43 mg cholesterol; 109 g water

Grilled Tuna with Honey Mustard Marinade

These tuna steaks can be grilled or broiled. If it's not good weather for outdoor grilling, they also work well on a contact grill like the George Foreman models.

$^1/_3$ cup (80 ml) red wine vinegar

1 tablespoon (15 g) spicy brown mustard

1 tablespoon (15 ml) honey

3 tablespoons (45 ml) extra-virgin olive oil

1 pound (455 g) tuna steaks

Combine the vinegar, mustard, honey, and olive oil in a jar or covered container; shake to mix well. Put tuna in a resealable plastic bag; add the mustard mixture. Seal the bag and let marinate for about 20 minutes. Heat the grill. Remove the tuna from the marinade and pour the marinade in a small saucepan. Bring marinade to a boil; remove from heat and set aside. Grill the tuna over high heat for about 2 minutes on each side, or to desired doneness. Drizzle with the hot marinade.

Yield: 4 servings

Per serving: 275 calories (53% from fat, 40% from protein, 7% from carbohydrate); 27 g protein; 16 g total fat; 3 g saturated fat; 9 g monounsaturated fat; 3 g polyunsaturated fat; 5 g carbohydrate; 0 g fiber; 4 g sugar; 294 mg phosphorus; 13 mg calcium; 1 mg iron; 89 mg sodium; 302 mg potassium; 2478 IU vitamin A; 743 mg ATE vitamin E; 0 mg vitamin C; 43 mg cholesterol; 100 g water

Marinated Tuna Steaks

Marinated in a southwestern-flavored sauce, these tuna steaks go well with Spanish rice and corn.

2 tablespoons (30 ml) olive oil

2 teaspoons (5 g) cumin

2 tablespoons (30 ml) lime juice

2 teaspoons (2.6 g) cilantro

1 pound (455 g) tuna steaks

Combine first 4 ingredients in a shallow dish; add fish and turn to coat. Marinate for 20 minutes, turning occasionally. Heat the grill. Remove the tuna from the marinade and grill the tuna over high heat for 2 minutes on each side, or until desired doneness.

Yield: 4 servings

Per serving: 229 calories (50% from fat, 48% from protein, 2% from carb); 27 g protein; 13 g total fat; 2 g saturated fat; 7 g monounsaturated fat; 2 g polyunsaturated fat; 1 g carbohydrate; 0 g fiber; 0 g sugar; 294 mg phosphorus; 20 mg calcium; 2 mg iron; 46 mg sodium; 315 mg potassium; 2521 IU vitamin A; 743 mg ATE vitamin E; 3 mg vitamin C; 43 mg cholesterol; 85 g water

Poached Salmon

Poaching fish is a healthy way to cook it, as well as making sure it stays moist and adding a little extra flavor.

4 cups (946 ml) water

2 tablespoons (30 ml) lemon juice

$^1/_4$ cup (30 g) carrot, thinly sliced

$^1/_2$ cup (80 g) onion, thinly sliced

1 bay leaf

1 tablespoon (4 g) fresh dill, chopped

$^1/_2$ pound (225 g) salmon fillets

Preheat oven to 350°F (180°C, or gas mark 4). Combine all ingredients except salmon in a saucepan and heat to boiling. Reduce heat and simmer 5 minutes. Place salmon in a glass baking dish large enough to hold salmon in a single layer; pour poaching liquid over. Cover and bake for 20 minutes, or until salmon flakes easily.

Yield: 2 servings

Per serving: 238 calories (47% from fat, 40% from protein, 13% from carbohydrate); 24 g protein; 12 g total fat; 3 g saturated fat; 4 g monounsaturated fat; 4 g polyunsaturated fat; 7 g carbohydrate; 1 g fiber; 3 g sugar; 291 mg phosphorus; 71 mg calcium; 1 mg iron; 97 mg sodium; 595 mg potassium; 2841 IU vitamin A; 17 mg ATE vitamin E; 16 mg vitamin C; 67 mg cholesterol; 614 g water

Maple Salmon

The sweetness of the maple syrup and the flavor of the balsamic vinegar go well with salmon.

$1/4$ cup (60 ml) balsamic vinegar

$1/4$ cup (60 ml) water

2 tablespoons (30 ml) olive oil

2 tablespoons (30 ml) maple syrup

$1/4$ teaspoon (0.8 g) garlic powder

$1/2$ pound (225 g) salmon fillets

Heat all ingredients except salmon in a large skillet, stirring to combine. Add salmon fillets. Cover and cook for 10 minutes, or until salmon is done, turning once.

Yield: 2 servings

Per serving: 387 calories (61% from fat, 24% from protein, 15% from carbohydrate); 23 g protein; 26 g total

fat; 4 g saturated fat; 14 g monounsaturated fat; 6 g polyunsaturated fat; 14 g carbohydrate; 0 g fiber; 12 g sugar; 268 mg phosphorus; 31 mg calcium; 1 mg iron; 71 mg sodium; 478 mg potassium; 57 IU vitamin A; 17 mg ATE vitamin E; 4 mg vitamin C; 67 mg cholesterol; 142 g water

Grilled Salmon and Vegetables

On hot days, it's sometimes a good idea to not use the stove at all. This recipe gives you protein, vegetables, and starch in one easy grilled packet.

1 cup (195 g) instant rice, uncooked

1 cup (235 ml) low sodium chicken broth

$1/2$ cup (56 g) zucchini, sliced

$1/2$ cup (60 g) carrot, shredded

$1/2$ pound (225 g) salmon fillets

$1/4$ teaspoon (0.5 g) black pepper

$1/2$ lemon, sliced

Heat grill to medium. Spray two large pieces of heavy-duty aluminum foil with nonstick vegetable oil spray. In a small bowl, mix together rice and broth. Let stand for 5 minutes, or until most of broth is absorbed. Stir in zucchini and carrots, and set aside. Place a salmon fillet in the center of each piece of foil. Sprinkle with pepper and place lemon slices on top. Place rice mixture around each fillet. Fold up foil and bring edges together. Fold over several times to seal. Fold in ends, allowing some room for the rice to expand during cooking. Place on the grill and cook for 10 to 15 minutes, or until salmon is done.

Yield: 2 servings

Per serving: 347 calories (35% from fat, 33% from protein, 32% from carbohydrate); 28 g protein; 14 g total fat; 3 g saturated fat; 5 g monounsaturated fat; 5 g polyunsaturated fat; 28 g carbohydrate; 2 g fiber; 3 g sugar; 369 mg phosphorus; 54 mg calcium; 2 mg iron; 130 mg sodium; 765 mg potassium; 5502 IU vitamin A; 17 mg ATE vitamin E; 19 mg vitamin C; 67 mg cholesterol; 320 g water

Grilled Salmon Fillets

You can use a whole salmon fillet for this recipe. It makes an impressive display, but it can be difficult to turn. I usually cut the fillet into serving-sized pieces, but then you need to be careful not to overcook them and dry them out. The sweetness of the sauce goes well with the salmon.

$1/4$ cup (60 g) brown sugar

2 tablespoons (30 ml) cider vinegar

2 tablespoons (30 ml) honey

$1/4$ teaspoon (1 ml) liquid smoke

$1/4$ teaspoon (0.5 g) black pepper

$1/4$ teaspoon (0.8 g) crushed garlic

2 pounds (905 g) salmon fillets

Preheat grill. In a small mixing bowl, combine the first 6 ingredients (through garlic). Mix well. Brush one side of the salmon with the basting sauce, then place the salmon (basted side down) on the grill. When the salmon is half finished cooking, baste the top portion of the salmon and flip the fillet so the fresh basting sauce is on the grill. When the fish is almost finished cooking, apply the basting sauce and flip the salmon again. Baste and flip the salmon once more and serve.

Yield: 6 servings

Per serving: 110 g water ; 334 calories (45% from fat, 37% from protein, 18% from carbohydrate); 30 g protein; 16 g total fat; 3 g saturated fat; 6 g monounsaturated fat; 6 g polyunsaturated fat; 15 g carbohydrate; 0 g fiber; 15 g sugar; 355 mg phosphorus; 27 mg calcium; 1 mg iron; 93 mg sodium; 587 mg potassium; 76 IU vitamin A; 23 mg ATE vitamin E; 6 mg vitamin C; 89 mg cholesterol

Tip: Be careful not to overcook the salmon; it will lose its juices and flavor if cooked too long.

Cedar Planked Salmon

Grilling salmon on a cedar plank gives it a marvelous smoky flavor. You can grill it plain, but we like this honey mustard sauce on it.

$1/4$ cup (60 g) Dijon mustard

1 tablespoon (15 ml) honey

1 teaspoon (1 g) dried dill

1 pound (455 g) salmon fillets

Mix mustard, honey, and dill. Pour over salmon in a glass baking dish and marinate while you prepare the grill. Preheat grill to medium and soak planks according to package directions. Place the plank on the heated grill and allow to preheat for 3 minutes. Turn the plank over and place salmon on plank. Close grill and cook for 12 minutes, or until fish flakes easily.

Yield: 4 servings

Per serving: 234 calories (50% from fat, 40% from protein, 9% from carbohydrate); 23 g protein; 13 g total

fat; 3 g saturated fat; 5 g monounsaturated fat; 5 g polyunsaturated fat; 5 g carbohydrate; 1 g fiber; 4 g sugar; 282 mg phosphorus; 27 mg calcium; 1 mg iron; 238 mg sodium; 443 mg potassium; 82 IU vitamin A; 17 mg ATE vitamin E; 5 mg vitamin C; 67 mg cholesterol; 91 g water

Tip: You can find cedar planks at stores with a large selection of grills and grilling equipment, such as Lowe's or The Home Depot.

Thyme Roasted Salmon

Simple in its preparation, with just three ingredients, this salmon doesn't lack for flavor.

1 pound salmon fillets

1 teaspoon dried thyme

$^1/_4$ teaspoon black pepper

Spray a baking sheet with non-stick cooking spray. Place the fillets on the sheet. Sprinkle with thyme and pepper. Cook at 350°F until fish flakes easily, about 20 minutes.

Yield: 4 servings

Per serving: 182 calories (55% from fat, 45% from protein , 1% from carb); 20 g protein ; 11 g total fat; 2 g saturated fat; 4 g monounsaturated fat; 4 g polyunsaturated fat; 0 g carb; 0 g fiber; 0 g sugar; 231 mg phosphorus; 17 mg calcium; 59 mg sodium; 362 mg potassium; 59 IU vitamin A; 15 mg ATE vitamin E; 4 mg vitamin C; 58 mg cholesterol

Salmon with Honey Mustard Glaze

Salmon is naturally sweet, making this honey mustard glaze especially appropriate.

1 pound salmon fillets

2 tablespoons honey

2 tablespoons Dijon mustard

$^1/_2$ teaspoon thyme

1 tablespoon olive oil

Heat oil over medium heat in a large non-stick skillet. Combine honey, mustard, and thyme. Brush on both sides of fish. Cook in oil until fish flakes easily, about 5 minutes per side.

Yield: 4 servings

Per serving: 249 calories (52% from fat, 32% from protein , 15% from carb); 20 g protein ; 14 g total fat; 3 g saturated fat; 6 g monounsaturated fat; 4 g polyunsaturated fat; 9 g carb; 0 g fiber; 9 g sugar; 238 mg phosphorus; 21 mg calcium; 147 mg sodium; 377 mg potassium; 65 IU vitamin A; 15 mg ATE vitamin E; 4 mg vitamin C; 58 mg cholesterol

Mediterranean Salmon

This complete meal makes a great presentation, not to mention that it tastes delicious.

1 pound (455 g) salmon fillets

1 cup (175 g) couscous

1 cup (113 g) zucchini, sliced

1 cup (160 g) red onion, peeled and sliced

4 ounces (115 g) mushrooms, sliced

1/2 cup (75 g) red bell pepper, cut in strips

2 tablespoons (30 ml) olive oil, divided

1 tablespoon (2.5 g) fresh basil

Prepare couscous according to package instructions. Meanwhile, preheat a skillet or griddle pan. Toss the zucchini, onion, mushrooms, and red bell pepper in 1 tablespoon (15 ml) oil. Sauté vegetables for 8 to 10 minutes, turning once. Remove from pan. Brush the salmon with the remaining 1 tablespoon (15 ml) oil and cook for 6 to 8 minutes, turning once. Add the vegetables and basil to the couscous and toss well. Serve the vegetable couscous topped with the salmon.

Yield: 4 servings

Per serving: 460 calories (39% from fat, 26% from protein, 35% from carbohydrate); 30 g protein; 20 g total fat; 4 g saturated fat; 9 g monounsaturated fat; 5 g polyunsaturated fat; 40 g carbohydrate; 4 g fiber; 3 g sugar; 392 mg phosphorus; 51 mg calcium; 2 mg iron; 78 mg sodium; 768 mg potassium; 752 IU vitamin A; 17 mg ATE vitamin E; 37 mg vitamin C; 67 mg cholesterol; 190 g water

Lemon Baked Salmon

This method will give you a little more intense lemon flavor than most. You can use this same preparation for a number of kinds of fish.

1 lemon

1 pound (455 g) salmon fillets

1/4 cup (60 ml) lemon juice

2 tablespoons (6 g) dill

2 teaspoons (10 ml) olive oil

Preheat oven to 350°F (180°C, or gas mark 4). Spray a 9 × 13-inch (23 × 33-cm) glass baking dish with nonstick vegetable oil spray. Slice lemon into 1/4-inch (0.6-cm) slices and place in bottom of pan. Lay fillets over slices. Combine lemon juice, dill, and oil and pour over fillets. Bake for 12 to 15 minutes, or until fish flakes easily.

Yield: 4 servings

Per serving: 213 calories (55% from fat, 38% from protein, 7% from carbohydrate); 20 g protein; 13 g total fat; 2 g saturated fat; 5 g monounsaturated fat; 4 g polyunsaturated fat; 4 g carbohydrate; 1 g fiber; 1 g sugar; 242 mg phosphorus; 44 mg calcium; 1 mg iron; 62 mg sodium; 449 mg potassium; 146 IU vitamin A; 15 mg ATE vitamin E; 19 mg vitamin C; 58 mg cholesterol; 95 g water

Salmon with Dill

This is a simple stick-it-in-the-oven-and-wait type of dish. It goes well with boiled potatoes (you could make a little extra of the sauce to put on them).

2 tablespoons (30 ml) olive oil

1 teaspoon (1 g) dried dill

1 teaspoon (3 g) onion powder

1/2 teaspoon (1 g) black pepper

1 pound (455 g) salmon fillets

Preheat oven to 400°F (200°C, or gas mark 6). Mix together oil, dill, onion powder, and pepper. Place salmon in a 9 × 13-inch (23 × 33-cm) baking dish that has been coated with nonstick vegetable oil spray. Brush all of the olive oil mixture on the fish. Bake for 20 minutes, or until fish flakes easily.

Yield: 4 servings

Per serving: 271 calories (65% from fat, 34% from protein, 1% from carbohydrate); 23 g protein; 19 g total fat; 3 g saturated fat; 9 g monounsaturated fat; 5 g polyunsaturated fat; 1 g carbohydrate; 0 g fiber; 0 g sugar; 268 mg phosphorus; 22 mg calcium; 1 mg iron; 68 mg sodium; 428 mg potassium; 73 IU vitamin A; 17 mg ATE vitamin E; 5 mg vitamin C; 67 mg cholesterol; 78 g water

Oven-Steamed Salmon and Vegetables

I've also cooked this on a gas grill.

8 ounces (225 g) salmon fillets

2 medium potatoes, diced

$^1/_2$ cup (56 g) yellow squash, thinly sliced

$^1/_2$ cup (65 g) carrot, thinly sliced

$^1/_4$ cup (25 g) scallions, thinly sliced

$^1/_2$ cup (35 g) mushrooms, sliced

2 teaspoons (10 ml) white wine

$^1/_2$ teaspoon (0.5 g) dried dill

$^1/_2$ teaspoon (1.5 g) minced garlic

$^1/_4$ teaspoon (0.5 g) black pepper, fresh ground

Preheat oven to 425°F (220°C, or gas mark 7). Place a baking sheet in the oven to preheat as well.

Meanwhile, spray the center of two 12-inch (30-cm) squares of aluminum foil with nonstick vegetable oil spray. Combine salmon, potatoes, squash, carrots, scallions, and mushrooms and divide evenly among the prepared foil sheets. Sprinkle with wine, dill, garlic, and pepper; fold diagonally to form a triangle; tightly seal edges. Place foil package on preheated baking sheet, then return to oven and bake 10 to 15 minutes, or until salmon is opaque and vegetables are tender.

Yield: 2 servings

Per serving: 498 calories (23% from fat, 25% from protein, 52% from carbohydrate); 31 g protein; 13 g total fat; 3 g saturated fat; 4 g monounsaturated fat; 5 g polyunsaturated fat; 65 g carbohydrate; 8 g fiber; 6 g sugar; 535 mg phosphorus; 82 mg calcium; 4 mg iron; 116 mg sodium; 2374 mg potassium; 5659 IU vitamin A; 17 mg ATE vitamin E; 46 mg vitamin C; 67 mg cholesterol; 464 g water

Mediterranean Tilapia

A tasty topping featuring sun-dried tomatoes and olives gives these simple fillets exceptional flavor.

$^1/_4$ cup sun dried tomatoes, oil packed, chopped

8 ripe olives, chopped

2 tablespoons pimento, diced

2 tablespoons fresh parsley

1 tablespoon fresh basil

1 tablespoon olive oil

4 tilapia fillets

$^1/_4$ teaspoon paprika

$^1/_8$ teaspoon cayenne

Spray a baking sheet with non-stick cooking spray. Combine tomatoes, olives, pimento, parsley, basil, and oil. Set aside. Place fillets on baking sheet. Sprinkle with paprika and cayenne. Bake at 400°F until fish flakes easily, about 15 minutes. Transfer to serving plates and spoon tomato mixture over top.

Yield: 4 servings

Per serving: 273 calories (58% from fat, 38% from protein, 4% from carb); 25 g protein ; 17 g total fat; 4 g saturated fat; 9 g monounsaturated fat; 3 g polyunsaturated fat; 3 g carb; 1 g fiber; 0 g sugar; 336 mg phosphorus; 40 mg calcium; 182 mg sodium; 626 mg potassium; 669 IU vitamin A; 24 mg ATE vitamin E; 16 mg vitamin C; 75 mg cholesterol

Greek Islands Fish

The flavor of this fish will whisk you away to a Mediterranean island. Serve with couscous.

6 tilapia fillets

1 cup no salt added tomatoes, diced

$^1/_2$ cup artichoke hearts, chopped

$^1/_2$ cup ripe olives, chopped

$^1/_2$ cup feta cheese, crumbled

Place fillets in a 9 × 13-inch baking pan coated with non-stick cooking spray. Top with remaining ingredients. Bake at 400°F for 15 to 20 minutes or until fish flakes easily.

Yield: 6 servings

Per serving: 274 calories (53% from fat, 40% from protein, 6% from carb); 27 g protein ; 16 g total fat; 5 g saturated fat; 7 g monounsaturated fat; 3 g

polyunsaturated fat; 4 g carb; 1 g fiber; 2 g sugar; 380 mg phosphorus; 101 mg calcium; 333 mg sodium; 612 mg potassium; 253 IU vitamin A; 39 mg ATE vitamin E; 7 mg vitamin C; 86 mg cholesterol

Grilled Swordfish

We don't have swordfish all that often, but occasionally I'll find it on sale and buy some. It works well for this simple barbecue recipe because it's dense enough to hold together.

$^1/_4$ cup (60 ml) barbecue sauce

1 tablespoon (15 ml) Worcestershire sauce

2 tablespoons (30 ml) fresh lime juice

2 tablespoons (20 g) chopped onion

$^1/_2$ teaspoon (1.5 g) minced garlic

2 swordfish steaks

Combine all ingredients except swordfish to make marinade. Marinate swordfish steaks for 6 hours or overnight, turning occasionally. When ready to grill, reserve marinade. Grill or cook as desired (do not overcook). Heat reserved marinade to boiling and pour over fish to serve.

Yield: 2 servings

Per serving: 242 calories (21% from fat, 47% from protein, 32% from carbohydrate); 28 g protein; 6 g total fat; 1 g saturated fat; 2 g monounsaturated fat; 1 g polyunsaturated fat; 19 g carbohydrate; 0 g fiber; 12 g sugar; 372 mg phosphorus; 11 mg calcium; 2 mg iron; 498 mg sodium; 487 mg potassium; 179 IU vitamin A; 49 mg ATE vitamin E; 20 mg vitamin C; 53 mg cholesterol; 147 g water

Baked Swordfish with Vegetables

This is a fairly simple recipe, with the flavor coming from the vegetables. It's good with pasta or plain brown rice.

4 ounces (115 g) mushrooms, sliced

1 cup (160 g) onion, sliced

2 tablespoons (19 g) green bell pepper, chopped

2 tablespoons (30 ml) lemon juice

$1/4$ teaspoon (0.3 g) dried dill

1 pound (455 g) swordfish steaks

4 small bay leaves

2 tomatoes, sliced

Preheat oven to 400°F (200°C, or gas mark 6). In a bowl, combine mushrooms, onions, green bell pepper, lemon juice, and dill. Line a shallow baking pan with foil. Spread vegetable mixture in bottom then arrange swordfish steaks on top. Place a bay leaf and 2 tomato slices on each swordfish steak. Cover pan with foil and bake for 45 to 55 minutes or until fish flakes easily with a fork.

Yield: 4 servings

Per serving: 165 calories (26% from fat, 59% from protein, 15% from carbohydrate); 24 g protein; 5 g total fat; 1 g saturated fat; 2 g monounsaturated fat; 1 g polyunsaturated fat; 6 g carbohydrate; 1 g fiber; 3 g sugar; 339 mg phosphorus; 18 mg calcium; 1 mg iron; 126 mg sodium; 529 mg potassium; 168 IU vitamin A; 41 mg ATE vitamin E; 12 mg vitamin C; 44 mg cholesterol; 159 g water

Brown Rice Tuna Bake

A variation on the traditional tuna casserole. Brown rice adds nutrients, and yogurt provides flavor and creaminess.

$1^1/4$ cups (238 g) uncooked brown rice

3 cups (710 ml) water

1 cup (100 g) chopped celery

$1/2$ cup (80 g) onion, finely diced

$1/2$ cup (115 g) plain fat-free yogurt

1 cup (235 ml) skim milk

$1/4$ teaspoon (0.3 g) red pepper flakes

$1/2$ teaspoon (0.3 g) dried tarragon

14 ounces (395 g) water-packed canned tuna, drained

2 cups (280 g) frozen peas, thawed

$3/4$ cup (90 g) low fat Cheddar cheese, shredded

Preheat oven to 350°F (180°C, or gas mark 4). Combine rice and water in large saucepan. Bring to a boil. Reduce heat, cover, and cook for 35 minutes. Remove from heat. Add celery, onion, yogurt, milk, red pepper flakes, and tarragon; mix well. Flake the tuna with a fork and add it and thawed peas to the rice mixture; mix well. Pour into 2-quart (1.9-L) casserole dish. Bake for 30 minutes. Top with shredded cheese.

Yield: 6 servings

Per serving: 321 calories (9% from fat, 37% from protein, 54% from carbohydrate); 29 g protein; 3 g total fat; 1 g saturated fat; 1 g monounsaturated fat; 1 g polyunsaturated fat; 42 g carbohydrate; 4 g fiber; 5 g sugar; 445 mg phosphorus; 209 mg calcium; 3 mg iron; 537 mg sodium; 526 mg potassium; 1231 IU vitamin A; 47 mg ATE vitamin E; 7 mg vitamin C; 25 mg cholesterol; 302 g water

Tuna Casserole

Ever have one of those nights where you can't think of a thing for dinner and end up pawing randomly through cookbooks looking for something that sounds good and that you have the ingredients for? This was the result. And it actually worked out well. The top layer is a quiche-like custard.

2 cups (330 g) cooked rice

4 eggs, divided

$^1/_2$ teaspoon (0.7 g) dried basil

1 tablespoon (10 g) onion, minced

7 ounces (200 g) water packed tuna

1 cup (235 ml) skim milk

4 ounces (115 g) Swiss cheese, shredded

Preheat oven to 350°F (180°C, or gas mark 4). Combine rice, 1 egg, basil, and onion. Press into the bottom of an 8 x 8-inch (20 x 20-cm) baking dish sprayed with nonstick vegetable oil spray. Spread tuna over the top. Combine remaining eggs, milk, and cheese and pour over the top. Bake for 40 to 45 minutes, or until a knife inserted near the center comes out clean.

Yield: 4 servings

Per serving: 285 calories (14% from fat, 48% from protein, 37% from carbohydrate); 33 g protein; 4 g total fat; 2 g saturated fat; 1 g monounsaturated fat; 1 g polyunsaturated fat; 26 g carbohydrate; 1 g fiber; 1 g sugar; 442 mg phosphorus; 417 mg calcium; 4 mg iron; 390 mg sodium; 419 mg potassium; 430 IU vitamin A; 57 mg ATE vitamin E; 1 mg vitamin C; 237 mg cholesterol; 219 g water

Tuna Noodle Casserole

This is traditional American comfort food.

1 tablespoon (15 ml) olive oil

2 tablespoons (16 g) flour

2 cups (470 ml) skim milk

$^1/_4$ cup (30 g) low fat Cheddar cheese, shredded

3 cups (450 g) cooked egg noodles

10-ounce (280 g) package frozen peas, thawed

7 ounces (200 g) water-packed tuna

4 ounces (115 g) mushrooms, sliced

$^1/_4$ cup (37 g) chopped green bell pepper

$^1/_8$ teaspoon (0.3 g) black pepper

$^1/_2$ cup (60 g) bread crumbs

Preheat oven to 375°F (190°C, or gas mark 5). Heat oil in a large skillet over low heat; add flour, stirring until smooth. Cook 1 minute, stirring constantly. Gradually add milk; cook over medium heat, stirring constantly, until mixture is thickened and bubbly. Stir in cheese; cook over low heat, stirring constantly, until cheese melts. Remove from heat. Combine cheese sauce, noodles, and next 5 ingredients (through black pepper). Spoon mixture into a 2-quart (1.9-L) casserole dish coated with nonstick vegetable oil spray. Sprinkle evenly with bread crumbs. Bake for 35 minutes, or until the casserole is bubbly and the top is browned.

Yield: 6 servings

Per serving: 277 calories (14% from fat, 28% from protein, 58% from carbohydrate); 19 g protein; 4 g total fat; 1 g saturated fat; 2 g monounsaturated fat; 1 g

polyunsaturated fat; 40 g carbohydrate; 7 g fiber; 3 g sugar; 303 mg phosphorus; 174 mg calcium; 2 mg iron; 414 mg sodium; 424 mg potassium; 1254 IU vitamin A; 59 mg ATE vitamin E; 11 mg vitamin C; 13 mg cholesterol; 211 g water

Herbed Fish

Simple baked fish made flavorful by a combination of herbs and spices.

2 pounds (905 g) perch, or other firm white fish

1 tablespoon (15 ml) olive oil

$^1/_2$ teaspoon (1.5 g) garlic powder

$^1/_2$ teaspoon (0.3 g) dried marjoram

$^1/_2$ teaspoon (0.5 g) dried thyme

$^1/_8$ teaspoon (0.3 g) white pepper

2 bay leaves

$^1/_2$ cup (80 g) onion, chopped

$^1/_2$ cup (120 ml) white wine

Preheat oven to 350°F (180°C, or gas mark 4). Wash fish, pat dry, and place in 9 × 13-inch (23 × 33-cm) dish. Combine oil with garlic powder, marjoram, thyme, and white pepper. Drizzle over fish. Top with bay leaves and onion. Pour wine over all. Bake, uncovered, for 20 to 30 minutes, or until fish flakes easily with a fork.

Yield: 4 servings

Per serving: 277 calories (26% from fat, 69% from protein, 5% from carbohydrate); 43 g protein; 7 g total fat; 1 g saturated fat; 4 g monounsaturated fat; 1 g polyunsaturated fat; 3 g carbohydrate; 0 g fiber; 1 g sugar; 503 mg phosphorus; 253 mg calcium; 2 mg iron; 173 mg sodium; 675 mg potassium; 100 IU vitamin A; 27 mg ATE vitamin E; 3 mg vitamin C; 95 mg cholesterol; 222 g water

Oven-Fried Fish

The nice crunchy coating is low in fat and sodium, and it goes really well with oven-fried potatoes.

1 egg

2 tablespoons (30 ml) skim milk

$^1/_2$ cup (30 g) dried mashed potato flakes

$^1/_4$ teaspoon (0.5 g) black pepper

1 pound (455 g) catfish fillets

Preheat oven to 325°F (170°C, or gas mark 3). Mix egg and milk together. Stir together potatoes and pepper. Dip fish in egg mixture, then potato flakes. Dip fish again in egg and then potato flakes. Place on baking sheet. Coat fish with nonstick vegetable oil spray. Bake for 15 minutes, or until fish flakes easily.

Yield: 4 servings

Per serving: 196 calories (43% from fat, 43% from protein, 14% from carbohydrate); 20 g protein; 9 g total fat; 2 g saturated fat; 4 g monounsaturated fat; 2 g polyunsaturated fat; 7 g carbohydrate; 1 g fiber; 0 g sugar; 269 mg phosphorus; 32 mg calcium; 1 mg iron; 100 mg sodium; 389 mg potassium; 130 IU vitamin A; 22 mg ATE vitamin E; 7 mg vitamin C; 104 mg cholesterol; 106 g water

Pecan-Crusted Catfish

A delightful southern treat. Serve with rice pilaf.

6 tablespoons (90 g) Dijon mustard

$^1/_4$ cup (60 ml) skim milk

1 cup (100 g) pecans, ground

1 pound (455 g) catfish fillets

Preheat oven to 450°F (230°C, or gas mark 8). Coat a baking sheet with nonstick vegetable oil spray. Mix mustard and milk in a shallow dish. Spread pecans in another dish. Dip fillets in mustard mixture, then roll in pecans to coat. Place on prepared pan. Bake 10 to 12 minutes, or until fish flakes easily.

Yield: 4 servings

Per serving: 364 calories (70% from fat, 23% from protein, 6% from carbohydrate); 22 g protein; 29 g total fat; 4 g saturated fat; 16 g monounsaturated fat; 8 g polyunsaturated fat; 6 g carbohydrate; 3 g fiber; 1 g sugar; 346 mg phosphorus; 64 mg calcium; 2 mg iron; 325 mg sodium; 510 mg potassium; 119 IU vitamin A; 26 mg ATE vitamin E; 1 mg vitamin C; 54 mg cholesterol; 119 g water

Baked Catfish

This easy-to-make catfish with a crunchy bread crumb topping goes with just about anything.

1 pound catfish fillets

$^1/_2$ teaspoon Italian seasoning

$^1/_4$ cup bread crumbs, soft

2 teaspoons unsalted butter, melted

Preheat oven to 425°F. Coat baking pan with non-stick cooking spray. Place fish in pan and sprinkle with Italian seasoning and bread crumbs. Drizzle with melted butter. Bake until fish flakes easily, about 20 minutes.

Yield: 4 servings

Per serving: 98 calories (50% from fat, 30% from protein, 21% from carb); 7 g protein ; 5 g total fat; 2 g saturated fat; 2 g monounsaturated fat; 1 g polyunsaturated fat; 5 g carb; 0 g fiber; 0 g sugar; 92 mg phosphorus; 18 mg calcium; 21 mg sodium; 135 mg potassium; 88 IU vitamin A; 22 mg ATE vitamin E; 0 mg vitamin C; 24 mg cholesterol

Salmon Patties

When I was growing up, canned salmon was cheaper than tuna. We had salmon patties fairly often because they were a quick and tasty meal. Salmon is no longer quite the bargain, but the patties still taste just as good.

14-ounce (400-g) can salmon, drained and flaked

2 eggs

$^3/_4$ **cup (90 g) bread crumbs**

$^1/_2$ **cup (80 g) onion, chopped**

Salt and pepper to taste

1 tablespoon (15 ml) olive oil

In a large bowl, combine salmon, eggs, bread crumbs, onion, salt, and pepper; shape into six equal-sized patties. Heat oil in a large frying pan over medium heat. Add salmon patties and brown on both sides.

Yield: 6 servings

Per serving: 217 calories (46% from fat, 33% from protein, 21% from carbohydrate); 18 g protein; 11 g total fat; 2 g saturated fat; 5 g monounsaturated fat; 3 g polyunsaturated fat; 11 g carbohydrate; 1 g fiber; 2 g sugar; 206 mg phosphorus; 47 mg calcium; 1 mg iron; 175 mg sodium; 254 mg potassium; 109 IU vitamin A; 10 mg ATE vitamin E; 4 mg vitamin C; 109 mg cholesterol; 76 g water

Linguine with Scallops

Seafood just seems to make any meal special. In this case, scallops turn an ordinary spaghetti dinner into something memorable.

1 tablespoon (15 ml) olive oil

1 tablespoon minced shallots

$^1/_2$ teaspoon crushed garlic

1 tablespoon minced fresh parsley

2 tablespoons minced fresh basil

$^1/_4$ teaspoon crushed red pepper flakes

2 cups (480 g) no-salt-added canned tomatoes

$^1/_2$ cup (120 ml) dry white wine

2 tablespoons (32 g) no-salt-added tomato paste

1 pound (455 g) scallops

9 ounces (255 g) artichoke hearts, thawed

8 ounces (225 g) whole wheat linguine

2 tablespoons (18 g) pine nuts, toasted

In 3-quart (3-L) saucepan, heat oil over medium heat. Add shallots and garlic and sauté 3 minutes. Add parsley, basil, pepper flakes, tomatoes, wine, and tomato paste. Bring to boil, stir to break tomatoes.

Cover and simmer 20 minutes. Slice large scallops crosswise in half. Add scallops and artichoke hearts to tomato mixture. Cook until scallops are cooked and artichokes are hot, about 5 minutes. Cook linguine as package label directs; drain. On platter, toss pasta with scallops mixture and sprinkle with pine nuts. If desired, garnish with basil leaf.

Yield: 4 servings

Per serving: 296 g water; 441 calories (17% from fat, 28% from protein, 54% from carb); 31 g protein; 8 g total fat; 1 g saturated fat; 3 g monounsaturated fat; 3 g polyunsaturated fat; 60 g carbohydrate; 5 g fiber; 5 g sugar; 500 mg phosphorus; 131 mg calcium; 5 mg iron; 247 mg sodium; 1058 mg potassium; 602 IU vitamin A; 17 mg vitamin E; 21 mg vitamin C; 37 mg cholesterol

Spaghetti with Fish

My daughter made this after seeing a similar recipe on a cooking program on TV. It turned out really well and is just different enough from the way we typically serve pasta that we tend to go back to it when we want something a little different, especially since it fits my daughter's rule that if you don't know what to have, make something Italian.

8 ounces (225 g) spaghetti

1 pound (455 g) perch, or other white fish

2 tablespoons (30 ml) olive oil

$^1/_2$ teaspoon (1.5 g) minced garlic

2 tablespoons (30 ml) lemon juice

1 tablespoon (2.5 g) Italian seasoning

$^1/_4$ teaspoon (0.5 g) black pepper

2 cups (360 g) canned no-salt-added tomatoes

1/4 cup (60 ml) white wine

2 tablespoons (8 g) fresh parsley

Cook spaghetti according to package directions, drain and set aside. Cut fish into 1-inch (2.5-cm) cubes. In a large skillet heat olive oil. Add garlic, lemon juice, Italian seasoning, and pepper. Cook until garlic starts to brown. Add fish and cook until nearly done. Add tomatoes and reheat to boiling. Remove from heat. Stir in spaghetti and wine and toss to coat spaghetti with sauce. Sprinkle with parsley.

Yield: 4 servings

Per serving: 276 calories (31% from fat, 35% from protein, 34% from carbohydrate); 24 g protein; 9 g total fat; 1 g saturated fat; 6 g monounsaturated fat; 1 g polyunsaturated fat; 22 g carbohydrate; 4 g fiber; 3 g sugar; 317 mg phosphorus; 177 mg calcium; 3 mg iron; 103 mg sodium; 599 mg potassium; 430 IU vitamin A; 14 mg ATE vitamin E; 19 mg vitamin C; 48 mg cholesterol; 263 g water

Linguine with Tuna

It's not scallops, but tuna can make a pretty fancy Italian meal too.

3/4 cup (175 ml) olive oil, divided

1 cup (150 g) sliced green bell pepper

1 cup (150 g) sliced red bell pepper

1 cup (150 g) sliced yellow bell pepper

1 cup (70 g) sliced mushrooms

1 cup (160 g) thinly sliced onion

1 teaspoon crushed garlic

1 can solid white tuna

3/4 cup (175 ml) dry white wine

4 ounces (115 g) romano cheese, grated

1/2 cup (30 g) chopped fresh parsley

1 pound (455 g) whole wheat linguine

Heat pan. Use enough olive oil to coat the bottom of the pan, about 1/4 cup. Add pepper, mushrooms, onion, and garlic. Sauté until crisp-tender. Add remaining oil. Add the tuna and the wine. Stir. Add cheese and parsley. Serve over linguine cooked according to package directions.

Yield: 8 servings

Per serving: 129 g water; 504 calories (46% from fat, 15% from protein, 39% from carb); 19 g protein; 26 g total fat; 6 g saturated fat; 16 g monounsaturated fat; 3 g polyunsaturated fat; 50 g carbohydrate; 1 g fiber; 3 g sugar; 335 mg phosphorus; 195 mg calcium; 3 mg iron; 192 mg sodium; 401 mg potassium; 1078 IU vitamin A; 14 mg vitamin E; 88 mg vitamin C; 24 mg cholesterol

Tuna Tacos

Looking for a quick lunch or dinner? These no-cook tacos are tasty and healthy, as well as being a snap to make.

6 1/2 ounces (184 g) tuna, drained and flaked

1/3 cup (33 g) chopped scallions

1/4 cup (65 g) salsa

2 cups (110 g) shredded lettuce

8 corn taco shells

1 cup (164 g) cooked chickpeas, drained

1 cup (180 g) chopped tomato

1/3 cup (33 g) ripe olives

In a medium bowl toss together tuna, scallions, and salsa until combined. To assemble tacos: Sprinkle lettuce into each taco shell. Divide tuna mixture among tacos, along with chickpeas, tomatoes, and olives. Garnish as desired with toppings.

Yield: 4 servings

Per serving: 180 g water; 359 calories (30% from fat, 20% from protein, 50% from carb); 18 g protein; 12 g total fat; 2 g saturated fat; 6 g monounsaturated fat; 3 g polyunsaturated fat; 45 g carbohydrate; 6 g fiber; 2 g sugar; 274 mg phosphorus; 97 mg calcium; 3 mg iron; 509 mg sodium; 512 mg potassium; 620 IU vitamin A; 3 mg vitamin E; 15 mg vitamin C; 19 mg cholesterol

Tip: Substitute 8 (6-inch) flour tortillas for the taco shells if soft tacos are preferred.

Sesame Fish

Sesame seeds add crunch as well as flavor to this Asian baked fish dish.

1 pound (455 g) halibut fillets

$^1/_2$ cup (120 ml) Dick's Reduced Sodium Teriyaki Sauce (see recipe page 25)

2 tablespoons (16 g) sesame seeds

1 tablespoon (8 g) flour

$^1/_2$ teaspoon (1 g) white pepper

Place fillets in a shallow baking dish. Pour teriyaki sauce over fish. Cover and refrigerate 30 minutes or overnight. Preheat oven to 450°F (230°C, or gas mark 8). Combine sesame seeds with flour and pepper. Dip each fillet in the flour mixture. Coat a nonstick baking pan with nonstick vegetable oil spray

and place fillets on the pan in a single layer. Lightly spray the top of each fillet with nonstick vegetable oil spray. Bake for 10 to 15 minutes, or until golden brown and fish flakes easily when pricked with a fork.

Yield: 4 servings

Per serving: 163 calories (15% from fat, 66% from protein, 19% from carbohydrate); 26 g protein; 3 g total fat; 0 g saturated fat; 1 g monounsaturated fat; 1 g polyunsaturated fat; 7 g carbohydrate; 0 g fiber; 5 g sugar; 310 mg phosphorus; 63 mg calcium; 2 mg iron; 86 mg sodium; 594 mg potassium; 178 IU vitamin A; 53 mg ATE vitamin E; 0 mg vitamin C; 36 mg cholesterol; 113 g water

Thai-Style Fish

A complex blend of flavors, this Asian fish stew will become a favorite.

2 pounds (905 g) catfish fillets, cut in 2-inch (5-cm) pieces

$^1/_4$ cup (60 ml) lime juice

$^1/_4$ teaspoon (0.3 g) red pepper flakes

1 tablespoon (15 ml) sesame oil

1 cup (160 g) onion, thinly sliced

1 cup (100 g) celery, sliced

1 cup (70 g) bok choy, shredded

1 teaspoon (1.8 g) ground ginger

1 teaspoon (3 g) minced garlic

1 tablespoon (6.3 g) curry powder

8 cups (1.9 L) low sodium chicken broth

2 cups (330 g) cooked rice

Mix catfish, lime juice, and red pepper flakes; set aside. Heat sesame oil in a large saucepan or Dutch oven. Sauté onion, celery, bok choy, ginger, and garlic for 1 minute. Sprinkle with curry powder. Reduce heat and sauté until onion is soft. Add chicken broth and bring to a boil. Stir in catfish mixture and simmer for 3 minutes, or until catfish is done. To serve, place rice in the center of soup bowls and ladle soup over.

Yield: 8 servings

Per serving: 275 calories (39% from fat, 35% from protein, 26% from carbohydrate); 24 g protein; 12 g total fat; 3 g saturated fat; 5 g monounsaturated fat; 3 g polyunsaturated fat; 18 g carbohydrate; 1 g fiber; 2 g sugar; 339 mg phosphorus; 47 mg calcium; 2 mg iron; 177 mg sodium; 668 mg potassium; 155 IU vitamin A; 17 mg ATE vitamin E; 6 mg vitamin C; 53 mg cholesterol; 393 g water

Tuna and Pasta Salad

A great main dish salad for those hot summer days when you don't feel like doing much cooking.

8 ounces (225 g) whole wheat pasta

$^1/_2$ pound (225 g) pea pods

1 can tuna

6 ounces (170 g) artichoke hearts

$^1/_2$ cup (50 g) sliced green olives

$^1/_2$ pound (35 g) sliced fresh mushrooms

$^1/_2$ cup (120 ml) Italian dressing

$^1/_2$ teaspoon lemon pepper

$^1/_4$ cup (25 g) grated Parmesan cheese

Cook pasta according to package directions; drain and let cool. Cook pea pods 1 minute in boiling water, remove, and let cool. Put shells and pea pods into a bowl. Drain water from tuna and add to bowl with pea pods. Add artichokes and artichoke liquid, olives, and mushrooms. Combine with pasta and pour dressing over it all. Add lemon pepper and mix well. Sprinkle with Parmesan cheese.

Yield: 4 servings

Per serving: 207 g water; 440 calories (28% from fat, 22% from protein, 49% from carb); 26 g protein; 15 g total fat; 3 g saturated fat; 4 g monounsaturated fat; 5 g polyunsaturated fat; 57 g carbohydrate; 9 g fiber; 6 g sugar; 394 mg phosphorus; 151 mg calcium; 5 mg iron; 782 mg sodium; 656 mg potassium; 801 IU vitamin A; 10 mg vitamin E; 38 mg vitamin C; 24 mg cholesterol

Pasta, White Bean, and Tuna Salad

A tasty main dish salad with two-thirds of your daily fiber requirements in one helping.

Vegetables

1 can artichoke hearts

6 ounces (170 g) green beans, blanched and drained

$^1/_2$ pound (225 g) beets, cooked or canned, drained and sliced

$1^1/_2$ cups (270 g) tomato, sliced in wedges

Pasta Mixture

$^1/_2$ pound (225 g) whole wheat pasta, cooked, rinsed, and drained

2 cups (200 g) cooked white beans, drained

1 can tuna, drained

Vinaigrette

$^1/_4$ cup (60 ml) olive oil

$^1/_2$ cup (120 ml) fresh lemon juice

$^1/_2$ teaspoon garlic, peeled and minced

1 teaspoon dried basil

$^1/_2$ teaspoon black pepper

Whisk all vinaigrette ingredients together. Using half the vinaigrette mixture, marinate the vegetables for at least 1 hour before serving. Stir together drained pasta, beans, and tuna and mix. Immediately before serving, toss vegetables and pasta mixture with the remaining vinaigrette.

Yield: 5 servings

Per serving: 216 g water; 629 calories (19% from fat, 22% from protein, 59% from carb); 37 g protein; 14 g total fat; 2 g saturated fat; 8 g monounsaturated fat; 2 g polyunsaturated fat; 97 g carbohydrate; 21 g fiber; 6 g sugar; 498 mg phosphorus; 255 mg calcium; 12 mg iron; 154 mg sodium; 2033 mg potassium; 628 IU vitamin A; 2 mg vitamin E; 33 mg vitamin C; 14 mg cholesterol

Shrimp and Spinach Pasta

Subtle flavor, but how can you go wrong with shrimp and spinach, either in taste or nutrition.

6 ounces whole wheat pasta

1 pound shrimp, peeled

$^1/_2$ cup dry white wine

2 tablespoons olive oil

1 cup onion, sliced

1 teaspoon garlic, minced

1 pound fresh spinach

Cook pasta according to package directions, omitting salt. Reserve one cup of pasta water. Drain pasta. Heat large skillet over medium heat. Add shrimp and wine. Cover and cook until shrimp are pink and opaque, about 1 to 2 minutes. Remove from skillet. Add oil to skillet and cook onions until tender. Add garlic and cook one minute longer. Stir in spinach, cover and cook until wilted, 2 to 3 minutes. Add shrimp and pasta. Stir to combine.

Yield: 4 servings

Per serving: 178 calories (39% from fat, 15% from protein , 46% from carb); 6 g protein ; 7 g total fat; 1 g saturated fat; 5 g monounsaturated fat; 1 g polyunsaturated fat; 20 g carb; 4 g fiber; 3 g sugar; 113 mg phosphorus; 132 mg calcium; 96 mg sodium; 738 mg potassium; 10638 IU vitamin A; 1 mg ATE vitamin E; 35 mg vitamin C; 2 mg cholesterol

Shrimp and Scallop Paella

Classic seafood paella, but made healthy.

1 cup red bell peppers, chopped

$^1/_2$ cup onion, chopped

1 tablespoon garlic, minced

$^1/_2$ teaspoon turmeric

$^1/_2$ teaspoon paprika

$3^1/_4$ cups water

$1^1/_2$ cups long grain rice, uncooked

1 cup artichoke hearts, halved

1 pound shrimp, peeled

$^1/_2$ pound scallops

$^1/_2$ cup frozen peas, thawed

Spray Dutch oven with non-stick cooking spray. Heat over medium-high heat. Add red pepper, onion, and garlic. Cook until crisp-tender, about 3 minutes. Add water, turmenic, and paprika. Bring to a boil. Stir in rice and artichokes. Cover, reduce heat to medium low and simmer for 18 minutes, Stir in shrimp, scallops and peas. Cover and simmer 5 minutes or until seafood is opaque. Let stand 5 minutes before serving.

Yield: 6 servings

Per serving: 321 calories (6% from fat, 34% from protein , 59% from carb); 27 g protein ; 2 g total fat; 0 g saturated fat; 0 g monounsaturated fat; 1 g polyunsaturated fat; 47 g carb; 3 g fiber; 3 g sugar; 332 mg phosphorus; 81 mg calcium; 203 mg sodium; 490 mg potassium; 1360 IU vitamin A; 46 mg ATE vitamin E; 54 mg vitamin C; 127 mg cholesterol

Quick and Easy Linguine with Scallops

Simple preparation and simply delicious.

1 pound linguine

2 tablespoons olive oil

1 teaspoon garlic, minced

28 ounces no salt added tomatoes, diced

1 pound scallops

$^1/_2$ cup dry white wine

2 tablespoons fresh parsley

Cook pasta according to package directions. Heat oil in large skillet. Add garlic and cook until beginning to brown, 1 to 2 minutes. Add tomatoes and scallops and cook until scallops are tender, about 5 minutes. Stir in wine and parsley. Serve over pasta.

Yield: 6 servings

Per serving: 473 calories (25% from fat, 21% from protein, 53% from carb); 25 g protein ; 13 g total fat; 2 g saturated fat; 8 g monounsaturated fat; 2 g polyunsaturated fat; 62 g carb; 3 g fiber; 5 g sugar; 356 mg phosphorus; 85 mg calcium; 153 mg sodium; 743 mg potassium; 363 IU vitamin A; 24 mg ATE vitamin E; 23 mg vitamin C; 97 mg cholesterol

10

Main Dishes:
Vegetarian

I f you are the kind of person who thinks they don't like meatless meals, you've come to the right place. Take a look through this chapter and I can almost guarantee you'll find something you like. If you want Indian or Italian or Mexican we have those here. If you want comfort food we have that too. If you just want a sandwich we can help you there, too. And the great thing is vegetarian recipes have to be heart-healthy. It's nearly impossible to create a high fat one. They contain a variety of the vegetables that most of us struggle to eat enough of. And many contain the fiber of legumes and whole grains. We've made one night a week a meatless night and it's amazing how many things we have discovered that we like. Start here to do the same.

Grilled Stuffed Portobellos

I discovered portobello mushrooms not too long ago. We like them grilled on a bun, but these Mediterranean-flavored ones are better served with pasta or rice.

$^2/_3$ cup (120 g) plum tomato, chopped

2 ounces (55 g) part-skim mozzarella, shredded

1 teaspoon (5 ml) olive oil, divided

$^1/_2$ teaspoon (0.4 g) fresh rosemary

$^1/_8$ teaspoon (0.3 g) coarsely ground black pepper

$^1/_4$ teaspoon (0.8 g) crushed garlic

4 portobello mushroom caps, about 4 to 5 inches (10 to 12.5 cm) each

2 tablespoons (30 ml) lemon juice

2 teaspoons (2.6 g) fresh parsley

Prepare grill. Combine the tomato, cheese, $^1/_2$ teaspoon (2.5 ml) oil, rosemary, pepper, and garlic in a small bowl. Remove brown gills from the undersides of mushroom caps using a spoon, and discard. Remove stems; discard. Combine remaining $^1/_2$ teaspoon oil (2.5 ml) and lemon juice in a small bowl. Brush over both sides of mushroom caps. Place the mushroom caps, stem sides down, on grill rack sprayed with nonstick vegetable oil spray, and grill for 5 minutes on each side or until soft. Spoon one-quarter of the tomato mixture into each mushroom cap. Cover and grill 3 minutes or until cheese is melted. Sprinkle with parsley.

Yield: 4 servings

Per serving: 75 calories (40% from fat, 29% from protein, 32% from carbohydrate); 6 g protein; 4 g total fat; 2 g saturated fat; 1 g monounsaturated fat; 0 g polyunsaturated fat; 6 g carbohydrate; 2 g fiber; 3 g sugar; 181 mg phosphorus; 122 mg calcium; 1 mg iron; 95 mg sodium; 490 mg potassium; 331 IU vitamin A; 18 mg ATE vitamin E; 8 mg vitamin C; 9 mg cholesterol; 115 g water

Grilled Portobello Mushrooms

This is a fairly simple recipe for grilled portobellos, but one that still provides a flavorful meat alternative.

4 portobello mushroom caps, cleaned and stems removed

$^1/_4$ cup (60 ml) balsamic vinegar

1 tablespoon (15 ml) olive oil

1 teaspoon (0.7 g) dried basil

1 teaspoon (1 g) dried oregano

$^1/_2$ teaspoon (1.5 g) minced garlic

4 ounces (115 g) low fat Provolone cheese, sliced

Place the mushroom caps smooth side up in a shallow dish. Mix together vinegar, oil, basil, oregano, and garlic. Pour over the mushrooms. Let stand at room temperature for 15 minutes, turning twice. Preheat grill to medium-high heat. Brush grate with oil. Place mushrooms on the grill, reserving marinade for basting. Grill for 5 to 8 minutes on each side, or until tender. Brush with marinade frequently. Top with cheese during the last 2 minutes of grilling.

Yield: 4 servings

Per serving: 156 calories (53% from fat, 30% from protein, 17% from carbohydrate); 9 g protein; 7 g total fat; 3 g saturated fat; 4 g monounsaturated fat; 1 g polyunsaturated fat; 5 g carbohydrate; 1 g fiber; 2 g sugar;

252 mg phosphorus; 230 mg calcium; 1 mg iron; 254 mg sodium; 466 mg potassium; 283 IU vitamin A; 65 mg ATE vitamin E; 0 mg vitamin C; 20 mg cholesterol; 102 g water

Hawaiian Portobello Burgers

We only recently started using portobello mushrooms, but they have quickly become a popular addition to our diet. This recipe gives you a sandwich so flavorful you won't miss the meat.

2 portobello mushrooms, cleaned and stems removed

2 tablespoons (30 ml) Dick's Reduced Sodium Teriyaki Sauce (see recipe page 25)

2 slices pineapple

2 slices low fat Monterey Jack cheese

2 lettuce leaves

2 slices tomato

2 hamburger buns

1 tablespoon (14 g) low fat mayonnaise

Place mushrooms in a shallow dish. Spread teriyaki sauce over the mushrooms and marinate for 15 minutes. Grill the mushrooms and pineapple slices over low heat until tender. Add the cheese on top of the mushrooms and continue to grill briefly to melt cheese. Assemble burgers by placing 1 lettuce leaf and tomato slice on each bottom bun, then top with the mushrooms and pineapple. Spread each top bun with half of the mayonnaise.

Yield: 2 servings

Per serving: 248 calories (19% from fat, 25% from protein, 56% from carbohydrate); 17 g protein; 6 g total fat; 2 g saturated fat; 1 g monounsaturated fat; 1 g polyunsaturated fat; 39 g carbohydrate; 11 g fiber; 26 g sugar; 441 mg phosphorus; 276 mg calcium; 4 mg iron; 329 mg sodium; 1671 mg potassium; 4191 IU vitamin A; 17 mg ATE vitamin E; 29 mg vitamin C; 9 mg cholesterol; 909 g water

Caribbean Vegetable Curry

A moderately spicy vegetarian curry meal. Adjust the amount of cayenne to your taste.

1 tablespoon (15 ml) olive oil

1 cup (160 g) thinly sliced onion

$^3/_4$ teaspoon crushed garlic

1 apple, peeled, cored, and chopped

$1^1/_2$ teaspoons curry powder

$1^1/_2$ teaspoons grated lemon peel

1 teaspoon ginger

1 teaspoon coriander

$^1/_8$ teaspoon turmeric

$^1/_8$ teaspoon cayenne pepper

2 cups (344 g) cooked black-eyed peas, drained

2 cups (200 g) cooked kidney beans

$^1/_3$ cup (50 g) raisins

1 cup (230 g) plain fat-free yogurt

3 eggs, hard boiled and halved

3 cups (495 g) cooked rice

6 radishes, thinly sliced

$^1/_4$ cup (25 g) sliced scallions

1/2 cup chopped fresh cilantro

1/4 cup (37 g) chopped peanuts

Heat oil in skillet. Sauté onion, garlic, and apple until soft. Combine curry powder, lemon peel, ginger, coriander, turmeric, and cayenne pepper. Stir into onion mixture. Add black-eyed peas, undrained kidney beans, and raisins. Cover; simmer 5 minutes. Remove from heat, stir in yogurt. Place egg halves on rice. Spoon curry over. Top with radishes, scallions, cilantro, and peanuts.

Yield: 6 servings

Per serving: 218 g water; 524 calories (12% from fat, 22% from protein, 66% from carb); 29 g protein; 7 g total fat; 2 g saturated fat; 3 g monounsaturated fat; 1 g polyunsaturated fat; 89 g carbohydrate; 22 g fiber; 16 g sugar; 513 mg phosphorus; 238 mg calcium; 9 mg iron; 119 mg sodium; 1465 mg potassium; 495 IU vitamin A; 40 mg vitamin E; 13 mg vitamin C; 119 mg cholesterol

Bean and Tomato Curry

This makes a good side dish with something like a grilled chicken breast or loin pork chop, but you can also use it for a vegetarian meal. In that case, serve over rice or with pita bread.

1 tablespoon (15 ml) canola oil

1 teaspoon (3.7 g) mustard seed

1 teaspoon (2.5 g) cumin seeds

1 cup (160 g) onion, chopped

1 tablespoon (6 g) fresh ginger, peeled and chopped

1/2 teaspoon (1.5 g) chopped garlic

4 cups (720 g) canned no-salt-added tomatoes

2 cups (450 g) kidney beans, drained and rinsed

1 teaspoon (2 g) curry powder

Heat oil in large pot over medium heat and stir-fry the mustard and cumin seeds until they pop. Add onion, ginger, and garlic, and stir-fry until lightly colored. Add tomatoes with juice, beans, and curry powder. Simmer for about 20 minutes or until thick and saucy.

Yield: 6 servings

Per serving: 140 calories (19% from fat, 19% from protein, 62% from carbohydrate); 7 g protein; 3 g total fat; 0 g saturated fat; 2 g monounsaturated fat; 1 g polyunsaturated fat; 23 g carbohydrate; 6 g fiber; 5 g sugar; 131 mg phosphorus; 81 mg calcium; 4 mg iron; 163 mg sodium; 598 mg potassium; 196 IU vitamin A; 0 mg ATE vitamin E; 18 mg vitamin C; 0 mg cholesterol; 215 g water

Tip: To lower the amount of sodium, use no-salt-added beans or cooked dried beans.

Garbanzo Curry

Indian vegetarian slow cooker recipes like this curry will warm you up on a cold day. It's so easy, but it tastes as good as vegetarian Indian recipes you get at a restaurant.

2 tablespoons (30 ml) canola oil

1 cup (160 g) onion, diced

1/2 teaspoon (1.5 g) minced garlic

1 teaspoon (2.7 g) fresh ginger, peeled and grated

1 teaspoon (2.5 g) cumin

1 teaspoon (2 g) coriander

1 teaspoon (2.2 g) turmeric

2 cups (480 g) canned garbanzo beans, drained and rinsed

2 cups (360 g) canned no-salt-added tomatoes

1/2 teaspoon (1.2 g) garam masala

Heat oil in a heavy skillet. Sauté onion, garlic, ginger, cumin, coriander, and turmeric until onion becomes soft. Place onion mixture and remaining ingredients in a slow cooker and cook on low for 8 to 10 hours or on high for 4 to 5 hours.

Yield: 4 servings

Per serving: 246 calories (31% from fat, 12% from protein, 57% from carbohydrate); 8 g protein; 9 g total fat; 1 g saturated fat; 5 g monounsaturated fat; 3 g polyunsaturated fat; 37 g carbohydrate; 7 g fiber; 5 g sugar; 148 mg phosphorus; 93 mg calcium; 4 mg iron; 377 mg sodium; 524 mg potassium; 185 IU vitamin A; 0 mg ATE vitamin E; 20 mg vitamin C; 0 mg cholesterol; 233 g water

Tip: Garam masala is an Indian spice blend that you can find at larger grocery or specialty stores.

Tofu Curry

This is one of the simplest vegetarian meals you'll find. Serve the curry over rice with whatever condiments you like.

3 tablespoons (45 ml) olive oil, divided

12 ounces (340 g) firm tofu, drained and cubed

1 cup (113 g) zucchini, sliced

1 cup (70 g) mushrooms, sliced

1 cup (235 ml) fat free evaporated milk

2 teaspoons (4 g) curry powder

Heat 1 tablespoon (15 ml) oil in a large skillet or work. Fry tofu until the bottom gets golden, then carefully turn and fry the other sides. Remove to a plate. Heat remaining oil and stir-fry zucchini and mushrooms until crisp-tender. Add milk and curry powder and continue cooking until slightly thickened. Stir in tofu.

Yield: 4 servings

Per serving: 204 calories (55% from fat, 23% from protein, 22% from carbohydrate); 12 g protein; 13 g total fat; 2 g saturated fat; 8 g monounsaturated fat; 2 g polyunsaturated fat; 12 g carbohydrate; 1 g fiber; 9 g sugar; 232 mg phosphorus; 223 mg calcium; 2 mg iron; 109 mg sodium; 531 mg potassium; 325 IU vitamin A; 76 mg ATE vitamin E; 7 mg vitamin C; 3 mg cholesterol; 171 g water

Tip: The possibilities for vegetable combinations are almost endless. Feel free to experiment.

Zucchini Frittata

During the summer when the garden is producing I'm often looking for uses for zucchini, and this one is popular.

2 cups (250 g) shredded zucchini

2 tablespoons (30 ml) olive oil

1/2 cup (35 g) mushrooms, sliced

4 eggs, beaten

1/3 cup (37 g) Swiss cheese, shredded

Place the zucchini in a paper towel and squeeze out any excess moisture. Heat oil in a 10-inch (25-cm)

skillet. Sauté the mushrooms briefly, then add the zucchini. Cook for 4 minutes, or until the squash is barely tender. Pour eggs over vegetables. Stir once quickly to coat vegetables. Cook over low heat until eggs begin to set. Sprinkle with the cheese. Place under the broiler until cheese browns. Let set for 2 to 3 minutes. Cut into wedges and serve.

Yield: 4 servings

Per serving: 144 calories (59% from fat, 32% from protein, 9% from carbohydrate); 12 g protein; 10 g total fat; 2 g saturated fat; 6 g monounsaturated fat; 2 g polyunsaturated fat; 3 g carbohydrate; 1 g fiber; 2 g sugar; 174 mg phosphorus; 149 mg calcium; 2 mg iron; 146 mg sodium; 310 mg potassium; 367 IU vitamin A; 4 mg ATE vitamin E; 11 mg vitamin C; 214 mg cholesterol; 125 g water

Pizza Omelet

When you have a taste for pizza, but don't have the time or want to make the effort to make it yourself, try this instead. This is a dinner-sized omelet for two.

4 eggs

2 tablespoons (30 g) fat free sour cream

2 tablespoons (30 ml) water

$1/2$ teaspoon (0.4 g) Italian seasoning

$1/2$ cup (35 g) mushrooms, sliced

$1/4$ cup (40 g) onion, sliced

$1/4$ cup (37 g) green bell pepper, coarsely chopped

$1/4$ cup (60 ml) spaghetti sauce, heated

2 ounces (55 g) part-skim mozzarella, shredded

Whisk together egg, sour cream, water, and Italian seasoning until fluffy. Sauté mushrooms, onion, and green bell pepper until onion begins to get soft. Pour egg mixture into a heated nonstick skillet or omelet pan sprayed with nonstick vegetable oil spray. Lift the edges as it cooks to allow uncooked egg to run underneath. When it is nearly set, cover half the omelet with the vegetables and fold the other half over the top. Remove to plate. Top with heated sauce and cheese.

Yield: 2 servings

Per serving: 232 calories (39% from fat, 45% from protein, 16% from carbohydrate); 24 g protein; 9 g total fat; 4 g saturated fat; 3 g monounsaturated fat; 2 g polyunsaturated fat; 9 g carbohydrate; 2 g fiber; 3 g sugar; 334 mg phosphorus; 323 mg calcium; 3 mg iron; 547 mg sodium; 599 mg potassium; 856 IU vitamin A; 51 mg ATE vitamin E; 20 mg vitamin C; 435 mg cholesterol; 224 g water

Ricotta Omelet

This makes a nice summer dinner, with a salad and bread. You could also add some vegetables if you like.

4 eggs

$1/4$ teaspoon (0.8 g) garlic powder

$1/4$ teaspoon (0.5 g) black pepper

$1/2$ cup (125 g) low fat ricotta cheese

2 tablespoons (30 ml) olive oil

Beat the eggs with the garlic powder, pepper, and ricotta. Heat the oil in a skillet or omelet pan. Add the egg mixture, and swirl to distribute evenly. Cook until nearly set, lifting edge to allow uncooked egg to run underneath. Fold over, cover, and cook until done.

Yield: 2 servings

Per serving: 311 calories (66% from fat, 29% from protein, 6% from carbohydrate); 22 g protein; 23 g total fat; 6 g saturated fat; 12 g monounsaturated fat; 4 g polyunsaturated fat; 4 g carbohydrate; 0 g fiber; 1 g sugar; 266 mg phosphorus; 235 mg calcium; 3 mg iron; 299 mg sodium; 398 mg potassium; 689 IU vitamin A; 65 mg ATE vitamin E; 0 mg vitamin C; 440 mg cholesterol; 150 g water

Tomato and Basil Quiche

A great meatless quiche. If you want, you can put it in a crust, but we like it just as well without it.

1 tablespoon (15 ml) olive oil

1 cup (160 g) onion, sliced

2 cups (360 g) tomatoes, sliced

2 tablespoons (16 g) flour

2 teaspoons (1.4 g) dried basil

3 eggs

$^1/_2$ cup (120 ml) skim milk

$^1/_2$ teaspoon (1 g) black pepper

1 cup (110 g) Swiss cheese, shredded

Preheat oven to 400°F (200°C, or gas mark 6). Heat olive oil in a large skillet over medium heat. Sauté onion until soft; remove from skillet. Sprinkle tomato slices with flour and basil, then sauté 1 minute on each side. In a small bowl, whisk together eggs and milk. Season with pepper. Spread half the cheese in the bottom of a pie pan sprayed with nonstick vegetable oil spray. Layer onions over the cheese and top with tomatoes. Pour the egg mixture over the vegetables. Sprinkle the remaining cheese over the top. Bake for 10 minutes. Reduce heat to 350°F (180°C, or gas mark 4), and bake for 15 to 20 minutes, or until filling is puffed and golden brown. Serve warm.

Yield: 4 servings

Per serving: 188 calories (33% from fat, 38% from protein, 29% from carbohydrate); 18 g protein; 7 g total fat; 2 g saturated fat; 3 g monounsaturated fat; 1 g polyunsaturated fat; 14 g carbohydrate; 2 g fiber; 2 g sugar; 327 mg phosphorus; 408 mg calcium; 2 mg iron; 196 mg sodium; 391 mg potassium; 781 IU vitamin A; 32 mg ATE vitamin E; 23 mg vitamin C; 173 mg cholesterol; 192 g water

Bean and Cheddar Cheese Pie

Beans and cheese combine to make a filling and tasty meatless main dish with a southwestern accent.

$^3/_4$ cup (93 g) flour

$1^1/_2$ cups (175 g) shredded Cheddar cheese, divided

$1^1/_2$ teaspoons baking powder

$^1/_3$ cup (80 ml) skim milk

1 egg, beaten

2 cups (328 g) cooked chickpeas, drained

2 cups (200 g) cooked kidney beans, drained

8 ounces (225 g) no-salt-added tomato sauce

$^1/_2$ cup (75 g) chopped green bell pepper

$^1/_4$ cup (40 g) chopped onion

2 teaspoons chili powder

$^1/_2$ teaspoon dried oregano leaves

$^1/_4$ teaspoon garlic powder

Heat oven to 375°F (190°C, gas mark 5). Spray a 10-inch (25-cm) pie plate with nonstick vegetable oil spray. Mix flour, $^1/_2$ cup (58 g) cheese, and baking powder in a medium bowl. Stir in milk and egg until blended. Spread over bottom and up sides of pie plate. Mix $^1/_2$ cup (58 g) of the remaining cheese and the remaining ingredients; spoon into pie plate. Sprinkle with remaining cheese. Bake about 25 minutes or until edges are puffy and light brown. Let stand 10 minutes before cutting.

Yield: 8 servings

Per serving: 109 g water; 400 calories (23% from fat, 23% from protein, 54% from carb); 23 g protein; 10 g total fat; 6 g saturated fat; 3 g monounsaturated fat; 1 g polyunsaturated fat; 55 g carbohydrate; 15 g fiber; 3 g sugar; 438 mg phosphorus; 343 mg calcium; 6 mg iron; 464 mg sodium; 957 mg potassium; 648 IU vitamin A; 81 mg vitamin E; 16 mg vitamin C; 52 mg cholesterol

Artichoke Pie

A nice meatless meal with a kind of Italian flavor.

3 eggs

3 ounces (85 g) cream cheese with chives, softened

$^3/_4$ teaspoon garlic powder

$^1/_4$ teaspoon black pepper

1$^1/_2$ cups (225 g) shredded mozzarella cheese, divided

1 cup (250 g) ricotta cheese

$^1/_2$ cup (115 g) low-fat mayonnaise

1 can artichoke hearts

1 cup (164 g) cooked chickpeas

$^1/_2$ cup (50 g) sliced black olives

2 ounces (55 g) pimento, drained and diced

2 tablespoons fresh parsley

1 9-inch (23-cm) pie shell, unbaked

$^1/_3$ cup (33 g) grated Parmesan cheese

In a mixing bowl, beat eggs. Stir in cream cheese, garlic powder, and pepper. Stir in 1 cup (150 g) of mozzarella, the ricotta, and the mayonnaise. Quarter 2 artichoke hearts and set aside. Chop remaining artichoke hearts; fold into cheese mixture. Fold in chickpeas, olives, pimento, and parsley. Turn mixture into pastry shell. Bake in a 350°F (180°C, gas mark 4) oven for 30 minutes. Top with remaining mozzarella and the Parmesan cheese. Bake about 15 minutes more until set. Let stand for 10 minutes. Top with quartered artichokes.

Yield: 8 servings

Per serving: 128 g water; 371 calories (56% from fat, 19% from protein, 26% from carb); 17 g protein; 22 g total fat; 8 g saturated fat; 7 g monounsaturated fat; 2 g polyunsaturated fat; 23 g carbohydrate; 3 g fiber; 2 g sugar; 283 mg phosphorus; 288 mg calcium; 2 mg iron; 697 mg sodium; 282 mg potassium; 841 IU vitamin A; 122 mg vitamin E; 10 mg vitamin C; 130 mg cholesterol

Cheese Pie

This is an ideal vegetarian main dish, needing only a salad to make it a complete meal.

4 ounces (115 g) feta cheese

16 ounces (455 g) low fat ricotta cheese

4 eggs

$^1/_4$ cup (30 g) flour

$^3/_4$ cup (180 ml) skim milk

$^1/_4$ teaspoon (0.5 g) black pepper

Preheat oven to 375°F (190°C, or gas mark 5). Spray an ovenproof skillet or glass baking dish with nonstick vegetable oil spray. Mix the cheeses together, then stir in the eggs, flour, milk, and pepper. Pour the batter into the prepared pan. Bake for 40 minutes, or until golden and set. Cut into wedges.

Yield: 4 servings

Per serving: 332 calories (47% from fat, 33% from protein, 20% from carbohydrate); 27 g protein; 17 g total fat; 10 g saturated fat; 5 g monounsaturated fat; 2 g polyunsaturated fat; 16 g carbohydrate; 0 g fiber; 2 g sugar; 439 mg phosphorus; 549 mg calcium; 2 mg iron; 597 mg sodium; 360 mg potassium; 875 IU vitamin A; 183 mg ATE vitamin E; 1 mg vitamin C; 272 mg cholesterol; 194 g water

Asparagus Strata

This can be either breakfast or dinner—fancy enough to serve guests, but easy enough to make often for family.

1 pound (455 g) asparagus

6 slices whole wheat bread

2 cups (225 g) shredded Cheddar cheese, divided

1 cup (150 g) cubed ham

5 eggs

$^3/_4$ teaspoon Worcestershire sauce

$^1/_4$ teaspoon garlic powder

$1^3/_4$ cups (410 ml) skim milk

2 tablespoons (20 g) minced onion

$^1/_8$ teaspoon cayenne

Cut asparagus into 1-inch (2.5-cm) pieces, drop into boiling, salted water and cook rapidly for 4 minutes. Drain. If using frozen asparagus, thaw and drain. Trim crusts from bread. Fit into 7 × 11-inch (28-cm) baking dish sprayed with nonstick vegetable oil spray. Sprinkle $1^1/_4$ cups (145 g) Cheddar cheese over the bread slices and distribute the asparagus and ham. Beat the remaining ingredients, except the reserved cheese, together until blended. Pour over the layered ingredients, cover, and refrigerate at least 8 hours or overnight. Bake uncovered in 350°F (180°C, gas mark 4) oven for 30 minutes. Top with remaining cheese and continue baking for 10 minutes until center is firm. Allow to stand for 5 minutes before cutting.

Yield: 8 servings

Per serving: 158 g water; 303 calories (50% from fat, 29% from protein, 21% from carb); 22 g protein; 17 g total fat; 9 g saturated fat; 5 g monounsaturated fat; 1 g polyunsaturated fat; 16 g carbohydrate; 2 g fiber; 3 g sugar; 398 mg phosphorus; 378 mg calcium; 3 mg iron; 576 mg sodium; 413 mg potassium; 1051 IU vitamin A; 167 mg vitamin E; 6 mg vitamin C; 191 mg cholesterol

Whole Wheat Apple Strata

This has become a traditional Christmas-morning breakfast. The original recipe called for ham, but no one seems to miss it. You could use any leftover bread, but I like honey wheat. If you can't find canned apples, you can use apple pie filling, although the result will be sweeter.

6 slices whole wheat bread, cubed

1 can (21-ounce, or 600 g) apples or apple pie filling

3 ounces (85 g) low fat Cheddar cheese, shredded

4 eggs

$^1/_4$ cup (60 ml) skim milk

Place bread in a 9-inch (23-cm) square pan coated with nonstick vegetable oil spray. Spoon apples over bread. Sprinkle with cheese. Combine eggs and milk and pour over bread mixture. Cover with plastic wrap and refrigerate overnight. Preheat oven to 350°F (180°C, or gas mark 4). Bake uncovered for 40 to 45 minutes, or until top is lightly browned and center is set.

Yield: 4 servings

Per serving: 232 calories (21% from fat, 31% from protein, 48% from carbohydrate); 18 g protein; 5 g total fat; 2 g saturated fat; 2 g monounsaturated fat; 2 g polyunsaturated fat; 28 g carbohydrate; 3 g fiber; 9 g sugar; 284 mg phosphorus; 189 mg calcium; 3 mg iron; 484 mg sodium; 276 mg potassium; 313 IU vitamin A; 22 mg ATE vitamin E; 2 mg vitamin C; 215 mg cholesterol; 125 g water

Fiber-Rich Casserole

This makes either a great side dish or a meatless meal. Serves 4 as a main dish, 6 as a side dish.

1$^1/_2$ cups (355 ml) chicken broth

1 cup (130 g) thinly sliced carrot

$^1/_2$ cup (100 g) pearl barley

2 cups (200 g) cooked kidney beans, drained

$^1/_4$ cup (40 g) chopped onion

$^1/_4$ cup fresh parsley

3 tablespoons (27 g) bulgur

$^1/_8$ teaspoon garlic powder

$^1/_4$ cup (30 g) shredded Cheddar cheese

Mix all together except cheese. Put in 1-quart (1-L) dish. Bake covered at 350°F (180°C, gas mark 4) for 50 minutes. Uncover; sprinkle on cheese. Return to oven to melt cheese.

Yield: 6 servings

Per serving: 96 g water; 318 calories (9% from fat, 24% from protein, 67% from carb); 20 g protein; 3 g total fat; 1 g saturated fat; 1 g monounsaturated fat; 1 g polyunsaturated fat; 55 g carbohydrate; 20 g fiber; 3 g sugar; 360 mg phosphorus; 148 mg calcium; 6 mg iron; 259 mg sodium; 1099 mg potassium; 3856 IU vitamin A; 14 mg vitamin E; 8 mg vitamin C; 6 mg cholesterol

Brown Rice and Beans

A simple but filling and good-tasting side dish or meal.

$^1/_2$ cup (95 g) brown rice

1$^1/_2$ cups (355 ml) water

$^1/_3$ cup (33 g) sliced celery

$^1/_3$ cup (55 g) chopped onion

$^1/_2$ cup (75 g) chopped green bell pepper

14 ounces (400 g) canned kidney beans, drained

2 cups (480 g) no-salt-added canned tomatoes

$^1/_4$ teaspoon garlic powder

$^1/_8$ teaspoon Tabasco sauce

Cook rice in water until water is absorbed. In a skillet, cook celery, onion, and bell pepper slowly over low heat about 10 minutes. Add beans, tomatoes, and seasoning. Bring to a boil and then simmer, uncovered, about 10 minutes. Add cooked rice and mix.

Yield: 4 servings

Per serving: 324 g water; 182 calories (3% from fat, 23% from protein, 74% from carb); 11 g protein; 1 g total fat; 0 g saturated fat; 0 g monounsaturated fat; 0 g polyunsaturated fat; 35 g carbohydrate; 12 g fiber; 4 g sugar; 189 mg phosphorus; 116 mg calcium; 4 mg iron; 32 mg sodium; 729 mg potassium; 253 IU vitamin A; 0 mg vitamin E; 29 mg vitamin C; 0 mg cholesterol

Bulgur Cheese Bake

This makes a great side dish and can also be used as a full meatless meal. It has a vaguely Italian flavor and is good with tomato sauce.

2 cups (475 ml) water

1 cup (140 g) bulgur

1 tablespoon (15 ml) olive oil

1 cup (160 g) finely chopped onion

$^{1}/_{2}$ teaspoon finely chopped garlic

$^{1}/_{2}$ cup (90 g) chopped, seeded plum tomatoes

2 eggs

$^{1}/_{2}$ cup (120 ml) skim milk

6 ounces (170 g) shredded Cheddar cheese

10 ounces (280 g) frozen chopped spinach, thawed and well drained

Preheat oven to 350°F (180°C, gas mark 4). Spray a 1$^{1}/_{2}$-quart (1.5-L) casserole dish with nonstick

vegetable oil spray. Bring water to boiling in a medium-size saucepan. Add bulgur, lower heat, and simmer, uncovered, 10 minutes or until liquid is absorbed. Set pan aside. Heat oil in a medium-size skillet over medium heat. Add the onion and the garlic to the skillet and sauté for 5 minutes. Stir in tomatoes and sauté for 5 minutes. Stir onion mixture into the bulgur. Beat together eggs and milk in large bowl. Stir together with cheese, spinach, and bulgur mixture until well mixed. Turn into the casserole dish. Bake in preheated oven for 30 minutes. Remove casserole and let stand for 15 minutes before serving.

Yield: 4 servings

Per serving: 302 g water; 416 calories (44% from fat, 21% from protein, 34% from carb); 23 g protein; 21 g total fat; 11 g saturated fat; 8 g monounsaturated fat; 2 g polyunsaturated fat; 37 g carbohydrate; 10 g fiber; 3 g sugar; 463 mg phosphorus; 501 mg calcium; 3 mg iron; 402 mg sodium; 598 mg potassium; 9332 IU vitamin A; 167 mg vitamin E; 7 mg vitamin C; 164 mg cholesterol

Broccoli Wild Rice Casserole

This is another of those recipes that can be used as either a side dish or as a vegetarian main course.

1$^{1}/_{2}$ cups (240 g) wild rice

6 cups (420 g) broccoli

2 cups (484 g) reduced-sodium cream of mushroom soup

2 cups (225 g) low fat Cheddar cheese, shredded

Preheat oven to 325°F (170°C, or gas mark 3). Prepare wild rice according to package directions. Layer rice in the bottom of a 9 × 9-inch (23 × 23-cm) casserole pan. Steam broccoli for 5 minutes and layer on top of rice. Mix soup and cheese together and spread on top of broccoli. Bake, uncovered, for 45 minutes.

Yield: 6 servings

Per serving: 293 calories (16% from fat, 27% from protein, 58% from carbohydrate); 20 g protein; 5 g total fat; 2 g saturated fat; 1 g monounsaturated fat; 1 g polyunsaturated fat; 44 g carbohydrate; 5 g fiber; 5 g sugar; 489 mg phosphorus; 245 mg calcium; 2 mg iron; 623 mg sodium; 800 mg potassium; 672 IU vitamin A; 28 mg ATE vitamin E; 81 mg vitamin C; 12 mg cholesterol; 185 g water

Potato and Winter Vegetable Casserole

A simple potato and vegetable casserole that's good for a winter's evening with rustic bread.

6 potatoes

2 tablespoons (30 ml) olive oil

1 cup (160 g) onion, sliced

2 cups (180 g) cabbage, chopped

2 cups (300 g) cauliflower, chopped

1 teaspoon (3 g) garlic, crushed

1 cup (230 g) plain fat free yogurt

2 cups (450 g) canned white kidney beans

$^1/_4$ cup (16 g) fresh dill, chopped

$^1/_2$ teaspoon (1.3 g) paprika

Preheat oven to 325°F (170°C, or gas mark 3). Boil or microwave the potatoes until nearly done. When cool enough, peel if desired. Heat the olive oil in a large skillet over medium-high heat. Sauté the onions until soft. Add the cabbage, cauliflower, and garlic, and fry until the cabbage and cauliflower are just tender. Add the yogurt to the vegetable mixture. Drain and rinse the white beans and add to the vegetable mixture. Mix thoroughly and set aside. Slice the potatoes into rounds and put half the slices on the bottom of a 9 × 13-inch (23 × 33-cm) baking dish sprayed with nonstick vegetable oil spray. Spread the vegetable mixture over the potatoes. Cover with the remaining potatoes. Sprinkle with dill and paprika. Bake for 20 minutes.

Yield: 6 servings

Per serving: 462 calories (11% from fat, 15% from protein, 74% from carbohydrate); 17 g protein; 6 g total fat; 1 g saturated fat; 3 g monounsaturated fat; 1 g polyunsaturated fat; 88 g carbohydrate; 12 g fiber; 11 g sugar; 400 mg phosphorus; 235 mg calcium; 6 mg iron; 89 mg sodium; 2352 mg potassium; 289 IU vitamin A; 1 mg ATE vitamin E; 70 mg vitamin C; 1 mg cholesterol; 415 g water

Mexican Bean Bake

This makes a great Mexican-flavored vegetarian meal. We usually have it with a simple salad topped with guacamole.

2 cups (460 g) refried beans

4 cups (660 g) cooked rice

2 cups (450 g) canned black beans, drained

1 cup (225 g) salsa

1 cup (120 g) low fat Cheddar cheese, shredded

Preheat oven to 375°F (190°C, or gas mark 5). In a 9 × 9-inch (23 × 23-cm) baking dish, spread out the refried beans. Layer cooked rice on top. Layer black beans on top of rice. Spread with salsa. Sprinkle with cheese. Bake for 15 to 20 minutes, or until heated through and cheese is melted.

Yield: 6 servings

Per serving: 334 calories (9% from fat, 22% from protein, 68% from carbohydrate); 19 g protein; 3 g total fat; 2 g saturated fat; 1 g monounsaturated fat; 0 g polyunsaturated fat; 57 g carbohydrate; 11 g fiber; 2 g sugar; 330 mg phosphorus; 168 mg calcium; 5 mg iron; 647 mg sodium; 630 mg potassium; 175 IU vitamin A; 13 mg ATE vitamin E; 6 mg vitamin C; 11 mg cholesterol; 228 g water

Eggplant and Fresh Mozzarella Bake

This again can be either a meal or a side dish with other Italian food. The fresh mozzarella adds a different flavor and has the benefit of being low in sodium.

6 ounces (170 g) fresh mozzarella

2 cups (470 ml) low sodium spaghetti sauce

1 eggplant, peeled and sliced

Preheat oven to 375°F (190°C, or gas mark 5). Slice mozzarella thinly and place on paper towels to soak up excess moisture. Cover the bottom of an 8 × 8-inch (20 × 20-cm) baking dish with spaghetti sauce, layer eggplant on top of sauce, then cheese on top of eggplant. Repeat layers, ending with a layer of sauce. Bake for 30 minutes or until bubbly and cheese is melted.

Yield: 6 servings

Per serving: 181 calories (41% from fat, 19% from protein, 39% from carbohydrate); 9 g protein; 9 g total fat; 3 g saturated fat; 4 g monounsaturated fat; 1 g polyunsaturated fat; 18 g carbohydrate; 5 g fiber; 12 g sugar; 180 mg phosphorus; 252 mg calcium; 1 mg iron; 202 mg sodium; 519 mg potassium; 669 IU vitamin A; 35 mg ATE vitamin E; 11 mg vitamin C; 18 mg cholesterol; 149 g water

Squash and Rice Bake

Another of those dishes that can be either a full meal or a side dish in a meal with meat. We like it both ways.

$1/2$ cup (95 g) rice

2 tablespoons (30 ml) olive oil

$1/4$ teaspoon (0.8 g) minced garlic

$1/2$ teaspoon (0.5 g) dried thyme

4 cups (450 g) yellow squash, sliced

2 ounces (55 g) low fat Swiss cheese, shredded

Preheat oven to 350°F (180°C, or gas mark 4). Cook rice according to package directions. Heat oil in a large skillet. Sauté garlic for a few minutes. Add thyme and squash. Sauté for a few minutes more. Stir the rice and cheese into the mixture. Turn into a 2-quart (1.9-L) baking dish that has been coated with nonstick vegetable oil spray. Bake for 25 minutes or until heated through.

Yield: 4 servings

Per serving: 128 calories (53% from fat, 18% from protein, 29% from carbohydrate); 6 g protein; 8 g total

fat; 1 g saturated fat; 5 g monounsaturated fat; 1 g polyunsaturated fat; 10 g carbohydrate; 1 g fiber; 3 g sugar; 140 mg phosphorus; 160 mg calcium; 1 mg iron; 40 mg sodium; 325 mg potassium; 252 IU vitamin A; 6 mg ATE vitamin E; 19 mg vitamin C; 5 mg cholesterol; 129 g water

Broccoli Pasta Sauce

A vegetable-based sauce for pasta, featuring fresh broccoli, peppers, and tomatoes.

2 cups (142 g) broccoli florets

$^1/_3$ cup (80 ml) olive oil

1 teaspoon minced garlic

4 ounces (120 ml) dry white wine

1 cup (150 g) green bell pepper, chopped small

2 cups (360 g) fresh tomato, chopped small

1 teaspoon black pepper, fresh ground

3 tablespoons grated Parmesan cheese

$^1/_2$ teaspoon Italian seasoning

$^3/_4$ cup (75 g) pitted, sliced black olives

$^1/_2$ pound (225 g) sliced mushrooms

Place broccoli in a pot of water; cover and let boil for 5 to 6 minutes. Drain water and set aside. Place oil and garlic in large skillet. Brown garlic on medium-low until light brown. Add wine and bell pepper and cook 6 to 7 minutes over medium heat. Add the tomato, black pepper, Parmesan cheese, and Italian seasoning. Cook 15 minutes, uncovered on medium heat, stirring often. Add the broccoli, olives, and mushrooms. Cook 5 minutes on medium heat, covered. Stir often. Remove and serve over whole wheat pasta.

Yield: 6 servings

Per serving: 157 g water; 185 calories (74% from fat, 9% from protein, 17% from carb); 4 g protein; 15 g total fat; 2 g saturated fat; 10 g monounsaturated fat; 2 g polyunsaturated fat; 8 g carbohydrate; 2 g fiber; 3 g sugar; 93 mg phosphorus; 75 mg calcium; 1 mg iron; 207 mg sodium; 385 mg potassium; 1304 IU vitamin A; 4 mg vitamin E; 50 mg vitamin C; 3 mg cholesterol

Tip: To remove skin from tomatoes, drop tomatoes in boiling water for 30 seconds to 1 minute. Place them in cold water for a couple minutes; then skin can be removed.

Ziti and Vegetables

An updated version of baked ziti that still tastes as good, but is healthier.

1 tablespoon (15 ml) olive oil

1 cup (130 g) thinly sliced carrot

1 cup (160 g) sliced onion

1 cup (113 g) sliced zucchini

1 cup (70 g) sliced mushrooms

1 cup (71 g) broccoli florets

4 ounces (115 g) shredded Muenster cheese, divided

1 cup (235 ml) tomato juice

1 cup (140 g) cooked whole wheat ziti

1 teaspoon chopped fresh basil

1 teaspoon chopped fresh parsley

$^1/_8$ teaspoon black pepper

In 10-inch (25-cm) skillet or a wok heat oil; add carrot and cook, stirring quickly and frequently, until carrot is tender, 1 to 2 minutes. Add onion, zucchini, mushrooms, and broccoli; continue stir-frying until vegetables are tender-crisp. Remove skillet (or wok) from heat and stir in 2 ounces (55 g) cheese, the tomato juice, ziti, basil, parsley, and pepper. Preheat oven to 350°F (180°C, gas mark 4). Transfer macaroni mixture to 2-quart (2-L) casserole dish and sprinkle with remaining cheese. Bake until cheese is melted and mixture is bubbly, about 20 minutes.

Yield: 4 servings

Per serving: 197 g water; 279 calories (39% from fat, 18% from protein, 44% from carb); 13 g protein; 13 g total fat; 6 g saturated fat; 5 g monounsaturated fat; 1 g polyunsaturated fat; 32 g carbohydrate; 5 g fiber; 7 g sugar; 274 mg phosphorus; 258 mg calcium; 2 mg iron; 219 mg sodium; 598 mg potassium; 6578 IU vitamin A; 84 mg vitamin E; 39 mg vitamin C; 27 mg cholesterol

Lentils and Pasta

We usually eat this as a side dish, but it also could be the start of a complete meal, just by adding salad and bread.

1 cup (225 g) lentils

$^1/_2$ cup (50 g) celery, sliced

1$^1/_2$ cups (240 g) onion, coarsely chopped, divided

2 tablespoons (30 ml) olive oil

$^1/_2$ teaspoon (1.3 g) cumin

1 tablespoon (4 g) cilantro

6 ounces (170 g) fresh spinach

8 ounces (225 g) pasta (small shapes like orzo are best)

Cook lentils in 6 cups (1.4 L) water with celery and $^1/_2$ cup (80 g) of the onion until soft, about 40 minutes. In a large skillet, heat the olive oil and sauté the remaining onions, cumin, and cilantro until onions are soft. Add spinach and sauté until wilted, another 4 to 5 minutes. Drain lentils and stir into onion-spinach mixture. Cook pasta according to package directions. Stir into mixture.

Yield: 6 servings

Per serving: 245 calories (20% from fat, 15% from protein, 65% from carbohydrate); 10 g protein; 5 g total fat; 1 g saturated fat; 3 g monounsaturated fat; 1 g polyunsaturated fat; 40 g carbohydrate; 6 g fiber; 4 g sugar; 160 mg phosphorus; 72 mg calcium; 2 mg iron; 39 mg sodium; 378 mg potassium; 3492 IU vitamin A; 0 mg ATE vitamin E; 5 mg vitamin C; 0 mg cholesterol; 96 g water

Pasta with Garbanzos

Again this could be a main dish or a fantastic side dish. I often take leftovers of dishes like this for lunch, skipping the meat.

1 tablespoon (15 ml) olive oil

$^1/_2$ cup (80 g) onion, diced

$^1/_8$ teaspoon (0.2 g) red pepper flakes

$^1/_2$ teaspoon (1.5 g) minced garlic

1$^1/_2$ cups (360 g) garbanzo beans, cooked

8 ounces (225 g) pasta

$^1/_4$ cup Parmesan, shredded

Heat oil in a large skillet over medium-high heat. Sauté onions, red pepper flakes, and garlic until onion is soft. Stir in cooked garbanzo beans. Cook pasta according to package directions and stir into mixture. Sprinkle with cheese.

Yield: 4 servings

Per serving: 383 calories (17% from fat, 15% from protein, 68% from carbohydrate); 15 g protein; 7 g total fat; 2 g saturated fat; 3 g monounsaturated fat; 1 g polyunsaturated fat; 65 g carbohydrate; 6 g fiber; 2 g sugar; 240 mg phosphorus; 115 mg calcium; 2 mg iron; 369 mg sodium; 321 mg potassium; 73 IU vitamin A; 7 mg ATE vitamin E; 5 mg vitamin C; 6 mg cholesterol; 88 g water

Macaroni and Ricotta Casserole

Easy Italian casserole that bakes while you find other things to do.

16 ounces no salt added crushed tomatoes

1 cup low sodium chicken broth

1 $^{1}/_{2}$ teaspoons Italian seasoning

$^{3}/_{4}$ teaspoon garlic powder, divided

15 ounces ricotta

$^{1}/_{2}$ teaspoon onion powder

8 ounces whole wheat pasta

2 ounces mozzarella, shredded

Preheat oven to 350°F. Spray an 8 inch square pan with non-stick cooking spray. Combine tomatoes, broth, Italian seasoning, and $^{1}/_{2}$ teaspoon garlic powder. In a separate bowl combine the ricotta, onion powder and remaining garlic powder. In the pan layer the following: 1 cup of tomato mixture, half the pasta, ricotta mixture, 1 cup of tomato mixture, remaining pasta, remaining tomato mixture. Cover and bake until pasta is at desired doneness, about an hour for al dente. Uncover, sprinkle with mozzarella and bake for 5 minutes more.

Yield: 5 servings

Per serving: 233 calories (35% from fat, 28% from protein , 37% from carb); 17 g protein ; 9 g total fat; 6 g saturated fat; 3 g monounsaturated fat; 1 g polyunsaturated fat; 22 g carb; 2 g fiber; 4 g sugar; 290 mg phosphorus; 356 mg calcium; 133 mg sodium; 396 mg potassium; 526 IU vitamin A; 104 mg ATE vitamin E; 13 mg vitamin C; 32 mg cholesterol

Spaghetti with Italian Vegetables

Fresh vegetables are all that's really needed to make a meal of spaghetti. This is a great summer dinner when the garden and farmer's market are overflowing.

12 ounces (340 g) spaghetti

2 tablespoons (30 ml) olive oil

1 cup (150 g) red bell pepper, cut in strips

1 cup (150 g) yellow bell pepper, cut in strips

1 cup (160 g) onion, thinly sliced

$^{1}/_{2}$ teaspoon (1.5 g) minced garlic

1 teaspoon (0.7 g) Italian seasoning

$^{1}/_{2}$ cup (120 ml) dry white wine

30 cherry tomatoes, halved

$^{1}/_{4}$ cup (20 g) Parmesan, shredded

Cook spaghetti according to package directions. Drain. Heat oil in large skillet or Dutch oven. Sauté peppers and onion until they begin to soften, then add the garlic, Italian seasoning, and wine and sauté a few minutes more, stirring to remove anything stuck to the pan. Add the tomatoes and sauté just until they begin to soften. Stir in the spaghetti. Top with cheese.

Yield: 4 servings

Per serving: 284 calories (32% from fat, 10% from protein, 58% from carbohydrate); 7 g protein; 10 g total fat; 2 g saturated fat; 6 g monounsaturated fat; 1 g polyunsaturated fat; 40 g carbohydrate; 7 g fiber; 4 g sugar; 149 mg phosphorus; 101 mg calcium; 1 mg iron; 101 mg sodium; 579 mg potassium; 2148 IU vitamin A; 7 mg ATE vitamin E; 160 mg vitamin C; 6 mg cholesterol; 198 g water

Vegetarian Lasagna

This recipe is the traditional way to assemble lasagna. It has no meat, but it still has lots of flavor. This is the kind of recipe that I like to tackle on the weekend when there's plenty of time, making a double batch and freezing the extra for a quick meal at some later date.

2 tablespoons (30 ml) olive oil

1 cup (160 g) onion, chopped

6 cups (1.4 L) low sodium spaghetti sauce

12 ounces (340 g) frozen spinach, thawed and drained

15 ounces (425 g) ricotta cheese

$^1/_2$ cup (40 g) Parmesan, shredded

4 ounces (115 g) part-skim mozzarella, shredded

2 tablespoons (0.8 g) dried parsley

2 eggs

12 ounces (340 g) lasagna noodles, cooked and drained

Preheat oven to 350°F (180°C, or gas mark 4). Heat olive oil in a large skillet over medium-high heat. Sauté onion until lightly browned. Add spaghetti sauce and stir to combine. In large bowl, mix the spinach, ricotta, Parmesan, mozzarella, parsley, and eggs. Spray a 9 × 13-inch (23 × 33-cm) baking pan with nonstick vegetable oil spray. Place a layer of tomato sauce in the bottom of the pan. Layer noodles, tomato sauce, and ricotta mixture in that order, making three layers of each. Add an additional layer of noodles and sauce on the top. Bake, covered with foil, for 60 to 75 minutes, or until bubbling and heated through. Remove the foil and bake 10 minutes longer.

Yield: 12 servings

Per serving: 376 calories (35% from fat, 17% from protein, 48% from carbohydrate); 16 g protein; 15 g total fat; 5 g saturated fat; 8 g monounsaturated fat; 1 g polyunsaturated fat; 46 g carbohydrate; 6 g fiber; 15 g sugar; 215 mg phosphorus; 309 mg calcium; 3 mg iron; 253 mg sodium; 626 mg potassium; 4477 IU vitamin A; 54 mg ATE vitamin E; 16 mg vitamin C; 61 mg cholesterol; 173 g water

Zucchini Lasagna

This simple vegetarian lasagna using no-boil noodles gets a flavor boost from zucchini. We make this often when the garden is producing more zucchini than we can use.

2 pounds (900 g) zucchini

8 ounces (225 g) low fat ricotta cheese

8 ounces (225 g) part-skim mozzarella, shredded

$^1/_2$ cup (40 g) Parmesan, shredded

$2^1/_2$ cups (570 ml) low sodium spaghetti sauce

8 ounces (225 g) no-boil lasagna noodles

Preheat oven to 350°F (180°C, or gas mark 4). Spray a 9 × 13-inch (23 × 33-cm) glass baking dish with nonstick vegetable oil spray. Slice zucchini lengthwise. Combine the ricotta, mozzarella, and Parmesan. Cover the bottom of the prepared dish with $^1/_2$ cup (120 ml) of the spaghetti sauce. Cover with 3 noodles. Layer with one-third of the ricotta mixture, $^1/_2$ cup (120 ml) sauce, and one-third of the zucchini. Repeat 3 times, ending with the remaining sauce. Bake for 40 minutes, or until bubbling and cheese is melted.

Yield: 6 servings

Per serving: 451 calories (34% from fat, 21% from protein, 45% from carbohydrate); 24 g protein; 17 g total fat; 8 g saturated fat; 7 g monounsaturated fat; 1 g polyunsaturated fat; 51 g carbohydrate; 5 g fiber; 14 g sugar; 374 mg phosphorus; 539 mg calcium; 3 mg iron; 451 mg sodium; 767 mg potassium; 1169 IU vitamin A; 96 mg ATE vitamin E; 26 mg vitamin C; 43 mg cholesterol; 207 g water

Tip: If you make multiple batches, this freezes well, so you can have it again without the same effort.

Roasted Vegetable Stuffed Pizza

My daughter found a picture of a recipe like this one in a bread book at Border's bookstore when she worked there part time. We set out with what she remembered to try to recreate it. I have to say I liked it better than anything new we've had in quite a while. But then, I've always thought that pizza is the perfect food.

1 cup (235 ml) water

4 teaspoons (20 ml) olive oil

$1^1/_2$ cups (190 g) bread flour

$1^1/_2$ cups (190 g) whole wheat flour

$1^1/_2$ teaspoons (3.5 g) yeast

3 cups (210 g) mushrooms, quartered

2 cups (226 g) zucchini, sliced

1 cup (160 g) onion, sliced

1 cup (150 g) red bell pepper, sliced

1 cup (150 g) green bell pepper, sliced

1 tablespoon (15 ml) olive oil

1 cup (235 ml) low sodium spaghetti sauce

3 ounces (85 g) part-skim mozzarella, shredded

Preheat oven to 450°F (230°C, or gas mark 8). Place first 5 ingredients (through yeast) in a bread machine pan in the order specified by the manufacturer. Process on the dough cycle. Meanwhile, combine mushrooms, zucchini, onion, red and green bell peppers, and olive oil in a large baking pan. Bake vegetable mixture for 20 minutes, or until tender and browned on the edges. Stir in spaghetti sauce and set aside. Reduce oven heat to 350°F (180°C, or gas mark 4). Grease the bottom and sides of a 9-inch (23-cm) springform pan. When dough is done, remove from bread machine, punch down, and allow to rest 10 minutes. Separate into two balls, with about three-quarters of the dough in the largest one. Roll the large ball out to a 16-inch (40-cm) circle. Place in bottom and up the sides of the pan. Sprinkle half the cheese on the bottom. Place the vegetable mixture on top of the cheese, then sprinkle the remaining cheese over. Roll the smaller ball to a 9-inch (23-cm) circle. Place over the mixture. Fold the edges of the bottom crust over the top and seal. Bake for 30 to 40 minutes, or until golden brown. Cool in pan 20 minutes, then remove sides and cut into six wedges.

Yield: 6 servings

Per serving: 393 calories (24% from fat, 15% from protein, 61% from carbohydrate); 15 g protein; 11 g total fat; 3 g saturated fat; 6 g monounsaturated fat; 1 g polyunsaturated fat; 62 g carbohydrate; 8 g fiber; 9 g sugar; 296 mg phosphorus; 157 mg calcium; 4 mg iron; 113 mg sodium; 702 mg potassium; 1280 IU vitamin A; 18 mg ATE vitamin E; 66 mg vitamin C; 9 mg cholesterol; 228 g water

Two-Bean Pita Pizzas

Not a pizza to make if you are looking for Italian flavor, but its preparation and the look of the finished product makes it one in my mind.

4 whole wheat pitas

2 tablespoons (28 ml) olive oil

1 cup (160 g) thinly sliced onion

$3/4$ teaspoon finely chopped garlic

16 ounces (455 g) kidney beans

16 ounces (455 g) chickpeas

12 ounces (340 g) salsa

1 teaspoon crumbled basil

$1/2$ teaspoon crumbled thyme

$1/2$ teaspoon crumbled oregano

4 ounces (113 g) shredded mozzarella cheese, divided

$1/4$ cup (25 g) grated Parmesan cheese

Preheat oven to 375°F (190°C, gas mark 5). Heat pitas on foil 8 to 10 minutes. Heat oil in skillet over medium heat. Sauté onion 3 minutes. Add garlic and sauté 2 more minutes. Drain and rinse beans. Add to skillet with salsa and herbs. Cook until heated. With serrated knife, slice pitas in half. Place pita rounds, inside facing up and overlapping slightly, around surface of 12-inch (30-cm) pizza pan. Sprinkle with $3/4$ cup (90 g) mozzarella. Spoon bean mixture on top and spread to cover. Sprinkle with remaining mozzarella and Parmesan cheese. Bake 10 to 15 minutes.

Yield: 8 servings

Per serving: 152 g water; 323 calories (22% from fat, 20% from protein, 58% from carb); 17 g protein; 8 g total fat; 3 g saturated fat; 4 g monounsaturated fat; 1 g polyunsaturated fat; 48 g carbohydrate; 11 g fiber; 3 g sugar; 295 mg phosphorus; 226 mg calcium; 4 mg iron; 577 mg sodium; 566 mg potassium; 237 IU vitamin A; 21 mg vitamin E; 5 mg vitamin C; 12 mg cholesterol

Bean Salad Burrito

A salad you can pick up and go with. Beans are layered with salad ingredients in a tortilla, giving a handy, tasty meal to go.

1 cup (100 g) cooked kidney beans

1 cup (182 g) cooked navy beans

1 cup (172 g) cooked black beans

1/4 cup (38 g) chopped green bell pepper

1/2 cup (50 g) sliced scallions

1/2 cup (90 g) chopped tomato

1 cup (260 g) salsa

3 cups (115 g) shredded lettuce

1 cup (230 g) plain fat-free yogurt

1 cup (115 g) shredded Cheddar cheese

6 flour tortillas

Drain and rinse beans and place in a large mixing bowl. Add bell pepper, scallions, tomato, and salsa; chill. Layer lettuce, beans, yogurt, and cheese on a tortilla and wrap like a burrito.

Yield: 6 servings

Per serving: 177 g water; 486 calories (20% from fat, 23% from protein, 58% from carb); 28 g protein; 11 g total fat; 5 g saturated fat; 3 g monounsaturated fat; 1 g polyunsaturated fat; 71 g carbohydrate; 18 g fiber; 9 g sugar; 548 mg phosphorus; 407 mg calcium; 7 mg iron; 400 mg sodium; 1359 mg potassium; 742 IU vitamin A; 58 mg vitamin E; 13 mg vitamin C; 24 mg cholesterol

3/4 cup (112 g) eggplant, sliced

1 cup (180 g) tomato, sliced

2 tablespoons (30 ml) olive oil

8 ounces (225 g) Swiss cheese, sliced

8 slices focaccia bread or 4 rolls

Preheat broiler. Brush onion, mushrooms, zucchini, eggplant, and tomato with oil. Grill or sauté until soft. Divide evenly between focaccia or rolls. Top each with a slice of Swiss cheese. Place under the broiler until cheese melts.

Yield: 4 servings

Per serving: 192 calories (46% from fat, 36% from protein, 18% from carbohydrate); 17 g protein; 10 g total fat; 3 g saturated fat; 6 g monounsaturated fat; 1 g polyunsaturated fat; 9 g carbohydrate; 2 g fiber; 4 g sugar; 381 mg phosphorus; 562 mg calcium; 0 mg iron; 153 mg sodium; 313 mg potassium; 432 IU vitamin A; 22 mg ATE vitamin E; 11 mg vitamin C; 20 mg cholesterol; 142 g water

Tip: Be prepared with extra napkins.

Grilled Veggie Subs

I particularly like these on focaccia bread, but they are also good on homemade rolls. You could add a slice of chicken or other leftover meat if you aren't into the all-veggie thing, but I don't see the need. Feel free to vary the vegetables as desired. I usually sprinkle a little homemade Italian dressing on them too.

4 slices red onion

1/2 cup (35 g) mushrooms, sliced

1/2 cup (56 g) zucchini, sliced

Zucchini Wraps

A nice change-of-pace zucchini dish, vegetarian and flavored with southwestern spices.

1 tablespoon (15 ml) olive oil

1 cup (160 g) onion, chopped

1 teaspoon (3 g) dry mustard

1 teaspoon (2.5 g) cumin

4 cups (500 g) zucchini, shredded

1/2 teaspoon (1.3 g) chili powder

¼ teaspoon (0.5 g) black pepper

4 tortillas

¼ cup (60 g) fat-free sour cream

In a medium wok or frying pan, heat the oil over medium-high heat. Add the onions, mustard, and cumin. Sauté until onions are soft. Add the shredded zucchini. Cook 5 to 10 minutes, stirring frequently, until the zucchini gets soft and well-cooked. Stir in the chili powder and pepper. Warm the tortillas and place on a flat surface. Spread 1 tablespoon (15 g) of sour cream on each. Place one-quarter of the zucchini filling in the center of each tortilla. Roll up each tortilla.

Yield: 4 servings

Per serving: 131 calories (32% from fat, 12% from protein, 56% from carbohydrate); 4 g protein; 4 g total fat; 1 g saturated fat; 3 g monounsaturated fat; 1 g polyunsaturated fat; 17 g carbohydrate; 3 g fiber; 4 g sugar; 135 mg phosphorus; 66 mg calcium; mg iron; 33 mg sodium; 456 mg potassium; 406 IU vitamin A; 15 mg ATE vitamin E; 24 mg vitamin C; 6 mg cholesterol; 174 g water

Bean Balls

A vegetarian alternative to meatballs. If you are skeptical, you really should try these.

1½ cups (265 g) cooked great northern beans, drained

1 cup (115 g) whole wheat bread crumbs

1 tablespoon grated Parmesan cheese

2 eggs

2 tablespoons parsley

2 teaspoons onion powder

Mash beans and add rest of ingredients. Form into balls and steam for 20 minutes. Serve with spaghetti as a substitute for meatballs.

Yield: 6 servings

Per serving: 62 g water; 180 calories (17% from fat, 22% from protein, 61% from carb); 10 g protein; 3 g total fat; 1 g saturated fat; 1 g monounsaturated fat; 1 g polyunsaturated fat; 28 g carbohydrate; 4 g fiber; 2 g sugar; 165 mg phosphorus; 94 mg calcium; 2 mg iron; 71 mg sodium; 306 mg potassium; 201 IU vitamin A; 27 mg vitamin E; 3 mg vitamin C; 80 mg cholesterol

Chickpea Sandwich Spread

Looking for something a little different for a sandwich? Try this along with lettuce and tomato on a whole grain bread.

1½ cups (246 g) cooked chickpeas, drained (save juice)

½ teaspoon onion powder

⅔ cup (30 g) chopped chives

1½ tablespoons (24 g) no-salt-added tomato paste

⅛ teaspoon lemon juice

Mash chickpeas and mix with rest of ingredients. Add ⅓ cup of the reserved juice and process in a blender or food processor. Use as sandwich spread.

Yield: 6 servings

Per serving: 50 g water; 77 calories (8% from fat, 17% from protein, 75% from carb); 3 g protein; 1 g total fat; 0 g saturated fat; 0 g monounsaturated fat; 0 g polyunsaturated fat; 15 g carbohydrate; 3 g fiber; 1 g sugar; 61 mg phosphorus; 26 mg calcium; 1 mg iron; 184 mg sodium; 162 mg potassium; 309 IU vitamin A; 0 mg vitamin E; 6 mg vitamin C; 0 mg cholesterol

Spinach-Stuffed Tomatoes

This is another of those recipes that would make a good side dish but could just as easily be the centerpiece of a vegetarian dinner.

10 ounces (280 g) fresh spinach

4 tomatoes

1 cup (115 g) part-skim mozzarella, divided

$^1/_4$ cup (40 g) onion, finely chopped

$^1/_4$ cup (25 g) Parmesan, grated

$^1/_8$ teaspoon (0.3 g) pepper

2 tablespoons (8 g) fresh parsley, minced

Preheat oven to 350°F (180°C, or gas mark 4). Steam or microwave spinach in a covered bowl until softened but still slightly crispy. Drain well and squeeze dry. Put in a large bowl. Slice and hollow out centers of tomatoes, reserving the pulp. Discard seeds. Chop pulp finely and add to spinach. Add $^1/_2$ cup (60 g) mozzarella cheese, onion, Parmesan, and pepper to spinach mixture and blend well. Spoon evenly into tomato shells. Sprinkle with remaining mozzarella and parsley. Arrange in an 8-inch (20 cm) round glass or ceramic baking dish and bake for 6 minutes, or until heated through.

Yield: 4 servings

Per serving: 158 calories (38% from fat, 32% from protein, 30% from carbohydrate); 14 g protein; 7 g total fat; 4 g saturated fat; 2 g monounsaturated fat; 1 g polyunsaturated fat; 13 g carbohydrate; 4 g fiber; 1 g sugar; 252 mg phosphorus; 412 mg calcium; 2 mg iron; 355 mg sodium; 602 mg potassium; 9802 IU vitamin A; 42 mg ATE vitamin E; 44 mg vitamin C; 24 mg cholesterol; 230 g water

Zucchini Patties

These taste like crab cakes but without the crab.

$2^1/_2$ cups (310 g) grated zucchini

1 egg, beaten

1 cup (115 g) bread crumbs

$^1/_4$ cup (60 g) minced onion

1 teaspoon (2.4 g) Old Bay Seasoning™

$^1/_4$ cup (30 g) flour

2 tablespoons (30 ml) olive oil

In a large bowl, combine zucchini and egg. Stir in bread crumbs, minced onion, and seasoning. Mix well. Shape mixture into patties. Dredge in flour. In a medium skillet, heat oil over medium-high heat until hot. Fry patties in oil until golden brown on both sides.

Yield: 6 servings

Per serving: 150 calories (36% from fat, 13% from protein, 51% from carbohydrate); 5 g protein; 6 g total fat; 1 g saturated fat; 4 g monounsaturated fat; 1 g polyunsaturated fat; 19 g carbohydrate; 2 g fiber; 2 g sugar; 70 mg phosphorus; 49 mg calcium; 2 mg iron; 156 mg sodium; 171 mg potassium; 141 IU vitamin A;

0 mg ATE vitamin E; 9 mg vitamin C; 35 mg cholesterol; 65 g water

Thai Spinach and Noodle Bowl

Great for a lunch or light dinner, this soup is bursting with flavor.

4 cups low sodium chicken broth

2 ounces whole wheat spaghetti

$1/8$ teaspoon red pepper flakes

2 cups fresh spinach, coarsely chopped

$1/4$ cup fresh basil

2 teaspoon ginger root, peeled and grated

In a medium saucepan bring the broth to a boil. Add the spaghetti and red pepper. Reduce the heat, cover and simmer until spaghetti is just tender. Remove from heat, stir in remaining ingredients, cover and let stand for 2 minutes.

Yield: 4 servings

Per serving: 97 calories (15% from fat, 28% from protein , 57% from carb); 8 g protein ; 2 g total fat; 0 g saturated fat; 1 g monounsaturated fat; 0 g polyunsaturated fat; 16 g carb; 2 g fiber; 0 g sugar; 127 mg phosphorus; 75 mg calcium; 86 mg sodium; 398 mg potassium; 1626 IU vitamin A; 0 mg ATE vitamin E; 6 mg vitamin C; 0 mg cholesterol

Vegetable Paella

This would be a good dish to try for those people who think they don't like vegetarian cooking. It has plenty of flavor and substance to satisfy.

2 tablespoons (30 ml) olive oil

$1^1/4$ cups (240 g) brown rice

1 cup (160 g) onion, sliced

2 cloves garlic, crushed

$1/8$ teaspoon (0.1 g) saffron

3 cups (710 ml) water

1 teaspoon (1.7 g) lemon peel

$1/4$ teaspoon (0.5 g) freshly ground black pepper

2 cups (240 g) leeks, cut in 1-inch (2.5-cm) pieces

$1/4$ cup (34 g) frozen peas, thawed

$1/4$ cup (25 g) black olives

Heat the oil in a large, deep pan. Add the brown rice and onion slices and stir until the rice is coated and begins to turn opaque. Add the garlic, saffron, water, lemon peel, and pepper. Mix well, then bring to a boil. Mix again to distribute the saffron. Arrange the leeks, peas, and olives on top of the rice. Bring to a boil. Cover and simmer for 45 minutes. Serve straight from the pan.

Yield: 4 servings

Per serving: 335 calories (25% from fat, 7% from protein, 67% from carbohydrate); 6 g protein; 10 g total fat; 1 g saturated fat; 6 g monounsaturated fat; 1 g polyunsaturated fat; 57 g carbohydrate; 4 g fiber; 4 g sugar; 230 mg phosphorus; 66 mg calcium; 2 mg iron; 126 mg sodium; 291 mg potassium; 987 IU vitamin A; 0 mg ATE vitamin E; 10 mg vitamin C; 0 mg cholesterol; 271 g water

Tip: To add even more flavor and protein, sprinkle with nuts.

11

Soups and Stews

What can we say about soups? They are almost always easy to cook, healthy, and delicious. In this chapter we have enough recipes that you could have a different one each week for a year and still have a number that you haven't tried. There are soups from around the country and around the world. There are spicy and refreshing ones. There are chowders and stews. And that's not to even mention all the extra heart-healthy bean and pea soups. So grab a soup and dig in. (By the way, a slice of one of the breads in Chapter 21 goes great with just about all of these.)

Chicken Corn Chowder

A good soup for a cool fall day. Add bread and you have a meal.

6 potatoes, peeled and diced

1¹/₂ cups (195 g) sliced carrot

1 cup (160 g) chopped onion

4 cups (950 ml) low-sodium chicken broth

12 ounces (340 g) frozen corn

2 cups (280 g) cooked, diced chicken

1 cup (235 ml) skim milk

¹/₄ teaspoon garlic powder

¹/₂ teaspoon black pepper

1 cup (225 g) instant mashed potatoes

Cook potatoes, carrot, and onion in broth until soft. Add corn and chicken. Cook 5 minutes longer. Add milk, garlic powder, pepper, and mashed potatoes. Stir until potatoes are dissolved. Heat through.

Yield: 6 servings

Per serving: 548 g water; 498 calories (10% from fat, 21% from protein, 69% from carb); 27 g protein; 6 g total fat; 2 g saturated fat; 2 g monounsaturated fat; 2 g polyunsaturated fat; 89 g carbohydrate; 9 g fiber; 8 g sugar; 391 mg phosphorus; 117 mg calcium; 2 mg iron; 169 mg sodium; 1716 mg potassium; 5617 IU vitamin A; 32 mg vitamin E; 39 mg vitamin C; 42 mg cholesterol

Italian Chicken Soup

One more cook-ahead meal for your slow cooker. This one is good either as a full meal or just to have on hand for lunches.

1 pound (455 g) boneless chicken breasts, cubed

4 cups (950 ml) low-sodium chicken broth

2 cups (480 g) low-sodium tomatoes

4 ounces (115 g) mushrooms, sliced

¹/₂ cup (65 g) sliced carrot

¹/₂ cup (56 g) sliced zucchini

¹/₂ cup (62 g) frozen green beans

6 ounces (170 g) frozen spinach

¹/₂ teaspoon garlic powder

1 teaspoon basil

¹/₂ teaspoon oregano

Combine ingredients and place in slow cooker. Cover and cook on low 8 to 10 hours or on high 4 to 5 hours.

Yield: 6 servings

Per serving: 305 g water; 78 calories (17% from fat, 40% from protein, 43% from carb); 9 g protein; 2 g total fat; 0 g saturated fat; 1 g monounsaturated fat; 0 g polyunsaturated fat; 10 g carbohydrate; 3 g fiber; 4 g sugar; 133 mg phosphorus; 73 mg calcium; 2 mg iron; 101 mg sodium; 568 mg potassium; 5706 IU vitamin A; 1 mg vitamin E; 23 mg vitamin C; 7 mg cholesterol

Mexican Chicken Soup

A flavorful Mexican chicken noodle soup. Serve with cornmeal bread for a complete meal.

1 1/2 pounds (675 g) boneless chicken breasts, cut in bite-size pieces

1 cup (150 g) green bell pepper, cut in strips

1 cup (160 g) diced onion

1/2 teaspoon minced garlic

2 cups (480 g) no-salt-added canned tomatoes

4 ounces (115 g) chopped green chiles

2 cups (475 ml) low-sodium chicken broth

2 tablespoons (28 ml) vinegar

1 teaspoon oregano

10 ounces (280 g) frozen corn

2 cups (342 g) cooked pinto beans, drained

2 ounces (55 g) egg noodles

Mix all ingredients together, except noodles, in Dutch oven. Simmer until chicken is cooked through and vegetables are tender, about 30 minutes. Add noodles and cook until they are done, about 10 minutes.

Yield: 6 servings

Per serving: 385 g water; 304 calories (8% from fat, 46% from protein, 46% from carb); 36 g protein; 3 g total fat; 1 g saturated fat; 1 g monounsaturated fat; 1 g polyunsaturated fat; 36 g carbohydrate; 9 g fiber; 5 g sugar; 395 mg phosphorus; 88 mg calcium; 4 mg iron; 188 mg sodium; 940 mg potassium; 252 IU vitamin A; 7 mg vitamin E; 39 mg vitamin C; 66 mg cholesterol

Smoked Chicken Minestrone

Not a very traditional minestrone. I was just looking for something with beans in it and a way to use up the last of a smoked chicken. If you don't have smoked chicken, regular chicken will also work.

1/2 pound (225 g) dry cannellini beans

1/2 pound (225 g) dry chickpeas

2 smoked chicken thighs

2 cups (475 ml) low-sodium chicken broth

1/4 cup (40 g) chopped onion

1/3 cup (43 g) sliced carrot

1 cup (113 g) sliced zucchini

1/2 teaspoon garlic powder

1 teaspoon basil

1 teaspoon oregano

2 cups (480 g) no-salt-added canned tomatoes

Soak beans and drain. Simmer chicken in broth and enough water to cover until meat separates from bones. Cool, skim off fat, and remove meat from bones. Return meat to broth. Add other ingredients and simmer 1 to 1 1/2 hours, until beans are tender. Add additional water as needed. Garnish with Parmesan cheese.

Yield: 4 servings

Per serving: 386 g water; 229 calories (8% from fat, 33% from protein, 59% from carb); 20 g protein; 2 g total fat; 1 g saturated fat; 1 g monounsaturated fat; 1 g polyunsaturated fat; 35 g carbohydrate; 9 g fiber; 5 g sugar; 353 mg phosphorus; 124 mg calcium; 4 mg iron; 781 mg sodium; 914 mg potassium; 2044 IU vitamin A; 0 mg vitamin E; 21 mg vitamin C; 17 mg cholesterol

Amish Chicken Soup

When I was growing up along the Maryland/Pennsylvania border, Amish chicken corn soup was always one of the highlights at volunteer fire company carnivals and suppers. This soup has a similar flavor.

4 cups (946 ml) low sodium chicken broth

2 cups (220 g) chicken, cooked and chopped

$^1/_2$ cup (50 g) celery, chopped

$^1/_2$ cup (65 g) carrot, sliced

$^1/_2$ cup (80 g) onion, chopped

1 tablespoon (0.4 g) dried parsley

$^1/_4$ teaspoon (0.8 g) garlic powder

2 cups (470 ml) water

12 ounces (340 g) egg noodles

Place all ingredients in a large kettle and simmer until noodles are tender (see package directions for approximate time).

Yield: 8 servings

Per serving: 148 calories (22% from fat, 37% from protein, 41% from carbohydrate); 14 g protein; 4 g total fat; 1 g saturated fat; 1 g monounsaturated fat; 1 g polyunsaturated fat; 15 g carbohydrate; 3 g fiber; 1 g sugar; 144 mg phosphorus; 20 mg calcium; 1 mg iron; 49 mg sodium; 262 mg potassium; 1456 IU vitamin A; 6 mg ATE vitamin E; 2 mg vitamin C; 31 mg cholesterol; 248 g water

Chicken Barley Soup

A nice change from chicken and noodle or rice soup featuring barley.

3 pound (1$^1/_4$ kg) chicken, cut up

2 quarts (1.9 L) water

1$^1/_2$ cups (195 g) diced carrot

1 cup (120 g) diced celery

1 cup (200 g) pearl barley

$^1/_2$ cup (60 g) chopped onion

1 bay leaf

$^1/_2$ teaspoon poultry seasoning

$^1/_2$ teaspoon black pepper

$^1/_2$ teaspoon dried sage

Cook chicken in water until tender. Cool broth and skim off fat. Bone chicken and cut into bite-size pieces; return to kettle along with remaining ingredients. Return to heat and bring to a boil. Simmer covered for at least 1 hour until vegetables are tender and barley is done, adding more water if needed. Remove bay leaf and serve.

Yield: 6 servings

Per serving: 546 g water; 400 calories (18% from fat, 54% from protein, 28% from carb); 53 g protein; 8 g total fat; 2 g saturated fat; 2 g monounsaturated fat; 2 g polyunsaturated fat; 27 g carbohydrate; 7 g fiber; 3 g sugar; 493 mg phosphorus; 69 mg calcium; 3 mg iron; 224 mg sodium; 829 mg potassium; 5595 IU vitamin A; 36 mg vitamin E; 9 mg vitamin C; 159 mg cholesterol

Chicken Vegetable Barley Soup

This soup is full of both flavor and nutrition, low in fat, and high in fiber.

4 cups (946 ml) low sodium chicken broth

4 cups (720 g) canned no-salt-added tomatoes

3 cups (710 ml) water

3 cups (480 g) onions, chopped

$^3/_4$ cup (98 g) carrot, chopped

1 $^2/_3$ cups (280 g) frozen corn, thawed

1 cup (150 g) red bell pepper, chopped

1 cup (165 g) frozen lima beans, thawed

$^1/_2$ cup (50 g) celery, chopped

$^1/_4$ cup (56 g) lentils

$^1/_4$ cup (50 g) pearl barley

$^1/_4$ cup (50 g) split peas

1 $^1/_2$ tablespoons (3 g) dried sage

2 cups (220 g) cooked chicken breast, diced

Combine all ingredients except chicken in large, heavy pot or Dutch oven. Bring to boil over medium-high heat. Reduce heat to medium. Simmer for 45 minutes, or until all vegetables and legumes are tender and soup is thick, stirring occasionally. Stir in chicken and heat through.

Yield: 8 servings

Per serving: 222 calories (11% from fat, 33% from protein, 55% from carbohydrate); 20 g protein; 3 g total fat; 1 g saturated fat; 1 g monounsaturated fat; 1 g polyunsaturated fat; 32 g carbohydrate; 7 g fiber; 9 g sugar; 256 mg phosphorus; 89 mg calcium; 3 mg iron; 109 mg sodium; 864 mg potassium; 2913 IU vitamin A; 2 mg ATE vitamin E; 44 mg vitamin C; 30 mg cholesterol; 479 g water

Chicken Barley Chowder

A simple, creamy soup of chicken and barley, perfect for a cold day.

2 tablespoons (28 ml) olive oil

$^1/_2$ cup (60 g) minced celery

$^3/_4$ cup (120 g) minced onion

1 tablespoon flour

$^1/_2$ teaspoon black pepper

6 cups (1.4 L) low-sodium chicken broth

1 cup (200 g) pearl barley

1 pound (455 g) cooked boneless chicken breast, shredded

$^1/_2$ cup (120 ml) fat-free evaporated milk

Heat oil in heavy saucepan. Sauté celery and onion; sprinkle with flour and pepper. Gradually stir in broth and barley. Add chicken. Simmer covered for about an hour, stirring occasionally until barley is tender. Remove from heat and add milk.

Yield: 4 servings

Per serving: 499 g water; 452 calories (23% from fat, 37% from protein, 41% from carb); 42 g protein; 12 g total fat; 2 g saturated fat; 6 g monounsaturated fat; 2 g polyunsaturated fat; 47 g carbohydrate; 9 g fiber; 6 g sugar; 528 mg phosphorus; 148 mg calcium; 4 mg iron; 236 mg sodium; 995 mg potassium; 218 IU vitamin A; 45 mg vitamin E; 4 mg vitamin C; 67 mg cholesterol

Chicken Minestrone

A richly flavored version of minestrone, with cubed chicken breast adding to the mix.

$^1/_2$ cup (80 g) onion, chopped

$^1/_2$ cup (65 g) carrot, diced

1 cup (113 g) zucchini, sliced

2 cloves garlic, crushed

3 boneless chicken breasts, cubed

2 cups (470 ml) low sodium chicken broth

2 cups (500 g) dried great northern beans

1 teaspoon (0.7 g) dried basil

1 teaspoon (1 g) dried oregano

2 cups (360 g) canned no-salt-added tomatoes

Parmesan cheese (optional)

Sauté onions, carrot, zucchini, and garlic until tender. Add to soup pot with remaining ingredients and simmer 1 to $1^1/_2$ hours. Add additional water if needed. Garnish with Parmesan cheese, if desired.

Yield: 6 servings

Per serving: 147 calories (6% from fat, 41% from protein, 53% from carbohydrate); 16 g protein; 1 g total fat; 0 g saturated fat; 0 g monounsaturated fat; 0 g polyunsaturated fat; 20 g carbohydrate; 5 g fiber; 4 g sugar; 197 mg phosphorus; 71 mg calcium; 3 mg iron; 229 mg sodium; 663 mg potassium; 1958 IU vitamin A; 2 mg ATE vitamin E; 14 mg vitamin C; 21 mg cholesterol; 260 g water

African Peanut Stew

A spicy vegetarian stew with sweet potatoes and other vegetables, flavored with peanut butter.

2 sweet potatoes, cubed

2 tablespoons (30 ml) canola oil

$^1/_2$ teaspoon (1.5 g) minced garlic

3 tablespoons fresh ginger, minced

2 tablespoons (12 g) ground coriander

$^1/_2$ teaspoon (0.9 g) cayenne pepper

4 cups (640 g) onion, chopped

1 cup (180 g) tomatoes, chopped

1 eggplant, cubed

$^1/_2$ cup (120 ml) water

1 cup (113 g) zucchini, chopped

1 cup (150 g) green bell pepper, chopped

2 cups (470 ml) low sodium tomato juice

$^1/_2$ cup (130 g) reduced-fat peanut butter

Steam or boil sweet potato cubes until tender. Heat oil in a large skillet over medium-high heat. Sauté garlic, ginger, coriander, and cayenne pepper for 1 minute. Add onions and cook until soft. Add tomatoes, eggplant, and water; simmer 10 minutes. Add zucchini and bell pepper; continue to simmer for 20 minutes, or until all vegetables are tender. Add sweet potatoes to stew along with tomato juice and peanut butter. Stir well and simmer on very low heat until sweet potatoes are cooked, about 15 minutes.

Yield: 6 servings

Per serving: 173 calories (25% from fat, 9% from protein, 66% from carbohydrate); 4 g protein; 5 g total fat; 0 g saturated fat; 3 g monounsaturated fat; 2 g polyunsaturated fat; 31 g carbohydrate; 7 g fiber; 13 g

sugar; 104 mg phosphorus; 69 mg calcium; 2 mg iron; 35 mg sodium; 829 mg potassium; 8694 IU vitamin A; 0 mg ATE vitamin E; 65 mg vitamin C; 0 mg cholesterol; 370 g water

Per serving: 856 g water; 302 calories (25% from fat, 33% from protein, 42% from carb); 23 g protein; 8 g total fat; 2 g saturated fat; 3 g monounsaturated fat; 2 g polyunsaturated fat; 28 g carbohydrate; 6 g fiber; 7 g sugar; 284 mg phosphorus; 90 mg calcium; 3 mg iron; 643 mg sodium; 790 mg potassium; 5468 IU vitaminA; 2 mg vitamin E; 16 mg vitamin C; 51 mg cholesterol

Turkey Carcass Soup

A great use for the last of the Thanksgiving turkey, flavorful and full of healthy things.

1 turkey carcass, most meat removed

3 quarts (2.8 L) water

1 tablespoon peppercorns

1 cup (100 g) chopped celery

2 cups (320 g) chopped onion

4 cups (950 ml) chicken broth

1 cup (235 ml) dry red wine

1 1/2 cups (195 g) chopped carrot

2 cups (300 g) chopped turnip

1/2 cup (97 g) rice

1/2 cup (100 g) pearl barley

In a large pot, barely cover turkey carcass with water. Add peppercorns and half of the chopped onion and celery. Simmer for 45 minutes. Drain, save liquid, and pick remaining meat from carcass. In saved liquid, add meat, chicken broth, and red wine; simmer 30 minutes. Add the rest of ingredients. Simmer until rice and barley are tender, at least 45 minutes and as much as 2 hours or more.

Yield: 6 servings

Beef Mushroom Soup with Barley

We have several recipes for beef vegetable soup that we make regularly, but this one is definitely a favorite. It just seems to be the kind of thing you want on a cold day.

1 pound (455 g) beef round steak, coarsely chopped

1 cup (160 g) onion, chopped

1 1/2 cups (105 g) mushrooms, sliced

2 cups (470 ml) reduced sodium beef broth

4 cups (946 ml) water

1 cup (200 g) pearl barley

1/2 teaspoon (1.5 g) garlic powder

2 teaspoons (10 ml) Worcestershire sauce

1/2 teaspoon (0.5 g) dried thyme

1 cup (130 g) carrots, shredded

1/2 cup (60 g) celery, sliced

1/2 teaspoon (1 g) black pepper

Brown beef and onion. When beef is almost done add mushrooms and cook a few minutes more. Transfer to a slow cooker, add remaining ingredients, and cook on low for 8 to 10 hours.

Yield: 6 servings

Per serving: 306 calories (14% from fat, 47% from protein, 39% from carbohydrate); 36 g protein; 5 g total fat; 1 g saturated fat; 2 g monounsaturated fat; 1 g polyunsaturated fat; 30 g carbohydrate; 7 g fiber; 3 g sugar; 309 mg phosphorus; 43 mg calcium; 4 mg iron; 176 mg sodium; 699 mg potassium; 3637 IU vitamin A; 0 mg ATE vitamin E; 8 mg vitamin C; 68 mg cholesterol; 348 g water

Beef Vegetable Soup

This is a pretty classic beef vegetable soup, the kind that country mothers have been making for years (except they probably didn't use the slow cooker).

1 $^1/_2$ pounds (680 g) round steak, cut in $^1/_2$-inch (1.3-cm) pieces

1 cup (160 g) onion, coarsely chopped

$^1/_2$ cup (50 g) celery, sliced

4 potatoes, cubed

4 cups (946 ml) reduced sodium beef broth

1 cup (70 g) cabbage, coarsely chopped

4 cups (750 g) frozen mixed vegetables, thawed

2 cups (360 g) canned no-salt-added tomatoes

Brown meat in a skillet and transfer to slow cooker. Add onion, celery, and potatoes. Pour broth over. Cook on low for 8 to 10 hours. Add cabbage, mixed vegetables, and tomatoes. Turn to high and cook for 30 minutes to 1 hour, or until vegetables are done.

Yield: 8 servings

Per serving: 373 calories (10% from fat, 39% from protein, 51% from carbohydrate); 37 g protein; 4 g total

fat; 1 g saturated fat; 2 g monounsaturated fat; 0 g polyunsaturated fat; 48 g carbohydrate; 8 g fiber; 8 g sugar; 367 mg phosphorus; 85 mg calcium; 5 mg iron; 446 mg sodium; 1525 mg potassium; 4015 IU vitamin A; 0 mg ATE vitamin E; 31 mg vitamin C; 49 mg cholesterol; 486 g water

Beef Goulash

This is the kind of stew that has been popular in the United States since colonial days. And with good reason—you couldn't ask for a better cold-weather meal.

5 tablespoons (40 g) flour, divided

$^1/_4$ teaspoon (0.5 g) black pepper

2 pounds (905 g) beef round steak, cut in 1-inch (2.5-cm) cubes

2 tablespoons (30 ml) olive oil

1 $^1/_2$ cups (240 g) onion, sliced

1 cup (235 ml) apple juice

1 $^1/_3$ cups (320 ml) water, divided

4 cups (560 g) rutabagas, cut in 1-inch (2.5-cm) cubes

3 cups (390 g) carrot, sliced

$^1/_2$ teaspoon (0.1 g) dried parsley

$^1/_2$ teaspoon (0.3 g) dried marjoram

$^1/_2$ teaspoon (0.5 g) dried thyme

6 potatoes, peeled, cooked, and mashed

Combine 2 tablespoons (16 g) of the flour with the pepper in a resealable plastic bag. Add meat a little at a time and shake to coat. Brown the meat in the oil in a Dutch oven, half at a time. Return all meat to Dutch oven, add onions, juice, and 1 cup (235 ml) of the water. Cover and simmer about 1 1/4 hours, or until meat is tender. Add rutabagas, carrot, parsley, marjoram, and thyme. Cover and simmer about 30 minutes more, until vegetables are done. Blend the remaining 1/3 cup (80 ml) water and the remaining 3 tablespoons (24 g) of the flour and stir into stew. Cook and stir until thickened and bubbly. Spoon mashed potatoes around the edge of the stew to serve.

Yield: 8 servings

Per serving: 538 calories (16% from fat, 36% from protein, 48% from carbohydrate); 48 g protein; 10 g total fat; 3 g saturated fat; 5 g monounsaturated fat; 1 g polyunsaturated fat; 64 g carbohydrate; 9 g fiber; 14 g sugar; 499 mg phosphorus; 94 mg calcium; 7 mg iron; 120 mg sodium; 2117 mg potassium; 8103 IU vitamin A; 0 mg ATE vitamin E; 47 mg vitamin C; 102 mg cholesterol; 489 g water

Savory Beef Stew

Here is the kind of meal you need as the weather starts to turn cooler (seems like I say that about a lot of recipes!). It has a wonderful aroma and flavor, thanks to a couple of unusual ingredients. And it can cook while you're away, so it's ready when you arrive home.

2 tablespoons (16 g) flour

1 pound (455 g) beef round steak, cubed

2 tablespoons (30 ml) olive oil

4 medium potatoes, cubed

1 cup (130 g) carrot, sliced

1/2 cup (80 g) onion, coarsely chopped

1 cup (235 ml) low sodium beef broth

2 cups (360 g) canned no-salt-added tomatoes

1/2 cup (120 ml) water

2 tablespoons (30 g) brown sugar

1 tablespoon (15 ml) Worcestershire sauce

1 tablespoon (15 ml) vinegar

1 1/2 teaspoons (1.5 g) instant coffee

1 teaspoon (2.5 g) cumin

1/2 teaspoon (0.9 g) ground ginger

1/4 teaspoon (0.5 g) ground allspice

Place flour in a plastic bag. Add beef and shake to coat. Heat oil in a large skillet over medium heat. Brown beef on all sides. Place potatoes, carrots, and onion in a slow cooker. Top with beef. Combine remaining ingredients and pour over meat and vegetables. Cover and cook on low for 8 to 10 hours or on high 4 to 5 hours.

Yield: 6 servings

Per serving: 424 calories (19% from fat, 32% from protein, 49% from carbohydrate); 34 g protein; 9 g total fat; 2 g saturated fat; 5 g monounsaturated fat; 1 g polyunsaturated fat; 53 g carbohydrate; 6 g fiber; 10 g sugar; 361 mg phosphorus; 74 mg calcium; 6 mg iron; 126 mg sodium; 1682 mg potassium; 3705 IU vitamin A; 0 mg ATE vitamin E; 35 mg vitamin C; 68 mg cholesterol; 413 g water

Vegetable and Ham Chowder

It's kind of hard to describe the flavor of this filling soup. The cumin gives it a bit of a southwestern style, but then I like cumin and add it to all kinds of things.

1 tablespoon unsalted butter

1 cup (150 g) coarsely chopped red bell pepper

1 cup (160 g) chopped onion

16 ounces (455 g) frozen corn

1 cup (235 ml) low-sodium chicken broth

4 ounces (113 g) ham, cubed

$^1/_2$ teaspoon ground cumin

$^1/_4$ teaspoon white pepper

3 cups (710 ml) fat-free evaporated milk, divided

$^1/_3$ cup (40 g) whole wheat pastry flour

$^1/_8$ teaspoon Tabasco sauce

In large saucepan, melt butter; sauté pepper and onion over medium heat for 5 minutes or until tender. Stir in corn, broth, ham, cumin, and white pepper. Cook for 5 more minutes, stirring occasionally, until corn is cooked. Pour $^1/_2$ cup (120 ml) evaporated milk into bowl; whisk in flour until well blended. Add remaining evaporated milk; mix well. Slowly pour into saucepan. Increase heat to medium-high; cook, stirring constantly, for 5 minutes until mixture comes to a boil and thickens. Boil for 1 minute; add Tabasco.

Yield: 6 servings

Per serving: 258 g water; 260 calories (17% from fat, 27% from protein, 56% from carb); 18 g protein; 5 g total fat; 2 g saturated fat; 2 g monounsaturated fat; 1 g polyunsaturated fat; 38 g carbohydrate; 4 g fiber; 19 g sugar; 410 mg phosphorus; 388 mg calcium; 2 mg iron; 376 mg sodium; 852 mg potassium; 1503 IU vitamin A; 167 mg vitamin E; 40 mg vitamin C; 18 mg cholesterol

Ham and Bean Soup

Bean soup is one of those classic comfort foods. Add a big slice of dark bread and everything is right with your world.

1 pound (455 g) dried navy beans

8 cups (1.9 L) water

$^1/_2$ pound (225 g) ham, cubed

2 medium potatoes, peeled and cubed

$^1/_2$ cup (50 g) celery, sliced

$^1/_2$ cup (65 g) carrots, sliced

$^1/_2$ cup (80 g) onion, chopped

$^1/_4$ teaspoon (0.5 g) black pepper

Soak beans in water overnight. Do not drain. Bring beans to a boil in the soaking liquid. Add ham, reduce heat, cover, and simmer for 1 hour or until beans are nearly done. Add remaining ingredients, cover, and simmer for 30 minutes more, or until vegetables are done.

Yield: 10 servings

Per serving: 148 calories (13% from fat, 26% from protein, 61% from carbohydrate); 10 g protein; 2 g total fat; 1 g saturated fat; 1 g monounsaturated fat; 0 g polyunsaturated fat; 23 g carbohydrate; 4 g fiber; 2 g sugar; 162 mg phosphorus; 42 mg calcium; 2 mg iron; 464 mg sodium; 594 mg potassium; 1104 IU vitamin A; 0 mg ATE vitamin E; 8 mg vitamin C; 9 mg cholesterol; 313 g water

Pork Stew

It's nice to have dinner finished when you get home once in a while. You can serve this over rice or noodles or just have it with a big slice of freshly baked bread (the delay bake option on the bread machine works *so* well with the slow cooker).

1 pound (455 g) pork loin

³/₄ cup (120 g) onion, sliced

2 cups (360 g) canned no-salt-added tomatoes

¹/₂ cup (75 g) green bell pepper, coarsely chopped

2 cups (470 ml) low sodium chicken broth

1 cup (70 g) mushrooms, quartered

1 tablespoon (0.4 g) dried parsley

1 teaspoon (1 g) dried thyme

¹/₄ cup (15 g) fresh cilantro, chopped

¹/₄ cup (30 g) flour

Cube pork. Layer all ingredients except the flour in a slow cooker, reserving half the chicken broth. Cook on low for 6 to 8 hours. Stir the flour into the remaining chicken broth. Add to slow cooker. Turn to high and cook an additional 30 minutes, or until slightly thickened.

Yield: 4 servings

Per serving: 242 calories (35% from fat, 35% from protein, 30% from carbohydrate); 22 g protein; 10 g total fat; 4 g saturated fat; 4 g monounsaturated fat; 1 g polyunsaturated fat; 18 g carbohydrate; 3 g fiber; 70 mg calcium; 3 mg iron; 91 mg sodium; 801 mg potassium; 1073 IU vitamin A; 54 mg vitamin C; 52 mg cholesterol

Chowder from the Sea

This one came about on a weekend when I didn't want to spend my day cooking and I knew everyone was going to be available for dinner at a different time. The answer: the slow cooker and a fish and shrimp soup that people could ladle up whenever they were ready.

¹/₂ pound (225 g) cod or other white fish, cubed

¹/₂ pound (225 g) shrimp, peeled

4 potatoes, shredded

1 cup (110 g) shredded carrot

¹/₂ cup (80 g) finely chopped onion

¹/₂ cup (75 g) finely chopped red bell pepper

¹/₂ cup (60 g) finely chopped celery

2 cups (475 ml) low-sodium chicken broth

1 cup (235 ml) skim milk

1 teaspoon seafood seasoning

Place fish and shrimp in slow cooker. Add potato and vegetables. Pour broth over meat and vegetables. Add milk and seasoning. Stir to mix. Cook on low 8 to 10 hours.

Yield: 6 servings

Per serving: 378 g water; 289 calories (5% from fat, 30% from protein, 65% from carb); 22 g protein; 2 g total fat; 0 g saturated fat; 0 g monounsaturated fat; 1 g polyunsaturated fat; 48 g carbohydrate; 5 g fiber; 4 g sugar; 295 mg phosphorus; 115 mg calcium; 2 mg iron; 186 mg sodium; 1161 mg potassium; 4209 IU vitamin A; 55 mg vitamin E; 35 mg vitamin C; 91 mg cholesterol

Greek Fish Stew

This is a soup to warm you on a cold night. A slice of bread is all that's needed to make it a meal.

4 ounces (115 g) orzo, or other small pasta

$^1/_2$ cup (80 g) onion, chopped

$^1/_2$ teaspoon (1.5 g) minced garlic

1 teaspoon (2 g) fennel seed

2 cups (360 g) canned no-salt-added tomatoes

2 cups (470 g) low sodium chicken broth

1 tablespoon (0.4 g) dried parsley

$^1/_2$ teaspoon (1 g) black pepper

$^1/_4$ teaspoon (0.6 g) turmeric

12 ounces (340 g) cod fillets, cut in 1-inch (2.5-cm) cubes

Cook pasta according to package directions. Drain and set aside. In a large nonstick saucepan coated with nonstick vegetable oil spray, cook onions, garlic, and fennel seed until onion is tender. Add tomatoes, broth, parsley, pepper, and turmeric. Reduce heat and simmer for 10 minutes. Add fish and simmer for 5 minutes, or until fish is cooked through. Divide pasta among four bowls. Ladle soup over pasta.

Yield: 4 servings

Per serving: 226 calories (8% from fat, 40% from protein, 53% from carbohydrate); 23 g protein; 2 g total fat; 0 g saturated fat; 1 g monounsaturated fat; 1 g polyunsaturated fat; 30 g carbohydrate; 3 g fiber; 5 g sugar; 295 mg phosphorus; 75 mg calcium; 3 mg iron; 101 mg sodium; 794 mg potassium; 255 IU vitamin A; 10 mg ATE vitamin E; 15 mg vitamin C; 37 mg cholesterol; 319 g water

Fish Wine Chowder

My daughter fixed this one rainy, cold night. Since she isn't a fish lover, I figured it must be the amount of wine in it that appealed to her. It turns out to be a liberal modification of a recipe in a *Better Homes and Gardens* soup cookbook. But it turned out quite well, and even she had to admit that fish isn't bad this way. You could use whatever fish you have on hand or prefer; the salmon and perch just happened to be what was in our freezer.

1 pound (455 g) salmon

1 pound (455 g) perch

4 slices low sodium bacon

$^1/_2$ cup (80 g) onion, chopped

$^1/_2$ cup (50 g) celery, chopped

$^1/_4$ teaspoon (0.8 g) minced garlic

$1^1/_2$ cups (355 ml) white wine

$1^1/_2$ cups (355 ml) water

2 potatoes, cubed

$^1/_4$ teaspoon (0.3 g) thyme

1 teaspoon (0.1 g) parsley

3 tablespoons (24 g) flour

3 tablespoons (45 ml) water

$^1/_2$ cup (60 ml) skim milk

Cut fish into cubes; set aside. Cook bacon in a Dutch oven; crumble and set aside. Drain grease from pan. Sauté onion, celery, and garlic until tender. Add wine, water, potatoes, thyme, and parsley. Simmer for 20 minutes, or until potatoes are almost done. Add fish, cover and simmer 10 minutes more. Mix together flour and water to form a paste. Stir into soup and simmer until thickened. Stir in milk and reserved bacon.

Yield: 8 servings

Per serving: 306 calories (30% from fat, 39% from protein, 31% from carbohydrate); 26 g protein; 9 g total fat; 2 g saturated fat; 3 g monounsaturated fat; 3 g polyunsaturated fat; 21 g carbohydrate; 2 g fiber; 2 g sugar; 368 mg phosphorus; 113 mg calcium; 2 mg iron; 142 mg sodium; 913 mg potassium; 133 IU vitamin A; 25 mg ATE vitamin E; 13 mg vitamin C; 62 mg cholesterol; 285 g water

Fish Stew

An Italian- or Mediterranean-flavored fish stew, great for a cold evening.

2 tablespoons (30 ml) olive oil

1 cup (160 g) onions, thinly sliced

1 teaspoon (3 g) minced garlic

$^1/_4$ cup (60 ml) dry sherry

$1^1/_2$ cups (270 g) tomatoes, chopped

3 potatoes, cubed

2 whole cloves

2 bay leaves

1 tablespoon (4 g) fresh parsley, minced

$^1/_2$ teaspoon dried tarragon

$^1/_2$ teaspoon (0.7 g) fresh marjoram

$^1/_4$ teaspoon (0.5 g) pepper

2 quarts (1.9 L) water

2 pounds (905 g) cod, halibut, or pollock fillets

$^1/_2$ cup (40 g) Parmesan cheese, shredded

Fresh parsley, for garnish

Heat oil in a large Dutch oven and sauté onion and garlic. Add sherry and next 9 ingredients (through water). Cover and simmer for 1 hour. Uncover and reduce liquid for two hours on a low simmer. Cut fish into large chunks. Add to stew and simmer for 10 minutes. Serve stew in soup bowls and top each with one tablespoon (5 g) Parmesan cheese. Garnish with parsley.

Yield: 8 servings

Per serving: 276 calories (21% from fat, 39% from protein, 40% from carbohydrate); 26 g protein; 6 g total fat; 2 g saturated fat; 3 g monounsaturated fat; 1 g polyunsaturated fat; 27 g carbohydrate; 3 g fiber; 3 g sugar; 371 mg phosphorus; 114 mg calcium; 2 mg iron; 182 mg sodium; 1196 mg potassium; 345 IU vitamin A; 21 mg ATE vitamin E; 26 mg vitamin C; 54 mg cholesterol; 466 g water

Fish Chowder

This makes a great chowder, thick and rich. You can substitute other fish, or a combination of different types of fish, for the cod.

2 tablespoons (30 ml) olive oil

2 cups (320 g) chopped onion

$^1/_2$ cup (35 g) mushrooms, sliced

$^1/_2$ cup (50 g) celery, chopped

5 cups (1.2 L) low sodium chicken broth, divided

4 medium potatoes, diced

2 pounds (905 g) cod, diced into $^1/_2$-inch (1.3-cm) cubes

$^1/_8$ teaspoon (0.3 g) seafood seasoning

$^1/_4$ teaspoon (0.5 g) black pepper

$^1/_2$ cup (60 g) flour

3 cups (710 ml) fat-free evaporated milk

In a large stockpot, heat oil over medium heat. Sauté onions, mushrooms, and celery until tender. Add 4 cups (946 ml) chicken broth and potatoes; simmer for 10 minutes. Add fish, and simmer another 10 minutes. Season to taste with seafood seasoning and pepper. Mix together remaining broth and flour until smooth; stir into soup. Cook until slightly thickened. Remove from heat and stir in evaporated milk.

Yield: 8 servings

Per serving: 397 calories (13% from fat, 35% from protein, 52% from carbohydrate); 35 g protein; 6 g total fat; 1 g saturated fat; 3 g monounsaturated fat; 1 g polyunsaturated fat; 52 g carbohydrate; 4 g fiber; 15 g sugar; 600 mg phosphorus; 334 mg calcium; 3 mg iron; 236 mg sodium; 1854 mg potassium; 468 IU vitamin A; 127 mg ATE vitamin E; 21 mg vitamin C; 53 mg cholesterol; 508 g water

Swedish Salmon Stew

This recipe turned up one night during a fairly desperate search for something different to do with fish.

1¹/₂ pounds (680 g) potatoes, peeled and sliced

1¹/₂ pounds (680 g) salmon fillets

1 tablespoon (4 g) fresh dill, chopped

¹/₄ cup (60 ml) olive oil, heated

¹/₂ cup (120 ml) white wine

¹/₄ cup (60 ml) sherry

¹/₂ cup (115 g) fat-free sour cream

2 tablespoons (30 g) horseradish, grated

Preheat oven to 350°F (180°C, or gas mark 4). Boil potatoes for 10 to 15 minutes, or until almost done. Layer potato slices in a large ovenproof casserole. Place the salmon on top. Sprinkle with the dill and drizzle with the olive oil. Cover and bake for 25 minutes. Remove from the oven and pour the wine and sherry over. Continue to cook uncovered until salmon flakes easily with a fork. Stir together sour cream and horseradish and pour over the top.

Yield: 6 servings

Per serving: 372 calories (50% from fat, 24% from protein, 26% from carbohydrate); 19 g protein; 18 g total fat; 3 g saturated fat; 6 g monounsaturated fat; 8 g polyunsaturated fat; 22 g carbohydrate; 2 g fiber; 3 g sugar; 288 mg phosphorus; 57 mg calcium; 1 mg iron; 82 mg sodium; 891 mg potassium; 154 IU vitamin A; 32 mg ATE vitamin E; 15 mg vitamin C; 56 mg cholesterol; 193 g water

Tuna Chowder

We like this for dinner with some freshly baked bread. It makes a nice warm meal on a cool evening, and it's the kind of thing you can throw together quickly when you haven't planned something for dinner.

2 cups (470 ml) water

2 cups (470 ml) low sodium chicken broth

6 potatoes, diced

14 ounces (400 g) water-packed tuna

¹/₂ cup (65 g) carrots, sliced

¹/₂ cup (50 g) celery, sliced

¹/₂ cup (80 g) onion, diced

¹/₂ cup (82 g) frozen corn, thawed

$^1/_2$ teaspoon (0.3 g) dried basil

$^1/_2$ teaspoon (0.5 g) dried dill

1 tablespoon (0.4 g) dried parsley

$^1/_2$ cup (120 ml) skim milk

In a large saucepan, mix water with broth. Add potatoes and simmer for 10 to 15 minutes, or until tender. Remove cooked potatoes from broth, reserving liquid. Purée cooked potatoes with $^1/_4$ cup (60 ml) reserved broth. Add tuna, carrots, celery, onion, corn, basil, dill, parsley, and puréed potatoes to remaining broth in saucepan. Simmer for 8 to 10 minutes, or until vegetables are tender. Stir in milk and heat to serving temperature, but do not boil.

Yield: 6 servings

Per serving: 379 calories (4% from fat, 28% from protein, 68% from carbohydrate); 27 g protein; 2 g total fat; 0 g saturated fat; 0 g monounsaturated fat; 1 g polyunsaturated fat; 66 g carbohydrate; 7 g fiber; 5 g sugar; 398 mg phosphorus; 93 mg calcium; 4 mg iron; 300 mg sodium; 2047 mg potassium; 2000 IU vitamin A; 24 mg ATE vitamin E; 35 mg vitamin C; 20 mg cholesterol; 562 g water

Shrimp and Corn Chowder

A soup that tastes richer than it is, with low fat and a nice dose of fiber.

2 slices low-sodium bacon, cut in $^1/_2$-inch (1-cm) pieces

1 cup (160 g) chopped onion

$^1/_4$ cup (25 g) sliced celery

6 potatoes, cut in $^1/_2$-inch (1-cm) pieces

12 ounces (340 g) frozen corn

4 cups (950 ml) low-sodium chicken broth

$^1/_4$ cup (30 g) whole wheat pastry flour

12 ounces (340 g) shrimp

$^1/_4$ teaspoon white pepper

$^1/_2$ teaspoon thyme

2 cups (475 ml) skim milk

Cook bacon in Dutch oven, stirring frequently, until crisp. Stir in onion, celery, potatoes, and corn. Cook 5 to 6 minutes, stirring often, until onion and celery are soft. Beat in broth and flour with whisk. Heat to boiling, reduce heat, and simmer about 15 minutes, until potatoes are soft. Stir in remaining ingredients and cook 5 to 6 minutes longer, until shrimp are pink and firm.

Yield: 6 servings

Per serving: 574 g water; 469 calories (8% from fat, 22% from protein, 70% from carb); 27 g protein; 4 g total fat; 1 g saturated fat; 1 g monounsaturated fat; 1 g polyunsaturated fat; 84 g carbohydrate; 8 g fiber; 6 g sugar; 467 mg phosphorus; 190 mg calcium; 3 mg iron; 236 mg sodium; 1614 mg potassium; 420 IU vitamin A; 81 mg vitamin E; 30 mg vitamin C; 91 mg cholesterol

Mock Crab Soup

This soup is typical of Maryland crab soup in flavor. The only big difference is the lack of crab meat, which is high in both sodium and cholesterol. In its place we have fish. I happened to have some flounder fillets available, but any white fish would do. This is also one of our spicier recipes. You can reduce the amount of pepper if you prefer a milder version.

1 pound (455 g) flounder

2 cups (470 ml) low sodium chicken broth

2 cups (360 g) canned no-salt-added tomatoes, diced

¹/₂ cup (82 g) frozen corn, thawed

¹/₂ cup (67 g) frozen peas, thawed

1¹/₂ teaspoons (3 g) seafood seasoning

¹/₂ teaspoon (1 g) black pepper

¹/₂ teaspoon (0.9 g) cayenne pepper

Shred the fish (processing in a food processor with a little of the broth does this easily). Place all ingredients in a large saucepan and simmer for 10 minutes, or until fish and vegetables are cooked.

Yield: 4 servings

Per serving: 178 calories (12% from fat, 58% from protein, 30% from carbohydrate); 26 g protein; 2 g total fat; 1 g saturated fat; 1 g monounsaturated fat; 1 g polyunsaturated fat; 14 g carbohydrate; 3 g fiber; 5 g sugar; 298 mg phosphorus; 70 mg calcium; 2 mg iron; 242 mg sodium; 810 mg potassium; 742 IU vitamin A; 11 mg ATE vitamin E; 16 mg vitamin C; 54 mg cholesterol; 350 g water

Florentine Soup

This spinach soup is a creamy delight. Cream cheese makes it thicker and richer.

1 cup (70 g) sliced mushrooms

¹/₂ cup (80 g) chopped onion

1 tablespoon unsalted butter

1 tablespoon flour

2 cups (475 ml) skim milk

12 ounces (340 g) fresh spinach

¹/₄ teaspoon garlic powder

8 ounces (225 g) cream cheese

Sauté mushrooms and onion in butter until onion is translucent. Stir in flour. Slowly add milk while stirring. Add spinach and garlic powder. Cook until spinach is tender. (Do not overcook!) Stir in cream cheese until melted and warm. You may want to thin with up to 1 cup more of milk. Serve warm.

Yield: 8 servings

Per serving: 125 g water; 160 calories (63% from fat, 16% from protein, 20% from carb); 7 g protein; 12 g total fat; 7 g saturated fat; 3 g monounsaturated fat; 1 g polyunsaturated fat; 8 g carbohydrate; 2 g fiber; 1 g sugar; 132 mg phosphorus; 179 mg calcium; 1 mg iron; 163 mg sodium; 319 mg potassium; 5680 IU vitamin A; 151 mg vitamin E; 3 mg vitamin C; 36 mg cholesterol

Gazpacho

A light and refreshing cold soup, perfect for a summer evening.

48 ounces (1.4 L) tomato juice

1 cup (100 g) chopped celery

1 cup (180 g) chopped tomato

1 cup (135 g) chopped cucumber

1 cup (150 g) chopped green bell pepper

¹/₂ cup (80 g) finely chopped onion

¹/₂ cup (50 g) finely chopped scallions

¹/₄ cup finely chopped fresh cilantro

¹/₄ cup (60 ml) white wine vinegar

¹/₄ cup (60 ml) lemon juice

2 teaspoons Tabasco sauce, to taste

1 tablespoon (15 ml) olive oil

Combine above in large container. Serve ice cold with croutons and grated Parmesan cheese.

Yield: 4 servings

Per serving: 500 g water; 130 calories (24% from fat, 11% from protein, 65% from carb); 4 g protein; 4 g total fat;
1 g saturated fat; 3 g monounsaturated fat; 1 g polyunsaturated fat; 24 g carbohydrate; 4 g fiber; 16 g sugar; 105 mg phosphorus; 74 mg calcium; 2 mg iron; 78 mg sodium; 1148 mg potassium; 2463 IU vitamin A; 0 mg vitamin E; 110 mg vitamin C; 0 mg cholesterol

New England Corn Chowder

A warming and filling soup. Add a nice slice of fresh-baked whole wheat bread and you couldn't ask for a better dinner.

3 slices low-sodium bacon, diced

$^2/_3$ cup (110 g) chopped onion

2 potatoes

3 cups (355 ml) skim milk

15 ounces (420 g) creamed corn

10 ounces (280 g) frozen corn

2 tablespoons (28 g) unsalted butter

Cook bacon pieces in large soup pot. Remove bacon and add onion. Sauté until translucent. Peel and dice potatoes. Bring to slow boil in separate pot for 20 minutes. Warm milk in separate pan. Add creamed corn to onion. Add corn and warm milk. Drain diced potatoes and combine all in original pot.

Yield: 4 servings

Per serving: 394 g water; 360 calories (24% from fat, 17% from protein, 60% from carb); 16 g protein; 10 g total fat; 5 g saturated fat; 3 g monounsaturated fat; 1 g polyunsaturated fat; 56 g carbohydrate; 6 g fiber; 5 g sugar; 424 mg phosphorus; 292 mg calcium; 2 mg iron; 194 mg sodium; 1441 mg potassium; 715 IU vitamin A; 161 mg vitamin E; 25 mg vitamin C; 26 mg cholesterol

Old-Fashioned Vegetable Soup

This is a summer vegetable soup, full of good things from the garden.

2 cups (480 g) no-salt-added canned tomatoes

1 quart (946 ml) low-sodium chicken broth

$^1/_2$ cup (80 g) chopped onion

$^1/_2$ cup (50 g) chopped celery

2 bay leaves

$2^1/_2$ teaspoons basil, divided

$^1/_2$ teaspoon black pepper

2 cups (140 g) coarsely chopped cabbage

$^1/_2$ cup (50 g) cauliflower

1 teaspoon parsley flakes

1 cup corn

1 cup (130 g) sliced carrot

1 cup (113 g) sliced zucchini

2 potatoes, peeled and diced

Place tomatoes in a large pot with broth. Bring to a boil. Add onion and celery, bay leaves, $1^1/_2$ teaspoons basil, and black pepper. Cover and simmer for 1 hour. Add cabbage, cauliflower, parsley, corn, carrot, zucchini, and potato. Cover and simmer until vegetables are tender, 45 to 60 minutes longer. Add remaining basil; simmer 5 minutes longer. Remove bay leaves before serving.

Yield: 8 servings

Per serving: 312 g water; 130 calories (8% from fat, 17% from protein, 75% from carb); 6 g protein; 1 g total fat; 0 g saturated fat; 0 g monounsaturated fat; 0 g polyunsaturated fat; 27 g carbohydrate; 4 g fiber; 4 g sugar; 138 mg phosphorus; 44 mg calcium; 2 mg iron; 70 mg sodium; 816 mg potassium; 3030 IU vitamin A; 0 mg vitamin E; 35 mg vitamin C; 0 mg cholesterol

Pumpkin Soup

This soup can be sipped from a mug or packed in a travel mug and taken with you.

$^1/_2$ cup (80 g) chopped onion

$^1/_2$ teaspoon minced garlic

1 teaspoon (5 ml) olive oil

$^1/_2$ cup (90 g) chopped tomato

2 cups (490 g) pumpkin

2 cups (475 ml) low-sodium chicken broth

$^1/_2$ teaspoon paprika

$1^1/_2$ teaspoons curry powder

In a large saucepan, cook the onion and garlic in the oil until tender, 2 to 3 minutes. Stir in the remaining ingredients and heat to boiling. Reduce heat, cover, and simmer 10 minutes, stirring occasionally, until vegetables are tender. Place in blender container and process until smooth.

Yield: 4 servings

Per serving: 261 g water; 86 calories (22% from fat, 18% from protein, 60% from carb); 4 g protein; 2 g total fat; 1 g saturated fat; 1 g monounsaturated fat; 0 g polyunsaturated fat; 15 g carbohydrate; 4 g fiber; 6 g sugar; 93 mg phosphorus; 48 mg calcium; 2 mg iron; 44 mg sodium; 449 mg potassium; 19380 IU vitamin A; 0 mg vitamin E; 9 mg vitamin C; 0 mg cholesterol

Pumpkin Vegetable Soup

This easy soup has a lot of flavor, both from the vegetables and the curry powder. To make it vegetarian, substitute vegetable broth for the chicken and omit the chicken breast.

$^1/_2$ cup (80 g) chopped onion

$^1/_2$ teaspoon minced garlic

1 teaspoon (5 ml) olive oil

2 cups (310 g) mixed vegetables, frozen

1 can pumpkin

1 can no-salt-added canned tomatoes

$^1/_2$ cup (120 ml) water

$1^1/_2$ teaspoons curry powder

$^1/_2$ teaspoon paprika

2 cups (475 ml) low-sodium chicken broth

1 cup (140 g) chopped cooked chicken breast

In a large saucepan, cook the onion and garlic in the oil until tender, 2 to 3 minutes. Stir in the remaining ingredients and heat to boiling. Reduce heat, cover, and simmer 10 minutes, stirring occasionally, until vegetables are tender.

Yield: 4 servings

Per serving: 261 g water; 158 calories (19% from fat, 42% from protein, 39% from carb); 16 g protein; 3 g total fat; 1 g saturated fat; 2 g monounsaturated fat; 1 g polyunsaturated fat; 15 g carbohydrate; 5 g fiber; 4 g sugar; 172 mg phosphorus; 43 mg calcium; 2 mg iron; 442 mg sodium; 396 mg potassium; 4059 IU vitamin A; 2 mg vitamin E; 5 mg vitamin C; 30 mg cholesterol

Tomato Vegetable Soup

This recipe starts with a cream of tomato–type soup then adds to it, and ends up with a really goodspicy vegetable soup.

1 cup (160 g) finely chopped onion

$^{1}/_{2}$ teaspoon finely chopped garlic

$^{1}/_{2}$ cup (75 g) finely chopped green bell pepper

1 cup (235 ml) low-sodium chicken broth

$^{1}/_{2}$ cup (115 g) canned corn

$^{1}/_{2}$ cup (113 g) canned peas

1 cup (105 g) macaroni

1 teaspoon low-sodium beef bouillon

2 cups (480 g) no-salt-added canned tomatoes

$^{1}/_{2}$ cup (34 g) nonfat dry milk powder

$^{1}/_{4}$ teaspoon salt-free seasoning blend, such as Mrs. Dash

$^{1}/_{4}$ teaspoon white pepper

1 $^{1}/_{2}$ cups (355 ml) water

$^{1}/_{4}$ cup (34 g) jalapeño peppers, roasted and minced

Sauté onion, garlic, and bell pepper until well cooked. Set aside. In a separate pot, combine chicken broth, juice from corn and peas, plus enough water to cook the macaroni (close to a quart). Bring to boil. Add macaroni. Cook for 12 minutes. Drain the macaroni. Puree the bouillon, tomatoes, dry milk, seasonings, water, and sautéed onion, garlic, and bell pepper. Combined pureed sauce, macaroni, peas, corn, and minced jalapeños and simmer for 30 minutes.

Yield: 4 servings

Per serving: 371 g water; 174 calories (6% from fat, 21% from protein, 73% from carb); 10 g protein; 1 g total fat; 0 g saturated fat; 0 g monounsaturated fat; 0 g polyunsaturated fat; 34 g carbohydrate; 5 g fiber; 12 g sugar; 196 mg phosphorus; 168 mg calcium; 2 mg iron; 108 mg sodium; 625 mg potassium; 926 IU vitamin A; 60 mg vitamin E; 36 mg vitamin C; 2 mg cholesterol

Country Vegetable Soup

We made this up as a mix to give for Christmas one year, packaging all the dry ingredients in a quart jar. It's a very tasty vegetarian soup as is, but you could also add chicken or beef if you like.

$^{1}/_{2}$ cup (98 g) split green peas

$^{1}/_{2}$ cup (100 g) barley

$^{1}/_{2}$ cup (96 g) lentils

$^{1}/_{2}$ cup (95 g) brown rice

2 tablespoons parsley

2 tablespoons onion flakes

$^{1}/_{2}$ teaspoon lemon pepper

2 tablespoons sodium-free beef bouillon

$^{1}/_{4}$ cup (23 g) alphabet noodles

1¹/₂ cups (157 g) macaroni

3 quarts (2.8 L) water

¹/₂ cup (50 g) chopped celery

¹/₂ cup (65 g) sliced carrot

1 cup (70 g) shredded cabbage

2 cups (480 g) low-sodium tomatoes

Combine all ingredients in a large soup pot and simmer until vegetables are tender, about 1 hour.

Yield: 8 servings

Per serving: 472 g water; 187 calories (4% from fat, 18% from protein, 78% from carb); 8 g protein; 1 g total fat; 0 g saturated fat; 0 g monounsaturated fat; 0 g polyunsaturated fat; 38 g carbohydrate; 8 g fiber; 4 g sugar; 151 mg phosphorus; 49 mg calcium; 2 mg iron; 96 mg sodium; 462 mg potassium; 1819 IU vitamin A; 0 mg vitamin E; 22 mg vitamin C; 0 mg cholesterol

Curried Vegetable Soup

This easy soup has a lot of flavor, from both the vegetables and the curry powder. To make it vegetarian, substitute vegetable broth for the chicken and omit the chopped chicken breast.

¹/₂ cup (80 g) chopped onion

¹/₂ teaspoon minced garlic

1 teaspoon (5 ml) olive oil

2 cups (310 g) mixed vegetables, frozen

2 cups (490 g) pumpkin

2 cups (480 g) no-salt-added canned tomatoes

¹/₂ cup (120 ml) water

1¹/₂ teaspoons curry powder

¹/₂ teaspoon paprika

2 cups (475 ml) low-sodium chicken broth

¹/₂ pound (225 g) boneless chicken breast, chopped

In a large saucepan, cook the onion and garlic in the oil until tender, 2 to 3 minutes. Stir in the remaining ingredients and heat to boiling. Reduce heat; cover and simmer 10 minutes, stirring occasionally, until vegetables are tender.

Yield: 4 servings

Per serving: 504 g water; 225 calories (13% from fat, 35% from protein, 52% from carb); 21 g protein; 3 g total fat; 1 g saturated fat; 1 g monounsaturated fat; 1 g polyunsaturated fat; 31 g carbohydrate; 9 g fiber; 11 g sugar; 269 mg phosphorus; 113 mg calcium; 5 mg iron; 129 mg sodium; 929 mg potassium; 23269 IU vitamin A; 3 mg vitamin E; 22 mg vitamin C; 33 mg cholesterol

Fiber-Rich Vegetable Soup

A meatless soup that could be made vegetarian by substituting vegetable broth for the beef. This makes a big pot of soup, but it freezes well if you don't need it all when you make it.

2 cups (300 g) chopped green bell pepper

2 cups (320 g) chopped onion

2 tablespoons (28 ml) olive oil

6 cups (1.4 L) water

4 cups (950 ml) low-sodium beef broth

4 cups (1 kg) no-salt-added canned tomatoes, with liquid

2 tablespoons (30 ml) lemon juice

2 cups (260 g) diced carrot

1 cup (164 g) corn

1 cup (90 g) chopped cabbage

2 cups (200 g) chopped celery

1 cup (113 g) diced yellow squash

1 large potato, diced

2 cups (200 g) green beans

1 bay leaf

2 teaspoons marjoram

1 teaspoon thyme

$1/2$ teaspoon black pepper

$1/4$ teaspoon crushed red pepper

$1/2$ cup (30 g) minced parsley

1 cup (200 g) pearl barley

In large pot, sauté green pepper and onion in oil about 2 to 3 minutes. Add water, broth, tomatoes, lemon juice, all vegetables, and all spices. Bring to low boil, reduce to simmer. Cover and simmer 20 minutes. Add barley and simmer 40 to 50 minutes longer. Remove bay leaf.

Yield: 8 servings

Per serving: 632 g water; 247 calories (16% from fat, 13% from protein, 70% from carb); 9 g protein; 5 g total fat;
1 g saturated fat; 3 g monounsaturated fat; 1 g polyunsaturated fat; 46 g carbohydrate; 11 g fiber; 10 g sugar; 196 mg phosphorus; 123 mg calcium; 4 mg iron; 151 mg sodium; 1066 mg potassium; 6347 IU vitamin A; 0 mg vitamin E; 70 mg vitamin C; 0 mg cholesterol

Beer Vegetable Soup

This soup has a lot of flavor. Good with just a simple bread like French or Italian.

1 pound (455 g) ground beef

$1^1/2$ cups (195 g) sliced carrot

1 cup (100 g) sliced celery

1 tablespoon (15 ml) Worcestershire sauce

4 cups (1 kg) no-salt-added canned tomatoes, chopped

2 cups (475 ml) vegetable juice, such as V8

2 cans beer

1 teaspoon onion powder

$1/2$ teaspoon black pepper

$1/2$ cup (100 g) pearl barley

3 large potatoes, diced

In a Dutch oven, brown beef. Drain and return to pot. Add next 8 ingredients. Bring to a boil; reduce heat, and simmer 1 hour. Add barley and potatoes. Simmer until barley is tender, about another hour.

Yield: 8 servings

Per serving: 435 g water; 354 calories (14% from fat, 24% from protein, 62% from carb); 17 g protein; 4 g total fat; 2 g saturated fat; 2 g monounsaturated fat; 0 g polyunsaturated fat; 44 g carbohydrate; 7 g fiber; 8 g sugar; 256 mg phosphorus; 83 mg calcium; 4 mg iron; 275 mg sodium; 1360 mg potassium; 4520 IU vitamin A; 0 mg vitamin E; 39 mg vitamin C; 39 mg cholesterol

Harvest Soup

Full of flavor from the garden, with a fiber boost from canned beans. This soup cooks quickly, making it easy to prepare when you get home from work.

1 tablespoon (15 ml) olive oil

2 cups (320 g) chopped onion

1¹/₂ cups (195 g) thinly sliced carrot

1 cup (100 g) thinly sliced celery

1 teaspoon minced garlic

2 teaspoons Italian seasoning

6 cups (1.4 L) low-sodium chicken broth

3 cups (710 ml) vegetable juice, such as V8

¹/₄ pound (115 g) green beans

1 bay leaf

¹/₈ teaspoon black pepper

2 cups (200 g) cooked kidney beans, drained

2 cups (364 g) cooked navy beans, drained

2 cups (226 g) coarsely chopped yellow squash

In 6-quart (6-L) Dutch oven over medium heat, in hot oil, cook onion, carrot, and celery with garlic and Italian seasoning until vegetables are tender. Stir in remaining ingredients except kidney beans, navy beans, and squash. Heat to boiling. Reduce heat to low; simmer 30 minutes. Add beans and squash; cook 5 minutes more or until squash is tender. Remove bay leaf.

Yield: 8 servings

Per serving: 379 g water; 427 calories (8% from fat, 24% from protein, 68% from carb); 27 g protein; 4 g total fat; 1 g saturated fat; 2 g monounsaturated fat; 1 g polyunsaturated fat; 75 g carbohydrate; 22 g fiber; 10 g sugar; 509 mg phosphorus; 195 mg calcium; 8 mg iron; 343 mg sodium; 1904 mg potassium; 4675 IU vitamin A; 0 mg vitamin E; 32 mg vitamin C; 0 mg cholesterol

Tip: If you have other fresh vegetables like tomatoes or zucchini, they make a great addition.

Winter Day Soup

This is just the kind of thing you need when you come in from shoveling snow. It's warm, filling, and delicious. Add a big slice of hot bread and you are set.

1 pound (455 g) ground beef

1¹/₂ cups (195 g) sliced carrot

1 cup (100 g) sliced celery

1 cup (160 g) diced onion

4 cups (1 kg) no-salt-added canned tomatoes, chopped

1 cup (200 g) pearl barley

4 cups (950 ml) low-sodium beef broth

¹/₂ teaspoon black pepper

2 tablespoons dried parsley

2 cups (475 ml) water

Brown ground beef in large soup pot. Skim off all fat. Add carrot, celery, and onion and sauté for a few minutes, until softened. Add tomatoes, barley, broth, pepper, parsley, and water. Simmer 1 hour until barley is fully cooked.

Yield: 4 servings

Per serving: 759 g water; 526 calories (20% from fat, 31% from protein, 49% from carb); 33 g protein; 9 g total fat; 3 g saturated fat; 4 g monounsaturated fat; 1 g

polyunsaturated fat; 53 g carbohydrate; 13 g fiber; 11 g sugar; 394 mg phosphorus; 153 mg calcium; 7 mg iron; 311 mg sodium; 1401 mg potassium; 8645 IU vitamin A; 0 mg vitamin E; 32 mg vitamin C; 78 mg cholesterol

Potato Leek Chowder

Warm and filling, this is the kind of soup you want to sip in front of a fire on a cold night.

1 cup leeks, sliced

1 cup (130 g) carrot, sliced

1 medium potato, cubed

1 cup (235 ml) low sodium chicken broth

2 cups (470 ml) fat-free evaporated milk

1 cup (170 g) frozen corn, thawed

2 tablespoons (8 g) fresh parsley, chopped

In medium saucepan, combine leeks, carrot, potato, and chicken broth. Cover and simmer 10 minutes or until vegetables are tender. Purée. Add milk and corn. Heat, without boiling, to serving temperature. Serve sprinkled with parsley.

Yield: 4 servings

Per serving: 240 calories (5% from fat, 24% from protein, 71% from carbohydrate); 15 g protein; 1 g total fat; 0 g saturated fat; 0 g monounsaturated fat; 0 g polyunsaturated fat; 44 g carbohydrate; 4 g fiber; 19 g sugar; 379 mg phosphorus; 407 mg calcium; 2 mg iron; 208 mg sodium; 1151 mg potassium; 6509 IU vitamin A; 151 mg ATE vitamin E; 21 mg vitamin C; 5 mg cholesterol; 297 g water

Vegetable Soup

A good cold-weather meal that makes use of the best late fall and winter vegetables. Feel free to vary the vegetables to meet availability and individual tastes.

1 1/2 pounds (680 g) beef round steak

6 cups (1.4 L) water

1/2 cup (80 g) onion, chopped

1 teaspoon (2 g) black pepper

1 teaspoon (0.7 g) dried basil

2 cups (360 g) canned no-salt-added tomatoes

3 medium potatoes, peeled and diced

2 medium turnips, peeled and diced

1/2 cup (65 g) carrot, peeled and sliced

1/2 cup (50 g) celery, sliced

12 ounces (340 g) frozen mixed vegetables, thawed

2 cups (140 g) cabbage, shredded

Trim fat from beef and cut into 1/2-inch (1.3-cm) cubes. Place beef, water, onion, pepper, and basil in a large pot. Simmer until beef is tender. Add remaining ingredients and continue cooking until vegetables are done.

Yield: 8 servings

Per serving: 334 calories (13% from fat, 43% from protein, 44% from carbohydrate); 36 g protein; 5 g total fat; 2 g saturated fat; 2 g monounsaturated fat; 0 g polyunsaturated fat; 36 g carbohydrate; 6 g fiber; 8 g sugar; 332 mg phosphorus; 81 mg calcium; 5 mg iron; 126 mg sodium; 1270 mg potassium; 3305 IU vitamin A; 0 mg ATE vitamin E; 40 mg vitamin C; 77 mg cholesterol; 490 g water

Indian Vegetable Soup

A great vegetarian meal. The amount of ginger gives it a sneaky sort of spiciness. I prefer mild curry powder, but if you want something even hotter you could use hot curry powder.

1 eggplant, peeled and cubed

1 pound (455 g) potatoes, cubed

2 cups (360 g) canned no-salt-added tomatoes

1 1/2 cups (360 g) cooked garbanzo beans

1 cup (160 g) onion, coarsely chopped

1 1/2 teaspoons (3 g) curry powder

1 1/2 teaspoons (2.7 g) ground ginger

1 teaspoon (2 g) ground coriander

1/4 teaspoon (0.5 g) black pepper

4 cups (946 ml) low sodium vegetable broth

In a slow cooker combine the eggplant, potatoes, tomatoes, garbanzo beans, and onion. Sprinkle curry powder, ginger, coriander, and pepper over top. Pour the broth over all. Cover and cook on low for 8 to 10 hours or on high for 4 to 5 hours.

Yield: 6 servings

Per serving: 196 calories (9% from fat, 18% from protein, 73% from carbohydrate); 9 g protein; 2 g total fat; 0 g saturated fat; 1 g monounsaturated fat; 1 g polyunsaturated fat; 38 g carbohydrate; 8 g fiber; 6 g sugar; 193 mg phosphorus; 76 mg calcium; 3 mg iron; 246 mg sodium; 969 mg potassium; 146 IU vitamin A; 0 mg ATE vitamin E; 21 mg vitamin C; 0 mg cholesterol; 426 g water

Winter Vegetable Soup

A good meal for a winter's evening. With no potatoes or pasta, it's also low in carbohydrates for an entire meal. Using a lean cut of meat like round steak also makes it low in fat.

1 pound (455 g) beef round steak

2 cups (470 ml) low sodium beef broth

2 cups (360 g) canned no-salt-added tomatoes

1 cup (150 g) turnips, diced

6 ounces (170 g) frozen green beans, thawed

6 ounces (170 g) frozen broccoli, thawed

6 ounces (170 g) frozen cauliflower, thawed

1/2 cup (65 g) carrot, sliced

1/2 cup (80 g) onion, diced

1/2 cup (50 g) celery, diced

Combine all ingredients in a slow cooker and cook on low for 8 to 10 hours or high 4 to 5 hours. Remove meat and cut into bite-sized pieces or shred. Return to slow cooker and stir until warmed through.

Yield: 4 servings

Per serving: 317 calories (19% from fat, 59% from protein, 23% from carbohydrate); 47 g protein; 7 g total fat; 2 g saturated fat; 2 g monounsaturated fat; 1 g polyunsaturated fat; 18 g carbohydrate; 7 g fiber; 8 g sugar; 377 mg phosphorus; 119 mg calcium; 6 mg iron; 188 mg sodium; 1135 mg potassium; 3451 IU vitamin A; 0 mg ATE vitamin E; 82 mg vitamin C; 102 mg cholesterol; 493 g water

Vegetarian Minestrone

You can either use canned beans for this or cook your own from dried beans.

$^1/_2$ cup (80 g) onion, chopped

$^1/_2$ cup (65 g) carrot, diced

1 cup (113 g) zucchini, sliced

2 cloves garlic, crushed

2 cups (470 ml) low sodium chicken broth

2 cups (450 g) canned great northern beans, no-salt-added

1 teaspoon (0.7 g) dried basil

1 teaspoon (1 g) dried oregano

2 cups (360 g) canned no-salt-added tomatoes

6 ounces (170 g) fresh spinach

Parmesan cheese (optional)

Sauté onions, carrot, zucchini, and garlic until tender. Add to a soup pot with the remaining ingredients and simmer for 1 to 1$^1/_2$ hours. Add additional water if needed. Garnish with Parmesan cheese, if desired.

Yield: 6 servings

Per serving: 149 calories (7% from fat, 26% from protein, 68% from carbohydrate); 10 g protein; 1 g total fat; 0 g saturated fat; 0 g monounsaturated fat; 0 g polyunsaturated fat; 27 g carbohydrate; 7 g fiber; 4 g sugar; 189 mg phosphorus; 133 mg calcium; 3 mg iron; 75 mg sodium; 727 mg potassium; 5370 IU vitamin A; 0 mg ATE vitamin E; 15 mg vitamin C; 0 mg cholesterol; 279 g water

Corn Chowder

This is great just the way it is, or you can add some cooked chicken or ground turkey if you like. We had it just like this, with breadsticks and nothing else.

1 tablespoon (15 ml) olive oil

1 cup (160 g) onion, chopped

$^1/_2$ cup (50 g) celery, sliced

$^1/_2$ cup (65 g) carrot, sliced

2 tablespoons (16 g) flour

2 cups (475 ml) low sodium chicken broth

4 cups (945 ml) skim milk

2 potatoes, peeled and diced

3 cups (410 g) frozen corn, thawed

$^1/_2$ teaspoon (1 g) black pepper

Heat the oil in a large Dutch oven. Add the onion, celery, and carrots and cook over medium heat until just soft. Sprinkle on the flour and cook for 3 minutes, stirring frequently. Stir in the broth and milk. Add the potatoes and corn. Simmer for 25 minutes or until potatoes are tender. Sprinkle with pepper.

Yield: 6 servings

Per serving: 278 calories (12% from fat, 18% from protein, 70% from carbohydrate); 13 g protein; 4 g total fat; 1 g saturated fat; 2 g monounsaturated fat; 1 g polyunsaturated fat; 52 g carbohydrate; 5 g fiber; 6 g sugar; 346 mg phosphorus; 268 mg calcium; 2 mg iron; 148 mg sodium; 1148 mg potassium; 2176 IU vitamin A; 100 mg ATE vitamin E; 18 mg vitamin C; 3 mg cholesterol; 427 g water

Cream of Broccoli Soup

I suppose this really should be called cream of vegetable, but the broccoli seems to dominate.

20 ounces (560 g) frozen mixed vegetables

10 ounces (280 g) frozen broccoli, chopped fine

8 slices low-sodium bacon

1/4 cup (40 g) chopped onion

1/4 cup (30 g) whole wheat pastry flour

4 cups (950 ml) skim milk

Boil frozen mixed vegetables and broccoli. Set aside to drain. Fry bacon until crispy. Set aside bacon. Pour enough bacon grease in soup pan to cover bottom of pan. Simmer onion until clear. Mix in flour, then add milk. Stir well. Add vegetables and bacon. Simmer until soup is thickened. Salt and pepper to taste. This soup has better flavor when eaten the next day.

Yield: 6 servings

Per serving: 276 g water; 219 calories (21% from fat, 28% from protein, 51% from carb); 15 g protein; 5 g total fat; 2 g saturated fat; 2 g monounsaturated fat; 1 g polyunsaturated fat; 28 g carbohydrate; 6 g fiber; 4 g sugar; 331 mg phosphorus; 278 mg calcium; 2 mg iron; 363 mg sodium; 616 mg potassium; 4907 IU vitamin A; 101 mg vitamin E; 24 mg vitamin C; 15 mg cholesterol

Borscht

A traditional Russian or eastern European soup, but one you don't see that often in the United States. Which is a shame, because it tastes good and is nutritious.

2 cups (140 g) finely shredded cabbage

1/2 cup (80 g) chopped onion

16 ounces (455 g) beets

3 cups (355 ml) low-sodium chicken broth

3 tablespoons (42 g) unsalted butter

2 teaspoons caraway seeds

1 teaspoon sugar

3 tablespoons (45 ml) lemon juice

Cook cabbage about 10 minutes in boiling water. Sauté onion in a soup pot a few minutes without browning. Drain and chop beets, reserving liquid. Add chicken broth to onion, and when it comes to a boil, add cabbage and the water in which it cooked. Add chopped beets, butter, beet juice, caraway seeds, and sugar and simmer for 10 minutes. Add lemon juice. Serve with sour cream.

Yield: 6 servings

Per serving: 231 g water; 113 calories (50% from fat, 13% from protein, 38% from carb); 4 g protein; 7 g total fat; 4 g saturated fat; 2 g monounsaturated fat; 0 g polyunsaturated fat; 12 g carbohydrate; 3 g fiber; 7 g sugar; 67 mg phosphorus; 38 mg calcium; 2 mg iron; 190 mg sodium; 306 mg potassium; 229 IU vitamin A; 48 mg vitamin E; 19 mg vitamin C; 15 mg cholesterol

Russian Vegetable Soup

This soup has a little bit of everything in it, and that really gives it a spark of flavor.

1 pound (455 g) mixed dried beans

1 pound (455 g) ham hocks

3 quarts (2.8 L) water

2 tablespoons (28 ml) olive oil

1 cup (160 g) diced onion

1 cup (120 g) diced celery

1/2 cup (75 g) diced green bell pepper

1 teaspoon crushed garlic

2 cups (260 g) diced carrot

2 cups (300 g) diced rutabaga

2 cups (142 g) diced broccoli

1 cup (200 g) pearl barley

2 tablespoons dried parsley

1 tablespoon black pepper

1 teaspoon basil

1 teaspoon coriander

1 teaspoon nutmeg

Soak beans overnight. Drain, then add the beans, ham, and water to the pot. Bring to a boil, then let it simmer for an hour. (Can be refrigerated overnight at this point to skin off grease.) Remove meat from ham bones and return to pot. Heat oil in a skillet and sauté onion, celery, bell pepper, and garlic until softened, about 5 minutes. Add to pot. Simmer for another hour. Add carrot, rutabaga, broccoli, barley, and herbs. Simmer for another hour.

Yield: 8 servings

Per serving: 522 g water; 421 calories (14% from fat, 29% from protein, 57% from carb); 32 g protein; 7 g total fat; 1 g saturated fat; 3 g monounsaturated fat; 1 g polyunsaturated fat; 62 g carbohydrate; 16 g fiber; 7 g sugar; 439 mg phosphorus; 215 mg calcium; 8 mg iron; 551 mg sodium; 1726 mg potassium; 5713 IU vitamin A; 0 mg vitamin E; 42 mg vitamin C; 35 mg cholesterol

Bean Soup with Dumplings

Whole wheat dumplings give this soup extra flavor and nutrition.

1 pound (455 g) dried navy beans

8 ounces (225 g) no-salt-added tomato sauce

2 cups (360 g) chopped tomato

1 cup (160 g) chopped onion

3 quarts (2.8 L) water

4 potatoes, diced

3/4 cup (90 g) whole wheat flour

2 teaspoons baking powder

1 egg, beaten

2 tablespoons (28 ml) skim milk

Use large soup pot. Add beans, tomato sauce, tomato, and onion. Cover with water and cook on low until beans are tender, about 2 hours. Add additional water if necessary. Add potatoes. Let cook about 1 additional hour. Sift the flour and baking powder together. Add the egg and milk and mix well. Drop in bean soup. Cover and cook at medium boil for 15 minutes. Do not take the lid off the pan until the 15 minutes are up.

Yield: 8 servings

Per serving: 630 g water; 271 calories (6% from fat, 16% from protein, 78% from carb); 11 g protein; 2 g total fat; 0 g saturated fat; 0 g monounsaturated fat; 1 g polyunsaturated fat; 55 g carbohydrate; 9 g fiber; 4 g sugar; 293 mg phosphorus; 146 mg calcium; 4 mg iron; 419 mg sodium; 1285 mg potassium; 394 IU vitamin A; 13 mg vitamin E; 31 mg vitamin C; 26 mg cholesterol

Pinto Bean and Squash Stew

An unexpected combination that makes a great meatless meal. Serve with crusty French bread or cornbread.

1 pound (455 g) dried pinto beans

$^1/_4$ cup (40 g) chopped onion

$^1/_2$ teaspoon minced garlic

4 slices bacon, cubed

1 jalapeño pepper, seeded and chopped

$^1/_4$ cup (25 g) minced scallions

1 butternut squash, peeled and diced

1 cup (235 ml) low-sodium beef broth

$^1/_2$ cup finely diced red onion

$^1/_4$ cup chopped fresh cilantro

$^3/_4$ cup (180 g) sour cream

Cover pinto beans with 3 inches (7.5 cm) of boiling water in large pot. Add onion and garlic. Cover and bake at 250°F (120°C, gas mark $^1/_2$) until beans are cooked, 2 to $2^1/_2$ hours. Keep warm. Cook bacon with jalapeño and scallions over low heat in large sauté pan until bacon is crisp. Add squash and broth. Cover and cook until squash is just tender, about 30 minutes. Combine beans and squash and mix gently but well. Spoon beans and squash into 6 serving bowls. Sprinkle each with red onion, cilantro, and 2 tablespoons (30 g) sour cream.

Yield: 6 servings

Per serving: 137 g water; 192 calories (16% from fat, 26% from protein, 58% from carb); 11 g protein; 3 g total fat; 1 g saturated fat; 1 g monounsaturated fat; 0 g polyunsaturated fat; 24 g carbohydrate; 7 g fiber; 1 g sugar; 183 mg phosphorus; 79 mg calcium; 2 mg iron; 163 mg sodium; 477 mg potassium; 293 IU vitamin A; 31 mg vitamin E; 5 mg vitamin C; 18 mg cholesterol

Senate Bean Soup

Bean soup is on the menu in the U.S. Senate's restaurant every day. According to the Senate website, there are several stories about the origin of that mandate. According to one story, the Senate's bean soup tradition began early in the 20th century at the request of Senator Fred Dubois of Idaho. Another story attributes the request to Senator Knute Nelson of Minnesota, who expressed his fondness for the soup in 1903. The recipe attributed to Dubois includes mashed potatoes (from his home state). The recipe served in the Senate today does not include mashed potatoes, but does include a braised onion. The recipe below has the mashed potatoes, because I like the way they thicken the soup.

1 pound (455 g) dried navy beans

$^1/_2$ pound (225 g) ham, diced

$1^1/_2$ cups (337 g) mashed potatoes

1 cup (160 g) chopped onion

$^1/_4$ cup (25 g) chopped celery

$^1/_2$ teaspoon chopped garlic

Clean the beans, then cover with water and cook until nearly done, about $1^1/_2$ hours. Drain. Add ham and 1 quart (946 ml) water and bring to a boil. Add potatoes and mix thoroughly. Add chopped vegetables and bring to a boil. Simmer for 1 hour before serving.

Yield: 6 servings

Per serving: 102 g water; 390 calories (15% from fat, 24% from protein, 61% from carb); 24 g protein; 7 g total

fat; 2 g saturated fat; 2 g monounsaturated fat; 1 g polyunsaturated fat; 60 g carbohydrate; 13 g fiber; 5 g sugar; 424 mg phosphorus; 135 mg calcium; 5 mg iron; 578 mg sodium; 1230 mg potassium; 88 IU vitamin A; 18 mg vitamin E; 8 mg vitamin C; 21 mg cholesterol

Spicy Bean Soup

If you like your bean soup with a little kick, this could be the recipe for you. (If not, just replace the spicy vegetable juice with regular and leave out the Tabasco.)

6 cups (1.4 L) water

1 cup (210 g) dried beans, assorted (navy, red, pinto, etc.)

$^1/_2$ cup (95 g) brown rice

1 cup (160 g) diced onion

1 cup (130 g) diced carrot

$^1/_2$ cup (75 g) diced green bell pepper

6 ounces (175 ml) spicy vegetable juice, such as V8

$^1/_4$ teaspoon Tabasco sauce

$^3/_4$ cup (90 g) diced celery

1 teaspoon black pepper

1 cup (150 g) diced ham

Combine all ingredients in a large pot. Simmer for at least 3 hours.

Yield: 6 servings

Per serving: 350 g water; 239 calories (11% from fat, 23% from protein, 66% from carb); 14 g protein; 3 g total fat; 1 g saturated fat; 1 g monounsaturated fat; 1 g polyunsaturated fat; 39 g carbohydrate; 7 g fiber; 4 g sugar; 256 mg phosphorus; 77 mg calcium; 3 mg iron; 426 mg sodium; 733 mg potassium; 3779 IU vitamin A; 0 mg vitamin E; 16 mg vitamin C; 10 mg cholesterol

White Bean Soup

A simple pureed bean soup that is both filling and tasty. Serve with multigrain bread and a salad.

$^1/_2$ cup (80 g) minced onion

$^1/_2$ cup (60 g) minced celery

$^1/_4$ cup (38 g) chopped green bell pepper

2 tablespoons (28 ml) olive oil

$^1/_2$ pound (225 g) smoked sausage, cut in $^1/_2$-inch (1-cm) slices

8 ounces (225 g) no-salt-added tomato sauce

4 cups (728 g) cooked navy beans

4 cups (950 ml) water

1 teaspoon black pepper

In large saucepan, cook onion, celery, and bell pepper in oil until soft. Add sausage and tomato sauce; simmer 15 to 20 minutes. In a separate saucepan, bring navy beans to boil. Puree beans and their liquid in a food processor or blender; add to vegetable mixture. Add the water and pepper and simmer for 1 hour.

Yield: 4 servings

Per serving: 477 g water; 477 calories (34% from fat, 19% from protein, 47% from carb); 24 g protein; 18 g total fat; 5 g saturated fat; 10 g monounsaturated fat; 3 g polyunsaturated fat; 57 g carbohydrate; 21 g fiber; 4 g sugar; 292 mg phosphorus; 154 mg calcium; 6 mg iron; 705 mg sodium; 1006 mg potassium; 290 IU vitamin A; 0 mg vitamin E; 25 mg vitamin C; 40 mg cholesterol

Winter Bean Soup

A flavorful soup with smoked sausage and just a hint of chili flavor.

2 cups (420 g) dried mixed beans

2 quarts (1.9 L) water

1/2 pound (225 g) smoked sausage, sliced

1 cup (160 g) chopped onion

1/2 teaspoon minced garlic

1 teaspoon chili powder

4 cups (1 kg) no-salt-added canned tomatoes

2 tablespoons (30 ml) lemon juice

Rinse beans and cover with water. Soak overnight. Drain and add 2 quarts (1.9 L) water and sausage and simmer until tender. Add onion, garlic, chili powder, tomatoes, and lemon juice and simmer 45 minutes more.

Yield: 6 servings

Per serving: 526 g water; 350 calories (19% from fat, 25% from protein, 57% from carb); 22 g protein; 8 g total fat; 3 g saturated fat; 3 g monounsaturated fat; 1 g polyunsaturated fat; 52 g carbohydrate; 12 g fiber; 7 g sugar; 243 mg phosphorus; 229 mg calcium; 9 mg iron; 500 mg sodium; 1567 mg potassium; 312 IU vitamin A; 0 mg vitamin E; 25 mg vitamin C; 26 mg cholesterol

Tip: Use a variety of beans (great northern, navy, black, chickpeas, split peas, pinto, red beans, or lentils, etc.).

Smoked Sausage and Bean Soup

A quick and easy soup to make for lunch or dinner. The bean, potato, and sausage mixture reminds me of the bean and ham meals we sometimes had when I was growing up.

3/4 teaspoon olive oil

1/3 cup (55 g) chopped onion

2/3 cup (87 g) sliced carrot

1 potato, peeled and cubed

1 cup (235 ml) low-sodium beef broth

5 ounces (142 g) smoked sausage, cut into 1/2-inch (1-cm) slices

10 ounces (280 g) great northern beans, undrained

10 ounces (180 g) green beans, frozen

Heat oil in a saucepan over medium heat. Sauté onion 4 to 5 minutes, stirring frequently, until tender. Add carrot, potato, and broth. Bring to a boil. Reduce heat to low, cover, and simmer about 15 minutes or until vegetables are tender. Add sausage and beans. Cook until thoroughly heated.

Yield: 4 servings

Per serving: 282 g water; 275 calories (25% from fat, 20% from protein, 56% from carb); 14 g protein; 8 g total fat; 3 g saturated fat; 4 g monounsaturated fat; 1 g polyunsaturated fat; 39 g carbohydrate; 8 g fiber; 4 g sugar; 196 mg phosphorus; 84 mg calcium; 3 mg iron; 492 mg sodium; 924 mg potassium; 4083 IU vitamin A; 0 mg vitamin E; 29 mg vitamin C; 25 mg cholesterol

Sausage and Bean Soup

A hearty soup with Italian flavors.

1 pound (455 g) Italian turkey sausage (see recipe in Chapter 13)

$^1/_2$ teaspoon minced garlic

1 cup (160 g) chopped onion

$^1/_3$ cup (20 g) chopped fresh parsley

$^3/_4$ cup (98 g) sliced carrot

1 cup (70 g) sliced mushrooms

2 cups (328 g) cooked chickpeas

3 cups (355 ml) low-sodium beef broth

$^1/_2$ teaspoon sage

$^1/_2$ teaspoon black pepper

Crumble sausage and cook in 3-quart (3-L) saucepan over medium-high heat, stirring often, until browned. Add garlic, onion, parsley, carrot, and mushrooms. Cook until limp. Add chickpeas and remaining ingredients. Bring to a boil, then lower heat and simmer covered, about 10 minutes. Skim off excess fat.

Yield: 4 servings

Per serving: 581 calories (25% from fat, 35% from protein, 40% from carb); 26 g protein; 9g total fat; 4 g saturated fat; 3 g monounsaturated fat; 1 g polyunsaturated fat; 35 g carbohydrate; 7 g fiber; 3 g sugar; 331 mg phosphorus; 97 mg calcium; 4 mg iron; 214 mg sodium; 845 mg potassium; 4491 IU vitamin A; 0 mg vitamin E; 18 mg vitamin C; 86 mg cholesterol

Mixed Bean Soup

This makes a really big batch of great-tasting soup. It's a good meal to feed a crowd, but it also freezes well, so you can store some for later.

$^1/_3$ cup (69 g) dried navy beans

$^1/_3$ cup (83 g) dried red kidney beans

$^1/_3$ cup (67 g) dried baby lima beans

$^1/_3$ cup (67 g) dried chickpeas

$^1/_3$ cup (64 g) dried pinto beans

$^1/_3$ cup (75 g) dried split peas

$^1/_3$ cup (64 g) dried lentils

$^1/_3$ cup (56 g) dried black-eyed peas

$^1/_3$ cup (65 g) pearl barley

$3^1/_2$ quarts (3.3 L) water

$^1/_2$ teaspoon red pepper flakes

4 cups (1 kg) no-salt-added canned tomatoes

$1^1/_2$ cups (240 g) diced onion

$^3/_4$ teaspoon minced garlic

$^1/_2$ cup (60 g) diced celery

1 cup (150 g) diced green bell pepper

2 tablespoons dried parsley

1 pound (455 g) boneless chicken breast, cut in 1-inch (2.5-cm) cubes

1 pound (455 g) smoked sausage, sliced

Wash beans and barley; drain and add water to cover. Soak overnight, then drain. Add the $3^1/_2$ quarts (3.3. L) water to the drained bean mixture. Cover and simmer until beans are tender, about $1^1/_2$ hours. Add all other ingredients except the chicken and sausage. Simmer uncovered $1^1/_2$ hours. Add chicken and sausage; simmer until chicken is done.

Per serving: 556 g water; 280 calories (29% from fat, 33% from protein, 38% from carb); 23 g protein; 9 g total fat; 3 g saturated fat; 4 g monounsaturated fat; 2 g polyunsaturated fat; 27 g carbohydrate; 7 g fiber; 5 g sugar; 222 mg phosphorus; 79 mg calcium; 4 mg iron; 662 mg sodium; 648 mg potassium; 316 IU vitamin A; 3 mg vitamin E; 32 mg vitamin C; 58 mg cholesterol

Tip: Packages of bean mixtures can be substituted for all the dry mix.

Multi-Bean Soup

Most large markets carry a bean mixture in their dried bean section. The one I found had 16 varieties. This is a meatless soup, but very filling. It could be made vegetarian by leaving out the chicken bouillon.

1 pound (455 g) mixed dried beans

1/2 cup (80 g) onion, chopped

1/2 cup (60 g) celery, sliced

1/2 cup (65 g) carrot, sliced

1 tablespoon (6 g) low sodium chicken bouillon

2 cups (360 g) canned no-salt-added tomatoes

1/2 teaspoon (1 g) black pepper

6 cups (1.4 L) water

Soak and drain beans. In a large saucepan or Dutch oven combine all ingredients. Bring to a boil. Reduce heat, cover, and simmer until beans are tender, about 1 1/2 hours.

Yield: 8 servings

Per serving: 215 calories (4% from fat, 22% from protein, 74% from carbohydrate); 12 g protein; 1 g total fat; 0 g saturated fat; 0 g monounsaturated fat; 1 g polyunsaturated fat; 41 g carbohydrate; 10 g fiber; 5 g sugar; 251 mg phosphorus; 117 mg calcium; 4 mg iron; 37 mg sodium; 848 mg potassium; 1449 IU vitamin A; 0 mg ATE vitamin E; 9 mg vitamin C; 0 mg cholesterol; 263 g water

Black Bean Soup

A flavorful Latin-style soup that's low in fat.

1 1/2 cups (375 g) dried black beans

4 cups (946 ml) water

1 tablespoon (15 ml) olive oil

1 cup (160 g) onion, finely chopped

1/2 cup (75 g) green bell pepper, finely chopped

1/2 teaspoon (1.5 g) garlic, minced

1/2 cup (65 g) carrot, finely chopped

1/2 cup (60 g) celery, finely chopped

1 teaspoon (2.5 g) cumin

1/4 teaspoon (0.5 g) cayenne pepper

1 tablespoon (15 ml) lime juice

1/4 cup (56 g) salsa

Soak beans in water overnight. Heat oil in a large Dutch oven over medium-high heat and sauté onion, green bell pepper, garlic, carrots, and celery until almost soft. Add cumin and cayenne pepper and sauté a few minutes more. Add beans, soaking water, lime juice, and salsa and simmer for 1 1/2 to 2 hours, or until beans begin to fall apart.

Yield: 6 servings

Per serving: 101 calories (23% from fat, 18% from protein, 60% from carbohydrate); 5 g protein; 3 g total fat; 0 g saturated fat; 2 g monounsaturated fat; 0 g polyunsaturated fat; 16 g carbohydrate; 5 g fiber; 2 g sugar; 82 mg phosphorus; 38 mg calcium; 1 mg iron; 86 mg sodium; 314 mg potassium; 1948 IU vitamin A; 0 mg ATE vitamin E; 14 mg vitamin C; 0 mg cholesterol; 251 g water

Bean and Barley Stew

This is a hearty meatless stew with a whopping 11 grams of fiber.

2 tablespoons (28 ml) olive oil

1 cup (160 g) chopped onion

1 cup (130 g) sliced carrot

1^1/$_2$ cups (105 g) sliced mushrooms

4 cups (684 g) cooked pinto beans, drained

2 cups (480 g) no-salt-added canned tomatoes

^{1}/$_8$ teaspoon Cajun seasoning

^{1}/$_4$ teaspoon basil

^{1}/$_4$ teaspoon tarragon

^{1}/$_4$ teaspoon oregano

^{1}/$_4$ teaspoon celery seed

^{1}/$_4$ teaspoon thyme

^{1}/$_4$ teaspoon marjoram

^{1}/$_4$ teaspoon sage

^{1}/$_4$ teaspoon black pepper

2 tablespoons (28 ml) Dick's Reduced Sodium Soy Sauce (see recipe page 25)

^{1}/$_2$ cup (95 g) brown rice

^{1}/$_3$ cup (65 g) pearl barley

6 cups (1.4 L) vegetable broth

Heat oil in a large kettle: Add onion, carrot, and mushrooms and sauté until softened, about 5 minutes. Add remaining ingredients. Bring to a boil. Reduce heat; simmer 1 to 2 hours until grains are tender.

Yield: 8 servings

Per serving: 337 g water; 333 calories (23% from fat, 15% from protein, 62% from carb); 13 g protein; 9 g total fat; 2 g saturated fat; 5 g monounsaturated fat; 2 g polyunsaturated fat; 53 g carbohydrate; 11 g fiber; 4 g sugar; 265 mg phosphorus; 102 mg calcium; 4 mg iron; 226 mg sodium; 753 mg potassium; 2773 IU vitamin A; 0 mg vitamin E; 12 mg vitamin C; 0 mg cholesterol

Dutch Pea Soup

A hearty pea soup with smoked sausage. We like this with a dark bread like pumpernickel.

2 cups (450 g) dried split peas

3^1/$_2$ quarts (3.3 L) water

4 leeks, chopped

1^1/$_2$ cups (150 g) chopped celery

^{1}/$_2$ pound (225 g) smoked sausage, sliced

Soak peas in 3 cups (710 ml) cold water for 12 hours; drain. Add water to make 3^1/$_2$ quarts (3.3 L) and bring to boil. Add leeks and celery, and simmer 3 to 5 hours until tender. Thirty minutes before soup is done, add sausage.

Yield: 6 servings

Per serving: 694 g water; 203 calories (31% from fat, 22% from protein, 47% from carb); 11 g protein; 7 g total

fat; 2 g saturated fat; 3 g monounsaturated fat; 1 g polyunsaturated fat; 24 g carbohydrate; 7 g fiber; 5 g sugar; 92 mg phosphorus; 71 mg calcium; 3 mg iron; 504 mg sodium; 415 mg potassium; 1107 IU vitamin A; 0 mg vitamin E; 14 mg vitamin C; 26 mg cholesterol

Green Pea Soup

If you are thinking split pea soup, think again. This chilled soup is made with green peas, yogurt, and dill. Perfect for a summer luncheon.

10 ounces (280 g) frozen peas

$^1/_4$ cup (25 g) chopped scallions

2 cups (475 ml) low-sodium chicken broth, divided

$^1/_2$ teaspoon dill

$^3/_4$ cup (180 g) plain fat-free yogurt

Place peas, scallions, 2 tablespoons (28 ml) of the chicken broth, and the dill in a heavy nonstick pan over medium-high heat. Cover and cook 5 to 6 minutes, or until peas are tender. Remove from heat and cool. Stir in remaining chicken broth. Working in batches, transfer pea mixture to a blender or food processor and process until smooth. Pour blended mixture into a bowl and repeat process until whole mixture is pureed. Cover and refrigerate until chilled. Just before serving, whisk yogurt into pea soup. Pour into individual serving bowls and top with an extra spoonful of yogurt, if desired.

Yield: 3 servings

Per serving: 288 g water; 137 calories (9% from fat, 33% from protein, 58% from carb); 12 g protein; 1 g total fat; 0 g saturated fat; 0 g monounsaturated fat; 0 g polyunsaturated fat; 21 g carbohydrate; 5 g fiber; 10 g

sugar; 233 mg phosphorus; 160 mg calcium; 2 mg iron; 402 mg sodium; 481 mg potassium; 2082 IU vitamin A; 1 mg vitamin E; 12 mg vitamin C; 1 mg cholesterol

Slow Cooker Split Pea Soup

I'm not sure what I like best about this soup, the great taste or the fact that it cooks while you are away.

1 pound (455 g) dried green split peas, rinsed

2 cups (300 g) diced ham

1$^1/_2$ cups (195 g) peeled, sliced carrot

1 cup (160 g) chopped onion

$^1/_2$ cup (50 g) chopped celery

$^1/_2$ teaspoon minced garlic

1 bay leaf

$^1/_4$ cup chopped fresh parsley

$^1/_2$ teaspoon black pepper

1$^1/_2$ quarts (1.4 L) water

Layer ingredients in slow cooker and pour in water. Do not stir. Cover and cook on high 4 to 5 hours or on low 8 to 10 hours until peas are very soft. Remove bay leaf before serving.

Yield: 6 servings

Per serving: 338 g water; 363 calories (12% from fat, 32% from protein, 56% from carb); 29 g protein; 5 g total fat; 1 g saturated fat; 2 g monounsaturated fat; 1 g polyunsaturated fat; 52 g carbohydrate; 21 g fiber; 9 g sugar; 403 mg phosphorus; 77 mg calcium; 4 mg iron; 548 mg sodium; 1088 mg potassium; 5742 IU vitamin A; 0 mg vitamin E; 9 mg vitamin C; 19 mg cholesterol

Tip: Serve garnished with croutons. Freezes well.

Chunky Pea Soup

Something a little more than most split pea soups, with turnips and lots of other vegetables adding more than the usual substance and flavor.

1 cup (225 g) dried yellow split peas

1 cup (225 g) dried green split peas

7 cups (1.6 L) cold water

2 cups (130 g) sliced carrot

2 cups (300 g) peeled, diced turnip

2 cups (320 g) peeled, chopped onion

1 cup (100 g) chopped celery

$^1/_2$ cup (97 g) rice

$^3/_4$ pound (340 g) ham

Sort and rinse peas. Add cold water, bring to boil. Cook for 1 hour. Add vegetables and rice and cook for 1 additional hour. Cut ham into small cubes and add for last 20 minutes of cooking.

Yield: 6 servings

Per serving: 471 g water; 388 calories (13% from fat, 30% from protein, 56% from carb); 30 g protein; 6 g total fat; 2 g saturated fat; 2 g monounsaturated fat; 1 g polyunsaturated fat; 56 g carbohydrate; 20 g fiber; 12 g sugar; 419 mg phosphorus; 97 mg calcium; 4 mg iron; 698 mg sodium; 1194 mg potassium; 7347 IU vitamin A; 0 mg vitamin E; 17 mg vitamin C; 23 mg cholesterol

Split Pea Soup

This soup has great flavor, even without the traditional ham, which adds more sodium than I can have. It also has a large helping of soluble fiber to help clean out your blood vessels.

1 cup (160 g) onion, chopped

$^1/_2$ cup (60 g) celery, chopped

$^1/_2$ cup (65 g) carrot, sliced

2 tablespoons (30 ml) olive oil

1$^1/_2$ cups (295 g) split peas

6 cups (1.4 L) low sodium chicken broth

$^1/_2$ teaspoon (0.5 g) dried thyme

$^1/_2$ teaspoon (0.4 g) dried basil

1 teaspoon (2 g) black pepper

Heat oil in a large Dutch oven over medium-high heat and sauté onion, celery, and carrot until onion is soft. Add remaining ingredients. Bring to a boil, then reduce heat and simmer for 1 hour, or until peas are very soft. Mash peas with a spoon against the side of the pot until you reach the desired consistency.

Yield: 8 servings

Per serving: 115 calories (34% from fat, 23% from protein, 43% from carbohydrate); 7 g protein; 5 g total fat; 1 g saturated fat; 3 g monounsaturated fat; 1 g polyunsaturated fat; 13 g carbohydrate; 4 g fiber; 3 g sugar; 101 mg phosphorus; 25 mg calcium; 1 mg iron; 66 mg sodium; 365 mg potassium; 1384 IU vitamin A; 0 mg ATE vitamin E; 2 mg vitamin C; 0 mg cholesterol; 229 g water

Tip: If you prefer a smoother soup, process in batches in a blender or food processor until smooth.

Lentil and Barley Soup

Lentil and barley make a great combination, both in terms of flavor and nutrition. This hearty soup proves that, tasting great and packing 10 grams of fiber while remaining low in sodium and saturated fat.

$^1/_4$ cup (60 ml) olive oil

$^1/_2$ teaspoon garlic

$^1/_2$ cup (80 g) diced onion

1 cup (110 g) shredded carrot

$^1/_2$ cup (50 g) sliced celery

1 teaspoon basil

3 quarts (2.8 L) water

1 pound (455 g) lentils

$^1/_2$ cup (100 g) pearl barley

$^1/_2$ teaspoon black pepper

$^1/_4$ teaspoon garlic powder

$^1/_4$ cup (60 ml) red wine

Heat oil in Dutch oven. Add garlic, onion, carrot, celery, and basil and cook until tender on low to medium heat, about 10 to 15 minutes. Add water, cover, and bring to boil. Add lentils, barley, pepper, garlic powder, and red wine. Reduce heat and simmer until beans are tender, about 1 hour.

Yield: 6 servings

Per serving: 566 g water; 245 calories (36% from fat, 15% from protein, 49% from carb); 9 g protein; 10 g total fat; 1 g saturated fat; 7 g monounsaturated fat; 1 g polyunsaturated fat; 30 g carbohydrate; 10 g fiber; 3 g sugar; 192 mg phosphorus; 48 mg calcium; 3 mg iron; 34 mg sodium; 462 mg potassium; 3608 IU vitamin A; 0 mg vitamin E; 4 mg vitamin C; 0 mg cholesterol

Lentil Brown Rice Soup

A hearty soup of lentils and rice.

$^3/_4$ cup (75 g) chopped celery

$^3/_4$ cup (120 g) chopped onion

2 tablespoons (28 ml) olive oil

6 cups (1.4 L) water

$^3/_4$ cup (144 g) lentils

4 cups (1 kg) no-salt-added canned tomatoes

$^1/_2$ teaspoon garlic powder

$^1/_4$ teaspoon black pepper

$^3/_4$ cup (142 g) brown rice

$^1/_2$ teaspoon rosemary

1 tablespoon (15 ml) Worcestershire sauce

$^1/_2$ cup (55 g) shredded carrot

Sauté celery and onion in oil in a Dutch oven. Add water and lentils. Cook 20 minutes. Add remaining ingredients, except carrot. Simmer 45 to 60 minutes. Add carrot. Cook 5 minutes more.

Yield: 6 servings

Per serving: 447 g water; 199 calories (24% from fat, 11% from protein, 64% from carb); 6 g protein; 6 g total fat; 1 g saturated fat; 4 g monounsaturated fat; 1 g polyunsaturated fat; 33 g carbohydrate; 5 g fiber; 6 g sugar; 168 mg phosphorus; 80 mg calcium; 3 mg iron; 73 mg sodium; 566 mg potassium; 2048 IU vitamin A; 0 mg vitamin E; 22 mg vitamin C; 0 mg cholesterol

Lentil Soup

This is a hearty soup, full of flavor. A dark multi-grain bread would go well with it.

1 tablespoon (15 ml) olive oil

1 cup (160 g) onion, diced

1 tablespoon (10 g) minced garlic

2 cups (360 g) canned no-salt-added tomatoes

1 cup (130 g) carrots, sliced

$1/4$ cup (30 g) celery, sliced

6 cups (1.4 L) water

2 cups (450 g) lentils

Heat oil in a Dutch oven over medium-high heat and sauté onion and garlic until onion starts to soften. Add tomatoes and sauté for 1 minute more. Add remaining ingredients. Bring to a boil, reduce heat to medium-low, and simmer for 1 hour or until lentils are soft.

Yield: 8 servings

Per serving: 99 calories (17% from fat, 21% from protein, 62% from carbohydrate); 5 g protein; 2 g total fat; 0 g saturated fat; 1 g monounsaturated fat; 0 g polyunsaturated fat; 16 g carbohydrate; 5 g fiber; 4 g sugar; 114 mg phosphorus; 46 mg calcium; 2 mg iron; 29 mg sodium; 390 mg potassium; 2779 IU vitamin A; 0 mg ATE vitamin E; 9 mg vitamin C; 0 mg cholesterol; 304 g water

12

Chilies

Chili is often thought of as Mexican, but it's an American invention. It originally started in Cincinnati as a meat sauce for spaghetti in a Greek restaurant. So we open this chapter with a version of Cincinnati chili, without beans and with the traditional cinnamon, allspice, and cocoa powder. But from there we move into the Tex-Mex variation that most people think of when you mention chili. We have a number of those here. And then we have some things that have chili flavor, but not the usual ingredients, such as chicken and barley or dumplings. All in all I think everyone will find something they like here, and many will find more than one.

Cincinnati-Style Chili

Cincinnati, Ohio, claims to be where chili was created. Cincinnati-style chili is quite different from the more familiar Tex-Mex variety. The chili is thinner and contains an unusual blend of spices that includes cinnamon, chocolate or cocoa, allspice, and Worcestershire sauce. It's usually served over spaghetti, although it's good in a bowl by itself or as a hot dog topping.

1 cup (160 g) onion, chopped

1 pound (455 g) extra-lean ground beef (93% lean)

$1/4$ teaspoon (0.8 g) minced garlic

1 tablespoon (7.5 g) chili powder

1 teaspoon (1.9 g) ground allspice

1 teaspoon (2.3 g) cinnamon

1 teaspoon (2.5 g) cumin

$1/2$ teaspoon (0.9 g) cayenne pepper

$1 1/2$ tablespoons (8 g) unsweetened cocoa powder

16 ounces (455 g) no-salt-added tomato sauce

1 tablespoon (15 ml) Worcestershire sauce

1 tablespoon (15 ml) cider vinegar

$1/2$ cup (120 ml) water

In a large frying pan over medium-high heat, sauté onion, ground beef, garlic, and chili powder until ground beef is slightly cooked. Add remaining ingredients. Reduce heat to low and simmer, uncovered, $1 1/2$ hours.

Yield: 6 servings

Per serving: 227 calories (32% from fat, 41% from protein, 27% from carbohydrate); 16 g protein; 6 g total fat; 2 g saturated fat; 2 g monounsaturated fat; 0 g polyunsaturated fat; 10 g carbohydrate; 3 g fiber; 4 g sugar; 156 mg phosphorus; 38 mg calcium; 3 mg iron; 98 mg sodium; 598 mg potassium; 688 IU vitamin A; 0 mg ATE vitamin E; 17 mg vitamin C; 52 mg cholesterol; 158 g water

Tip: To serve the traditional Cincinnati way, ladle chili over cooked spaghetti and serve with toppings of your choice. Oyster crackers are served on the side. Cincinnati chili is ordered by number: Two-, Three-, Four-, or Five-Way.

Two-Way Chili: Chili served on spaghetti

Three-Way Chili: Additionally topped with shredded Cheddar cheese

Four-Way Chili: Additionally topped with chopped onions

Five-Way Chili: Additionally topped with kidney beans

Chili with Beans

This makes a nice thick, moderately spicy chili. The preparation isn't difficult, but like most chili it's best if it's simmered for a while.

2 pounds (900 g) ground beef

1 tablespoon (15 ml) olive oil

1 cup (160 g) chopped onion

1 cup (150 g) chopped red bell pepper

$1/2$ teaspoon minced garlic

$1/2$ teaspoon black pepper, fresh ground

1 teaspoon ground cumin

1 ounce (28 g) dried ground chipotle pepper

1 teaspoon cayenne pepper

1 tablespoon chili powder

3 cups (710 ml) water

6 ounces (170 g) no-salt-added tomato paste

4 cups (1 kg) no-salt-added canned tomatoes

4 cups (1 kg) dried kidney beans

Brown beef in 2 batches in thick-bottomed soup kettle. Drain off fat and set browned beef aside. Heat oil in kettle over medium-high heat, adding onion when hot. Sauté for 4 to 5 minutes, stirring often. Add bell pepper and garlic, continuing to cook 2 to 3 more minutes. Add black pepper, cumin, chipotle, and cayenne to taste plus chili powder. Stir continually until spices begin to stick to bottom of kettle and brown. Quickly add water. Add tomato paste and tomatoes with the juice they were packed in. Add kidney beans. Add the beef but try not to include any fat that may have accumulated. Stir. When chili begins to boil, reduce heat to low and cover. Ideally chili should be simmered 3 hours to let all the flavors blend together. Stir about every 15 minutes, while checking to make sure heat is not too high, causing chili to stick to the bottom of kettle. If you don't have 3 hours to cook the chili, use less chipotle and cayenne or else they will overpower the other flavors.

Per serving: 375 g water; 486 calories (38% from fat, 34% from protein, 28% from carb); 42 g protein; 21 g total fat; 7 g saturated fat; 9 g monounsaturated fat; 1 g polyunsaturated fat; 34 g carbohydrate; 12 g fiber; 7 g sugar; 425 mg phosphorus; 130 mg calcium; 8 mg iron; 274 mg sodium; 1365 mg potassium; 2149 IU vitamin A; 0 mg vitamin E; 43 mg vitamin C; 98 mg cholesterol

Basic Chili

I never seem to make chili the same way twice, so I keep coming up with new recipes. One thing that's become fairly constant, though, is sautéing the spices, which seems to give it a deeper flavor.

1 pound (455 g) dried kidney beans

2 pounds (905 g) beef round steak

1 tablespoon (15 ml) olive oil

$^1/_2$ cup (80 g) onion, coarsely chopped

$^1/_2$ teaspoon (1.5 g) minced garlic

$^1/_2$ cup (75 g) green bell pepper, coarsely chopped

4 ounces (115 g) canned jalapeño peppers

2 tablespoons (15 g) chili powder

1 tablespoon (7 g) cumin

1 teaspoon (1 g) dried oregano

1 tablespoon (4 g) cilantro

2 cups (360 g) canned no-salt-added tomatoes

2 cups (360 g) canned no salt added crushed tomatoes

Soak kidney beans overnight. Drain and add fresh water. Simmer for $1^1/_2$ hours, or until almost tender. Coarsely grind beef or chop into small cubes no bigger than $^1/_2$ inch (1.3 cm). Heat oil in a skillet and sauté beef, onion, garlic, green bell pepper, and jalapeños until beef is browned on all sides. Add chili powder, cumin, oregano, and cilantro and sauté an additional 5 minutes. Transfer to slow cooker. Stir in tomatoes. Drain beans and add to slow cooker. Stir to mix, cover, and cook on low 4 to 5 hours.

Yield: 8 servings

Per serving: 353 calories (22% from fat, 54% from protein, 24% from carbohydrate); 48 g protein; 8 g total fat; 2 g saturated fat; 4 g monounsaturated fat; 1 g polyunsaturated fat; 21 g carbohydrate; 6 g fiber; 4 g sugar; 379 mg phosphorus; 77 mg calcium; 8 mg iron; 223 mg sodium; 948 mg potassium; 884 IU vitamin A; 0 mg ATE vitamin E; 28 mg vitamin C; 102 mg cholesterol; 249 g water

Healthy Chili

A healthier version of chili that doesn't suffer at all in the taste department. Low in fat, high in fiber, but still just as tasty.

1 pound (455 g) ground turkey

4 cups (684 g) cooked pinto beans, undrained

18 ounces (510 g) no-salt-added tomato sauce

6 ounces (170 g) no-salt-added tomato paste

2 cups (475 ml) vegetable juice, such as V8

2 tablespoons chili powder

1 teaspoon cumin

1 teaspoon cinnamon

$^1/_2$ cup (70 g) bulgur

Brown turkey and drain. Add remaining ingredients. Simmer 30 minutes. Stir often.

Yield: 6 servings

Per serving: 295 g water; 410 calories (12% from fat, 35% from protein, 53% from carb); 37 g protein; 6 g total fat; 2 g saturated fat; 1 g monounsaturated fat; 2 g polyunsaturated fat; 56 g carbohydrate; 16 g fiber; 11 g sugar; 438 mg phosphorus; 120 mg calcium; 7 mg iron; 337 mg sodium; 1614 mg potassium; 1840 IU vitamin A; 0 mg vitamin E; 35 mg vitamin C; 57 mg cholesterol

Tip: Serve with grated cheese if desired and cornbread.

Black Bean Chili

This could be the perfect chili. Not only does it taste great, but it's good for you, high in fiber, and low in fat. And it cooks in only about 20 minutes. Plus, it makes a great, different-tasting way to use up leftover turkey.

1 cup (250 g) dried black beans

1 tablespoon (15 ml) canola oil

1 cup (160 g) onion, chopped

$^1/_2$ cup (75 g) red bell pepper, cubed

1 teaspoon (3 g) minced garlic

2 jalapeño peppers, seeded and chopped

2 cups (360 g) canned no-salt-added tomatoes

2 tablespoons (15 g) chili powder

1 teaspoon (2.5 g) cumin

1 teaspoon (2 g) coriander

1 teaspoon (0.6 g) dried marjoram

$^1/_4$ teaspoon (0.3 g) red pepper flakes

$^1/_4$ teaspoon (0.6 g) cinnamon

2 cups (225 g) cooked turkey breast, cubed

$^1/_3$ cup fresh (20 g) cilantro, coarsely chopped

4 teaspoons (8 g) low fat Cheddar cheese, shredded

Soak and cook black beans according to package directions. Heat oil in a 3-quart (2.8-L) saucepan and sauté onion, bell pepper, garlic, and jalapeño peppers until crisp-tender. Add all other ingredients except turkey, cilantro, and cheese. Bring to a boil, then simmer for 10 to 15 minutes. Stir in turkey and cilantro and cook until heated throughout. To serve, ladle into bowls and top with cheese.

Yield: 4 servings

Per serving: 153 calories (27% from fat, 17% from protein, 56% from carbohydrate); 7 g protein; 5 g total fat; 1 g saturated fat; 2 g monounsaturated fat; 2 g polyunsaturated fat; 23 g carbohydrate; 8 g fiber; 6 g sugar; 133 mg phosphorus; 97 mg calcium; 3 mg iron; 77 mg sodium; 608 mg potassium; 2208 IU vitamin A; 2 mg ATE vitamin E; 46 mg vitamin C; 1 mg cholesterol; 207 g water

Steak Chili

This is a guy's kind of chili—spicy and full of just meat, with no beans for filler.

2 tablespoons (30 ml) canola oil

3 pounds (1.4 kg) beef round steak

2 cups (470 ml) low sodium beef broth

8 ounces (225 g) no-salt-added tomato sauce

2 cups (360 g) canned no-salt-added tomatoes

4 ounces (115 g) canned chile peppers

$^3/_4$ cup (175 ml) beer

2 tablespoons (15 g) chili powder

1 teaspoon (3 g) garlic powder

1 tablespoon (9 g) onion powder

1 teaspoon (5 ml) hot pepper sauce

1 tablespoon (7 g) cumin

Heat oil in a skillet and sauté beef until done; drain well. Put beef and broth in a large pot and bring to a slow simmer. Add remaining ingredients and simmer slowly for about 1$^1/_2$ hours, or until meat is tender.

Yield: 10 servings

Per serving: 370 calories (27% from fat, 58% from protein, 15% from carbohydrate); 52 g protein; 11 g total fat; 3 g saturated fat; 5 g monounsaturated fat; 2 g polyunsaturated fat; 14 g carbohydrate; 5 g fiber; 7 g sugar; 362 mg phosphorus; 45 mg calcium; 7 mg iron; 129 mg sodium; 921 mg potassium; 3599 IU vitamin A; 0 mg ATE vitamin E; 12 mg vitamin C; 122 mg cholesterol; 209 g water

Black Bean and Squash Chili

Winter squash adds color and a seasonal twist to this vegetarian chili.

1 medium butternut squash

1 tablespoon (15 ml) olive oil

1 cup (160 g) onion, chopped

$^1/_2$ teaspoon (1.5 g) minced garlic

$^3/_4$ cup (112 g) green bell pepper, chopped

4 cups (900 g) canned black beans, drained and rinsed

4 cups (720 g) canned no-salt-added tomatoes

4 ounces (115 g) canned chile peppers

1 teaspoon (2.5 g) ground cumin

$^1/_2$ teaspoon (0.5 g) dried oregano

Cut squash in half and scoop out and discard seeds. Place squash in a microwave-safe container with $^1/_4$-inch (63 mm) of water. Cover and microwave until tender, allowing 2 to 3 minutes per squash half. Remove squash and let cool, then peel and cut into chunks. In a large pot, heat oil over medium heat. Add onion and cook, stirring often, for 5 minutes or until soft. Add remaining ingredients except squash and mix well. Bring to a boil. Reduce heat and simmer gently for 15 minutes. Stir in squash and heat through.

Yield: 10 servings

Per serving: 199 calories (11% from fat, 17% from protein, 72% from carbohydrate); 9 g protein; 3 g total fat; 0 g saturated fat; 1 g monounsaturated fat; 1 g polyunsaturated fat; 39 g carbohydrate; 12 g fiber; 10 g

sugar; 167 mg phosphorus; 92 mg calcium; 4 mg iron; 28 mg sodium; 951 mg potassium; 9267 IU vitamin A; 0 mg ATE vitamin E; 66 mg vitamin C; 0 mg cholesterol; 247 g water

Three-Bean Chili

Okay, you all have figured out by now that I get bored and start experimenting. Actually, we have been making baked beans with a mixture of beans for a number of years, so a similar chili seemed like a natural extension. Other than the beans, it's a pretty standard recipe.

$1/2$ cup (125 g) dried kidney beans

$1/2$ cup (125 g) dried black beans

$1/2$ cup (125 g) dried white beans

7 cups (1.64 L) water, divided

1 pound (455 g) extra-lean ground beef (93% lean)

1 cup (160 g) onion, chopped

$1/2$ cup (75 g) green bell pepper, chopped

4 cups (720 g) canned no-salt-added tomatoes

12 ounces (340 g) no-salt-added tomato sauce

1 cup (235 ml) water

2 tablespoons (15 g) chili powder

$1/2$ teaspoon (1.3 g) cumin

$1/2$ teaspoon (1.5 g) garlic powder

$1/2$ teaspoon (0.5 g) dried oregano

1 tablespoon (15 ml) vinegar

Place beans in 6 cups (1.4 L) water in a large pan. Bring to a boil; boil for 1 minute. Remove from heat and let stand for 1 hour. Return beans to heat and simmer about 30 minutes, or until almost tender. Meanwhile brown beef, onion, and green bell pepper in a skillet. Drain beans. Add beans, beef mixture, and remaining ingredients to a large pot. Simmer for 1 to 1$1/2$ hours, or until beans are done and chili is desired consistency. Stir occasionally and add more water if needed.

Yield: 6 servings

Per serving: 374 calories (18% from fat, 33% from protein, 49% from carbohydrate); 26 g protein; 6 g total fat; 2 g saturated fat; 2 g monounsaturated fat; 1 g polyunsaturated fat; 38 g carbohydrate; 12 g fiber; 9 g sugar; 308 mg phosphorus; 155 mg calcium; 7 mg iron; 119 mg sodium; 1415 mg potassium; 1180 IU vitamin A; 0 mg ATE vitamin E; 37 mg vitamin C; 52 mg cholesterol; 576 g water

Vegetarian Chili

This is a different kind of chili, but it's still very good. Garnish with fresh cilantro, crushed corn chips, shredded low fat cheese, or fat-free sour cream (or all of them!).

$1/4$ cup (60 ml) dry sherry

1 tablespoon (15 ml) olive oil

2 cups (320 g) onion, chopped

$1/2$ cup (50 g) celery, chopped

$1/2$ cup (65 g) carrot, sliced

$1/2$ cup (75 g) red bell pepper, chopped

4 cups (900 g) cooked black beans

2 cups (475 ml) water

$1/2$ teaspoon (1.5 g) minced garlic

1 cup (180 g) plum tomato, chopped

2 teaspoons (5 g) ground cumin

4 teaspoons (10 g) chili powder

$1/2$ teaspoon (0.5 g) dried oregano

1/4 cup (15 g) chopped fresh cilantro

2 tablespoons (30 ml) honey

2 tablespoons (30 ml) no-salt-added tomato paste

In a large, heavy pot over medium heat, combine sherry and oil and heat to simmering. Add onions and sauté 8 to 10 minutes. Add celery, carrots, and bell pepper and sauté 5 minutes more, stirring frequently. Add remaining ingredients and bring to a boil. Lower heat and simmer, covered, for 45 minutes to 1 hour. Mixture should be thick, with all water absorbed.

Yield: 8 servings

Per serving: 192 calories (12% from fat, 18% from protein, 69% from carbohydrate); 9 g protein; 3 g total fat; 0 g saturated fat; 1 g monounsaturated fat; 1 g polyunsaturated fat; 34 g carbohydrate; 10 g fiber; 9 g sugar; 155 mg phosphorus; 55 mg calcium; 3 mg iron; 35 mg sodium; 563 mg potassium; 2358 IU vitamin A; 0 mg ATE vitamin E; 20 mg vitamin C; 0 mg cholesterol; 201 g water

White Chili

A delicious, mildly spicy chili with white beans and chicken. You could also use leftover turkey breast.

1 pound (455 g) dried large white beans

6 cups (1.4 L) low sodium chicken broth

1/2 teaspoon (1.5 g) minced garlic

1 cup (160 g) chopped onion, divided

1 tablespoon (15 ml) olive oil

8 ounces (225 g) canned chile peppers

2 teaspoons (5 g) ground cumin

1 1/2 teaspoons (1.5 g) dried oregano

1/4 teaspoon (0.5 g) cayenne pepper

4 cups (440 g) cooked chicken breast, diced

1 1/2 cups (170 g) low fat Monterey Jack cheese, grated

Soak beans overnight in water. Drain. Combine beans, chicken broth, garlic, and 1/2 cup (80 g) onions in a large soup pot and bring to a boil. Reduce heat and simmer for at least 3 hours, or until beans are very soft. Add additional water if necessary. Heat oil in a skillet over medium-high heat and sauté remaining 1/2 cup (80 g) onions until tender. Add chiles, cumin, oregano, and cayenne pepper and mix thoroughly. Add to bean mixture. Add chicken and continue to simmer for 1 hour. Serve topped with grated cheese.

Yield: 8 servings

Per serving: 407 calories (17% from fat, 44% from protein, 39% from carbohydrate); 45 g protein; 8 g total fat; 3 g saturated fat; 3 g monounsaturated fat; 1 g polyunsaturated fat; 40 g carbohydrate; 10 g fiber; 3 g sugar; 519 mg phosphorus; 272 mg calcium; 8 mg iron; 269 mg sodium; 1461 mg potassium; 213 IU vitamin A; 19 mg ATE vitamin E; 25 mg vitamin C; 65 mg cholesterol; 285 g water

Chicken Chili

This is not like any chili you've had before. I suppose it's a stretch to call it chili at all. But the flavor is great, even if a bit unexpected, and it tastes like chili, so. . . .

1 tablespoon (15 ml) olive oil

1 cup (160 g) onion, chopped

1/2 teaspoon (1.5 g) minced garlic

2 cups (470 ml) water

³/₄ cup (140 g) quick-cooking barley

4 cups (720 g) canned no-salt-added tomatoes

2 cups (470 ml) low sodium chicken broth

6 ounces (170 g) frozen corn, thawed

6-ounce (170-g) can jalapenos, chopped

1 tablespoon (7.5 g) chili powder

¹/₂ teaspoon (1.3 g) cumin

3 cups (330 g) cooked chicken breast, cubed

Heat oil in a Dutch oven and cook onion and garlic until onion is tender. Add remaining ingredients except chicken. Bring to a boil. Reduce heat, cover, and simmer for 10 minutes, stirring occasionally. Add chicken and continue simmering an additional 5 to 10 minutes, or until chicken is heated through and barley is tender.

Yield: 9 servings

Per serving: 143 calories (24% from fat, 47% from protein, 30% from carbohydrate); 17 g protein; 4 g total fat; 1 g saturated fat; 2 g monounsaturated fat; 1 g polyunsaturated fat; 11 g carbohydrate; 2 g fiber; 4 g sugar; 162 mg phosphorus; 52 mg calcium; 2 mg iron; 76 mg sodium; 442 mg potassium; 396 IU vitamin A; 3 mg ATE vitamin E; 13 mg vitamin C; 40 mg cholesterol; 267 g water

Chicken Chili Verde

Yet another chili variation. "Green chili" in Spanish, it does not contain tomatoes and has chicken instead of the more traditional beef. If you can't find cannellini beans, which are an Italian white kidney bean, you can substitute any other white bean, such as navy or great northern beans.

3 cups (300 g) cooked cannellini beans, drained

1 cup (160 g) chopped onion

¹/₂ teaspoon minced garlic

4 ounces (115 g) chopped chiles

2 teaspoons oregano

1¹/₂ teaspoons cumin

¹/₄ teaspoon ground cloves

¹/₄ teaspoon cayenne

3 cups (420 g) cooked diced chicken

Combine all ingredients in a large pot and simmer gently about 1 hour.

Yield: 6 servings

Per serving: 146 g water; 259 calories (20% from fat, 44% from protein, 36% from carb); 28 g protein; 6 g total fat; 2 g saturated fat; 2 g monounsaturated fat; 1 g polyunsaturated fat; 24 g carbohydrate; 7 g fiber; 2 g sugar; 303 mg phosphorus; 91 mg calcium; 4 mg iron; 66 mg sodium; 637 mg potassium; 322 IU vitamin A; 11 mg vitamin E; 49 mg vitamin C; 62 mg cholesterol

Chili-Chicken Stew

It may have a Mexican flavor, but make no mistake—this is real comfort food. It will raise your spirits even faster than Grandma's chicken noodle soup.

6 boneless chicken breasts, cut in 1-inch (2.5-cm) cubes

1 cup (160 g) chopped onion

1 cup (150 g) chopped green bell pepper

¹/₂ teaspoon minced garlic

1 tablespoon (15 ml) vegetable oil

4 cups (1 kg) no-salt-added stewed tomatoes, undrained and chopped

2 cups (342 g) cooked pinto beans, drained

2/3 (173 g) cup salsa

1 teaspoon ground cumin

2 tablespoons chili powder

3/4 cup (180 g) fat-free sour cream

1/2 cup (50 g) sliced scallions

1/2 cup (58 g) shredded Cheddar cheese

1 avocado, diced

Cook chicken, onion, bell pepper, and garlic in hot oil in a Dutch oven until lightly browned. Add tomatoes, beans, salsa, cumin, and chili powder. Cover, reduce heat, and simmer 20 minutes. Top individual servings with remaining ingredients.

Yield: 6 servings

Per serving: 214 g water; 338 calories (32% from fat, 35% from protein, 33% from carb); 27 g protein; 11 g total fat; 4 g saturated fat; 4 g monounsaturated fat; 2 g polyunsaturated fat; 26 g carbohydrate; 9 g fiber; 3 g sugar; 355 mg phosphorus; 181 mg calcium; 3 mg iron; 175 mg sodium; 840 mg potassium; 1276 IU vitamin A; 63 mg vitamin E; 29 mg vitamin C; 65 mg cholesterol

Black Bean Turkey Chili

This makes a rather mild chili, but you can easily add more chili powder or some red pepper flakes to spice it up if that's the way you like your chili.

1 pound (455 g) ground turkey

1 tablespoon (15 ml) olive oil

3/4 cup (120 g) chopped onion

1/2 cup (75 g) seeded and chopped green bell pepper

1/2 teaspoon minced garlic

4 cups (688 g) cooked no-salt-added black beans, rinsed and drained

2 cups (510 g) no-salt-added stewed tomatoes

8 ounces (225 g) no-salt-added tomato sauce

1 cup (235 ml) dark beer, or low-sodium beef broth

1 tablespoon chili powder

1 tablespoon ground cumin

1 teaspoon ground coriander

1 teaspoon dried oregano, crushed

Heat large, heavy saucepan or Dutch oven to medium-high. Brown the turkey until done. Drain meat and set aside. In the saucepan, add the oil and bring to medium heat. Add the onion, bell pepper, and garlic, and cook until vegetables are tender, about 5 to 6 minutes. Return meat to pan. Add remaining ingredients. Bring chili to a boil; then reduce heat and simmer for 30 to 45 minutes or until thickened, stirring occasionally. Taste to adjust seasonings.

Yield: 6 servings

Per serving: 301 g water; 368 calories (18% from fat, 39% from protein, 44% from carb); 35 g protein; 7 g total fat; 2 g saturated fat; 3 g monounsaturated fat; 2 g polyunsaturated fat; 40 g carbohydrate; 14 g fiber; 5 g sugar; 374 mg phosphorus; 134 mg calcium; 6 mg Iron; 92 mg sodium; 1108 mg potassium; 733 IU vitamin A; 0 mg vitamin E; 25 mg vitamin C; 57 mg cholesterol

Chili Beans

These are good either by themselves or as an addition to chili or other dishes.

1 cup (194 g) dried black beans

1 cup (167 g) dried black-eyed peas

1 ham hock

3 cups (355 ml) low-sodium chicken broth

1 1/2 tablespoons chili powder

1 tablespoon cumin

The night before, cover beans and peas with water and let stand to soften. Preheat oven to 275°F (140°C, gas mark 1). Combine beans, ham hock, broth, and spices in a heavy 2-quart (2-L) ovenproof pot, over medium heat. Cover, bring to a boil, and place in the oven. Check the beans every 30 minutes and add 1/2 cup more broth each time if all the liquid has been absorbed. Cook for 1 1/2 hours or until beans are soft.

Yield: 6 servings

Per serving: 155 g water; 113 calories (17% from fat, 28% from protein, 55% from carb); 8 g protein; 2 g total fat; 1 g saturated fat; 1 g monounsaturated fat; 1 g polyunsaturated fat; 17 g carbohydrate; 5 g fiber; 2 g sugar; 127 mg phosphorus; 34 mg calcium; 2 mg iron; 102 mg sodium; 376 mg potassium; 592 IU vitamin A; 0 mg vitamin E; 2 mg vitamin C; 2 mg cholesterol

Beef with Chili Dumplings

A great southwestern meal in a pot. With the dumplings, nothing else is even needed.

2 pound (900 g) beef round steak

1/4 cup (31 g) flour

1 teaspoon chili powder

1/2 teaspoon cumin

1/4 teaspoon black pepper

2 tablespoons (28 ml) olive oil

1 cup (160 g) chopped onion

2 cups (200 g) cooked kidney beans

10 ounces (280 g) frozen corn

Dumplings

1 tablespoon unsalted butter

1 teaspoon chili powder

3/4 cup (175 ml) skim milk

2 cups (128 g) biscuit baking mix

Trim fat from beef and cut into 1-inch (2.5-cm) cubes. Shake meat with flour, chili powder, cumin, and pepper in a resealable plastic bag to coat well. Heat oil in a large Dutch oven. Add beef cubes to oil, a few at a time, and brown. Remove beef from pot. Stir onion into the pot and sauté until soft. Return beef to pot. Drain liquid from beans into a large measuring container and add water to make 3 cups. Stir into beef mixture and cover. Heat to boiling. Lower heat and simmer for 2 hours or until beef is tender. Stir in corn and beans; heat to boiling again. To make chili dumplings, heat butter with chili powder in a small saucepan until bubbly. In large bowl add milk and chili-butter mix to baking mix all at once and stir with a fork until evenly moist. Drop batter by tablespoon on top of boiling stew to make 12 mounds. Cook uncovered, 10 minutes. Cover. Cook 10 minutes longer or until dumplings are done.

Yield: 8 servings

Per serving: 143 g water; 624 calories (21% from fat, 37% from protein, 42% from carb); 58 g protein; 15 g total fat; 4 g saturated fat; 7 g monounsaturated fat; 2 g polyunsaturated fat; 65 g carbohydrate; 14 g fiber; 3 g sugar; 678 mg phosphorus; 201 mg calcium; 10 mg iron; 118 mg sodium; 1438 mg potassium; 486 IU vitamin A; 56 mg vitamin E; 7 mg vitamin C; 106 mg cholesterol

13

Italian

I like Italian cooking maybe even more than my wife does, who is half Italian. And that is reflected in the fact that we have 60 recipes in this chapter, plus other Italian flavored dishes scattered throughout the rest of the book. We start with a homemade version of low fat, low sodium turkey Italian sausage, then get in sauces, all kinds of pasta dishes, meat dishes, pizzas, and soups. So take your pick and enjoy a good meal like an Italian would.

Turkey Italian Sausage

This makes a very nice-flavored sausage, not really hot, but with a little kick. You can vary the amount of red pepper depending on how hot you like your sausage. A serving is 2 ounces (55 g), which may be less than you'd use in a main dish.

2 pounds (905 g) ground turkey

1 tablespoon (5.8 g) fennel seed

2 bay leaves, ground

1 tablespoon (0.4 g) dried parsley

³/₄ teaspoon (2.3 g) minced garlic

¹/₂ teaspoon (1.5 g) onion powder

¹/₈ teaspoon (0.2 g) red pepper flakes

¹/₂ teaspoon (0.5 g) black pepper

¹/₄ cup (60 ml) water

Combine all ingredients and mix well. Pan fry, grill, or broil to desired doneness.

Yield: 16 servings

Per serving: 98 calories (28% from fat, 71% from protein, 2% from carbohydrate); 17 g protein; 3 g total fat; 1 g saturated fat; 1 g monounsaturated fat; 1 g polyunsaturated fat; 0 g carbohydrate; 0 g fiber; 0 g sugar; 123 mg phosphorus; 20 mg calcium; 1 mg iron; 40 mg sodium; 179 mg potassium; 26 IU vitamin A; 0 mg ATE vitamin E; 0 mg vitamin C; 43 mg cholesterol; 41 g water

Italian Meat Sauce

Use this sauce over spaghetti or other pasta or as a cooking sauce for lasagna. The olives and artichokes give it more flavor than many Italian sauces, as well as a big increase in fiber.

1 pound (455 g) ground beef

1 tablespoon Italian seasoning

1 teaspoon minced garlic

1 teaspoon minced onion

1¹/₂ cups (105 g) sliced mushrooms

4 cups (1 kg) crushed tomatoes

¹/₄ cup (25 g) sliced black olives

14 ounces (400 g) artichoke hearts, drained

Brown meat with seasoning, garlic, onion, and mushrooms. Drain grease. Add all other ingredients. Heat to boiling; simmer 30 minutes.

Yield: 4 servings

Per serving: 321 g water; 447 calories (63% from fat, 21% from protein, 16% from carb); 24 g protein; 32 g total fat; 13 g saturated fat; 14 g monounsaturated fat; 2 g polyunsaturated fat; 18 g carbohydrate; 7 g fiber; 1 g sugar; 269 mg phosphorus; 59 mg calcium; 4 mg iron; 218 mg sodium; 952 mg potassium; 1177 IU vitamin A; 0 mg vitamin E; 45 mg vitamin C; 96 mg cholesterol

Italian Beef Sauce

A hearty sauce to serve over pasta or rice. This one cooks all day in the slow cooker, so dinner is ready in no time when you get home.

1 pound (455 g) beef round steak, cubed

2 cups (360 g) canned no-salt-added tomatoes

2 tablespoons (30 ml) red wine

$1/4$ teaspoon garlic powder

2 teaspoons (1.4 g) dried Italian seasoning

1 cup (160 g) onion, coarsely chopped

$1/2$ cup (35 g) mushrooms, sliced

6 ounces (170 g) no-salt-added tomato paste

Place beef in the bottom of a slow cooker. Stir together remaining ingredients except tomato paste. Pour over beef. Cover and cook on low for 8 to 10 hours. Turn to high. Stir in tomato paste and cook until thickened, 10 to 15 minutes.

Yield: 4 servings

Per serving: 307 calories (18% from fat, 59% from protein, 23% from carbohydrate); 45 g protein; 6 g total fat; 2 g saturated fat; 2 g monounsaturated fat; 0 g polyunsaturated fat; 18 g carbohydrate; 4 g fiber; 10 g sugar; 337 mg phosphorus; 75 mg calcium; 7 mg iron; 111 mg sodium; 1141 mg potassium; 824 IU vitamin A; 0 mg ATE vitamin E; 24 mg vitamin C; 102 mg cholesterol; 261 g water

Fresh Tomato Meat Sauce

A little different variation on spaghetti sauce. This makes a large batch. You can freeze the leftovers if you like. As you might guess, this was developed when the tomatoes in the garden were producing in quantity.

1 pound (455 g) ground beef

$1/2$ pound (225 g) Italian sausage

1 onion, chopped

1 green bell pepper, chopped

$1/2$ pound (225 g) mushrooms, sliced

15 tomatoes

1 tablespoon minced garlic

2 tablespoons (28 ml) olive oil

6 cans no-salt-added tomato paste

2 tablespoons oregano

1 tablespoon basil

2 tablespoons parsley

$1/2$ cup (120 ml) red wine

Crumble beef and sausage into a large skillet. Add onion, pepper, and mushrooms. Cook until meat is done. Immerse tomatoes in boiling water for about 30 seconds. Drain, peel, and chop finely. In a large Dutch oven, sauté garlic in olive oil until lightly browned, about 2 minutes. Add tomatoes, tomato paste, spices, wine, and meat/veggie mixture. Simmer slowly until desired thickness, 1 to 2 hours.

Yield: 8 servings

Per serving: 180 g water; 404 calories (48% from fat, 26% from protein, 26% from carb); 26 g protein; 22 g total fat; 7 g saturated fat; 10 g monounsaturated fat; 2 g polyunsaturated fat; 27 g carbohydrate; 6 g fiber; 16 g sugar; 299 mg phosphorus; 79 mg calcium; 6 mg iron; 1253 mg sodium; 1689 mg potassium; 2100 IU vitamin A; 0 mg vitamin E; 31 mg vitamin C; 70 mg cholesterol

Vegetable Pasta Sauce

Low in calories, fat free, 3 grams of fiber, and great Italian flavor on top of all that.

1 cup (160 g) finely chopped onion

1 teaspoon crushed garlic

2 teaspoons basil

1 1/2 teaspoons oregano

1 bay leaf

28 ounces (800 g) no-salt-added canned tomatoes

16 ounces (455 g) no-salt-added tomato sauce

1/4 teaspoon black pepper, fresh ground

4 tablespoons (16 g) chopped fresh parsley

In a large pot, heat onion, garlic, basil, oregano, bay leaf, tomatoes, tomato sauce, pepper, and parsley. Mix well, mashing tomatoes with a fork. Bring to boiling, reduce heat, and simmer, uncovered, stirring occasionally for 1 1/2 hours. Remove bay leaf. Serve over whole wheat pasta.

Yield: 6 servings

Per serving: 218 g water; 64 calories (5% from fat, 14% from protein, 81% from carb); 2 g protein; 0 g total fat; 0 g saturated fat; 0 g monounsaturated fat; 0 g polyunsaturated fat; 14 g carbohydrate; 3 g fiber; 8 g sugar; 61 mg phosphorus; 71 mg calcium; 2 mg iron; 28 mg sodium; 597 mg potassium; 668 IU vitamin A; 0 mg vitamin E; 28 mg vitamin C; 0 mg cholesterol

Fish Sauce for Pasta

Even though this recipe may seem higher in fat than most of the others, it's the good kind of fat that comes from olive oil and fish. So enjoy it guilt-free.

1/4 cup (60 ml) olive oil

12 ounces (340 g) salmon fillets, cubed

12 ounces (340 g) cod fillets, cubed

1 teaspoon (3 g) minced garlic

1/2 cup (120 ml) white wine

1/2 teaspoon (0.5 g) dried oregano

1/2 teaspoon (0.6 g) dried rosemary

1 teaspoon (0.1 g) dried parsley

1 tablespoon (10 g) onion, minced

Heat oil in a heavy skillet. Add salmon, cod, and garlic and sauté for a minute or two, until nearly cooked through. Add wine and remaining ingredients and continue cooking until sauce has been reduced by about half. Serve over pasta.

Yield: 6 servings

Per serving: 248 calories (61% from fat, 37% from protein, 2% from carbohydrate); 21 g protein; 16 g total fat; 3 g saturated fat; 9 g monounsaturated fat; 3 g polyunsaturated fat; 1 g carbohydrate; 0 g fiber; 0 g sugar; 252 mg phosphorus; 21 mg calcium; 1 mg iron; 66 mg sodium; 461 mg potassium; 76 IU vitamin A; 15 mg ATE vitamin E; 3 mg vitamin C; 58 mg cholesterol; 104 g water

Sun-Dried Tomato Alfredo Sauce

I saw a jar of this on the supermarket shelf and decided to try to get creative and see if I could come up with something similar, but healthier. I was quite happy with the way it turned out. By the way, my $1/3$ cup (80 ml) serving size is bigger than the USDA's standard $1/4$ cup (60 ml) serving of pasta sauce, but I think it seems closer to what people are likely to eat in reality.

2 cups (470 ml) skim milk

2 tablespoons (16 g) cornstarch

$1/2$ cup (40 g) Parmesan cheese, shredded

$1/2$ cup (55 g) oil-packed sun-dried tomatoes, finely chopped

$1/2$ teaspoon (1.5 g) garlic powder

$1/2$ teaspoon (0.5 g) dried oregano

Shake milk and cornstarch together in a jar. Place in saucepan. Cook over medium heat and stir for 10 minutes, or until thickened and beginning to boil. Add cheese, tomatoes, garlic powder, and oregano and stir until cheese is melted.

Yield: 6 servings

Per serving: 100 calories (34% from fat, 27% from protein, 38% from carbohydrate); 7 g protein; 4 g total fat; 2 g saturated fat; 2 g monounsaturated fat; 0 g polyunsaturated fat; 10 g carbohydrate; 1 g fiber; 0 g sugar; 167 mg phosphorus; 216 mg calcium; 0 mg iron; 200 mg sodium; 307 mg potassium; 327 IU vitamin A; 60 mg ATE vitamin E; 10 mg vitamin C; 9 mg cholesterol; 80 g water

Tuna Alfredo Sauce

If you're looking for something a little different to put over pasta, this could be just the thing.

2 tablespoons (28 g) butter

4 ounces (115 g) mushrooms, sliced

2 tablespoons (16 g) flour

1 cup (235 ml) skim milk

1 can (6-ounce, or 170-g) tuna

2 tablespoons (10 g) Parmesan cheese, grated

Melt butter in a saucepan and sauté mushrooms. Stir in flour, then slowly add milk and tuna, cooking and stirring until thickened and bubbly. Remove from heat and stir in cheese.

Yield: 4 servings

Per serving: 114 calories (20% from fat, 54% from protein, 27% from carbohydrate); 15 g protein; 2 g total fat; 2 g saturated fat; 0 g monounsaturated fat; 0 g polyunsaturated fat; 7 g carbohydrate; 0 g fiber; 1 g sugar; 214 mg phosphorus; 130 mg calcium; 1 mg iron; 107 mg sodium; 312 mg potassium; 147 IU vitamin A; 44 mg ATE vitamin E; 1 mg vitamin C; 32 mg cholesterol; 114 g water

Lower-Fat Pesto Sauce

I really like pesto sauce. It is an easy treat in the summer when the basil is growing in the garden. But while traditional recipes contain a lot of oil, this version is very tasty, and you needn't feel guilty at all!

2 tablespoons (30 ml) low sodium chicken broth

$1/2$ teaspoon (1.5 g) minced garlic

1 cup (40 g) fresh basil

$^1/_3$ cup (33 g) Parmesan cheese, freshly grated

2 tablespoons (18 g) pine nuts

Combine broth and garlic and heat in the microwave on high for 5 minutes (or heat on the stove). Allow to cool. Chop basil in food processor. Add cooled broth mixture, Parmesan cheese, and pine nuts. Process until everything is finely chopped and blended. Serve over pasta with additional Parmesan cheese, if desired.

Yield: 6 servings

Per serving: 58 calories (53% from fat, 21% from protein, 26% from carbohydrate); 3 g protein; 4 g total fat; 1 g saturated fat; 1 g monounsaturated fat; 1 g polyunsaturated fat; 4 g carbohydrate; 2 g fiber; 0 g sugar; 86 mg phosphorus; 181 mg calcium; 3 mg iron; 88 mg sodium; 221 mg potassium; 550 IU vitamin A; 7 mg ATE vitamin E; 4 mg vitamin C; 5 mg cholesterol; 7 g water

Whole Wheat Linguine with White Clam Sauce

Simple to make and great taste.

$^1/_2$ cup (120 ml) olive oil

1 cup (160 g) chopped onion

1 teaspoon minced garlic

6 ounces (170 g) minced clams, including liquid

6 ounces (170 g) whole clams, drained

$^1/_2$ cup (120 ml) water

1 tablespoon parsley

$^1/_2$ teaspoon oregano

$^1/_4$ teaspoon black pepper

8 ounces (225 g) mushrooms, sliced

1 pound (455 g) whole wheat linguine, cooked and drained

Heat oil in skillet. Simmer onion and garlic until golden. Add clams, water, parsley, oregano, pepper, and mushrooms. Simmer for 15 minutes. Pour sauce over linguine.

Yield: 6 servings

Per serving: 121 g water; 526 calories (34% from fat, 20% from protein, 47% from carb); 27 g protein; 20 g total fat; 3 g saturated fat; 13 g monounsaturated fat; 3 g polyunsaturated fat; 64 g carbohydrate; 1 g fiber; 2 g sugar; 428 mg phosphorus; 93 mg calcium; 19 mg iron; 74 mg sodium; 685 mg potassium; 386 IU vitamin A; 97 mg vitamin E; 16 mg vitamin C; 38 mg cholesterol

Fettuccine with Vegetables

Fresh vegetables and Romano cheese make the pasta dish special.

$^1/_2$ pound (225 g) asparagus

2 tablespoons (28 g) unsalted butter

2 tablespoons (28 ml) olive oil

$^1/_2$ teaspoon minced garlic

1 cup (113 g) zucchini, seeds removed, diced small

$^1/_4$ cup (25 g) thinly sliced scallions

$^1/_2$ cup (65 g) frozen peas, defrosted and drained

1/4 teaspoon black pepper

8 ounces (225 g) whole wheat fettuccine

1/4 cup minced fresh parsley

3 tablespoons minced fresh chives

2 ounces (55 g) grated Romano cheese

Cut the asparagus on the diagonal into 1/2-inch (1-cm) pieces. Bring a pot of water to a boil, add asparagus, and time for 2 minutes. Drain, rinse with cold water and pat dry. In a large skillet, heat butter and oil over medium heat. Add garlic and sauté for 1 minute. Stir in zucchini and scallions, sautéing for 2 minutes. Add asparagus, peas, and pepper, heating for 2 minutes. After cooking fettuccine, drain it and put back into hot pan. Add vegetables, parsley, chives, and cheese, stirring to coat.

Yield: 4 servings

Per serving: 119 g water; 402 calories (37% from fat, 15% from protein, 48% from carb); 16 g protein; 17 g total fat; 7 g saturated fat; 8 g monounsaturated fat; 1 g polyunsaturated fat; 50 g carbohydrate; 3 g fiber; 3 g sugar; 322 mg phosphorus; 211 mg calcium; 4 mg iron; 248 mg sodium; 413 mg potassium; 1623 IU vitamin A; 60 mg vitamin E; 18 mg vitamin C; 30 mg cholesterol

Rigatoni with Artichoke Sauce

A nice pasta sauce flavored with marinated artichoke hearts.

1 pound (455 g) whole wheat rigatoni

6 ounces (170 g) artichoke hearts, drained

1/4 cup (60 ml) olive oil

3/4 teaspoon minced garlic

2 tablespoons chopped fresh parsley

3 cups (720 g) no-salt-added canned tomatoes, drained and chopped

1/8 teaspoon red pepper flakes

1/4 cup (25 g) grated Parmesan cheese

1/4 teaspoon black pepper, fresh ground

Cook pasta according to directions. Meanwhile, slice artichokes thinly. In large saucepan, heat oil and sauté garlic 2 minutes. Add artichoke hearts, parsley, tomatoes, and pepper flakes. Cook 20 minutes, stirring occasionally. Drain rigatoni and place in serving dish. Top pasta with sauce and sprinkle with cheese and black pepper.

Yield: 6 servings

Per serving: 145 g water; 395 calories (25% from fat, 14% from protein, 61% from carb); 15 g protein; 12 g total fat; 2 g saturated fat; 7 g monounsaturated fat; 2 g polyunsaturated fat; 65 g carbohydrate; 3 g fiber; 3 g sugar; 267 mg phosphorus; 123 mg calcium; 4 mg iron; 101 mg sodium; 478 mg potassium; 326 IU vitamin A; 5 mg vitamin E; 14 mg vitamin C; 4 mg cholesterol

Whole Wheat Pasta with Pesto

Quick and easy pasta meal with fresh pesto.

1 tablespoon (15 ml) olive oil

1 teaspoon (5 ml) water

1/8 teaspoon salt

$^1/_2$ teaspoon minced garlic

3 tablespoons minced fresh basil

3 tablespoons minced fresh parsley

$^1/_4$ cup (25 g) grated Parmesan cheese

2 cups (210 g) whole wheat pasta, cooked

Combine oil, water, salt, garlic, basil, parsley, and cheese in container of an electric blender. Cover and process until smooth pesto is formed. Combine pasta and pesto mixture in a medium bowl, and toss gently.

Yield: 4 servings

Per serving: 9 g water; 245 calories (21% from fat, 16% from protein, 63% from carb); 10 g protein; 6 g total fat; 2 g saturated fat; 3 g monounsaturated fat; 1 g polyunsaturated fat; 41 g carbohydrate; 5 g fiber; 0 g sugar; 191 mg phosphorus; 128 mg calcium; 3 mg iron; 176 mg sodium; 192 mg potassium; 412 IU vitamin A; 7 mg vitamin E; 5 mg vitamin C; 6 mg cholesterol

Lower Fat Chicken Tetrazzini

This recipe is proof that you can have rich-tasting dishes without the sodium and fat.

1 tablespoon (15 ml) olive oil

1 cup (160 g) onion, chopped

$^1/_2$ cup (35 g) mushrooms, sliced

1 tablespoon (8 g) flour

$^1/_4$ cup (60 ml) white wine

3 cups (330 g) cooked chicken breast, cubed

12 ounces (340 g) macaroni, cooked

2 cups (470 ml) low sodium chicken broth

Dash nutmeg

4 ounces (115 g) low fat Swiss cheese, diced

2 tablespoons (30 ml) skim milk

Preheat oven to 350°F (180°C, or gas mark 4). In a skillet, heat the oil over low heat. Add onions and cook for 15 minutes, or until golden brown, stirring often. Add mushrooms and cook 5 minutes longer. Stir in flour, blending thoroughly. Stir in remaining ingredients except milk. Transfer to ovenproof casserole dish. Cover and bake for 30 minutes. Stir in milk. Re-cover and bake 5 minutes longer.

Yield: 6 servings

Per serving: 289 calories (19% from fat, 48% from protein, 34% from carbohydrate); 33 g protein; 6 g total fat; 2 g saturated fat; 2 g monounsaturated fat; 1 g polyunsaturated fat; 23 g carbohydrate; 2 g fiber; 2 g sugar; 353 mg phosphorus; 214 mg calcium; 2 mg iron; 130 mg sodium; 369 mg potassium; 54 IU vitamin A; 15 mg ATE vitamin E; 2 mg vitamin C; 66 mg cholesterol; 211 g water

Pasta with Meat Sauce

An updated, healthier version of a typical Hamburger Helper–type meal. This is one that's sure to please young people as well as adults.

8 ounces (255 g) pasta

2 tablespoons (30 ml) olive oil

2 cups (320 g) onion, chopped

1 teaspoon (0.7 g) dried Italian seasoning

$^1/_2$ teaspoon (1.5 g) chopped garlic

1 pound (455 g) extra-lean ground beef (93% lean)

2 cups (360 g) canned no-salt-added crushed tomatoes

$^1/_2$ teaspoon (0.4 g) dried basil

Cook pasta according to package directions, omitting the salt. Drain. Heat olive oil in a large skillet on medium heat. Add the chopped onion and Italian seasoning. Cook for 5 minutes, stirring occasionally, until the onions are softened. Add the garlic. Cook for an additional minute. Remove onion mixture and add meat to pan, breaking it up as you add it. Brown the meat on one side, then turn over to brown the other side. When meat is browned, return the onions to the pan. Add tomatoes and basil. Simmer, uncovered, for 15 minutes. Stir in the cooked pasta. Serve immediately.

Yield: 4 servings

Per serving: 589 calories (29% from fat, 25% from protein, 46% from carbohydrate); 30 g protein; 15 g total fat; 4 g saturated fat; 8 g monounsaturated fat; 1 g polyunsaturated fat; 55 g carbohydrate; 5 g fiber; 8 g sugar; 315 mg phosphorus; 82 mg calcium; 4 mg iron; 97 mg sodium; 800 mg potassium; 167 IU vitamin A; 0 mg ATE vitamin E; 17 mg vitamin C; 78 mg cholesterol; 262 g water

Pasta with Vegetables

It doesn't get any easier than this when you are looking for a quick, easy dinner. By the time the pasta cooks, everything else will be ready too.

$^1/_2$ pound (225 g) linguine

1 tablespoon (15 ml) olive oil

$^1/_2$ cup (66 g) zucchini, sliced

4 ounces (115 g) mushrooms, sliced

$^1/_2$ cup (75 g) green bell pepper, sliced

$^1/_2$ cup (90 g) tomato, chopped

$^1/_2$ cup (80 g) onion, sliced

$^1/_2$ teaspoon (1.5 g) garlic powder

$^1/_2$ teaspoon (0.5 g) dried oregano

1 teaspoon (0.7 g) dried basil

2 tablespoons (10 g) Parmesan cheese, grated

Cook linguine according to package directions. Heat olive oil in a large skillet over medium-high heat. Sauté zucchini, mushrooms, green bell pepper, tomato, onion, garlic powder, oregano, and basil. Toss with pasta. Sprinkle with cheese.

Yield: 4 servings

Per serving: 287 calories (22% from fat, 15% from protein, 63% from carbohydrate); 11 g protein; 7 g total fat; 2 g saturated fat; 3 g monounsaturated fat; 1 g polyunsaturated fat; 46 g carbohydrate; 3 g fiber; 4 g sugar; 206 mg phosphorus; 72 mg calcium; 2 mg iron; 65 mg sodium; 391 mg potassium; 329 IU vitamin A; 13 mg ATE vitamin E; 22 mg vitamin C; 50 mg cholesterol; 100 g water

Pasta with Portobello Mushrooms

A delicious meatless version of pasta primavera. You can use whatever shape pasta you happen to have on hand.

16 ounces (455 g) pasta

2 tablespoons (30 ml) olive oil

$^1/_2$ teaspoon (1.5 g) minced garlic

$^1/_2$ pound (225 g) Portobello mushroom caps, chopped

$^3/_4$ cup (113 g) red bell pepper, diced

1 cup (113 g) zucchini, cut into $^1/_2$-inch (1.3-cm) slices

$^1/_4$ cup (60 ml) red wine vinegar

2 tablespoons (10 g) Parmesan cheese, grated

In a large pot cook pasta until al dente. Drain. Heat the oil in a large nonstick skillet over medium heat and cook the garlic, mushrooms, red bell pepper, and zucchini for 10 minutes, or until soft, stirring frequently. Stir in red wine vinegar. Toss cooked pasta with mushroom mixture. Top with grated Parmesan cheese. Serve warm.

Yield: 6 servings

Per serving: 359 calories (22% from fat, 14% from protein, 64% from carbohydrate); 13 g protein; 9 g total fat; 2 g saturated fat; 4 g monounsaturated fat; 2 g polyunsaturated fat; 58 g carbohydrate; 4 g fiber; 3 g sugar; 260 mg phosphorus; 58 mg calcium; 2 mg iron; 54 mg sodium; 468 mg potassium; 681 IU vitamin A; 15 mg ATE vitamin E; 27 mg vitamin C; 65 mg cholesterol; 88 g water

Vegetable "Lasagna"

You could use this as a side dish with something like a grilled chicken breast, or just serve it as a vegetarian main dish. I used a George Foreman grill to grill the vegetables, but you could also use a regular grill or roast them in the oven.

4 cups (450 g) zucchini, sliced lengthwise

1 eggplant, sliced

8 ounces (225 g) mushrooms, sliced

1 cup (180 g) onion, sliced

2 cups (470 ml) low sodium spaghetti sauce

8 ounces (225 g) part-skim mozzarella, shredded

Preheat oven to 400°F (200°C, or gas mark 6). Slice zucchini, eggplant, mushrooms, and onion and coat with olive oil spray. Grill until crisp-tender. Place a small amount of spaghetti sauce in an 8 × 12 (20 × 30-cm) baking dish. Layer vegetables and sauce in this order: zucchini, eggplant, sauce, onion, and mushrooms, sauce, eggplant, and zucchini. Top with remaining sauce and sprinkle with cheese. Bake for 15 minutes, or until cheese is melted and starts to brown.

Yield: 6 servings

Per serving: 237 calories (38% from fat, 22% from protein, 40% from carbohydrate); 14 g protein; 10 g total fat; 4 g saturated fat; 4 g monounsaturated fat; 1 g polyunsaturated fat; 25 g carbohydrate; 7 g fiber; 15 g sugar; 296 mg phosphorus; 345 mg calcium; 1 mg iron; 272 mg sodium; 903 mg potassium; 880 IU vitamin A; 47 mg ATE vitamin E; 28 mg vitamin C; 24 mg cholesterol; 291 g water

Italian Chicken and Mushroom Sauce

This looks like it would be a high-calorie, high-fat meal, but it's not. Add a salad and you have a complete meal.

3 boneless chicken breasts

2 tablespoons (30 ml) olive oil

$^1/_2$ teaspoon (1.5 g) minced garlic

$^1/_2$ pound (225 g) fresh mushrooms, sliced

2 cups (470 ml) skim milk

$^1/_4$ cup (30 g) flour

2 teaspoons (1.4 g) dried Italian seasoning

Cut chicken into 1-inch (2.5-cm) cubes. Heat olive oil in a skillet over medium-high heat. Sauté garlic, chicken, and mushrooms until chicken is done. Remove from skillet. Shake milk and flour together in a jar with a tight-fitting lid and add to skillet. Stir in Italian seasoning. Cook and stir until thickened and beginning to boil. Stir chicken mixture into sauce. Serve over pasta.

Yield: 6 servings

Per serving: 141 calories (34% from fat, 37% from protein, 28% from carbohydrate); 13 g protein; 5 g total fat; 1 g saturated fat; 3 g monounsaturated fat; 1 g polyunsaturated fat; 10 g carbohydrate; 1 g fiber; 1 g sugar; 201 mg phosphorus; 129 mg calcium; 1 mg iron; 74 mg sodium; 372 mg potassium; 197 IU vitamin A; 52 mg ATE vitamin E; 2 mg vitamin C; 22 mg cholesterol; 136 g water

Baked Italian Chicken Breasts

This is really "oven fried" chicken. Using boneless breasts cuts way back on the saturated fat, and the sun-dried tomatoes and Italian seasoning give it a different flavor. We had this recently with roasted vegetables that we also sprinkled with Italian seasoning.

2 boneless chicken breasts

$^1/_2$ cup (60 g) bread crumbs

$^1/_4$ cup (28 g) oil-packed sun-dried tomatoes

$^1/_4$ teaspoon (0.8 g) garlic powder

1 teaspoon (0.7 g) Italian seasoning

1 egg, beaten

Preheat oven to 400°F (200°C, or gas mark 6). Split each chicken breast in half to make two thin cutlets. Combine bread crumbs, tomatoes, garlic powder, and Italian seasoning in a food processor. Process until well blended. Dip chicken in egg and then in crumb mixture to coat thoroughly. Place in an ovenproof casserole dish. Bake for 20 minutes, or until chicken is cooked through.

Yield: 2 servings

Per serving: 243 calories (20% from fat, 41% from protein, 39% from carbohydrate); 25 g protein; 5 g total fat; 1 g saturated fat; 2 g monounsaturated fat; 2 g polyunsaturated fat; 23 g carbohydrate; 2 g fiber; 2 g sugar; 243 mg phosphorus; 88 mg calcium; 3 mg iron; 336 mg sodium; 465 mg potassium; 339 IU vitamin A; 4 mg ATE vitamin E; 15 mg vitamin C; 151 mg cholesterol; 88 g water

Chicken with Red Pepper Sauce

This was a recipe that sat in my "I need to try that" file for a while. It had a great flavor, but wasn't overly hot.

For Chicken:

$^1/_4$ cup (30 g) flour

$^1/_2$ teaspoon (1.3 g) paprika

$^1/_4$ teaspoon (0.5 g) black pepper

2 pounds (905 g) boneless chicken breasts

For Sauce:

1 tablespoon (15 ml) canola oil

$^3/_4$ cup (113 g) red bell pepper, cut in 1-inch (2.5-cm) cubes

$^1/_4$ cup (25 g) scallions, sliced

2 tablespoons (16 g) flour

1 cup (235 ml) low sodium chicken broth

2 tablespoons (26 g) sugar

$^1/_2$ tablespoon (2.5 g) cayenne pepper

$^1/_3$ cup (80 ml) cider vinegar

Preheat oven to 375°F (190°C, or gas mark 5).

To make the chicken: In a plastic bag, combine flour, paprika, and pepper. Add chicken, a few pieces at a time, to the bag, shaking to coat well. Arrange chicken in a shallow baking pan. Coat with nonstick vegetable oil spray to moisten the flour. Bake for 20 minutes.

To make the sauce: Heat the oil in a medium saucepan; cook red bell pepper and scallions until tender. Stir in flour. Add chicken broth, sugar, and cayenne pepper. Cook and stir until thickened and bubbly. Cook and stir for 1 minute more. Remove from heat, stir in vinegar, and cool slightly. Spoon sauce over chicken. Bake for 20 minutes more, or until done, basting with the sauce 2 or 3 times during baking.

Yield: 6 servings

Per serving: 249 calories (18% from fat, 61% from protein, 21% from carbohydrate); 37 g protein; 5 g total fat; 1 g saturated fat; 2 g monounsaturated fat; 1 g polyunsaturated fat; 13 g carbohydrate; 1 g fiber; 5 g sugar; 326 mg phosphorus; 26 mg calcium; 2 mg iron; 113 mg sodium; 503 mg potassium; 942 IU vitamin A; 9 mg ATE vitamin E; 27 mg vitamin C; 88 mg cholesterol; 186 g water

Tip: If you want something a little spicier, just increase the amount of cayenne pepper.

Chicken Breasts Cacciatore

This made a great-tasting sauce with no extra work. And it's always nice to come home to a meal that's done and has filled the house with such an aroma.

1 cup (160 g) onion, sliced

4 boneless chicken breasts

12 ounces (340 g) no-salt-added tomato paste

$^1/_4$ teaspoon (0.5 g) black pepper

$^1/_2$ teaspoon (1.5 g) garlic powder

1 teaspoon (1 g) dried oregano

1 teaspoon (0.7 g) dried basil

$^1/_4$ cup (60 ml) dry white wine

$^1/_4$ cup (60 ml) water

Place onion in the bottom of a slow cooker. Place chicken on top. Combine remaining ingredients and pour over. Cook on low for 8 to 10 hours.

Yield: 6 servings

Per serving: 119 calories (7% from fat, 46% from protein, 47% from carbohydrate); 14 g protein; 1 g total fat; 0 g saturated fat; 0 g monounsaturated fat; 0 g polyunsaturated fat; 14 g carbohydrate; 3 g fiber; 8 g sugar; 151 mg phosphorus; 39 mg calcium; 2 mg iron; 88 mg sodium; 752 mg potassium; 898 IU vitamin A; 3 mg ATE vitamin E; 15 mg vitamin C; 27 mg cholesterol; 119 g water

Italian Baked Chicken Breasts

A variation on oven-baked chicken recipes, this one with an Italian flavor. Great with pasta and a salad for dinner.

12 low sodium saltines, crushed

1 teaspoon (5 g) brown sugar

$^1/_2$ teaspoon (1.4 g) sesame seeds

1 tablespoon (7 g) wheat germ

$^1/_2$ teaspoon (0.5 g) dried oregano

$^1/_4$ teaspoon (0.5 g) celery seed

$^1/_4$ teaspoon (0.8 g) garlic powder

1 teaspoon (3 g) onion, minced

$^1/_2$ teaspoon (0.1 g) dried parsley

1 teaspoon (0.7 g) dried Italian seasoning

4 boneless chicken breasts

1 egg, beaten

Preheat oven to 350°F (180°C, or gas mark 4). Combine all ingredients except chicken and egg. Dip the chicken in the egg and then in the crumb mixture, turning to cover on all sides. Place in a 9 × 13-inch (23 × 33-cm) baking dish coated with nonstick vegetable oil spray. Spray chicken with vegetable oil spray until crumbs are moistened. Bake for 30 to 40 minutes, or until done.

Yield: 4 servings

Per serving: 164 calories (11% from fat, 52% from protein, 38% from carbohydrate); 20 g protein; 2 g total fat; 0 g saturated fat; 0 g monounsaturated fat; 1 g polyunsaturated fat; 15 g carbohydrate; 1 g fiber; 1 g sugar; 198 mg phosphorus; 30 mg calcium; 2 mg iron; 170 mg sodium; 183 mg potassium; 112 IU vitamin A; 4 mg ATE vitamin E; 1 mg vitamin C; 96 mg cholesterol; 68 g water

Italian Burgers

A little added flavor for the meat accompaniment to your pasta. The sun-dried tomatoes add moistness as well as flavor.

1 pound (455 g) extra-lean ground beef (93% lean)

$^1/_2$ cup (55 g) oil-packed sun-dried tomatoes, chopped

$^1/_4$ teaspoon (0.8 g) garlic powder

$^1/_2$ teaspoon (0.7 g) dried basil

$^1/_2$ teaspoon (0.5 g) dried oregano

Mix all ingredients together. Form into patties and grill or fry to desired doneness.

Yield: 4 servings

Per serving: 296 calories (45% from fat, 47% from protein, 7% from carbohydrate); 22 g protein; 9 g total fat; 3 g saturated fat; 4 g monounsaturated fat; 1 g polyunsaturated fat; 3 g carbohydrate; 1 g fiber; 0 g sugar; 180 mg phosphorus; 18 mg calcium; 3 mg iron; 112 mg sodium; 544 mg potassium; 194 IU vitamin A; 0 mg ATE vitamin E; 14 mg vitamin C; 78 mg cholesterol; 79 g water

Steak Cacciatore

Serve this over pasta or just stir some pre-cooked pasta in along with the zucchini.

2 pounds (905 g) beef round steak

$^1/_4$ teaspoon (0.5 g) black pepper

$^1/_2$ cup (80 g) onion, sliced

$^1/_2$ cup (75 g) green bell pepper, cut in strips

1 jar (28 ounces, 795 g) low sodium spaghetti sauce

1 cup (113 g) zucchini, sliced

Cut beef into serving-sized pieces. Sprinkle with pepper. Layer beef, onion, and green pepper in slow cooker. Pour spaghetti sauce over. Cover and cook on low for 8 to 10 hours. Stir in zucchini, cover, turn heat to high and cook 15 to 20 minutes more, or until zucchini is tender.

Yield: 6 servings

Per serving: 456 calories (28% from fat, 51% from protein, 21% from carbohydrate); 58 g protein; 14 g total fat; 3 g saturated fat; 7 g monounsaturated fat; 1 g polyunsaturated fat; 24 g carbohydrate; 5 g fiber; 17 g sugar; 404 mg phosphorus; 51 mg calcium; 6 mg iron; 111 mg sodium; 1110 mg potassium; 900 IU vitamin A; 0 mg ATE vitamin E; 29 mg vitamin C; 136 mg cholesterol; 232 g water

Italian Beef Roast

Not only does this make a great meal with spaghetti or other pasta, but when it's cold it's also easy to cut into thin slices that make wonderful sandwiches.

$^{1}/_{2}$ cup (120 ml) dry red wine

2 tablespoons (4.2 g) Italian seasoning

4 pounds (1.8 kg) beef round tip roast

1 cup (235 ml) low sodium spaghetti sauce

1 cup (160 g) onion, sliced

1 cup (100 g) celery, sliced

1 cup (70 g) mushrooms, sliced

$^{1}/_{2}$ cup (115 g) fat free sour cream

$^{1}/_{4}$ cup (60 ml) water

$^{1}/_{4}$ cup (30 g) flour

Combine wine and Italian seasoning. Marinate roast in mixture overnight. In a Dutch oven, combine

marinade and spaghetti sauce. Add roast. Cover and simmer for $1^{1}/_{2}$ hours. Add onion, celery, and mushrooms, cover, and simmer for 1 hour, or until meat is tender. Remove roast and vegetables. Skim fat off pan juices and return 2 cups (470 ml) liquid to pan. Combine sour cream and water. Stir in flour. Stir sour cream mixture into the pan juices and simmer until thickened. Serve sauce with meat.

Yield: 10 servings

Per serving: 298 calories (25% from fat, 61% from protein, 14% from carbohydrate); 40 g protein; 7 g total fat; 2 g saturated fat; 3 g monounsaturated fat; 0 g polyunsaturated fat; 10 g carbohydrate; 2 g fiber; 4 g sugar; 409 mg phosphorus; 75 mg calcium; 4 mg iron; 128 mg sodium; 823 mg potassium; 286 IU vitamin A; 12 mg ATE vitamin E; 5 mg vitamin C; 101 mg cholesterol; 212 g water

Italian Breaded Pork Chops

You can easily vary the flavor of these chops by changing the seasonings. I was looking for a sort of Italian flavor, but you could just as easily make them southern, Mexican, barbecue, or whatever you want.

4 pork loin chops

$^{1}/_{2}$ cup (60 g) bread crumbs

1 tablespoon (0.4 g) dried parsley

1 tablespoon (2.1 g) Italian seasoning

1 teaspoon (2 g) black pepper

1 teaspoon (3 g) onion powder

Preheat oven to 350°F (180°C, or gas mark 4). Moisten chops with water. Combine bread crumbs and remaining ingredients in a plastic bag. Add chops and shake until evenly covered. Coat a baking sheet with nonstick vegetable oil spray. Place the chops on the sheet and spray the tops with more of the vegetable oil spray. Bake for 20 to 30 minutes depending on thickness of chops, or until done.

Yield: 4 servings

Per serving: 189 calories (25% from fat, 51% from protein, 24% from carbohydrate); 23 g protein; 5 g total fat; 2 g saturated fat; 2 g monounsaturated fat; 1 g polyunsaturated fat; 11 g carbohydrate; 1 g fiber; 1 g sugar; 247 mg phosphorus; 55 mg calcium; 2 mg iron; 152 mg sodium; 430 mg potassium; 139 IU vitamin A; 2 mg ATE vitamin E; 3 mg vitamin C; 64 mg cholesterol; 76 g water

Italian Pork Skillet

There's enough sauce here to serve over rice or pasta to make a complete meal.

2 tablespoons (30 ml) olive oil

4 pork loin chops

1 cup (160 g) onion, chopped

$^1/_2$ cup (75 g) green bell pepper, chopped

$^1/_2$ teaspoon (1.5 g) minced garlic

2 cups (360 g) canned no-salt-added tomatoes

1 teaspoon (0.7 g) Italian seasoning

$^1/_4$ teaspoon (0.5 g) black pepper

In a large skillet, heat the oil and brown the pork chops for 2 to 3 minutes per side. Remove the chops from the skillet and cover to keep warm. Add the onion, green bell pepper, and garlic to the skillet and

sauté for 3 to 5 minutes, until tender and lightly browned. Stir in the tomatoes, Italian seasoning, and black pepper. Return the pork chops to the skillet; reduce the heat to low, cover, and simmer for 30 minutes, or until the chops are cooked through.

Yield: 4 servings

Per serving: 227 calories (44% from fat, 40% from protein, 16% from carbohydrate); 23 g protein; 11 g total fat; 2 g saturated fat; 7 g monounsaturated fat; 1 g polyunsaturated fat; 9 g carbohydrate; 2 g fiber; 5 g sugar; 256 mg phosphorus; 65 mg calcium; 2 mg iron; 69 mg sodium; 665 mg potassium; 166 IU vitamin A; 2 mg ATE vitamin E; 15 mg vitamin C; 64 mg cholesterol; 223 g water

Italian Pork Roast

This can be part of a great Italian meal, but it also makes the best Italian pork sub sandwiches that you will ever have.

$^1/_2$ teaspoon (1 g) ground allspice

1 teaspoon (2 g) fennel seed, crushed

1 teaspoon (1.2 g) dried rosemary

1 teaspoon (2 g) black pepper

$2^1/_2$ pound (1.1 kg) pork loin roast

Preheat oven to 325°F (170°C, or gas mark 3). Combine allspice, fennel, rosemary, and pepper and mix well. Rub this mixture thoroughly into all sides of the roast. Marinate in the refrigerator overnight. Bake for 30 to 40 minutes per pound, until internal temperature is 170°F (77°C).

Yield: 8 servings

Per serving: 42 calories (31% from fat, 66% from protein, 4% from carbohydrate); 7 g protein; 1 g total fat; 0 g saturated fat; 1 g monounsaturated fat; 0 g polyunsaturated fat; 0 g carbohydrate; 0 g fiber; 0 g sugar; 71 mg phosphorus; 9 mg calcium; 0 mg iron; 17 mg sodium; 126 mg potassium; 6 IU vitamin A; 1 mg ATE vitamin E; 0 mg vitamin C; 20 mg cholesterol; 23 g water

Portobello Pizzas

Pizza-flavored snacks with Portobello mushroom "crusts." These proved to be an unexpected hit with young people.

5 ounces (140 g) frozen chopped spinach

6 ounces (170 g) part-skim mozzarella, shredded

4 ounces (115 g) turkey pepperoni, coarsely chopped

1 teaspoon (0.7 g) dried basil, crushed

$^1/_4$ teaspoon (0.5 g) coarsely ground black pepper

12 Portobello mushroom caps, 3- to 4-inches (7.5- to 10-cm) diameter

2 tablespoons (30 ml) olive oil

Fresh basil, for garnish

Preheat oven to 350°F (180°C, or gas mark 4). Thaw spinach; press out liquid; finely chop. Combine spinach, cheese, pepperoni, basil, and pepper. Clean mushrooms; remove stems. Place open side up on lightly greased baking sheet; brush with olive oil. Spoon 2 tablespoons spinach mixture into each. Bake for 12 minutes or broil 4 inches (10 cm) from heat for 3 to 4 minutes. Garnish with fresh basil.

Yield: 12 servings

Per serving: 105 calories (47% from fat, 32% from protein, 20% from carbohydrate); 9 g protein; 6 g total

fat; 2 g saturated fat; 3 g monounsaturated fat; 1 g polyunsaturated fat; 6 g carbohydrate; 2 g fiber; 2 g sugar; 180 mg phosphorus; 140 mg calcium; 1 mg iron; 280 mg sodium; 497 mg potassium; 1503 IU vitamin A; 19 mg ATE vitamin E; 0 mg vitamin C; 21 mg cholesterol; 99 g water

French Bread Pizza

Our version of French bread pizza has much less fat and sodium than anything you can get commercially.

1 cup (235 ml) water

$2^3/_4$ cups (345 g) bread flour

1 tablespoon (13 g) sugar

$1^1/_2$ teaspoons (3.5 g) yeast

1 cup (235 ml) low sodium spaghetti sauce

4 ounces (115 g) part-skim mozzarella, shredded

Place water, flour, sugar, and yeast in bread machine pan in order specified by the manufacturer and process on dough cycle. Remove dough from pan and place in a bowl sprayed with nonstick vegetable oil spray. Turn to coat all sides. Cover and let rise in a warm place until doubled, about 30 minutes. Spray a large baking sheet with nonstick vegetable oil spray. Gently push a fist into the dough to deflate. Roll dough into a 16 × 12-inch (40 × 30-cm) rectangle. Cut in half to form two 8 × 12-inch (20 × 30-cm) rectangles. Fold each 12-inch (30-cm) side of the rectangle over the center. Flatten and place on prepared baking sheet. Cover and let rise until doubled again, about 30 to 40 minutes. Bake at 375°F (190°C, or gas mark 5) for 20 to 25 minutes, or until golden brown. Turn oven up to 400°F (200°C, or gas mark 6). Cut the top half off of each loaf, forming four half-loaves. Spread each with sauce. Add cheese. Bake for 10 to 12 minutes, or until cheese melts and starts to brown.

Yield: 4 servings

Per serving: 497 calories (17% from fat, 16% from protein, 67% from carbohydrate); 20 g protein; 9 g total fat; 4 g saturated fat; 4 g monounsaturated fat; 1 g polyunsaturated fat; 83 g carbohydrate; 4 g fiber; 11 g sugar; 264 mg phosphorus; 256 mg calcium; 5 mg iron; 199 mg sodium; 389 mg potassium; 522 IU vitamin A; 35 mg ATE vitamin E; 7 mg vitamin C; 18 mg cholesterol; 134 g water

Veggie Pizza

There is nothing like hot pizza, fresh from the oven.

1 cup (120 g) whole wheat flour

1 teaspoon yeast

$^1/_2$ cup (120 ml) hot water

1 tablespoon (15 ml) olive oil

1 cup (160 g) minced onion

8 ounces (225 g) mushrooms, coarsely chopped

2 tablespoons (28 ml) olive oil

$^1/_4$ teaspoon black pepper

$^1/_2$ teaspoon crumbled oregano

6 ounces (170 g) pizza sauce

4 ounces (115 g) shredded mozzarella cheese

2 cups (360 g) sliced tomato

2 ounces (55 g) grated Parmesan cheese

To make the crust: In a small bowl mix flour and yeast. With fork, stir in water and 1 tablespoon olive oil to form a soft dough. Cover lightly with plastic wrap. Let rise in warm place for about 30 minutes. Fit into a 12-inch (30-cm) pizza pan coated with nonstick vegetable oil spray, building up edges slightly. Bake at 425°F (220°C, gas mark 7) for 10 minutes. Sauté onion and mushrooms in oil in small skillet for 10 minutes or until mushroom liquid is evaporated. Sprinkle with pepper and oregano. Spread partially baked pizza shell with the pizza sauce. Distribute onion mixture evenly over sauce. Sprinkle with mozzarella. Top with sliced tomato. Sprinkle with Parmesan. Bake at 425°F (220°C, gas mark 7) for 10 minutes or until hot and bubbly and crust is browned.

Yield: 4 servings

Per serving: 245 g water; 403 calories (47% from fat, 19% from protein, 35% from carb); 19 g protein; 22 g total fat; 8 g saturated fat; 11 g monounsaturated fat; 2 g polyunsaturated fat; 36 g carbohydrate; 7 g fiber; 6 g sugar; 415 mg phosphorus; 335 mg calcium; 3 mg iron; 641 mg sodium; 758 mg potassium; 1075 IU vitamin A; 66 mg vitamin E; 29 mg vitamin C; 35 mg cholesterol

Vegetarian Pizza

A good way to use fresh tomatoes—and a very tasty one at that.

$^1/_2$ recipe Whole Wheat Pizza Dough (see recipe page 489)

1 cup (180 g) roma tomatoes, sliced $^1/_4$-inch (63-cm) thick

$^1/_2$ cup (75 g) green bell pepper, thinly sliced

$^1/_2$ cup (80 g) onion, thinly sliced

$^1/_2$ cup (66 g) zucchini, thinly sliced

8 ounces (225 g) part-skim mozzarella, shredded

Prepare dough and bake according to directions. Cover with slices of roma tomatoes, then green bell pepper, onion, zucchini, and cheese. Return to oven and bake for 5 minutes, or until vegetables are softened and cheese is melted.

Yield: 6 servings

Per serving: 122 calories (46% from fat, 33% from protein, 21% from carbohydrate); 10 g protein; 6 g total fat; 4 g saturated fat; 2 g monounsaturated fat; 0 g polyunsaturated fat; 7 g carbohydrate; 1 g fiber; 2 g sugar; 191 mg phosphorus; 304 mg calcium; 0 mg iron; 238 mg sodium; 159 mg potassium; 456 IU vitamin A; 47 mg ATE vitamin E; 16 mg vitamin C; 24 mg cholesterol; 79 g water

Pizza Primavera

Yes, you read that right. Not pasta, but pizza primavera. A white-sauced pizza with the traditional primavera vegetables. Try this the next time you really don't want pepperoni.

2 cups (142 g) broccoli florets

1 cup (130 g) julienned carrot

$^1/_2$ cup snow pea pods, halved crosswise

2 tablespoons (16 g) cornstarch

8 ounces (235 ml) fat-free evaporated milk

$^1/_2$ cup (50 g) grated Parmesan cheese, divided

$^1/_4$ cup (60 ml) dry white wine

$^1/_8$ teaspoon garlic powder

$^1/_3$ cup (33 g) sliced scallions

2 tablespoons chopped fresh basil

$^1/_2$ cup (60 g) shredded Provolone cheese

1 whole wheat pizza crust

Cook broccoli and carrot in boiling water 2 minutes. Add snow peas; cook 1 minute. Drain and rinse under cold running water; set aside. Combine cornstarch and milk in a large saucepan; stir well. Bring to a boil, and cook 2 minutes or until thickened, stirring constantly. Remove from heat; stir in $^1/_4$ cup (25 g) Parmesan cheese and next 4 ingredients. Add broccoli mixture, tossing gently; set aside. Sprinkle Provolone cheese over prepared crust, leaving a $^1/_2$-inch (1-cm) border. Spoon vegetable mixture on top of cheese. Sprinkle with remaining Parmesan cheese. Bake at 500°F (250°C, gas mark 10) for 12 minutes on bottom rack of oven. Remove pizza to a cutting board; let stand 5 minutes.

Yield: 6 servings

Per serving: 98 g water; 363 calories (22% from fat, 19% from protein, 59% from carb); 17 g protein; 9 g total fat; 4 g saturated fat; 3 g monounsaturated fat; 1 g polyunsaturated fat; 52 g carbohydrate; 2 g fiber; 6 g sugar; 224 mg phosphorus; 327 mg calcium; 1 mg iron; 841 mg sodium; 360 mg potassium; 4789 IU vitamin A; 80 mg vitamin E; 30 mg vitamin C; 16 mg cholesterol

Deep Dish Pizza

This makes a huge amount of pizza, somewhere around eight or nine meal-size servings. It also makes *good* pizza—my wife, Ginger, says it's the best homemade I've made. The recipe here is for a veggie pizza, so if you add meat you'll need to take that into account when looking at the nutritional values.

1$^1/_3$ cups (315 ml) water

2 tablespoons (30 ml) olive oil

4 cups (500 g) flour

$1/4$ cup (24 g) nonfat dry milk powder

1 tablespoon (13 g) sugar

$2^1/4$ teaspoons (5.3 g) yeast

2 tablespoons (30 ml) olive oil

1 cup (235 ml) low sodium spaghetti sauce

$1/2$ cup (80 g) onion, coarsely chopped

$1/2$ cup (75 g) green bell pepper, coarsely chopped

1 cup (70 g) mushrooms, sliced

8 ounces (225 g) part-skim mozzarella shredded

Place first 6 ingredients (through yeast) in bread machine pan in the order specified by the manufacturer. Process on the dough cycle. At the end of the kneading cycle, turn off machine and remove dough. Separate into 3 balls. Put 2 teaspoons (10 ml) of oil in each of three 9-inch (23-cm) round cake pans and rotate pan to coat the entire bottom. Roll each dough ball into a 9-inch (23-cm) circle and place in pan. Spray with nonstick vegetable oil spray, cover, and let rise until doubled, 1 to $1^1/2$ hours. Preheat oven to 475°F (240°C, or gas mark 9). Spread $1/3$ cup (80 ml) of spaghetti sauce over the dough in each pan. Place onion, green bell pepper, and mushrooms on sauce and cover with cheese. Bake for 20 minutes, or until cheese is bubbly and edges of crust are brown.

Yield: 9 servings

Per serving: 372 calories (29% from fat, 15% from protein, 56% from carbohydrate); 14 g protein; 12 g total fat; 4 g saturated fat; 7 g monounsaturated fat; 1 g polyunsaturated fat; 52 g carbohydrate; 3 g fiber; 7 g sugar; 229 mg phosphorus; 241 mg calcium; 3 mg iron; 178 mg sodium; 292 mg potassium; 367 IU vitamin A; 45 mg ATE vitamin E; 11 mg vitamin C; 16 mg cholesterol; 99 g water

Tip: If you don't happen to have 3 round cake pans, as I didn't, you can buy a pack of 3 foil ones for about $1.

Veggie White Pizza

The cheese is the main ingredient adding fat to pizza (unless you go with the pepperoni lover's variety), so you need to limit it to less than Pizza Hut uses. But that doesn't mean that you can't have a good-tasting treat.

For Dough:
$1^1/2$ teaspoons (3.5 g) yeast

$1^3/4$ cups (220 g) bread flour

$3/4$ cup (180 ml) water

1 tablespoon (15 ml) honey

1 tablespoon (15 ml) olive oil

For Sauce:
$1^1/2$ cups (355 ml) skim milk

3 tablespoons (24 g) flour

$1/2$ teaspoon (1.5 g) garlic powder

$1/2$ teaspoon (1.5 g) onion powder

1 teaspoon (0.7 g) dried Italian seasoning

For Toppings:
1 tomato, sliced

$1/2$ cup (75 g) green bell pepper, cut in rings

$1/2$ cup (80 g) onion, coarsely chopped

1 cup (70 g) broccoli florets

1 cup (115 g) part-skim mozzarella, shredded

$1/4$ cup (25 g) Parmesan cheese, grated

Place dough ingredients in bread machine pan in the order specified by the manufacturer and process on the dough cycle. Turn out the dough onto a floured board. At this point you may form the pizza or refrigerate the dough for several hours, well-wrapped in plastic so it won't dry out. (Although a refrigerator rest is not necessary, it makes the dough easier to handle.) Preheat oven to 400°F (200°C, or gas mark 6). Stretch dough into a 12-inch (30-cm) circle on a pizza pan or baking sheet. Bake for 10 minutes, or until lightly browned around the edges. Shake sauce ingredients together in a jar. Cook in a saucepan over medium heat and stir for 10 to 15 minutes, or until thickened. Spread sauce over crust; arrange vegetables on top. Sprinkle cheese over all. Return to oven and bake for 5 to 10 minutes, or until cheese is melted and starting to brown.

Yield: 8 servings

Per serving: 186 calories (16% from fat, 17% from protein, 67% from carbohydrate); 8 g protein; 3 g total fat; 1 g saturated fat; 2 g monounsaturated fat; 0 g polyunsaturated fat; 31 g carbohydrate; 1 g fiber; 3 g sugar; 129 mg phosphorus; 117 mg calcium; 2 mg iron; 80 mg sodium; 203 mg potassium; 418 IU vitamin A; 32 mg ATE vitamin E; 17 mg vitamin C; 4 mg cholesterol; 95 g water

Italian Bean Bake

A really nice Italian side dish. If you can't find cannellini beans, which are a white kidney bean, you can substitute other white beans such as navy or great northern.

3 cups (300 g) cooked cannellini beans, drained

³/₄ cup (90 g) whole wheat bread crumbs

¹/₂ cup (80 g) chopped onion

2 tablespoons grated Romano cheese

1 teaspoon minced garlic

¹/₂ teaspoon basil

¹/₄ teaspoon oregano

¹/₈ teaspoon thyme

¹/₈ teaspoon black pepper

3 tablespoons grated Parmesan cheese

Preheat oven to 350°F (180°C, gas mark 4). Coat a 2-quart (2-L) casserole dish with nonstick vegetable oil spray. In a bowl, combine all ingredients except Parmesan. Turn into prepared dish. Cover and bake 30 minutes. Sprinkle with Parmesan; cook uncovered 30 minutes more until cheese is melted.

Yield: 8 servings

Per serving: 57 g water; 147 calories (15% from fat, 24% from protein, 61% from carb); 9 g protein; 2 g total fat; 1 g saturated fat; 1 g monounsaturated fat; 0 g polyunsaturated fat; 23 g carbohydrate; 5 g fiber; 1 g sugar; 174 mg phosphorus; 132 mg calcium; 2 mg iron; 94 mg sodium; 304 mg potassium; 33 IU vitamin A; 6 mg vitamin E; 2 mg vitamin C; 6 mg cholesterol

Italian Baked Beans

An Italian-flavored version of baked beans.

1 pound (455 g) navy beans

8 cups (1.9 L) water

1 pound (455 g) hot Italian sausage links, sliced

1 cup (160 g) chopped onion

¹/₃ cup (50 g) green bell pepper, cut in 1-inch (2.5-cm) pieces

¹/₂ cup (35 g) halved mushrooms

2 bay leaves

$^1/_3$ cup (80 ml) ketchup

$^1/_3$ cup (113 g) molasses

1 tablespoon dry mustard

2 teaspoons crushed oregano

$^1/_2$ teaspoon black pepper

$^1/_4$ teaspoon garlic salt

Rinse beans; place in large saucepan. Add water. Bring to boil; reduce heat and simmer, covered, for 1 hour. Transfer to bowl; cover, and refrigerate overnight. Drain beans, reserving $1^1/_2$ cups of the liquid. In slow cooker, combine drained beans, sausage, onion, bell pepper, mushrooms, and bay leaves. Blend reserved bean liquid with ketchup, molasses, mustard, oregano, pepper, and garlic salt; stir into bean mixture. Cover and cook on high heat for 6 hours, or on low heat for 12 hours.

Yield: 8 servings

Per serving: 310 g water; 452 calories (37% from fat, 17% from protein, 45% from carb); 20 g protein; 19 g total fat; 7 g saturated fat; 8 g monounsaturated fat; 3 g polyunsaturated fat; 52 g carbohydrate; 9 g fiber; 13 g sugar; 331 mg phosphorus; 142 mg calcium; 5 mg iron; 433 mg sodium; 1125 mg potassium; 141 IU vitamin A; 0 mg vitamin E; 11 mg vitamin C; 43 mg cholesterol

Tip: Serve over rice and top with a sprinkling of Parmesan cheese.

Italian Potato Bake

Although we don't usually think of potatoes as Italian food, this potato casserole will change your mind. It's a great side dish with a piece of grilled meat.

6 large potatoes

2 tablespoons (30 ml) canola oil

$^1/_2$ cup (80 g) chopped onions

$^1/_2$ teaspoon (0.4 g) dried basil

$^1/_4$ teaspoon (0.5 g) black pepper

1 tablespoon (2.1 g) Italian seasoning

8 ounces (225 g) part-skim mozzarella, shredded

2 eggs, beaten

Preheat oven to 400°F (200°C, or gas mark 6). Peel potatoes and dice into large pieces. Boil potatoes until almost done. Heat oil in a frying pan over medium-high heat. Add potatoes, onion, basil, pepper, and Italian seasoning. Sauté and stir until potatoes are tender and lightly browned, like hash browns. Spray a casserole dish with nonstick vegetable oil spray. Layer potatoes in the bottom of the dish. Sprinkle mozzarella over the top. Pour eggs into casserole dish to cover the potatoes. Bake for approximately 40 minutes, or until eggs are done in the middle. Remove from oven and serve hot.

Yield: 8 servings

Per serving: 355 calories (26% from fat, 22% from protein, 52% from carbohydrate); 20 g protein; 11 g total fat; 4 g saturated fat; 4 g monounsaturated fat; 2 g polyunsaturated fat; 46 g carbohydrate; 5 g fiber; 4 g sugar; 380 mg phosphorus; 292 mg calcium; 4 mg iron; 304 mg sodium; 1413 mg potassium; 415 IU vitamin A; 35 mg ATE vitamin E; 25 mg vitamin C; 69 mg cholesterol; 300 g water

Italian Orzo

This is kind of the quick-and-easy alternative to risotto. Made with rice-shaped orzo pasta, it has the same creaminess as risotto but doesn't require a half hour of stirring.

1 tablespoon (15 ml) olive oil

8 ounces (225 g) orzo

1 1/4 cups (300 ml) low sodium chicken broth

1 1/4 cups (300 ml) water

1/4 cup (20 g) Parmesan cheese, shredded

1 teaspoon (0.7 g) dried basil

1/4 teaspoon (0.5 g) black pepper

1/4 cup (35 g) pine nuts, toasted

Heat oil in a saucepan over medium heat. Add orzo and cook for 3 minutes, stirring constantly. Stir in broth and water; bring to a boil. Reduce heat and simmer for 15 minutes, or until liquid is absorbed and orzo is done. Remove from heat; stir in Parmesan, basil, and pepper. Sprinkle with pine nuts. Serve immediately.

Yield: 6 servings

Per serving: 224 calories (32% from fat, 15% from protein, 53% from carbohydrate); 8 g protein; 8 g total fat; 2 g saturated fat; 3 g monounsaturated fat; 2 g polyunsaturated fat; 30 g carbohydrate; 1 g fiber; 1 g sugar; 150 mg phosphorus; 61 mg calcium; 2 mg iron; 83 mg sodium; 172 mg potassium; 31 IU vitamin A; 5 mg ATE vitamin E; 0 mg vitamin C; 4 mg cholesterol; 102 g water

Risotto

Risotto is a traditional Italian rice dish. It's a little more work than just putting rice to simmer or steam, but the creamy texture and flavor are worth it.

2 cups (470 ml) low sodium chicken broth

4 cups (946 ml) water

2 tablespoons (30 ml) olive oil

1/2 cup (80 g) onion, chopped

1 1/2 cups (300 g) Arborio rice

3/4 cup (180 ml) white wine

1 cup (70 g) mushrooms, sliced

1 cup (134 g) frozen peas, thawed

1 cup (110 g) cooked chicken breast, cubed

Bring broth and water to a simmer in two separate saucepans. Heat the oil in a large skillet or Dutch oven and sauté the onion. Add the rice and sauté until translucent, but not brown. Add the wine and simmer until liquid is almost completely absorbed. Add 1 cup (235 ml) of the broth and simmer until liquid is almost completely absorbed. Alternate adding 1 cup (235 ml) water and then broth, allowing it to cook after each addition until liquid is absorbed and rice is tender. Stir in mushrooms, peas, and chicken with 1/2 cup (120 ml) of water and simmer until heated through.

Yield: 6 servings

Per serving: 193 calories (32% from fat, 28% from protein, 41% from carbohydrate); 12 g protein; 6 g total fat; 1 g saturated fat; 4 g monounsaturated fat; 1 g polyunsaturated fat; 17 g carbohydrate; 2 g fiber; 2 g sugar; 142 mg phosphorus; 31 mg calcium; 2 mg iron; 136 mg sodium; 275 mg potassium; 565 IU vitamin A;

1 mg ATE vitamin E; 4 mg vitamin C; 20 mg cholesterol; 347 g water

Sun-Dried Tomato Rice

I guess I just get bored easily, but I'm always looking for a way to make things a little different. Don't get me wrong, I love plain rice. I could make a meal of a nice bowlful fresh from the steamer with nothing on it at all. But somehow that seems too plain for a meal. So we added a few Italian things to give you a different side dish. I serve it with a grilled piece of fish that I've marinated in Italian dressing.

2 tablespoons (30 ml) olive oil

$^1/_4$ cup (40 g) onion, chopped

1 cup (185 g) rice

$^1/_4$ teaspoon (0.8 g) garlic powder

$^1/_4$ cup (14 g) sun-dried tomatoes, chopped

$2^1/_4$ cups (530 ml) water

Heat oil in a large saucepan and sauté onion and rice for 2 minutes or until rice begins to brown. Add remaining ingredients, cover, reduce heat, and simmer for 20 minutes, or until rice is tender.

Yield: 6 servings

Per serving: 85 calories (55% from fat, 5% from protein, 40% from carbohydrate); 1 g protein; 5 g total fat; 1 g saturated fat; 4 g monounsaturated fat; 1 g polyunsaturated fat; 9 g carbohydrate; 1 g fiber; 0 g sugar; 23 mg phosphorus; 11 mg calcium; 1 mg iron; 16 mg sodium; 98 mg potassium; 59 IU vitamin A; 0 mg ATE vitamin E; 5 mg vitamin C; 0 mg cholesterol; 116 g water

Italian Oven Chowder

This Italian dish, halfway between a soup and a casserole, cooks in the oven while you do other things. The cheese and cream make it very rich tasting.

1 cup (113 g) sliced zucchini

$1^1/_2$ cups (240 g) sliced onion

2 cups (328 g) cooked chickpeas

2 cups (480 g) no-salt-added canned tomatoes, chopped

$1^1/_2$ cups (355 ml) dry white wine

2 teaspoons minced garlic

1 teaspoon basil

1 bay leaf

2 ounces (55 g) shredded Monterey Jack cheese

2 ounces (55 g) grated Romano cheese

1 cup (235 ml) whipping cream

Combine zucchini, onion, chickpeas, tomatoes and their liquid, wine, garlic, basil, and bay leaf in 3-quart (3-L) baking dish. Cover and bake at 400°F (200°C, gas mark 6) for 1 hour, stirring once halfway through. Season to taste with salt and pepper. Stir in cheeses and cream. Bake 10 minutes longer. Remove bay leaf.

Yield: 6 servings

Per serving: 258 g water; 309 calories (42% from fat, 16% from protein, 42% from carb); 11 g protein; 13 g total fat; 7 g saturated fat; 4 g monounsaturated fat; 1 g polyunsaturated fat; 29 g carbohydrate; 5 g fiber; 5 g sugar; 245 mg phosphorus; 257 mg calcium; 2 mg iron; 427 mg sodium; 485 mg potassium; 480 IU vitamin A; 81 mg vitamin E; 17 mg vitamin C; 40 mg cholesterol

Minestrone with Italian Sausage

A hearty version of the classic Italian soup. Great flavor—I think it tastes even better the next day.

1 cup (208 g) dried navy beans

4 cups (950 ml) low-sodium chicken broth

2 quarts (1.9 L) water

1 pound (455 g) Italian turkey sausage (see page 266)

1¹/₂ pounds (675 g) cabbage

1¹/₂ cups (195 g) sliced carrot

2 medium potatoes, diced

2 cups (480 g) no-salt-added canned tomatoes

¹/₄ cup (60 ml) olive oil

1¹/₂ cups (240 g) diced onion

¹/₂ cup (60 g) diced celery

1 cup (113 g) sliced zucchini

¹/₂ teaspoon minced garlic

¹/₄ teaspoon black pepper

¹/₄ cup chopped fresh parsley

4 ounces (115 g) whole wheat pasta

¹/₂ cup (50 g) grated Parmesan cheese

1¹/₂ teaspoons Italian seasoning

Cover beans with cold water. Soak overnight. Drain. Pour chicken broth and water into an 8-quart (8-L) kettle. Add the beans. Bring to boiling. Reduce heat and simmer, covered, 1 hour. In medium skillet, simmer sausage gently in water to cover until cooked through, about 20 minutes. Drain well. Sauté over medium heat until browned all over. Slice sausage ¹/₄ inch (0.5 cm) thick on the diagonal; set aside. Wash cabbage and quarter; remove core and slice ¹/₄ inch (0.5 cm) thick. Add to soup along with carrot, potatoes, and tomatoes. Cover; cook 30 minutes longer. Heat oil in medium skillet. Sauté onion, stirring, about 5 minutes. Add celery, zucchini, garlic, and black pepper to skillet and sauté over low heat, stirring occasionally, 20 minutes. Add to bean mixture with parsley, pasta, and Italian seasoning. Cook slowly, covered and stirring occasionally, 30 minutes. Add sausage; heat through. Serve hot sprinkled with Parmesan cheese.

Yield: 10 servings

Per serving: 358 calories (35% from fat, 24% from protein, 40% from carb); 18 g protein; 10 g total fat; 3 g saturated fat; 6 g monounsaturated fat; 1 g polyunsaturated fat; 39 g carbohydrate; 7 g fiber; 7 g sugar; 269 mg phosphorus; 163 mg calcium; 3 mg iron; 298 mg sodium; 974 mg potassium; 3566 IU vitamin A; 6 mg vitamin E; 43 mg vitamin C; 18 mg cholesterol

Italian Garden Vegetable Soup

A vegetarian soup with Italian flavor.

2 tablespoons (28 ml) olive oil

1 cup (160 g) chopped onion

¹/₂ teaspoon minced garlic

¹/₂ cup (65 g) peeled and sliced carrot

¹/₂ cup (50 g) sliced celery

1 cup (113 g) sliced zucchini

2 cups (475 ml) low-sodium chicken broth

2 cups (480 g) no-salt-added canned tomatoes

2 cups ((328 g) cooked chickpeas

$^1/_2$ teaspoon basil

$^1/_2$ teaspoon oregano

$^1/_2$ teaspoon black pepper

In large saucepan, heat oil. Add onion, cooking until soft. Add garlic; cook for 1 minute, stirring often. Add carrot, celery, and zucchini. Cook 3 minutes. Add broth, tomatoes, chickpeas, and spices. Stir. Cover and simmer for 10 minutes. Taste for seasonings. Serve with grated cheese on top and croutons, if desired.

Yield: 6 servings

Per serving: 269 g water; 182 calories (29% from fat, 15% from protein, 57% from carb); 7 g protein; 6 g total fat;
1 g saturated fat; 4 g monounsaturated fat; 1 g polyunsaturated fat; 27 g carbohydrate; 6 g fiber; 4 g sugar; 134 mg phosphorus; 74 mg calcium; 2 mg iron; 291 mg sodium; 513 mg potassium; 1998 IU vitamin A; 0 mg vitamin E; 17 mg vitamin C; 0 mg cholesterol

Italian Lentil Soup

A rich and hearty soup, full of flavor. Serve with Italian bread for a complete meal.

$^3/_4$ cup (120 g) chopped onion

$^3/_4$ cup (75 g) chopped celery

$^1/_2$ teaspoon minced garlic

2 tablespoons (28 ml) olive oil

4 cups (950 ml) vegetable broth

2 cups (475 ml) water

4 cups (1 kg) no-salt-added canned tomatoes

$^3/_4$ cup (144 g) dry lentils, rinsed and drained

$^3/_4$ cup (150 g) pearl barley

$^1/_2$ teaspoon dried rosemary, crushed

$^1/_2$ teaspoon dried oregano, crushed

$^1/_4$ teaspoon black pepper

1 cup (130 g) thinly sliced carrot

In 4-quart (4-L) Dutch oven, cook onion, celery, and garlic in oil until tender. Add broth, water, tomatoes, lentils, barley, rosemary, oregano, and pepper. Bring to boil; reduce heat. Cover and simmer 45 minutes. Add carrot and simmer for 15 minutes or until carrot is tender.

Yield: 5 servings

Per serving: 547 g water; 321 calories (30% from fat, 12% from protein, 59% from carb); 10 g protein; 11 g total fat; 2 g saturated fat; 6 g monounsaturated fat; 2 g polyunsaturated fat; 49 g carbohydrate; 11 g fiber; 8 g sugar; 227 mg phosphorus; 125 mg calcium; 5 mg iron; 999 mg sodium; 834 mg potassium; 4616 IU vitamin A; 0 mg vitamin E; 25 mg vitamin C; 0 mg cholesterol

Italian Vegetable Soup

A hearty Italian-flavored soup, full of vegetables and beans.

1 pound (455 g) sweet Italian sausage

1 cup (160 g) diced onion

2 cups (480 g) no-salt-added canned tomatoes, chopped

8 ounces (225 g) no-salt-added tomato sauce

2 cups (475 ml) water

2 cups (475 ml) low-sodium beef broth

$^1/_2$ teaspoon basil

2 cups (328 g) cooked chickpeas

2 cups (200 g) cooked kidney beans

$1^1/_2$ cups (169 g) sliced zucchini

Brown sausage, breaking up into small pieces. Drain. Cook onion until transparent. Put sausage and onion in large kettle. Add tomatoes, sauce, water, broth, and basil. Drain beans and add to soup. Bring to boil. Simmer and cook 30 minutes. Add zucchini and cook another 15 minutes.

Yield: 6 servings

Per serving: 436 g water; 461 calories (16% from fat, 28% from protein, 56% from carb); 33 g protein; 8 g total fat; 3 g saturated fat; 3 g monounsaturated fat; 1 g polyunsaturated fat; 66 g carbohydrate; 21 g fiber; 7 g sugar; 457 mg phosphorus; 181 mg calcium; 8 mg iron; 753 mg sodium; 1603 mg potassium; 313 IU vitamin A; 0 mg vitamin E; 26 mg vitamin C; 23 mg cholesterol

Tip: Serve with grated Parmesan cheese.

Pasta e Fagioli

In Italian, pasta and beans. A traditional Italian soup.

$1^1/_2$ cups (312 g) dried navy beans

$^1/_2$ pound (225 g) whole wheat pasta

3 tablespoons (45 ml) olive oil

1 cup (160 g) chopped onion

1 cup (130 g) sliced carrot

1 cup (100 g) sliced celery

$^1/_2$ teaspoon crushed garlic

2 cups (360 g) tomato, peeled and diced

1 teaspoon dried sage

$^1/_2$ teaspoon dried oregano

$^1/_4$ teaspoon black pepper

In large bowl, combine beans with 6 cups (1.4 L) cold water. Refrigerate overnight. Next day, turn beans and water into 6-quart (6-L) kettle. Bring to a boil, reduce heat, and simmer, covered, about 3 hours or until beans are tender. Stir several times during cooking; drain, reserving about 2 cups of liquid. Cook pasta. Heat oil in a large skillet. Sauté onion, carrot, celery, and garlic until soft (about 20 minutes). Do not brown. Add tomato, sage, oregano, and pepper. Cover and cook over medium heat, 15 minutes. In large saucepan or kettle, combine beans, pasta, and sautéed vegetables. Add $1^1/_2$ cups (355 ml) of reserved bean liquid. Bring to a boil and cover; simmer 35 to 40 minutes, stirring several times and adding more liquid if needed.

Yield: 6 servings

Per serving: 115 g water; 400 calories (18% from fat, 16% from protein, 66% from carb); 17 g protein; 8 g total fat; 1 g saturated fat; 5 g monounsaturated fat; 1 g polyunsaturated fat; 69 g carbohydrate; 13 g fiber; 6 g sugar; 341 mg phosphorus; 120 mg calcium; 5 mg iron; 38 mg sodium; 971 mg potassium; 4089 IU vitamin A; 0 mg vitamin E; 12 mg vitamin C; 0 mg cholesterol

Tip: Serve garnished with parsley and Parmesan cheese.

Italian Kitchen Sink Soup

Okay, so the name's kind of strange. But it sure seems like it has everything in it. In truth, it's a heartier version of the Italian Wedding Soup that's become popular in recent years. This one is truly a meal in a bowl. And it's low in fat, sodium, and potassium, but high in fiber and vitamins.

4 cups (946 ml) water

2 cups (320 g) onion, chopped

2 red potatoes, diced

1 cup (250 g) dried great northern beans

$1/2$ cup (65 g) carrot, sliced

$1/2$ cup (35 g) mushrooms, sliced

$1/2$ cup (100 g) uncooked pearl barley

$1/2$ pound (225 g) round steak, cubed

2 cups (360 g) canned no-salt-added tomatoes

2 cups (470 ml) low sodium beef broth

1 tablespoon (2.1 g) Italian seasoning

$1/2$ teaspoon (1.5 g) minced garlic

1 cup (113 g) zucchini, sliced

1 cup (20 g) fresh spinach, torn into bite-sized pieces

$1/2$ cup (75 g) small pasta

1 tablespoon (3.3 g) dried rosemary

$1/2$ teaspoon (1 g) black pepper

Combine first 12 ingredients (through garlic) in a large electric slow cooker. Cover with lid, and cook on high for 6 hours or low for 10 to 12 hours. Add remaining ingredients, cover and cook on high-heat setting for an additional 30 minutes, or until beans are tender.

Yield: 8 servings

Per serving: 209 calories (9% from fat, 30% from protein, 61% from carbohydrate); 16 g protein; 2 g total fat; 1 g saturated fat; 1 g monounsaturated fat; 0 g polyunsaturated fat; 33 g carbohydrate; 8 g fiber; 4 g sugar; 203 mg phosphorus; 112 mg calcium; 4 mg iron; 256 mg sodium; 689 mg potassium; 4349 IU vitamin A; 0 mg ATE vitamin E; 15 mg vitamin C; 18 mg cholesterol; 366 g water

Italian Fish Stew

A fish stew in the tradition of southern Italy.

2 tablespoons (30 ml) olive oil

1 cup (160 g) red onion, chopped

$1/2$ teaspoon (1.5 g) chopped garlic

1 cup (60 g) fresh parsley, chopped

2 teaspoons (1.4 g) dried basil

$1 1/2$ cups (270 g) tomatoes, peeled, seeded, and finely chopped

1 cup (235 ml) water

$1/2$ cup (120 ml) dry white wine

1 pound (455 g) cod fillets, cut into 1-inch cubes

$1/4$ cup (25 g) Parmesan cheese, grated

Heat the olive oil in a wide, heavy pot over medium heat. Add the onions and garlic and cook, stirring occasionally, for 5 minutes, or until onions are translucent. Add the parsley, basil, and tomatoes. Raise the heat and bring to a simmer. Add water and wine. Cook, partially covered, for 10 minutes. Add the fish, cover, and simmer for 12 to 15 minutes. Ladle into bowls and top with grated cheese.

Yield: 4 servings

Per serving: 239 calories (40% from fat, 44% from protein, 16% from carbohydrate); 24 g protein; 10 g total fat; 2 g saturated fat; 6 g monounsaturated fat; 1 g polyunsaturated fat; 9 g carbohydrate; 2 g fiber; 2 g sugar; 317 mg phosphorus; 133 mg calcium; 2 mg iron; 175 mg sodium; 777 mg potassium; 1718 IU vitamin A; 21 mg ATE vitamin E; 39 mg vitamin C; 54 mg cholesterol; 279 g water

Italian Winter Vegetable Soup

When the weather gets cooler, the slow cooker gets more use in my house. This is a different variation on minestrone, with fall or winter vegetables predominating.

1 cup (250 g) dried kidney beans

1 pound (455 g) beef round steak, cut in $^1/_2$-inch (1.3-cm) cubes

$2^1/_2$ cups (350 g) butternut squash, peeled and cubed

2 medium potatoes, peeled and cubed

2 pounds (905 g) fennel bulbs, cut in 1-inch (2.5-cm) cubes

1 cup (160 g) onion, coarsely chopped

$^1/_2$ teaspoon (1.5 g) minced garlic

4 cups (120 g) spinach, chopped

1 tablespoon (4.5 g) dried Italian seasoning

4 cups (946 ml) low sodium chicken broth

1 cup (235 ml) white wine

Cook beans according to package directions until almost done. In a skillet, brown the beef. Drain. In a large slow cooker, place squash, potatoes, fennel, onion, garlic, and spinach on the bottom. Sprinkle Italian seasoning over top. Add beans and beef. Pour broth and wine over all. Cook on low for 8 to 10 hours.

Yield: 8 servings

Per serving: 346 calories (12% from fat, 38% from protein, 50% from carbohydrate); 32 g protein; 5 g total fat; 1 g saturated fat; 1 g monounsaturated fat; 1 g polyunsaturated fat; 42 g carbohydrate; 11 g fiber; 4 g sugar; 380 mg phosphorus; 255 mg calcium; 7 mg iron; 278 mg sodium; 1756 mg potassium; 16294 IU vitamin A; 0 mg ATE vitamin E; 36 mg vitamin C; 51 mg cholesterol; 489 g water

Italian-Style Mixed Vegetables

We originally had this as a side dish with meat loaf. It started out as a toss-together of vegetables we had from the most recent garden harvesting, but it turned out well and has become a regular on our menu.

1 tablespoon (15 ml) olive oil

$^1/_2$ cup (75 g) green bell pepper, chopped

$^1/_2$ cup (80 g) onion, chopped

1 cup (113 g) zucchini, sliced

$^1/_2$ cup (75 g) eggplant, peeled and cubed

1 large potato, cubed

8 ounces (225 g) no-salt-added tomato sauce

1 teaspoon (0.7 g) dried Italian seasoning

$^1/_4$ teaspoon (0.8 g) minced garlic

Heat oil in a large skillet over medium heat. Sauté green bell pepper, onion, zucchini, and eggplant in oil until just softened. Boil potato until soft. Add potato to vegetable mixture. Stir in tomato sauce, Italian seasoning, and garlic and heat through.

Yield: 6 servings

Per serving: 92 calories (24% from fat, 10% from protein, 66% from carbohydrate); 2 g protein; 3 g total fat; 0 g saturated fat; 2 g monounsaturated fat; 0 g polyunsaturated fat; 16 g carbohydrate; 2 g fiber; 4 g sugar; 64 mg phosphorus; 21 mg calcium; 1 mg iron; 13 mg sodium; 526 mg potassium; 237 IU vitamin A; 0 mg ATE vitamin E; 26 mg vitamin C; 0 mg cholesterol; 121 g water

Italian Vegetable Bake

A tasty side dish that's almost a meal in itself. Just add a simple piece of meat and you are done.

2 potatoes, sliced $1/4$-inch (63-mm) thick

12 ounces (340 g) frozen winter vegetable mix, thawed

2 cups (360 g) canned no-salt-added tomatoes, drained

1 teaspoon (0.7 g) dried Italian seasoning

1 teaspoon (0.1 g) dried parsley

1 cup (250 g) low fat ricotta cheese

2 eggs

Preheat oven to 350°F (180°C, or gas mark 4). Cook potatoes and vegetables until crisp-tender.

Drain and combine with tomatoes. Place in an ovenproof casserole. Stir together remaining ingredients until well combined. Pour over vegetables. Bake for 30 minutes, or until mixture is set.

Yield: 6 servings

Per serving: 211 calories (19% from fat, 22% from protein, 60% from carbohydrate); 12 g protein; 5 g total fat; 2 g saturated fat; 1 g monounsaturated fat; 1 g polyunsaturated fat; 33 g carbohydrate; 5 g fiber; 3 g sugar; 224 mg phosphorus; 177 mg calcium; 3 mg iron; 133 mg sodium; 854 mg potassium; 3243 IU vitamin A; 43 mg ATE vitamin E; 24 mg vitamin C; 83 mg cholesterol; 270 g water

Italian Vegetable Casserole

A meatless Italian meal, relatively low in the things most people should be avoiding anyway. Summer would probably be the best time for this, when fresh vegetables are plentiful.

2 cups (300 g) eggplant, sliced

1 cup (150 g) red bell pepper, cut in rings

1 cup (160 g) onion, sliced

16 ounces (455 g) mushrooms, sliced

4 cups (450 g) zucchini, sliced

2 tablespoons (30 ml) olive oil

3 cups (710 ml) low sodium spaghetti sauce

4 ounces (115 g) part-skim mozzarella shredded

Preheat oven to 400°F (200°C, or gas mark 6). Brush eggplant, red bell pepper, onions, mushrooms, and zucchini with olive oil. Grill or pan-fry until soft. Coat a 9 × 13-inch (23 × 33-cm) baking dish with nonstick vegetable oil spray. Spoon enough spaghetti sauce in the bottom to cover. Layer vegetables, adding sauce every couple of layers. Finish with sauce and then top with cheese. Bake for 20 to 25 minutes, or until heated through and cheese is browned.

Yield: 6 servings

Per serving: 278 calories (43% from fat, 15% from protein, 42% from carbohydrate); 11 g protein; 14 g total fat; 3 g saturated fat; 8 g monounsaturated fat; 1 g polyunsaturated fat; 31 g carbohydrate; 7 g fiber; 20 g sugar; 250 mg phosphorus; 208 mg calcium; 2 mg iron; 169 mg sodium; 1107 mg potassium; 1809 IU vitamin A; 23 mg ATE vitamin E; 64 mg vitamin C; 12 mg cholesterol; 324 g water

Tortellini Salad

A delightful Italian salad based on packaged tortellini. Delicious as either a main dish or a side dish.

7 ounces cheese tortellini

1 cup (71 g) broccoli florets

$^1/_2$ cup (30 g) finely chopped fresh parsley

1 tablespoon chopped pimento

6 ounces (170 g) marinated artichoke hearts, undrained

$^1/_4$ cup (25 g) chopped scallions

2$^1/_2$ teaspoons chopped fresh basil

$^1/_2$ teaspoon garlic powder

$^1/_2$ cup (120 ml) Italian dressing

8 cherry tomatoes, halved

$^1/_4$ cup (25 g) sliced ripe olives

$^1/_4$ cup (25 g) grated Parmesan cheese

Cook tortellini according to package directions. Drain and cool. In large bowl combine all ingredients except tomatoes, olives, and cheese. Cover; refrigerate 4 to 6 hours. Just before serving, add tomatoes and mix lightly. Garnish with olives and sprinkle with Parmesan cheese.

Yield: 4 servings

Per serving: 91 g water; 298 calories (41% from fat, 16% from protein, 42% from carb); 13 g protein; 14 g total fat; 4 g saturated fat; 4 g monounsaturated fat; 5 g polyunsaturated fat; 32 g carbohydrate; 5 g fiber; 3 g sugar; 108 mg phosphorus; 189 mg calcium; 3 mg iron; 898 mg sodium; 389 mg potassium; 1706 IU vitamin A; 7 mg vitamin E; 41 mg vitamin C; 39 mg cholesterol

Sicilian-Style Pasta Salad

Italian pasta salad, but with a deeper set of flavors than the usual one.

12 ounces (340 g) whole wheat pasta

$^1/_3$ cup (80 ml) olive oil

$^1/_2$ teaspoon finely minced garlic

1 cup (160 g) chopped onion

1 tablespoon chopped fresh parsley

1 tablespoon (16 g) no-salt-added tomato paste

$^1/_4$ cup (60 ml) water

4 tablespoons (60 ml) dry white wine

1 teaspoon basil

$^1/_4$ teaspoon ground rosemary

$^1/_8$ teaspoon ground marjoram

$^1/_8$ teaspoon black pepper

$^1/_8$ teaspoon ground thyme

$^1/_8$ teaspoon ground oregano

$^1/_2$ cup (75 g) chopped green bell pepper

$^1/_2$ cup (75 g) chopped red bell pepper

6 ounces (170 g) black olives

Cook pasta according to package directions. In a large skillet simmer oil, garlic, onion, and parsley until tender. Combine tomato paste and water. Add the tomato mixture, wine, and seasonings. Continue to simmer 5 to 7 minutes. Add bell peppers. Simmer an additional 2 minutes until tender. Pour over pasta and blend. Garnish with black olives. Chill approximately 1 to 2 hours. Serve cold.

Yield: 6 servings

Per serving: 95 g water; 364 calories (38% from fat, 10% from protein, 52% from carb); 9 g protein; 16 g total fat; 2 g saturated fat; 11 g monounsaturated fat; 2 g polyunsaturated fat; 49 g carbohydrate; 7 g fiber; 2 g sugar; 166 mg phosphorus; 63 mg calcium; 3 mg iron; 258 mg sodium; 256 mg potassium; 659 IU vitamin A; 0 mg vitamin E; 30 mg vitamin C; 0 mg cholesterol

Italian Pasta Salad

A quick and zesty salad with the flavor of Italy. We like this with barbecued chicken.

1 pound (455 g) tricolored pasta

$^1/_2$ cup (50 g) chopped black olives

$^1/_2$ cup (90 g) chopped roasted red pepper

$^1/_2$ cup (150 g) chopped artichoke hearts

1 cup (71 g) broccoli

4 ounces (120 ml) Italian dressing

Cook pasta according to directions on box. Add other ingredients and salad dressing to cooked pasta while it's still warm. Refrigerate.

Yield: 6 servings

Per serving: 63 g water; 359 calories (19% from fat, 12% from protein, 69% from carb); 11 g protein; 8 g total fat; 1 g saturated fat; 2 g monounsaturated fat; 3 g polyunsaturated fat; 62 g carbohydrate; 5 g fiber; 2 g sugar; 111 mg phosphorus; 52 mg calcium; 4 mg iron; 615 mg sodium; 327 mg potassium; 351 IU vitamin A; 0 mg vitamin E; 20 mg vitamin C; 0 mg cholesterol

Tip: For a more flavorful pasta, prepare it 1 day before you plan to eat it so the flavors have time to develop.

Italian Salad

Try this salad with your next Italian meal. Or add some tuna or salami and make it a meal.

2 cups (110 g) Romaine lettuce, torn into bite-size pieces

2 cups (110 g) iceberg lettuce, torn into bite-size pieces

1 cup (160 g) red onion, separated into rings

1 can artichoke hearts, drained and separated

1 cup (71 g) broccoli florets

1 cup (150 g) shredded mozzarella cheese

$^1/_2$ cup (120 ml) Italian dressing

Toss all ingredients together.

Yield: 4 servings

Per serving: 191 g water; 227 calories (57% from fat, 16% from protein, 26% from carb); 10 g protein; 15 g total

fat; 5 g saturated fat; 4 g monounsaturated fat; 4 g polyunsaturated fat; 16 g carbohydrate; 4 g fiber; 6 g sugar; 176 mg phosphorus; 188 mg calcium; 1 mg iron; 706 mg sodium; 419 mg potassium; 2,375 IU vitamin A; 49 mg vitamin E; 29 mg vitamin C; 22 mg cholesterol

Italian Dinner Salad

A meal on a plate. This may be "only" a salad, but I guarantee you won't walk away from the table hungry.

4 cups(220 g) finely chopped Romaine lettuce

2 cups (180 g) finely chopped cabbage

1 cup (150 g) chopped green bell pepper

1 cup (150 g) chopped red bell pepper

8 ounces (225 g) dry salami, cut up

2 cups (328 g) cooked chickpeas, drained

4 ounces (115 g) black olives

4 ounces (115 g) Swiss cheese, cut up

$^1/_2$ cup (50 g) thinly sliced celery

6 ounces (170 g) boneless chicken breast, cooked and chopped

Dressing

$^1/_2$ cup (160 ml) olive oil

2 tablespoons (28 ml) red wine vinegar

1 teaspoon (5 ml) balsamic vinegar

$^1/_2$ teaspoon minced garlic

1 teaspoon lemon juice

1 tablespoon (15 ml) Dijon mustard

1 teaspoon sugar

2 tablespoons Italian seasoning

$^1/_8$ teaspoon black pepper, fresh ground

Divide lettuce between 6 plates. Arrange other vegetables, meats, and cheese over lettuce. Shake dressing ingredients together and drizzle over salads.

Yield: 6 servings

Per serving: 233 g water; 552 calories (61% from fat, 20% from protein, 20% from carb); 27 g protein; 38 g total fat; 11 g saturated fat; 22 g monounsaturated fat; 4 g polyunsaturated fat; 28 g carbohydrate; 7 g fiber; 4 g sugar; 347 mg phosphorus; 280 mg calcium; 4 mg iron; 1218 mg sodium; 638 mg potassium; 3092 IU vitamin A; 43 mg vitamin E; 75 mg vitamin C; 70 mg cholesterol

14

Asian

I was about to say I liked Asian food, but then I realized I said that about Italian food, and would probably want to say it about Mexican and Cajun food when we get to them. Maybe I just like to eat! At any rate Asian food was one of the things I missed the most when I first started on a low sodium diet. It is almost impossible to find low sodium Asian food with all the high sodium sauces the recipes tend to use. Eventually after much experimentation I came up with the reduced sodium versions of soy and teriyaki sauce that are in Chapter 2 and things got easier. That led to the collection of recipes in this chapter, low in sodium, high in the nutrition of fresh vegetables, and altogether good.

Szechuan Chicken

A spicy Szechuan dish made with diced chicken, peanuts, and chile peppers.

For Marinade:

1 1/2 tablespoons (22 ml) water

1 tablespoon (15 ml) Dick's Reduced Sodium Soy Sauce (see recipe page 25)

1 1/2 tablespoons (12 g) cornstarch

1 tablespoon (15 ml) rice wine

For Chicken:

1 pound (455 g) boneless chicken breasts

2 tablespoons (30 ml) oil

8 dried chile peppers

1/2 teaspoon (1.5 g) minced garlic

1/2 cup (75 g) green bell pepper, cut in 1/2-inch (1.3-cm) pieces

1/2 cup (75 g) dry-roasted peanuts

For Sauce:

2 tablespoons (30 ml) Dick's Reduced Sodium Soy Sauce (see recipe page 25)

1 tablespoon (15 ml) sherry

1 tablespoon (13 g) sugar

1 teaspoon (3 g) cornstarch

1/4 teaspoon (1 ml) sesame oil

To make the marinade: Mix together marinade ingredients.

To make the chicken: Marinate chicken for at least 20 minutes. Heat wok. When hot, add 2 tablespoons (30 ml) oil. When oil is hot, add dried chile peppers and garlic and stir-fry until brown and fragrant. Add the green pepper cubes. After approximately two minutes, push the peppers up the side of the wok and add the chicken cubes in the middle of the wok. Stir-fry until the chicken cubes are thoroughly cooked.

To make the sauce: Combine sauce ingredients and add into the wok. Stir until thickened. Add peanuts just before removing the chicken mixture from the wok.

Yield: 4 servings

Per serving: 288 calories (17% from fat, 22% from protein, 61% from carbohydrate); 31 g protein; 11 g total fat; 2 g saturated fat; 5 g monounsaturated fat; 5 g polyunsaturated fat; 87 g carbohydrate; 2 g fiber; 7 g sugar; 304 mg phosphorus; 32 mg calcium; 1 mg iron; 156 mg sodium; 499 mg potassium; 383 IU vitamin A; 7 mg ATE vitamin E; 17 mg vitamin C; 66 mg cholesterol; 129 g water

Lemon Chicken

A lemon chicken recipe similar to what you get from your favorite Chinese carryout. This version is pan-fried, rather than deep-fried, to reduce the fat content.

For Chicken:

1/4 cup (32 g) cornstarch

1/8 teaspoon black pepper

2 tablespoons (30 ml) water

2 eggs

4 boneless chicken breasts, cut into bite-sized pieces

2 tablespoons (30 ml) oil

1/4 cup (25 g) scallions, sliced

For Lemon Sauce:

3/4 cup (180 ml) water

1/4 cup (60 ml) lemon juice

2 tablespoons (30 g) brown sugar

1¹/₂ tablespoons (12 g) cornstarch

1¹/₂ tablespoons (22 ml) honey

1 tablespoon (6 g) low sodium chicken bouillon

¹/₄ teaspoon (0.5 g) ground ginger

To make the chicken: Combine cornstarch and pepper. Blend in water and eggs. Dip chicken pieces into cornstarch mixture. Heat oil in a wok or frying pan. Fry chicken in oil for 5 minutes, or until golden. Drain. Sprinkle with scallions.

To make the sauce: Combine all the sauce ingredients in a saucepan. Cook over medium heat, stirring, for 5 minutes, or until sauce boils and thickens. Pour sauce over chicken.

Yield: 4 servings

Per serving: 302 calories (27% from fat, 28% from protein, 45% from carbohydrate); 21 g protein; 9 g total fat; 1 g saturated fat; 2 g monounsaturated fat; 5 g polyunsaturated fat; 34 g carbohydrate; 0 g fiber; 14 g sugar; 42 mg calcium; 2 mg iron; 129 mg sodium; 257 mg potassium; 9 mg vitamin C; 142 mg cholesterol

Sesame Chicken

Just like you get at your local Chinese restaurant, except it's healthy.

¹/₄ cup (32 g) flour

¹/₈ teaspoon (0.3 g) black pepper

4 boneless chicken breasts, cut into strips

2 tablespoons (30 ml) olive oil

¹/₄ cup (60 ml) Dick's Reduced Sodium Soy Sauce (see recipe page 25)

¹/₄ cup (50 g) sugar

¹/₂ teaspoon (3 ml) sesame oil

2 tablespoons (16 g) sesame seeds, toasted

¹/₄ cup (12 g) chives, chopped

Combine the flour and pepper in a resealable plastic bag. Add the chicken and shake to coat. Heat the olive oil in a large skillet. Add the chicken and cook until no longer pink. Remove from skillet. Add the soy sauce and sugar to the skillet; cook and stir until the sugar is melted. Stir in the sesame oil and sesame seeds. Add the chicken and chives and stir to coat.

Yield: 4 servings

Per serving: 241 calories (13% from fat, 11% from protein, 75% from carbohydrate); 17 g protein; 9 g total fat; 2 g saturated fat; 6 g monounsaturated fat; 3 g polyunsaturated fat; 117 g carbohydrate; 0 g fiber; 15 g sugar; 141 mg phosphorus; 20 mg calcium; 1 mg iron; 143 mg sodium; 190 mg potassium; 147 IU vitamin A; 3 mg ATE vitamin E; 2 mg vitamin C; 44 mg cholesterol; 58 g water

Tip: Don't try to get by without the sesame oil. It should be available in the Asian food section of any large grocery store, and it really is critical to the flavor of the dish. Toast the sesame seeds by placing in a dry skillet and cooking over medium heat for 2 to 3 minutes, or until golden brown. Stir and shake the pan frequently to keep them from burning.

Sweet and Sour Chicken

A simple, quick-to-prepare version that has a very nice sauce.

8$^1/_2$ ounces (240 g) pineapple chunks, undrained

$^1/_2$ cup (120 ml) duck sauce, divided

2 tablespoons (30 g) brown sugar

$^1/_4$ cup (60 ml) rice vinegar

$^1/_4$ cup (60 ml) orange juice

1 pound (455 g) boneless chicken breasts, cut in $^1/_2$-inch (1.3-cm) pieces

1 teaspoon (5 ml) Dick's Reduced Sodium Soy Sauce (see recipe page 25)

1 pound (455 g) frozen oriental vegetable mix, thawed

$^1/_4$ teaspoon (0.5 g) ground ginger

2 teaspoons (3 g) cornstarch

1 tablespoon (15 ml) water

Mix juice from pineapple with $^1/_4$ cup (60 ml) duck sauce, brown sugar, vinegar, soy sauce, and orange juice. Set aside. In a large skillet with a tight-fitting lid, add chicken and sauté for 5 minutes, or until no longer pink on the outside. Add soy sauce mixture, pineapple chunks, vegetables, and ginger. Cover and simmer until chicken is done and vegetables are crisp-tender. Stir together water and cornstarch. Add to pan with remaining $^1/_4$ cup (60 ml) duck sauce. Cook until mixture is thickened and bubbly. Serve over rice.

Yield: 4 servings

Per serving: 330 calories (5% from fat, 34% from protein, 61% from carbohydrate); 30 g protein; 2 g total fat; 0 g saturated fat; 0 g monounsaturated fat; 1 g polyunsaturated fat; 54 g carbohydrate; 6 g fiber; 15 g sugar; 297 mg phosphorus; 64 mg calcium; 3 mg iron; 332 mg sodium; 725 mg potassium; 4926 IU vitamin A; 7 mg ATE vitamin E; 15 mg vitamin C; 66 mg cholesterol; 288 g water

Cashew Chicken

This is Chinese food that doesn't taste like you are watching your diet. It has become one of our favorite Asian meals with plain white or brown rice.

3 boneless chicken breasts

$^1/_4$ cup (60 ml) Dick's Reduced Sodium Soy Sauce (see recipe page 25)

2 tablespoons (16 g) cornstarch

$^1/_2$ teaspoon (2 g) sugar

2 tablespoons (30 ml) canola oil, divided

4 ounces (115 g) dry-roasted cashews

$^1/_2$ pound (225 g) snow pea pods, ends and strings removed

1 cup (70 g) mushrooms, sliced

1 cup (235 ml) low sodium chicken broth

2 cups (260 g) bamboo shoots, drained

$^1/_4$ cup (25 g) scallions, sliced

Slice breasts horizontally into very thin slices and cut into 1-inch (2.5-cm) pieces. Mix soy sauce, cornstarch, and sugar; set aside. Heat 1 tablespoon (15 ml) of the oil in a skillet over moderate heat. Add the cashews and cook for 1 minute, shaking the pan to toast the nuts lightly. Remove cashews and set aside. Pour remaining oil in the pan and fry chicken quickly, turning often until it looks opaque. Add pea pods, mushrooms, and broth. Reduce heat, cover, and cook for 2 minutes. Add soy sauce mixture and bamboo shoots and cook until thickened, stirring constantly. Add scallions and cashews and serve immediately.

Yield: 6 servings

Per serving: 248 calories (25% from fat, 11% from protein, 63% from carbohydrate); 15 g protein; 14 g total fat; 2 g saturated fat; 8 g monounsaturated fat; 4 g polyunsaturated fat; 81 g carbohydrate; 3 g fiber; 6 g sugar; 244 mg phosphorus; 46 mg calcium; 3 mg iron; 112 mg sodium; 650 mg potassium; 474 IU vitamin A; 2 mg ATE vitamin E; 26 mg vitamin C; 21 mg cholesterol; 173 g water

Quick Asian Chicken

About as "real Chinese" as the chow mein you can buy on your grocer's shelves or frozen food case, but it still tastes good.

1 cup (110 g) chicken breast, cubed

12 ounces (340 g) frozen oriental vegetable mix, thawed

4 ounces (115 g) water chestnuts

2 cups (470 ml) low sodium chicken broth

$1/4$ cup (60 ml) Dick's Reduced Sodium Soy Sauce (see recipe page 25)

2 tablespoons (16 g) cornstarch

Stir-fry chicken in a wok or heavy skillet sprayed with nonstick vegetable oil spray. Remove chicken. Stir-fry

vegetables and water chestnuts until crisp-tender. Shake broth, soy sauce, and cornstarch together in a jar with a tight-fitting lid. Add broth mixture to wok and cook until thickened and bubbly. Stir in chicken. Serve over rice.

Yield: 4 servings

Per serving: 161 calories (4% from fat, 12% from protein, 85% from carbohydrate); 16 g protein; 2 g total fat; 1 g saturated fat; 1 g monounsaturated fat; 2 g polyunsaturated fat; 114 g carbohydrate; 4 g fiber; 5 g sugar; 172 mg phosphorus; 40 mg calcium; 1 mg iron; 196 mg sodium; 381 mg potassium; 3651 IU vitamin A; 2 mg ATE vitamin E; 3 mg vitamin C; 30 mg cholesterol; 230 g water

Chinese Chicken Meatballs

There was a place where I used to get lunch in the pre-diet days that had a Chinese meatball dish that I was quite fond of. I've never been able to duplicate the flavor, but this is my favorite of the ways I've tried. You can use these meatballs in place of the meat in any of the Asian recipes in this cookbook.

1 pound (455 g) ground chicken breast

1 tablespoon (6 g) sodium free beef bouillon

$1/4$ teaspoon (0.5 g) ground ginger

$1/8$ teaspoon (0.4 g) garlic powder

$1/8$ teaspoon (0.3 g) black pepper

1 tablespoon (15 ml) sherry

1 egg

Preheat oven to 350°F (180°C, or gas mark 4). Combine all ingredients. Shape into 1-inch (2.5-cm) balls. Place in a roasting pan that has been well coated with nonstick vegetable oil spray. Roast for 30 to 40 minutes, or until done, turning once.

Yield: 4 servings

Per serving: 153 calories (14% from fat, 80% from protein, 6% from carbohydrate); 28 g protein; 2 g total fat; 1 g saturated fat; 1 g monounsaturated fat; 1 g polyunsaturated fat; 2 g carbohydrate; 0 g fiber; 1 g sugar; 245 mg phosphorus; 25 mg calcium; 1 mg iron; 123 mg sodium; 254 mg potassium; 90 IU vitamin A; 7 mg ATE vitamin E; 1 mg vitamin C; 116 mg cholesterol; 100 g water

Chicken Egg Foo Young

This can also be made meatless or, as I like to do, with some leftover chicken.

For Sauce:

2 tablespoons (30 ml) Dick's Reduced Sodium Soy Sauce (see recipe page 25)

$^1/_2$ cup (120 ml) low sodium chicken broth

1 teaspoon (4 g) sugar

1 teaspoon (5 ml) rice vinegar

1 teaspoon (3 g) cornstarch

For Chicken:

6 eggs, beaten

2 cups Chinese mixed vegetables

1 cup (110 g) cooked chicken breast, diced

2 tablespoons (30 ml) canola oil

To make the sauce: In a jar with a tight-fitting lid, shake together the sauce ingredients until cornstarch is dissolved. Pour into a saucepan and heat until just boiling. Simmer 5 minutes. Set aside.

To make the chicken: Mix the eggs, mixed vegetables, and chicken. Heat the oil in a heavy skillet. Spoon the egg mixture into the skillet to form small patties. Turn, browning both sides. Serve with sauce.

Yield: 4 servings

Per serving: 274 calories (23% from fat, 22% from protein, 55% from carbohydrate); 25 g protein; 11 g total fat; 2 g saturated fat; 3 g monounsaturated fat; 7 g polyunsaturated fat; 64 g carbohydrate; 4 g fiber; 6 g sugar; 255 mg phosphorus; 83 mg calcium; 3 mg iron; 285 mg sodium; 500 mg potassium; 4241 IU vitamin A; 2 mg ATE vitamin E; 3 mg vitamin C; 171 mg cholesterol; 216 g water

Chicken Stir-Fry

This recipe has a very nice light sauce, without the usual soy sauce. We like it over fried rice.

$^1/_4$ teaspoon (0.5 g) ground ginger

$^1/_4$ teaspoon (0.5 g) garlic powder

$^1/_4$ teaspoon (0.5 g) black pepper

2 tablespoons (30 ml) olive oil, divided

$^1/_2$ cup (75 g) carrot, sliced

$^1/_2$ cup (80 g) onion, chopped

1 cup (70 g) mushrooms, sliced

1 cup (70 g) bok choy, chopped

2 boneless chicken breasts, thinly sliced

1 tablespoon (15 ml) sherry

1 tablespoon (15 ml) chile sauce

1 cup (235 ml) low sodium chicken broth

1 tablespoon (8 g) cornstarch

In a small bowl, combine the ginger, garlic powder, and black pepper; set aside. In a wok heat 1 tablespoon (15 ml) oil. Add the carrots and onion and half the spice mixture and stir-fry for 2 minutes. Add the mushrooms and bok choy and stir-fry 1 minute. Remove vegetables. Add the remaining oil to the wok and heat. Add chicken and remaining spice mixture and stir-fry until chicken is no longer pink. Return the vegetables to the wok. Stir together the sherry, chile sauce, broth, and cornstarch. Add to wok and heat until mixture thickens and begins to bubble.

Yield: 4 servings

Per serving: 151 calories (46% from fat, 28% from protein, 26% from carbohydrate); 11 g protein; 8 g total fat; 1 g saturated fat; 5 g monounsaturated fat; 1 g polyunsaturated fat; 10 g carbohydrate; 1 g fiber; 3 g sugar; 120 mg phosphorus; 27 mg calcium; 1 mg iron; 144 mg sodium; 309 mg potassium; 2773 IU vitamin A; 2 mg ATE vitamin E; 5 mg vitamin C; 21 mg cholesterol; 162 g water

Chicken with Snow Peas and Asian Vegetables

This is a fairly traditional Chinese-type recipe, similar to dishes like moo goo gai pan.

1 pound (455 g) boneless chicken breasts

2 tablespoons (16 g) cornstarch, divided

1 egg white

1 tablespoon sherry

$1/2$ teaspoon white pepper

8 ounces (225 g) mushrooms, sliced

$1 1/2$ cups (355 ml) low-sodium chicken broth

1 tablespoon sliced gingerroot

2 tablespoons (28 ml) cold water

5 tablespoons (75 ml) olive oil, divided

$1/4$ cup (25 g) sliced scallions

$1/4$ cup (25 g) sliced celery

4 ounces (115 g) snow peas

$1/4$ cup (31 g) sliced water chestnuts

1 cup (70 g) coarsely shredded napa cabbage

In a bowl, combine the chicken, 1 tablespoon of the cornstarch, the egg white, sherry, and pepper. Marinate at least 15 minutes. Simmer mushrooms in broth 15 minutes. Drain and reserve liquid. Simmer gingerroot in broth until ready to use. Mix remaining cornstarch with water. Shake well to thoroughly dissolve. Heat 3 tablespoons (45 ml) oil in a wok or heavy skillet. Add chicken and cook, stirring, just until pieces separate and chicken is no longer pink. Drain into a sieve over a bowl. Add remaining oil to wok. Add scallions, celery, snow peas, water chestnuts, mushrooms, and cabbage and stir-fry for 2 minutes. Remove ginger pieces from chicken broth. Add broth to wok. Bring to a boil. Return chicken to wok. Add water–cornstarch mixture. Cook, stirring, until thickened. Serve over steamed rice.

Yield: 4 servings

Per serving: 235 g water; 251 calories (64% from fat, 16% from protein, 20% from carb); 10 g protein; 18 g total fat; 3 g saturated fat; 13 g monounsaturated fat; 2 g polyunsaturated fat; 13 g carbohydrate; 2 g fiber; 3 g sugar; 137 mg phosphorus; 38 mg calcium; 2 mg iron; 66 mg sodium; 474 mg potassium; 473 IU vitamin A; 1 mg vitamin E; 21 mg vitamin C; 11 mg cholesterol

Chicken Fried Rice

This is similar to the fried rice flavor of Rice-a-Roni. I don't know if any of you have been missing that kind of boxed convenience or not, but this is very nearly as easy to make (there's just a little extra measuring) and a whole lot better for you.

1 tablespoon (15 ml) olive oil

1 cup (185 g) long-grain rice

$^1/_2$ cup (90 g) orzo, or other small pasta

$3^1/_2$ cups (825 ml) water

$^1/_2$ teaspoon (1.5 g) onion powder

$^1/_4$ teaspoon (0.5 g) garlic powder

1 teaspoon (0.1 g) dried parsley

1 tablespoon (6 g) oriental seasoning

$^1/_4$ cup (60 ml) Dick's Reduced Sodium Soy Sauce (see recipe page 25)

Heat oil in a skillet over medium-high heat and sauté rice and pasta for 2 minutes, or until pasta is golden brown. Add remaining ingredients, cover, reduce heat, and simmer for 20 minutes or until rice is tender.

Yield: 6 servings

Per serving: 213 calories (5% from fat, 4% from protein, 91% from carbohydrate); 5 g protein; 3 g total fat; 0 g saturated fat; 2 g monounsaturated fat; 2 g polyunsaturated fat; 105 g carbohydrate; 1 g fiber; 2 g

sugar; 81 mg phosphorus; 24 mg calcium; 2 mg iron; 77 mg sodium; 112 mg potassium; 22 IU vitamin A; 0 mg ATE vitamin E; 0 mg vitamin C; 0 mg cholesterol; 159 g water

Tip: If water is not all absorbed (it will depend on the kind of pasta you use), you may need to remove the lid for the last five minutes of cooking time.

Chinese Pepper Steak

This looks particularly nice if you use a mixture of pepper colors. Using beef round steak helps to keep the fat level down while giving you the traditional flavor.

$1^1/_2$ pounds (680 g) beef round steak, sliced thinly

$^1/_3$ cup (80 ml) red wine

2 teaspoons (8 g) sugar

2 tablespoons (30 ml) olive oil, divided

1 tablespoon (10 g) minced garlic

1 cup (160 g) onion, sliced

1 cup (150 g) green bell pepper, sliced

1 cup (150 g) red bell pepper, sliced

1 cup (70 g) mushrooms, sliced

Dash ground ginger

$^1/_2$ cup (120 ml) boiling water

1 teaspoon (2 g) low sodium beef bouillon

2 tablespoons (30 ml) water

1 tablespoon (8 g) cornstarch

In a large bowl combine first 3 ingredients. Cover and marinate overnight, turning beef occasionally. Drain, reserving marinade. In a wok, heat 1 tablespoon (15 ml) of the oil. Add beef and garlic and stir-fry for 2 minutes. Transfer to a platter. In the wok, heat the remaining oil. Add onions, bell peppers, mushrooms, and ginger. Stir-fry for 2 minutes. In a bowl combine $^1/_2$ cup (120 ml) boiling water and bouillon and set aside. In second bowl, combine 2 tablespoons (30 ml) water and cornstarch. Set aside. Increase heat under wok. Add beef and bouillon mixture and cook until mixture starts to bubble around the edges. Stir in cornstarch mixture. Cook and stir until sauce thickens.

Yield: 8 servings

Per serving: 235 calories (31% from fat, 57% from protein, 12% from carbohydrate); 32 g protein; 8 g total fat; 2 g saturated fat; 4 g monounsaturated fat; 1 g polyunsaturated fat; 7 g carbohydrate; 1 g fiber; 3 g sugar; 218 mg phosphorus; 15 mg calcium; 3 mg iron; 42 mg sodium; 430 mg potassium; 652 IU vitamin A; 0 mg ATE vitamin E; 41 mg vitamin C; 77 mg cholesterol; 138 g water

Asian Grilled Burgers

There used to be a packaged mix for these, as well as a number of other Asian dishes, but they seem to have faded from the scene before I had a chance to banish them because of the sodium content. The oriental vegetable mix I use contains bean sprouts, mushrooms, water chestnuts, bamboo shoots, and red peppers, but you can use whatever vegetable mix you like.

$1^1/_2$ pounds (680 g) extra-lean ground beef (93% lean)

1 can (15 ounces, or 420 g) oriental vegetable mix

$^1/_2$ teaspoon (1 g) oriental seasoning

$^1/_4$ teaspoon (0.5 g) ground ginger

$^1/_4$ cup (60 ml) Dick's Reduced Sodium Soy Sauce (see recipe page 25)

Combine all ingredients. Shape into 6 patties. Grill or fry to desired doneness.

Yield: 6 servings

Per serving: 274 calories (16% from fat, 21% from protein, 63% from carbohydrate); 21 g protein; 7 g total fat; 3 g saturated fat; 3 g monounsaturated fat; 2 g polyunsaturated fat; 65 g carbohydrate; 0 g fiber; 1 g sugar; 168 mg phosphorus; 13 mg calcium; 2 mg iron; 144 mg sodium; 349 mg potassium; 4 IU vitamin A; 0 mg ATE vitamin E; 0 mg vitamin C; 78 mg cholesterol; 85 g water

Steak and Vegetable Stir-Fry

This Asian dish is similar to pepper steak, but with a greater variety of vegetables.

$1^1/_2$ pounds (680 g) beef round steak

3 tablespoons (45 ml) Dick's Reduced Sodium Soy Sauce (see recipe page 25)

2 tablespoons (30 ml) olive oil, divided

$^1/_4$ teaspoon (0.5 g) black pepper

$^1/_4$ teaspoon (0.8 g) minced garlic

$^1/_2$ teaspoon (0.9 g) ground ginger

1 cup (150 g) green bell pepper, cut in strips

2 cups (140 g) mushrooms, sliced

1 cup (160 g) onion, sliced

$^1/_2$ cup (120 ml) low sodium beef broth

1 tablespoon (8 g) cornstarch

1 cup (180 g) tomatoes, cut in wedges

Partially freeze beef to make it easier to slice. Slice diagonally into $^1/_4$ inch (63 cm)–thick slices. In a large bowl combine soy sauce, 1 tablespoon (15 ml) oil, and pepper. Add beef. Toss to coat well and marinate for several hours in the refrigerator. Heat the remaining 1 tablespoon (15 ml) oil in a wok or large skillet and stir-fry the garlic and ginger for 1 minute. Add beef and stir-fry for 4 minutes, or until browned. Remove beef. Add green bell pepper, mushrooms, and onions and stir-fry for 2 minutes, or until crisp-tender. Return beef to wok. Combine remaining marinade, broth, and cornstarch. Pour over beef. Cook and stir until thickened. Add tomatoes and heat through.

Yield: 6 servings

Per serving: 305 calories (19% from fat, 35% from protein, 46% from carbohydrate); 43 g protein; 10 g total fat; 3 g saturated fat; 6 g monounsaturated fat; 2 g polyunsaturated fat; 56 g carbohydrate; 1 g fiber; 3 g sugar; 304 mg phosphorus; 21 mg calcium; 4 mg iron; 120 mg sodium; 624 mg potassium; 251 IU vitamin A; 0 mg ATE vitamin E; 29 mg vitamin C; 102 mg cholesterol; 188 g water

Asian Pork Chops

These are good either as an Asian-style meal with stir-fried vegetables and rice or in a more American setting with pasta or potatoes.

1 tablespoon (15 ml) vegetable oil

4 pork loin chops

$^1/_4$ teaspoon (0.5 g) black pepper

1 teaspoon (1.8 g) ground ginger

$^1/_4$ cup (60 ml) orange juice

Heat oil in a large skillet over medium heat. Brown chops on both sides. Sprinkle with pepper and ginger and pour orange juice over. Cover and cook for 10 to 15 minutes, or until done.

Yield: 4 servings

Per serving: 168 calories (43% from fat, 53% from protein, 5% from carbohydrate); 21 g protein; 8 g total fat; 2 g saturated fat; 3 g monounsaturated fat; 2 g polyunsaturated fat; 2 g carbohydrate; 0 g fiber; 0 g sugar; 223 mg phosphorus; 16 mg calcium; 1 mg iron; 52 mg sodium; 411 mg potassium; 20 IU vitamin A; 2 mg ATE vitamin E; 6 mg vitamin C; 64 mg cholesterol; 88 g water

Oriental Grilled Pork Chops

Using loin chops reduces the amount of fat in this Asian-flavored dish. Good with steamed mixed vegetables and rice.

$^1/_4$ cup (60 ml) sweet and sour sauce

2 tablespoons (30 ml) Dick's Reduced Sodium Soy Sauce (see recipe page 25)

4 pork loin chops

Combine sauces and brush on chops. Grill over medium heat for 15 minutes, or until done, turning once.

Yield: 4 servings

Per serving: 170 calories (11% from fat, 24% from protein, 64% from carbohydrate); 21 g protein; 4 g total fat; 2 g saturated fat; 2 g monounsaturated fat; 2 g polyunsaturated fat; 57 g carbohydrate; 0 g fiber; 1 g sugar; 230 mg phosphorus; 19 mg calcium; 1 mg iron; 206 mg sodium; 442 mg potassium; 18 IU vitamin A; 2 mg ATE vitamin E; 1 mg vitamin C; 64 mg cholesterol; 95 g water

Twice-Cooked Pork

A Szechuan dish in which pork is boiled, then stir-fried with vegetables in a spicy sauce.

$^3/_4$ pound (340 g) pork loin

2 tablespoons (30 ml) olive oil

1 cup (120 g) leeks, sliced

1 jalapeno pepper, chopped

$^1/_2$ cup (75 g) red bell pepper, cut in $^1/_2$-inch (1.3-cm) pieces

1 tablespoon (15 g) chile paste

1 tablespoon (15 ml) Dick's Reduced Sodium Soy Sauce (see recipe page 25)

Cook pork in boiling water for 20 minutes. Remove and let cool. Cut the pork into thin matchbox slices. Heat wok. When hot, add olive oil. Add, one at a time, leeks, jalapeno peppers, and red bell peppers to wok and stir-fry, taking care not to overcook. Add the chile paste and soy sauce, followed by the pork slices. Blend and cook together for 1 to 2 minutes.

Yield: 4 servings

Per serving: 192 calories (33% from fat, 26% from protein, 41% from carbohydrate); 19 g protein; 11 g total fat; 2 g saturated fat; 4 g monounsaturated fat; 5 g

polyunsaturated fat; 29 g carbohydrate; 1 g fiber; 2 g sugar; 202 mg phosphorus; 28 mg calcium; 1 mg iron; 96 mg sodium; 411 mg potassium; 1007 IU vitamin A; 2 mg ATE vitamin E; 29 mg vitamin C; 54 mg cholesterol; 110 g water

Sweet-and-Sour Pork

This sweet-and-sour pork recipe is healthier than most, trading the usual breaded, deep-fried pork pieces for lean chunks of pork that still taste great in the zesty sauce.

$^1/_2$ pound (225 g) pork loin

1 tablespoon (15 ml) canola oil

2 teaspoons (10 ml) sesame oil

$^1/_4$ cup (37 g) carrot, sliced thinly on the diagonal

$^1/_2$ cup (75 g) green bell pepper strips

$^1/_4$ cup (25 g) scallions, sliced

$^1/_4$ cup (60 g) brown sugar, packed

2 teaspoons (16 g) cornstarch

2 tablespoons (30 ml) water

2 tablespoons (30 ml) red wine vinegar

1 teaspoon (5 ml) Dick's Reduced Sodium Soy Sauce (see recipe page 25)

$^1/_8$ teaspoon (0.2 g) ground ginger

8 ounces (225 g) pineapple chunks, drained

Partially freeze pork and thinly slice into bite-sized strips. Heat a work or heavy frying pan. Add canola oil and sesame oil to pan. Add the pork. Cook and stir for 2 to 3 minutes, or until pork is no longer pink. Stir in sliced carrot, green bell pepper strips, and scallions. Cook for 2 to 4 minutes more or until the vegetables are crisp-tender. Stir together the brown sugar and cornstarch. Stir in water, red wine vinegar, soy sauce, and ground ginger. Add to pan and cook until thickened and bubbly. Stir in drained pineapple chunks. Cook for about 45 seconds more, or until pineapple is heated through. Serve with rice.

Yield: 2 servings

Per serving: 420 calories (31% from fat, 21% from protein, 49% from carbohydrate); 25 g protein; 17 g total fat; 3 g saturated fat; 8 g monounsaturated fat; 5 g polyunsaturated fat; 59 g carbohydrate; 2 g fiber; 37 g sugar; 279 mg phosphorus; 76 mg calcium; 2 mg iron; 103 mg sodium; 824 mg potassium; 3004 IU vitamin A; 2 mg ATE vitamin E; 43 mg vitamin C; 71 mg cholesterol; 280 g water

Chinese Pork Stir-Fry

Has anyone out there gotten the impression that I'm fond of Asian food? You would be right. I used to say that I could eat it six nights a week. And if you are careful with the preparation, it doesn't have to be bad for you

1 pound (455 g) pork loin

1/4 cup (60 ml) olive oil

2 cups (140 g) cabbage, shredded

1/2 cup (65 g) carrots, shredded

1 cup (160 g) onion, cut in strips

1/2 teaspoon (1 g) oriental seasoning

1/4 cup (60 ml) Dick's Reduced Sodium Soy Sauce (see recipe page 25)

Slice pork thinly, then shred the strips. Heat 2 tablespoons (30 ml) of the oil in a wok or heavy skillet. Stir-fry the pork until cooked through. Remove from wok. Add the remaining 2 tablespoons (30 ml) oil and stir-fry the cabbage, carrots, and onion until crisp-tender. Return the pork to the wok. Add the oriental seasoning and soy sauce. Heat through. Serve over rice.

Yield: 4 servings

Per serving: 251 calories (17% from fat, 16% from protein, 67% from carbohydrate); 25 g protein; 12 g total fat; 3 g saturated fat; 7 g monounsaturated fat; 3 g polyunsaturated fat; 106 g carbohydrate; 2 g fiber; 6 g sugar; 288 mg phosphorus; 55 mg calcium; 1 mg iron; 183 mg sodium; 644 mg potassium; 2748 IU vitamin A; 2 mg ATE vitamin E; 21 mg vitamin C; 71 mg cholesterol; 195 g water

Stir-Fried Pork with Vegetables

I like stir-frying for a number of reasons. Not only is it a healthy way to cook, but also it's quick and easy when you are looking for a meal that doesn't take much time and effort to get on the table.

3/4 pound (340 g) pork tenderloin

3 tablespoons (45 ml) Dick's Reduced Sodium Soy Sauce (see recipe page 25)

1 tablespoon (15 ml) dry sherry

2 1/2 teaspoons (7 g) cornstarch

1 1/4 teaspoons (5 g) sugar

1/8 teaspoon (0.2 g) ground ginger

2 tablespoons (30 ml) canola oil, divided

1 cup (70 g) broccoli, cut into bite-sized pieces

1 cup (70 g) sliced mushrooms

$^1/_2$ cup (65 g) carrot, thinly sliced

$^1/_2$ cup (50 g) scallions, sliced

Cut pork crosswise into $^1/_8$-inch (31-mm) slices. In a medium bowl, mix pork with soy sauce, sherry, cornstarch, sugar, and ginger. Marinate for 30 minutes to 1 hour. Heat 1 tablespoon (15 ml) oil in a skillet or wok over high heat and stir-fry broccoli, mushrooms, carrot, and scallions until vegetables are tender-crisp. Remove vegetables from wok and keep warm. Cook pork in remaining 1 tablespoon (15 ml) oil, stirring constantly, for 3 minutes, or until pork loses its pink color. Return vegetables to wok and stir-fry until heated through. Serve over rice.

Yield: 3 servings

Per serving: 283 calories (18% from fat, 16% from protein, 66% from carbohydrate); 26 g protein; 13 g total fat; 2 g saturated fat; 7 g monounsaturated fat; 5 g polyunsaturated fat; 108 g carbohydrate; 2 g fiber; 6 g sugar; 323 mg phosphorus; 48 mg calcium; 2 mg iron; 190 mg sodium; 743 mg potassium; 3954 IU vitamin A; 2 mg ATE vitamin E; 33 mg vitamin C; 74 mg cholesterol; 191 g water

Asian Marinated Tuna Steaks

Marinating tuna steaks helps to keep them moist and avoid their tendency to dry out and be tough. Plus, it adds a nice extra bit of flavor. The other thing to remember to keep them juicy is to avoid cooking them too long.

1 tablespoon (15 ml) lemon juice

1 teaspoon (3 g) minced garlic

2 tablespoons (12 g) fresh ginger, peeled and minced

$^1/_4$ cup (60 ml) Dick's Reduced Sodium Teriyaki Sauce (see recipe page 25)

$^1/_4$ cup (60 ml) olive oil

1 teaspoon (1.2 g) red pepper flakes

$^1/_4$ teaspoon (0.5 g) black pepper

3 tablespoons (12 g) fresh cilantro, chopped

2 pounds (905 g) tuna steaks

Mix all ingredients except the tuna in a bowl or baking dish that is just big enough to hold the steaks in one layer. Add the steaks and turn them to coat. Marinate for 30 minutes. Grill or pan-fry the steaks, turning once, until medium to medium-rare, about 4 minutes per side.

Yield: 4 servings

Per serving: 392 calories (39% from fat, 56% from protein, 6% from carbohydrate); 53 g protein; 16 g total fat; 2 g saturated fat; 10 g monounsaturated fat; 2 g polyunsaturated fat; 5 g carbohydrate; 0 g fiber; 3 g sugar; 442 mg phosphorus; 42 mg calcium; 2 mg iron; 245 mg sodium; 1057 mg potassium; 453 IU vitamin A; 41 mg ATE vitamin E; 6 mg vitamin C; 102 mg cholesterol; 180 g water

Hong Kong Tuna Steaks

Tuna steaks are better if they marinate before cooking to help keep them moist. The marinade gives them a new Asian flavor.

2 tablespoons (30 ml) orange juice

1 tablespoon (15 ml) sesame oil

1 tablespoon (8 g) sesame seeds

2 tablespoons (30 ml) Dick's Reduced Sodium Soy Sauce (see recipe page 25)

2 teaspoons (5.4 g) fresh ginger, grated, or 1 1/4 teaspoons (2.3 g) ground ginger

1/4 cup (25 g) scallions, chopped

1 pound (455 g) tuna steaks

In a resealable plastic bag, combine first 6 ingredients (through scallions). Add the tuna and let marinate for 20 minutes. Broil or grill the tuna 6 inches (15 cm) from the heat source for 4 to 5 minutes per side. Cook until done as desired.

Yield: 4 servings

Per serving: 208 calories (21% from fat, 27% from protein, 52% from carbohydrate); 27 g protein; 9 g total fat; 2 g saturated fat; 3 g monounsaturated fat; 4 g polyunsaturated fat; 51 g carbohydrate; 0 g fiber; 1 g sugar; 299 mg phosphorus; 19 mg calcium; 1 mg iron; 98 mg sodium; 349 mg potassium; 2548 IU vitamin A; 743 mg ATE vitamin E; 4 mg vitamin C; 43 mg cholesterol; 100 g water

Teriyaki Fish

Serve this Asian-flavored dish with steamed rice and broccoli.

1/4 cup (30 g) flour

1/8 teaspoon (0.3 g) black pepper

12 ounces (340 g) catfish fillets, cut in 1-inch (2.5-cm) cubes

2 tablespoons (30 ml) olive oil

1/4 cup (60 ml) Dick's Reduced Sodium Soy Sauce (see recipe page 25)

1/4 cup (50 g) sugar

1/2 teaspoon (2.5 ml) sesame oil

1/4 cup (12 g) chives, chopped

Combine the flour and pepper in a resealable plastic bag. Add the fish and shake to coat. Heat the olive oil in a large skillet. Add the fish and cook until done. Remove from skillet. And the soy sauce and sugar to the pan. Cook and stir until the sugar is melted. Stir in the sesame oil. Add the fish and chives and stir to coat.

Yield: 4 servings

Per serving: 222 calories (21% from fat, 9% from protein, 70% from carbohydrate); 14 g protein; 14 g total fat; 3 g saturated fat; 8 g monounsaturated fat; 4 g polyunsaturated fat; 104 g carbohydrate; 0 g fiber; 2 g sugar; 194 mg phosphorus; 20 mg calcium; 1 mg iron; 149 mg sodium; 310 mg potassium; 179 IU vitamin A; 13 mg ATE vitamin E; 2 mg vitamin C; 40 mg cholesterol; 88 g water

Teriyaki Salmon

A nice Asian dish with a sweet-and-sour kind of flavor. Serve over plain rice.

1/4 cup (60 ml) Dick's Reduced Sodium Soy Sauce (see recipe page 25)

1/4 cup (60 ml) rice wine vinegar

1/4 cup (50 g) sugar

1/4 teaspoon (0.8 g) garlic powder

1/2 teaspoon (0.9 g) ground ginger

1/4 teaspoon (0.5 g) black pepper

1 pound (455 g) salmon fillets, cubed

$^1/_2$ cup (66 g) zucchini, sliced

$^1/_2$ cup (80 g) onion, quartered

$^1/_2$ cup (75 g) red bell peppers, cubed

1 cup (70 g) mushrooms, sliced in half

2 tablespoons (30 ml) canola oil

2 tablespoons (16 g) cornstarch

Combine soy sauce, vinegar, sugar, garlic powder, ginger, and black pepper. Stir until sugar is dissolved; set aside. Place fish in one resealable plastic bag and zucchini, onion, red bell pepper, and mushrooms in another. Divide soy sauce mixture between the two bags. Seal and marinate in the refrigerator for at least 1 hour, turning occasionally. Drain, reserving marinade. Heat oil in wok, add vegetables, and stir-fry for 5 minutes. Add fish and stir-fry for 1 minute. Stir cornstarch into reserved marinade, add to wok, and cook and stir until thickened.

Yield: 4 servings

Per serving: 374 calories (23% from fat, 13% from protein, 64% from carbohydrate); 24 g protein; 19 g total fat; 3 g saturated fat; 6 g monounsaturated fat; 10 g polyunsaturated fat; 120 g carbohydrate; 2 g fiber; 18 g sugar; 318 mg phosphorus; 34 mg calcium; 1 mg iron; 177 mg sodium; 686 mg potassium; 1494 IU vitamin A; 17 mg ATE vitamin E; 66 mg vitamin C; 67 mg cholesterol; 202 g water

Sweet-and-Sour Fish

This recipe produces a great tasting sweet-and-sour dish, with the health benefits of fish. Serve over plain brown rice to add even more healthy food to the menu.

1 pound (455 g) catfish fillets

2 tablespoons (30 ml) olive oil

$^3/_4$ cup (113 g) green bell pepper, chopped

$^1/_2$ cup (65 g) carrot, sliced

$^1/_4$ teaspoon (0.8 g) minced garlic

$1^1/_2$ cups (355 ml) low sodium chicken broth

$^3/_4$ cup (150 g) sugar

$^1/_2$ cup (120 ml) red wine vinegar

1 tablespoon (15 ml) Dick's Reduced Sodium Soy Sauce (see recipe page 25)

3 tablespoons (24 g) cornstarch

$^1/_4$ cup (60 ml) water

Preheat oven to 350°F (180°C, or gas mark 4). Place fish fillets in a glass baking dish that has been coated with nonstick vegetable oil spray. Bake for 12 minutes, or until done. Meanwhile, heat oil in a large saucepan over medium-high heat and sauté green bell peppers, carrots, and garlic until tender. Add broth, sugar, vinegar, and soy sauce. Bring to a boil and cook for 1 minute. Stir cornstarch into cold water until dissolved. Stir into hot mixture. Cook and stir until thickened. Cut fish into bite-sized pieces. Stir into sauce.

Yield: 6 servings

Per serving: 278 calories (28% from fat, 16% from protein, 56% from carbohydrate); 13 g protein; 11 g total fat; 2 g saturated fat; 6 g monounsaturated fat; 2 g polyunsaturated fat; 48 g carbohydrate; 1 g fiber; 27 g sugar; 182 mg phosphorus; 18 mg calcium; 1 mg iron; 86 mg sodium; 360 mg potassium; 1901 IU vitamin A; 11 mg ATE vitamin E; 16 mg vitamin C; 36 mg cholesterol; 174 g water

Spinach and Mushroom Stir-Fry

A vegetable stir-fry, this makes an excellent accompaniment to one of the Asian-flavored fish recipes.

2 tablespoons (30 ml) olive oil

$^1/_2$ teaspoon (1.5 g) minced garlic

1 teaspoon (2 g) fresh ginger, minced

$^1/_4$ teaspoon (0.3 g) red pepper flakes

1 cup (150 g) red bell pepper, cut in 1-inch (2.5 cm) pieces

$^1/_2$ cup (35 g) mushrooms, sliced

10 ounces (280 g) fresh spinach, washed, stemmed, and coarsely chopped

Heat wok over high heat 1 minute or until hot. Drizzle oil into wok; heat 30 seconds. Add garlic, ginger, and red pepper flakes; stir-fry for 30 seconds. Add red bell pepper and mushrooms; stir-fry for 2 minutes. Add spinach; stir-fry for 1 to 2 minutes or until spinach is wilted.

Yield: 4 servings

Per serving: 96 calories (62% from fat, 13% from protein, 25% from carbohydrate); 4 g protein; 7 g total fat; 1 g saturated fat; 5 g monounsaturated fat; 1 g polyunsaturated fat; 7 g carbohydrate; 4 g fiber; 2 g sugar; 54 mg phosphorus; 113 mg calcium; 2 mg iron; 71 mg sodium; 330 mg potassium; 9761 IU vitamin A; 0 mg ATE vitamin E; 50 mg vitamin C; 0 mg cholesterol; 106 g water

Lo Mein

Who says you can't have healthy Chinese food? This version is vegetarian, but you could add a little shredded chicken breast or leftover pork loin without blowing the fat content. Tofu would work well too. I find that something like that makes a great lunch for those days you are home, because it's quick to prepare and very healthy.

1 tablespoon (15 ml) canola oil

$^1/_4$ cup (40 g) onion, chopped

$^1/_4$ cup (38 g) green bell pepper, chopped

$^1/_2$ cup (65 g) carrots, sliced

12 ounces (340 g) spaghetti, cooked and drained

$^1/_4$ cup (60 ml) Dick's Reduced Sodium Soy Sauce (see recipe page 25)

1 teaspoon (2 g) oriental seasoning

Heat oil in a wok or large skillet. Stir-fry onion, green bell pepper, and carrots until crisp-tender. Add spaghetti and soy sauce. Mix together and continue cooking until heated through. Sprinkle with oriental seasoning.

Yield: 6 servings

Per serving: 126 calories (7% from fat, 4% from protein, 90% from carbohydrate); 4 g protein; 3 g total fat; 0 g saturated fat; 1 g monounsaturated fat; 3 g polyunsaturated fat; 85 g carbohydrate; 2 g fiber; 3 g sugar; 48 mg phosphorus; 15 mg calcium; 1 mg iron; 78 mg sodium; 106 mg potassium; 1820 IU vitamin A; 0 mg ATE vitamin E; 6 mg vitamin C; 0 mg cholesterol; 71 g water

Pan-Fried Noodles

This lets you get that Chinese flavor while still staying heart-healthy. The sesame oil adds a nice flavor if you have it.

6 ounces (170 g) ramen noodles, without the seasoning

2 tablespoons (30 ml) sesame oil, divided

2 tablespoons (30 ml) Dick's Reduced Sodium Teriyaki Sauce (see recipe page 25)

Cook the noodles according to package directions. Heat a wok or large nonstick frying pan over high heat until hot. Add 1 tablespoon (15 ml) of the sesame oil and swirl it around to cover the bottom. Spread the noodles over the oil. Sprinkle the teriyaki sauce over the noodles. Cook until the noodles start to get crisp on the bottom. Turn over all in one piece. Sprinkle the remaining 1 tablespoon (15 ml) sesame oil over the top and cook until that side crisps. Remove from heat and cut in wedges to serve.

Yield: 4 servings

Per serving: 260 calories (48% from fat, 7% from protein, 45% from carbohydrate); 4 g protein; 14 g total fat; 4 g saturated fat; 5 g monounsaturated fat; 3 g polyunsaturated fat; 29 g carbohydrate; 0 g fiber; 1 g sugar; 14 mg phosphorus; 2 mg calcium; 2 mg iron; 27 mg sodium; 20 mg potassium; 0 IU vitamin A; 0 mg ATE vitamin E; 0 mg vitamin C; 0 mg cholesterol; 8 g water

Tip: The tricks are to have the pan nice and hot before you put anything in it and to let the noodles cook without stirring until the teriyaki sauce caramelizes and the noodles start to get crisp.

Japanese-Style Eggplant

Asian eggplant is usually long and thin, but I had an abundance of the more traditional American round ones from the garden, so that's what I used for this Japanese-flavored recipe.

1 eggplant

1 tablespoon (15 g) brown sugar

3 tablespoons (45 ml) Dick's Reduced Sodium Soy Sauce (see recipe page 25)

1 tablespoon (5.5 g) ground ginger

1 tablespoon (15 ml) rice vinegar

$1/2$ teaspoon (2.5 ml) sesame oil

$1/2$ teaspoon (1.5 g) minced garlic

Peel and cut eggplant into $1/2$-inch (1.3-cm) cubes. Coat a skillet with nonstick vegetable oil spray. Sauté eggplant in skillet until it starts to soften. Mix together remaining ingredients. Stir into eggplant. Cook and stir until eggplant is soft and evenly coated with sauce.

Yield: 4 servings

Per serving: 60 calories (2% from fat, 1% from protein, 96% from carbohydrate); 1 g protein; 1 g total fat; 0 g saturated fat; 0 g monounsaturated fat; 2 g polyunsaturated fat; 84 g carbohydrate; 4 g fiber; 8 g sugar; 41 mg phosphorus; 22 mg calcium; 1 mg iron; 82 mg sodium; 326 mg potassium; 37 IU vitamin A; 0 mg ATE vitamin E; 3 mg vitamin C; 0 mg cholesterol; 125 g water

Tofu and Broccoli Stir-Fry

This makes a quick and hearty meal with just rice as a base.

12 ounces (340 g) firm tofu

6 tablespoons (90 ml) Dick's Reduced Sodium Soy Sauce (see recipe page 25)

2 tablespoons (30 ml) mirin wine

1 teaspoon (5 ml) sesame oil

$^1/_4$ teaspoon (0.8 g) minced garlic

$^1/_2$ teaspoon (0.9 g) ground ginger

1 tablespoon (15 ml) olive oil

6 cups (420 g) broccoli florets

$^1/_2$ cup (35 g) mushrooms, sliced

Remove tofu from package and drain under a plate or other weight. Combine soy sauce, mirin, sesame oil, garlic, and ginger. Remove tofu from weight, cut into $^3/_4$-inch (2-cm) cubes, and place in soy sauce mixture. Heat olive oil in a wok or large skillet. Stir-fry broccoli and mushrooms until broccoli is crisp-tender. Remove from wok. Add tofu and cook until it begins to turn golden, then carefully turn and cook the other sides. Return vegetables to wok. Add remaining marinade. Cook and stir carefully until heated through.

Yield: 4 servings

Per serving: 155 calories (9% from fat, 5% from protein, 86% from carbohydrate); 9 g protein; 7 g total fat; 1 g saturated fat; 3 g monounsaturated fat; 5 g polyunsaturated fat; 156 g carbohydrate; 0 g fiber; 5 g sugar; 174 mg phosphorus; 92 mg calcium; 2 mg iron; 217 mg sodium; 606 mg potassium; 3204 IU vitamin A; 0 mg ATE vitamin E; 100 mg vitamin C; 0 mg cholesterol; 214 g water

Asian Noodles

A great Asian side dish.

8 ounces (225 g) angel hair pasta

1 tablespoon (15 ml) olive oil

$^1/_2$ tablespoon (8 ml) sesame oil

2 cups (140 g) cabbage, shredded

$^1/_2$ cup (50 g) scallions, sliced

$^1/_4$ cup (60 ml) Dick's Reduced Sodium Soy Sauce (see recipe page 25)

1 cup (104 g) bean sprouts, drained

Cook pasta according to package directions. Drain. Heat olive oil and sesame oil in a skillet. Sauté cabbage and scallions for 5 minutes. Add pasta, soy sauce, and bean sprouts and heat through.

Yield: 4 servings

Per serving: 147 calories (9% from fat, 2% from protein, 89% from carbohydrate); 3 g protein; 6 g total fat; 1 g saturated fat; 3 g monounsaturated fat; 3 g polyunsaturated fat; 118 g carbohydrate; 4 g fiber; 4 g sugar; 81 mg phosphorus; 40 mg calcium; 1 mg iron; 158 mg sodium; 174 mg potassium; 209 IU vitamin A; 0 mg ATE vitamin E; 19 mg vitamin C; 0 mg cholesterol; 141 g water

Tip: You can add meat to the dish to make a complete meal.

Asian Pork Salad

Another main dish salad for those hot days. This one uses fresh Asian-style vegetables and marinated pork chops to give you a taste of Asia in a cool meal.

For Marinade:

4 boneless pork loin chops

$^1/_4$ cup (60 ml) Dick's Reduced Sodium Soy Sauce (see recipe page 25)

1 tablespoon (15 ml) sesame oil

1 tablespoon (15 ml) rice vinegar

1 tablespoon (13 g) sugar

For Salad:

$^1/_2$ pound (225 g) lettuce, shredded

4 ounces (115 g) snow peas

$^1/_2$ cup (65 g) carrot, sliced

1 cup (70 g) cabbage, shredded

4 ounces (115 g) mushrooms, sliced

$^1/_2$ cup (75 g) red bell pepper, sliced

4 ounces (115 g) mung bean sprouts

For Dressing:

$^1/_4$ cup (60 ml) Dick's Reduced Sodium Soy Sauce (see recipe page 25)

2 tablespoons (30 ml) rice vinegar

2 tablespoons (30 ml) mirin wine

$^1/_2$ teaspoon (0.9 g) ground ginger

1 tablespoon (8 g) sesame seeds

Thinly slice chops. Combine soy sauce, sesame oil, vinegar, and sugar. Place pork and marinade in a resealable plastic bag and marinate for 1 to 2 hours. Drain and stir-fry until cooked through. Toss salad ingredients, top with pork slices. Combine all dressing ingredients and spoon dressing over salad to serve.

Yield: 6 servings

Per serving: 173 calories (7% from fat, 10% from protein, 83% from carbohydrate); 17 g protein; 5 g total fat; 1 g saturated fat; 2 g monounsaturated fat; 4 g polyunsaturated fat; 140 g carbohydrate; 2 g fiber; 9 g sugar; 222 mg phosphorus; 52 mg calcium; 2 mg iron; 191 mg sodium; 564 mg potassium; 2634 IU vitamin A; 1 mg ATE vitamin E; 37 mg vitamin C; 42 mg cholesterol; 209 g water

Asian-Flavored Chicken Salad

A great use for leftover chicken, whether roasted, grilled, or smoked.

6 cups (120 g) iceberg lettuce, torn into bite-sized pieces

$^1/_4$ cup (25 g) scallions, sliced

$^1/_2$ cup (30 g) cilantro, chopped

$^1/_2$ cup (30 g) fresh parsley, chopped

$^1/_2$ cup (50 g) celery, sliced

$^1/_4$ cup (60 ml) rice vinegar

1 tablespoon (15 ml) sesame oil

$^1/_4$ cup (60 ml) Dick's Reduced Sodium Soy Sauce (see recipe page 25)

1 tablespoon (8 g) sesame seeds

2 cups (220 g) cooked chicken breast, chopped

$^1/_2$ cup (100 g) mandarin oranges

$^1/_4$ cup (31 g) slivered almonds

Chop lettuce, scallions, cilantro, parsley, and celery and toss together. For dressing, combine vinegar, sesame oil, soy sauce, and sesame seeds. Marinate the chopped chicken in the dressing for a few hours or overnight. Just before serving, add oranges, almonds, and chicken with dressing to salad. Toss well.

Yield: 4 servings

Per serving: 247 calories (15% from fat, 16% from protein, 68% from carbohydrate); 25 g protein; 11 g total fat; 2 g saturated fat; 5 g monounsaturated fat; 5 g polyunsaturated fat; 108 g carbohydrate; 3 g fiber; 8 g sugar; 253 mg phosphorus; 89 mg calcium; 2 mg iron; 188 mg sodium; 608 mg potassium; 1935 IU vitamin A; 4 mg ATE vitamin E; 27 mg vitamin C; 60 mg cholesterol; 241 g water

Japanese Salad

A great side dish with a plain piece of meat marinated in a little more of the dressing.

For Salad:

$^1/_2$ pound (225 g) lettuce, shredded

4 ounces (115 g) snow peas

$^1/_2$ cup (65 g) carrot, sliced

1 cup (70 g) cabbage, shredded

4 ounces (115 g) mushrooms, sliced

$^1/_2$ cup (75 g) red bell pepper, sliced

4 ounces (115 g) mung bean sprouts

For Dressing:

$^1/_4$ cup (60 ml) Dick's Reduced Sodium Soy Sauce (see recipe page 25)

2 tablespoons (30 ml) rice vinegar

2 tablespoons (30 ml) mirin wine

$^1/_2$ teaspoon (0.9 g) ground ginger

1 tablespoon (8 g) sesame seeds

To make the salad: Toss all salad ingredients.

To make the dressing: Mix all dressing ingredients until well combined. Spoon dressing over salad.

Yield: 6 servings

Per serving: 50 calories (1% from fat, 3% from protein, 95% from carbohydrate); 3 g protein; 0 g total fat; 0 g saturated fat; 0 g monounsaturated fat; 2 g polyunsaturated fat; 72 g carbohydrate; 2 g fiber; 5 g sugar; 67 mg phosphorus; 38 mg calcium; 1 mg iron; 87 mg sodium; 287 mg potassium; 2625 IU vitamin A; 0 mg ATE vitamin E; 36 mg vitamin C; 0 mg cholesterol; 144 g water

Asian Chicken Soup

This is an easy-to-make soup that can cook while you are running errands. It's a little different flavor than most soups, which can be a welcome change if you are tired of the same old thing. (Or am I the only one who gets bored?)

2 cups (140 g) sliced mushrooms

$1^1/_2$ cups sliced bok choy

1 cup (160 g) chopped onion

1 cup (130 g) sliced carrot

1 pound (455 g) boneless skinless chicken breasts, cut in 1-inch (2.5-cm) pieces

1 cup (190 g) brown rice

4 cups (950 ml) low-sodium chicken broth

$^1/_4$ cup (60 ml) Dick's Reduced Sodium Soy Sauce (see recipe page 25)

1 tablespoon (15 ml) sesame oil

$^1/_2$ teaspoon garlic powder

1 teaspoon ground ginger

Place vegetables in bottom of slow cooker. Place chicken pieces on top. Sprinkle rice over top. Combine remaining ingredients and pour over. Cook on low for 8 to 10 hours or on high for 4 to 5 hours.

Yield: 6 servings

Per serving: 322 g water; 199 calories (21% from fat, 47% from protein, 32% from carb); 24 g protein; 5 g total fat; 1 g saturated fat; 2 g monounsaturated fat; 2 g polyunsaturated fat; 16 g carbohydrate; 2 g fiber; 3 g sugar; 278 mg phosphorus; 53 mg calcium; 2 mg iron; 181 mg sodium; 596 mg potassium; 4385 IU vitamin A; 5 mg vitamin E; 13 mg vitamin C; 44 mg cholesterol

15

Mexican and Latin American

This is another chapter where the variety of possibilities led to a lot of recipes. We have everything here from traditional Mexican fajitas and enchiladas to Cuban style pork roasts to a large selection of soups and stews. If you are looking to be carried away to somewhere where the sun is warmer and the pace is slower, these recipes are a good place to start. And since beans are such an integral part of many Mexican dishes, we get a nice fiber boost as an added bonus.

Turkey Chorizo

This will give an authentic Mexican flavor to any dish you add it to, without adding a lot of saturated fat that pork sausage contains. I prefer to cook them in the oven and then freeze them as individual pre-cooked patties so I can pull one out and heat it in the microwave for a minute and it's ready to go.

1 pound (455 g) ground turkey

$^1/_4$ cup (60 ml) cider vinegar

$^1/_2$ teaspoon (1.5 g) garlic powder

2 tablespoons (14 g) cumin

$^1/_2$ teaspoon (0.7 g) cilantro

$^1/_8$ teaspoon (0.3 g) cayenne pepper

Combine all ingredients and mix well. Shape into 2-ounce (55-g) patties and cook or freeze for later use as desired.

Yield: 8 servings

Per serving: 104 calories (29% from fat, 68% from protein, 4% from carbohydrate); 17 g protein; 3 g total fat; 1 g saturated fat; 1 g monounsaturated fat; 1 g polyunsaturated fat; 1 g carbohydrate; 0 g fiber; 0 g sugar; 130 mg phosphorus; 29 mg calcium; 2 mg iron; 43 mg sodium; 204 mg potassium; 34 IU vitamin A; 0 mg ATE vitamin E; 0 mg vitamin C; 43 mg cholesterol; 44 g water

Chili Chicken Breasts

These make a good meal with some Spanish-style rice.

2 tablespoons (30 ml) olive oil

$^1/_3$ cup (80 ml) lime juice

2 tablespoons (6 ml) chopped green chiles

$^1/_4$ teaspoon (0.8 g) garlic powder

4 boneless chicken breasts

4 ounces (115 g) low-fat Swiss cheese

Salsa, for serving

In a 9-inch (23-cm) square baking pan stir together the olive oil, lime juice, chiles, and garlic powder. Add chicken breasts; marinate in the refrigerator for at least 45 minutes, turning once. Remove chicken from marinade; drain. Grill or sauté chicken for 7 minutes; turn over and continue cooking for 6 to 8 minutes, or until done. Top each chicken breast with a slice of cheese. Continue cooking until cheese begins to melt. Serve with salsa.

Yield: 4 servings

Per serving: 195 calories (43% from fat, 51% from protein, 6% from carbohydrate); 25 g protein; 9 g total fat; 2 g saturated fat; 6 g monounsaturated fat; 1 g polyunsaturated fat; 3 g carbohydrate; 0 g fiber; 1 g sugar; 315 mg phosphorus; 285 mg calcium; 1 mg iron; 138 mg sodium; 243 mg potassium; 74 IU vitamin A; 15 mg ATE vitamin E; 8 mg vitamin C; 51 mg cholesterol; 92 g water

Grilled Southwestern Chicken Breasts

The cilantro and lime give these chicken breasts a nice southwestern flavor.

4 boneless chicken breasts

$^1/_4$ cup (60 ml) olive oil

2 tablespoons (30 g) Dijon mustard

1 tablespoon (15 ml) rice wine vinegar

1 teaspoon (2 g) black pepper

dash hot pepper sauce

$^1/_4$ cup (60 ml) lime juice

2 tablespoons (8 g) cilantro

Pound the chicken breasts to $^1/_2$-inch (1.3-cm) thickness and place all ingredients in a 1-gallon (3.8-L) resealable plastic bag or a bowl and cover. Marinate in the refrigerator for at least 30 minutes. Grill over medium heat for 20 minutes, or until done.

Yield: 4 servings

Per serving: 209 calories (64% from fat, 32% from protein, 4% from carbohydrate); 17 g protein; 15 g total fat; 2 g saturated fat; 10 g monounsaturated fat; 2 g polyunsaturated fat; 2 g carbohydrate; 0 g fiber; 0 g sugar; 151 mg phosphorus; 18 mg calcium; 1 mg iron; 133 mg sodium; 226 mg potassium; 117 IU vitamin A; 4 mg ATE vitamin E; 6 mg vitamin C; 41 mg cholesterol; 78 g water

Tip: Serve with rice and grilled corn.

Jerk Chicken Breasts

A simple recipe for jerk-flavored chicken. You could also cook this on the grill or a rotisserie, if desired.

$^1/_2$ cup (80 g) onion, finely chopped

6 boneless chicken breasts

1 teaspoon (2.5 g) paprika

2 teaspoons (6 g) garlic powder

3 tablespoons (19 g) jerk seasoning

Preheat oven to 350°F (180°C, or gas mark 4). Rub the onion into the chicken, inside and out. Combine the paprika, garlic powder, and jerk seasoning. Rub all over the chicken and allow the chicken to marinate for at least 2 hours. Roast in oven for 45 minutes to an hour, or until done.

Yield: 6 servings

Per serving: 88 calories (10% from fat, 80% from protein, 10% from carbohydrate); 17 g protein; 1 g total fat; 0 g saturated fat; 0 g monounsaturated fat; 0 g polyunsaturated fat; 2 g carbohydrate; 0 g fiber; 1 g sugar; 148 mg phosphorus; 12 mg calcium; 1 mg iron; 47 mg sodium; 220 mg potassium; 217 IU vitamin A; 4 mg ATE vitamin E; 2 mg vitamin C; 41 mg cholesterol; 65 g water

Carne Asada

Most recipes call for skirt or flank steak for this, but any cut of beef will do. The London broil, or round steak, is relatively inexpensive and low in fat.

2 pounds (905 g) beef round steak

$^1/_4$ cup (60 ml) lime juice

$^1/_2$ teaspoon (1.5 g) minced garlic

2 tablespoons (5.3 g) Mexican seasoning

Place steak in resealable plastic bag with lime juice and garlic. Marinate 2 hours, turning occasionally. Remove from marinade; rub 1 tablespoon (2.6 g) of Mexican seasoning on each side. Grill over medium heat until desired doneness. Slice thinly to serve.

Yield: 6 servings

Per serving: 304 calories (23% from fat, 75% from protein, 1% from carbohydrate); 55 g protein; 8 g total

fat; 3 g saturated fat; 3 g monounsaturated fat; 0 g polyunsaturated fat; 1 g carbohydrate; 0 g fiber; 0 g sugar; 343 mg phosphorus; 8 mg calcium; 5 mg iron; 68 mg sodium; 518 mg potassium; 5 IU vitamin A; 0 mg ATE vitamin E; 3 mg vitamin C; 136 mg cholesterol; 98 g water

Low Fat Carnitas

Carnitas is crispy spiced pork that can be used for tacos, burritos, tostadas, or sandwiches.

2 pounds (905 g) pork loin

$^1/_2$ cup (80 g) onion, sliced

$^1/_2$ teaspoon (1.5 g) minced garlic

$^1/_2$ teaspoon (0.5 g) dried oregano

$^1/_2$ teaspoon (1.3 g) cumin

$^1/_2$ teaspoon (1.5 g) garlic powder

In a 3-quart (2.8-L) saucepan combine pork, onion, garlic, oregano, and cumin; add enough water to cover. Bring to a boil, reduce heat, cover, and simmer for 2 hours. Preheat oven to 350°F (180°C, or gas mark 4). Drain meat and place in a baking pan. Sprinkle meat with garlic powder. Bake for 45 minutes. Remove from oven. While meat is still warm, use forks to shred meat.

Yield: 8 servings

Per serving: 151 calories (30% from fat, 67% from protein, 3% from carbohydrate); 24 g protein; 5 g total fat; 2 g saturated fat; 2 g monounsaturated fat; 1 g polyunsaturated fat; 1 g carbohydrate; 0 g fiber; 0 g sugar; 252 mg phosphorus; 20 mg calcium; 1 mg iron; 59 mg sodium; 440 mg potassium; 14 IU vitamin A; 2 mg ATE vitamin E; 2 mg vitamin C; 71 mg cholesterol; 92 g water

Caribbean Grilled Pork

Grilled pork, seasoned with a spicy sauce. The pork tenderloin is low in fat, but still very tender. Be careful not to overcook.

2 pounds (905 g) pork tenderloin

$^1/_2$ cup (120 ml) bottled jerk sauce

Make shallow cuts in the roast and rub in the sauce. Marinate overnight. Grill at lowest possible setting for 15 to 20 minutes, or until done. Adding apple or other aromatic wood to the fire will add to the flavor.

Yield: 4 servings

Per serving: 307 calories (24% from fat, 65% from protein, 11% from carbohydrate); 48 g protein; 8 g total fat; 3 g saturated fat; 4 g monounsaturated fat; 1 g polyunsaturated fat; 8 g carbohydrate; 0 g fiber; 6 g sugar; 516 mg phosphorus; 14 mg calcium; 3 mg iron; 144 mg sodium; 878 mg potassium; 68 IU vitamin A; 5 mg ATE vitamin E; 2 mg vitamin C; 147 mg cholesterol; 184 g water

Lechon Asado Roast Pork

Lechon asado is a Cuban pork disk. It would typically use sour orange juice, but it can be difficult to find, so I substitute a combination of lime and orange juice here.

3 pounds (1.4 kg) pork loin roast

1 tablespoon (3 g) minced garlic

1 bay leaf, ground

$^1/_2$ teaspoon (0.5 g) dried oregano

$^1/_2$ teaspoon (1.3 g) cumin

1 tablespoon (15 ml) olive oil

$^1/_2$ teaspoon (1 g) freshly ground black pepper

$^1/_4$ cup (60 ml) orange juice

$^1/_4$ cup (60 ml) lime juice

$^1/_4$ cup (60 ml) dry white wine

$1^1/_2$ cups (240 g) onion, sliced

4 medium potatoes, peeled and quartered

Stick pork all over with the tip of a knife. Mash the garlic into a paste, then add the ground bay leaf, oregano, cumin, and olive oil and mix together. Rub spice mixture all over the roast. Place roast in a large glass baking dish, then sprinkle with pepper and pour orange and lime juice and wine over the roast. Scatter the onions over the roast, then wrap the entire roast in plastic and refrigerate. Marinate at least one hour or overnight, turning several times. Preheat oven to 350°F (180°C, or gas mark 4). Put the meat in a roasting pan, save the marinade, and place roast in the oven. Cook for 1 hour. Turn roast over, add marinade and potatoes, and reduce heat to 325°F (170°C, or gas mark 3). Baste frequently with the pan juices and continue cooking until done (30 to 35 minutes per pound, until roast reaches 180°F (82°C) internal temperature). Add water or wine if necessary to keep drippings from burning. Let sit before carving.

Yield: 10 servings

Per serving: 310 calories (22% from fat, 42% from protein, 36% from carbohydrate); 32 g protein; 7 g total fat; 2 g saturated fat; 4 g monounsaturated fat; 1 g polyunsaturated fat; 27 g carbohydrate; 3 g fiber; 3 g sugar; 398 mg phosphorus; 44 mg calcium; 2 mg iron; 80 mg sodium; 1241 mg potassium; 33 IU vitamin A; 3 mg ATE vitamin E; 20 mg vitamin C; 86 mg cholesterol; 258 g water

Latin-Style Pork Roast

Many years ago I had a lunch in a little Cuban restaurant in a multi-ethnic neighborhood in Washington, DC. The main course was an absolutely marvelous roast pork, crispy on the outside, juicy inside, slightly sour and spicy. I've never forgotten it, and I've never had a recipe or even an idea of the name of the dish. This is as close as I've come so far, but my family knows I'll keep trying. I cooked this on the rotisserie, but you could also grill or roast it.

$^1/_2$ cup (120 ml) cider vinegar

1 tablespoon (7 g) cumin

1 teaspoon (3 g) onion powder

$^1/_2$ teaspoon (0.9 g) cayenne pepper

2 pounds (905 g) pork loin

2 tablespoons (30 g) brown sugar

Combine vinegar, cumin, onion powder, and cayenne pepper. Place in a resealable plastic bag with pork roast, turning to coat on all sides. Marinate overnight in refrigerator, turning occasionally. When ready to cook remove roast from marinade, discarding excess. Rub with brown sugar. Prepare grill or preheat oven to 350°F (180°C, or gas mark 4). Roast for 1 hour, or until done.

Yield: 6 servings

Per serving: 221 calories (28% from fat, 61% from protein, 10% from carbohydrate); 32 g protein; 7 g total fat; 2 g saturated fat; 3 g monounsaturated fat; 1 g polyunsaturated fat; 5 g carbohydrate; 0 g fiber; 5 g sugar; 339 mg phosphorus; 36 mg calcium; 2 mg iron; 82 mg sodium; 614 mg potassium; 85 IU vitamin A; 3 mg ATE vitamin E; 2 mg vitamin C; 95 mg cholesterol; 130 g water

Mexican Baked Fish

Depending on the salsa you use, this dish can be either mild or hot.

1 1/2 pounds (680 g) cod fillets

1 cup (225 g) salsa

1 cup (115 g) low fat Cheddar cheese, shredded

1 cup (28 g) corn chips, crushed

1 avocado, peeled, pitted, and sliced

1/4 cup (58 g) fat-free sour cream

Preheat oven to 400°F (200°C, or gas mark 6). Spray an 8 × 12-inch (20 × 30-cm) baking dish with nonstick vegetable oil spray. Lay fillets side by side in the prepared baking dish. Pour the salsa over the top and sprinkle evenly with the shredded cheese. Top with the crushed corn chips. Bake, uncovered, for 15 minutes, or until fish is opaque and flakes with a fork. Serve topped with sliced avocado and sour cream.

Yield: 6 servings

Per serving: 243 calories (33% from fat, 47% from protein, 20% from carbohydrate); 28 g protein; 9 g total fat; 2 g saturated fat; 4 g monounsaturated fat; 2 g polyunsaturated fat; 11 g carbohydrate; 3 g fiber; 2 g sugar; 387 mg phosphorus; 150 mg calcium; 1 mg iron; 519 mg sodium; 751 mg potassium; 288 IU vitamin A; 37 mg ATE vitamin E; 4 mg vitamin C; 57 mg cholesterol; 169 g water

Island Fish Grill

Although jalapeno peppers aren't really island fare, they add the heat necessary to make this dish taste Caribbean.

2 tablespoons (30 ml) olive oil

1 teaspoon (3 g) minced garlic

1 1/2 tablespoons (22 ml) lime juice

1 tablespoon (6 g) fresh ginger, peeled and minced

2 tablespoons (18 g) jalapeño peppers, seeded and sliced

1 pound (455 g) cod fillets

1/2 teaspoon (1 g) black pepper

Combine the olive oil with the garlic, lime juice, ginger, and jalapeño peppers in a mixing bowl. Add the fish fillets and turn to coat them well. Cover and refrigerate for 1 hour. Prepare grill. Remove the fillets from the marinade and scrape off most of the garlic and ginger pieces. Season the fish with black pepper and grill until done.

Yield: 4 servings

Per serving: 161 calories (43% from fat, 52% from protein, 5% from carbohydrate); 20 g protein; 8 g total fat; 1 g saturated fat; 5 g monounsaturated fat; 1 g polyunsaturated fat; 2 g carbohydrate; 0 g fiber; 0 g sugar; 235 mg phosphorus; 23 mg calcium; 1 mg iron; 62 mg sodium; 505 mg potassium; 73 IU vitamin A; 14 mg ATE vitamin E; 4 mg vitamin C; 49 mg cholesterol; 100 g water

Bean and Corn Burritos

Not only are these burritos delicious, but also they provide almost your whole day's fiber requirement in one dish.

$^1/_2$ cup (80 g) chopped onion

$^1/_4$ cup (38 g) diced green bell pepper

1 teaspoon minced jalapeño pepper

$^1/_2$ teaspoon minced garlic

1 teaspoon ground cumin

$^1/_8$ teaspoon white pepper

2 cups (200 g) cooked kidney beans, drained and mashed

$^1/_2$ cup frozen corn, thawed and drained

4 flour tortillas

$^3/_4$ cup (90 g) shredded Cheddar cheese

1 cup (260 g) salsa

$^1/_4$ cup (60 g) fat-free sour cream

$^1/_4$ cup chopped fresh cilantro

Spray a nonstick skillet with nonstick vegetable oil spray. Place over medium heat until hot. Add onion, bell pepper, jalapeño, and garlic. Sauté until tender. Stir in cumin and white pepper. Cook 1 minute, stirring constantly. Remove from heat; stir in mashed beans and corn. Spread $^1/_2$ cup (50 g) bean mixture evenly over surface of each tortilla. Sprinkle 3 tablespoons cheese down center of each tortilla. Roll up tortillas and place seam side down on a baking sheet. Bake at 425°F (220°C, gas mark 7) for 7 to 8 minutes or until thoroughly heated. For each serving, top each burrito with $^1/_4$ cup (65 g) salsa and 1 tablespoon sour cream. Garnish with fresh cilantro.

Yield: 4 servings

Per serving: 129 g water; 551 calories (19% from fat, 24% from protein, 57% from carb); 32 g protein; 12 g total fat; 6 g saturated fat; 4 g monounsaturated fat; 1 g polyunsaturated fat; 78 g carbohydrate; 26 g fiber; 6 g sugar; 585 mg phosphorus; 394 mg calcium; 9 mg iron; 414 mg sodium; 1646 mg potassium; 715 IU vitamin A; 79 mg vitamin E; 16 mg vitamin C; 32 mg cholesterol

Black Bean Burritos

I love Mexican food. And I love it even more when it's good for you. Unlike many burritos, these are low in saturated fat and sodium.

Two 10-inch (25-cm) flour tortillas

1 tablespoon (15 ml) canola oil

1 cup (160 g) onion, chopped

$^1/_2$ cup (75 g) red bell pepper, chopped

1 teaspoon (3 g) minced garlic

1 teaspoon (2.5 g) canned jalapeño

15 ounces (510 g) canned black beans, rinsed and drained

3 ounces (85 g) fat-free cream cheese

2 tablespoons (8 g) chopped fresh cilantro

Preheat oven to 350°F (180°C, or gas mark 4). Wrap tortillas in foil and bake for 15 minutes, or until heated through. Heat oil in a skillet over medium heat. Place onion, bell pepper, garlic, and jalapeño in skillet; cook for 2 minutes, stirring occasionally. Add beans to skillet and cook 3 minutes more, stirring. Cut cream cheese into cubes and add to skillet. Cook for 2 minutes, stirring occasionally. Stir cilantro into mixture. Spoon mixture evenly down the center of warmed tortillas and roll tortillas up.

Yield: 2 servings

Per serving: 481 calories (20% from fat, 18% from protein, 62% from carbohydrate); 23 g protein; 11 g total fat; 1 g saturated fat; 5 g monounsaturated fat; 3 g polyunsaturated fat; 76 g carbohydrate; 22 g fiber; 6 g sugar; 372 mg phosphorus; 122 mg calcium; 6 mg iron; 200 mg sodium; 1019 mg potassium; 1364 IU vitamin A; 0 mg ATE vitamin E; 55 mg vitamin C; 0 mg cholesterol; 259 g water

Chicken Enchiladas

We make this fairly often, sometimes with different meat. In fact, it's one of our favorite uses of leftover Thanksgiving turkey.

$^1/_2$ cup (80 g) onion, sautéed

2 cups (220 g) cooked chicken breast, chopped

1 small jalapeno, chopped

4 ounces (115 g) fat-free cream cheese

6 flour tortillas

$^1/_2$ cup (115 g) fat-free sour cream

$^1/_2$ cup (120 ml) skim milk

$^1/_4$ cup (30 g) low fat Monterey Jack cheese, shredded

Preheat oven to 350°F (180°C, or gas mark 4). Combine the first 4 ingredients (through cream cheese). Roll in tortillas. Place in a 9 × 13-inch (23 × 33-cm) baking dish. Combine the sour cream and milk. Pour over tortillas. Bake for 30 minutes. Sprinkle cheese on top for the last 10 minutes of baking time.

Yield: 6 servings

Per serving: 266 calories (20% from fat, 41% from protein, 38% from carbohydrate); 22 g protein; 5 g total fat; 1 g saturated fat; 2 g monounsaturated fat; 1 g polyunsaturated fat; 20 g carbohydrate; 1 g fiber; 1 g sugar; 245 mg phosphorus; 143 mg calcium; 2 mg iron; 336 mg sodium; 289 mg potassium; 285 IU vitamin A; 73 mg ATE vitamin E; 2 mg vitamin C; 60 mg cholesterol; 104 g water

Tofu Enchiladas

Is this what they call "fusion," a blending of cultures? Bear with me here, this is one of those mad-chemist-type of things that came to me as I was trying to find something for dinner. It's basically a cheese enchilada, but with less fat and sodium and more protein.

12 ounces (340 g) tofu

4 ounces (115 g) fat-free cream cheese

$^1/_4$ cup (30 g) low fat Monterey Jack cheese, shredded

5 flour tortillas

$^1/_2$ teaspoon (0.9 g) Mexican seasoning

1 cup (235 ml) skim milk

$^1/_2$ cup (115 g) fat-free sour cream

Preheat oven to 350°F (180°C, or gas mark 4). Cut tofu into small cubes. Mix with cream cheese and jack cheese. Divide among tortillas. Roll up and place in a 9 × 13-inch (23 × 33-cm) baking dish coated with nonstick vegetable oil spray. Combine Mexican seasoning, milk, and sour cream and pour over rolled tortillas. Bake for 30 minutes.

Yield: 5 servings

Per serving: 248 calories (25% from fat, 26% from protein, 49% from carbohydrate); 12 g protein; 5 g total fat; 1 g saturated fat; 2 g monounsaturated fat; 2 g polyunsaturated fat; 23 g carbohydrate; 1 g fiber; 2 g sugar; 223 mg phosphorus; 208 mg calcium; 2 mg iron; 350 mg sodium; 332 mg potassium; 371 IU vitamin A; 99 mg ATE vitamin E; 1 mg vitamin C; 25 mg cholesterol; 152 g water

Baja Chipotle Fish Tacos

Grilled fish and a creamy smoked pepper sauce for that authentic Baja flavor.

1 pound (455 g) boneless fillets of your choice white fish

$^1/_4$ cup (60 ml) Chipotle Marinade (see recipe page 30)

8 corn tortillas, warmed

2 cups (140 g) cabbage, shredded

$^1/_4$ cup (60 ml) Chipotle Sauce (see recipe pages 30–31)

Grill fish, turning and brushing with marinade. Heat tortillas in microwave until warm, but not crisp. To serve, divide fish among tortillas. Top with cabbage and drizzle with Chipotle Sauce.

Yield: 4 servings

Per serving: 293 calories (22% from fat, 48% from protein, 29% from carbohydrate); 35 g protein; 7 g total fat; 1 g saturated fat; 1 g monounsaturated fat; 2 g polyunsaturated fat; 21 g carbohydrate; 4 g fiber; 3 g

sugar; 472 mg phosphorus; 122 mg calcium; 2 mg iron; 376 mg sodium; 858 mg potassium; 498 IU vitamin A; 61 mg ATE vitamin E; 22 mg vitamin C; 46 mg cholesterol; 162 g water

Chicken Fajitas

Making fajitas out of chicken breast greatly reduces the fat and cholesterol over the beef or shrimp version, with no loss of flavor.

2 tablespoons (30 ml) oil

1 pound (455 g) boneless chicken breasts, thinly sliced

1 cup (160 g) onion, cut in strips

1 cup (150 g) green bell pepper, cut in strips

1 tablespoon (2.6 g) taco seasoning

8 flour tortillas

$^1/_2$ cup (115 g) fat free sour cream

$^1/_2$ cup (112 g) salsa

Heat oil in a large skillet and sauté chicken, onion, green bell pepper, and taco seasoning for 5 minutes, or until chicken is done. Place tortillas between 2 wet paper towels. Microwave on high for 30 seconds. Place chicken mixture in the center of the tortillas; garnish with sour cream and salsa. Fold in one side, the bottom, and then the other side.

Yield: 4 servings

Per serving: 449 calories (29% from fat, 32% from protein, 39% from carbohydrate); 33 g protein; 13 g total fat; 2 g saturated fat; 5 g monounsaturated fat; 5 g polyunsaturated fat; 40 g carbohydrate; 4 g fiber; 5 g sugar; 355 mg phosphorus; 143 mg calcium; 3 mg iron;

730 mg sodium; 641 mg potassium; 471 IU vitamin A; 37 mg ATE vitamin E; 35 mg vitamin C; 78 mg cholesterol; 227 g water

Bean Chalupa

Kind of like a super pot of nachos, pork and pinto beans are slow cooked until falling apart, then served over corn chips, topped with cheese, lettuce, tomato, avocado, and hot sauce.

1 pound (455 g) dried pinto beans

3 pound (1 $^1/_4$ kg) pork loin roast

7 cups (1.6 L) water

$^1/_2$ cup (80 g) chopped onion

$^1/_2$ teaspoon minced garlic

2 tablespoons chili powder

1 tablespoon cumin

1 teaspoon oregano

4 ounces (115 g) chopped green chiles

Mix all together in heavy pan and cook, covered, on low heat for 5 hours. Break up roast and cook uncovered 30 minutes more.

Yield: 12 servings

Per serving: 241 g water; 287 calories (18% from fat, 46% from protein, 36% from carb); 32 g protein; 6 g total fat; 2 g saturated fat; 2 g monounsaturated fat; 1 g polyunsaturated fat; 26 g carbohydrate; 7 g fiber; 1 g sugar; 412 mg phosphorus; 76 mg calcium; 4 mg iron; 118 mg sodium; 1003 mg potassium; 403 IU vitamin A; 2 mg vitamin E; 8 mg vitamin C; 71 mg cholesterol

Mexican Pitas

Another "fusion" recipe . . . a mixing of cultures and tastes. Whatever you call it, these Mexican-flavored pocket sandwiches are a hit with everyone who tries them.

$^1/_2$ pound (225 g) ground turkey

$^1/_2$ cup (80 g) chopped onion

2 teaspoons taco seasoning

2 cups (342 g) cooked pinto beans, drained

$^1/_2$ cup (130 g) salsa

3 whole wheat pitas, halved

2 cups (110 g) shredded lettuce

1 cup (180 g) shredded tomato

$^1/_2$ cup (58 g) shredded Cheddar cheese

Brown turkey and onion in skillet. Drain. Add taco seasoning, beans, and salsa and heat. Spoon mixture into each pita pocket. Add lettuce, tomato, and cheese.

Yield: 3 servings

Per serving: 304 g water; 591 calories (20% from fat, 30% from protein, 49% from carb); 46 g protein; 14 g total fat; 6 g saturated fat; 3 g monounsaturated fat; 2 g polyunsaturated fat; 74 g carbohydrate; 17 g fiber; 6 g sugar; 599 mg phosphorus; 271 mg calcium; 6 mg iron; 622 mg sodium; 1206 mg potassium; 1093 IU vitamin A; 57 mg vitamin E; 11 mg vitamin C; 81 mg cholesterol

Texas Cornbread Skillet Meal

This makes a nice meal-in-a-pot sort of dinner. I've also made a meatless variation of it for lunch that was every bit as good.

1 pound (455 g) ground beef

1 cup (160 g) chopped onion

1 tablespoon minced garlic clove

2 cups (480 g) no-salt-added canned tomatoes

2 cups (344 g) cooked black-eyed peas, drained

1 1/2 teaspoons Cajun seasoning

1/2 cup (70 g) cornmeal

1/2 cup (62 g) flour

1 tablespoon baking powder

1 egg

1/2 cup (120 ml) skim milk

In a large cast-iron or ovenproof skillet, brown ground beef, onion, and garlic. Add undrained tomatoes, black-eyed peas, and seasoning. Stir well. In a separate bowl, combine cornmeal, flour, and baking powder. Stir egg and milk together, then stir into dry ingredients. Top meat mixture with cornbread batter and cook in 425°F (220°C, gas mark 7) oven about 20 to 25 minutes, or until cornbread is golden brown.

Yield: 4 servings

Per serving: 311 g water; 608 calories (32% from fat, 28% from protein, 39% from carb); 43 g protein; 22 g total fat; 8 g saturated fat; 9 g monounsaturated fat; 2 g polyunsaturated fat; 60 g carbohydrate; 9 g fiber; 9 g sugar; 494 mg phosphorus; 334 mg calcium; 8 mg iron; 510 mg sodium; 1086 mg potassium; 394 IU vitamin A; 41 mg vitamin E; 17 mg vitamin C; 145 mg cholesterol

Mexican Chicken and Black Beans

This is a quick one-pan meal. All you need is a little leftover rice to have it on the table in less than half an hour.

1 pound (455 g) boneless chicken breast, cut in 1-inch (2.5-cm) cubes

1/2 cup (80 g) chopped onion

1 teaspoon crushed garlic

2 cups (344 g) cooked black beans, rinsed, drained

1 cup (180 g) chopped tomato

3 tablespoons (48 g) salsa, mild or hot

1/2 cup (115 g) fat-free sour cream

1 cup (220 g) cooked brown rice

1 avocado, sliced

Spray large skillet with nonstick vegetable oil spray; heat over medium heat until hot. Sauté chicken, onion, and garlic until chicken is cooked, 5 to 8 minutes. Stir in beans, tomato, salsa, and sour cream. Cook until hot, 1 to 2 minutes. Season to taste with salt and pepper. Serve over rice, garnished with avocado.

Yield: 4 servings

Per serving: 290 g water; 410 calories (25% from fat, 36% from protein, 39% from carb); 37 g protein; 11 g total fat; 4 g saturated fat; 5 g monounsaturated fat; 1 g polyunsaturated fat; 40 g carbohydrate; 12 g fiber; 2 g sugar; 450 mg phosphorus; 87 mg calcium; 3 mg iron; 125 mg sodium; 977 mg potassium; 459 IU vitamin A; 37 mg vitamin E; 16 mg vitamin C; 78 mg cholesterol

Mexican Skillet Meal

This is one of those one-pan meals that you used to buy in a box. I have to say I think the flavor of this one is better than anything Hamburger Helper ever did.

1 pound (455 g) extra-lean ground beef (93% lean)

$^1/_2$ cup (80 g) onion, chopped

$^1/_4$ cup (37 g) green bell peppers, chopped

$^1/_4$ cup (37 g) red bell pepper, chopped

$^1/_2$ teaspoon (1.5 g) minced garlic

1$^1/_2$ cups (290 g) rice

3 cups (710 ml) water

2 teaspoons (4 g) low sodium beef bouillon

2 cups (360 g) canned no-salt-added tomatoes

1 tablespoon (7.5 g) chili powder

$^1/_2$ teaspoon (1.3 g) cumin

$^1/_4$ teaspoon (0.3 g) dried oregano

12 ounces (340 g) frozen corn, thawed

Sauté beef, onion, green and red bell peppers, and garlic in a large skillet until beef is browned and vegetables are tender. Add rice and sauté 2 minutes longer. Stir in remaining ingredients. Bring to boil. Reduce heat, cover, and simmer for 20 minutes, or until rice is tender and liquid is absorbed.

Yield: 5 servings

Per serving: 357 calories (22% from fat, 31% from protein, 47% from carbohydrate); 22 g protein; 7 g total fat; 2 g saturated fat; 3 g monounsaturated fat; 1 g polyunsaturated fat; 33 g carbohydrate; 4 g fiber; 6 g sugar; 225 mg phosphorus; 64 mg calcium; 4 mg iron; 98 mg sodium; 653 mg potassium; 826 IU vitamin A; 0 mg ATE vitamin E; 29 mg vitamin C; 63 mg cholesterol; 404 g water

Southwestern Pie

A kind of Mexican quiche. Lots of flavor and good nutrition. Serve topped with salsa with cornbread on the side.

1 cup (160 g) chopped onion

1 tablespoon (15 ml) olive oil

1 teaspoon chili powder

1 teaspoon cumin

$^1/_2$ teaspoon garlic powder

2 cups (200 g) cooked kidney beans

1$^1/_2$ cups (330 g) cooked brown rice

1 cup (115 g) shredded Cheddar cheese

$^3/_4$ cup (175 ml) skim milk

2 eggs, beaten

In saucepan, cook onion in oil. Stir in chili powder, cumin, and garlic powder. Cook 1 minute. Cool. Stir in beans, rice, cheese, milk, and eggs. Spray a 10-inch (25-cm) microwave-safe pie plate with nonstick vegetable oil spray. Add rice mixture. Bake to 350°F (180°C, gas mark 4) until heated through, about 20 minutes. Serve garnished with chopped green pepper if desired.

Yield: 6 servings

Per serving: 86 g water; 537 calories (22% from fat, 20% from protein, 57% from carb); 28 g protein; 14 g total fat; 6 g saturated fat; 5 g monounsaturated fat; 2 g polyunsaturated fat; 78 g carbohydrate; 18 g fiber; 3 g sugar; 598 mg phosphorus; 321 mg calcium; 7 mg iron; 205 mg sodium; 1123 mg potassium; 502 IU vitamin A; 101 mg vitamin E; 5 mg vitamin C; 103 mg cholesterol

Mexican Layered Casserole

A Mexican version of lasagna, with tortillas layered with meat, beans, and cheese.

1 pound (455 g) ground beef

1 cup (160 g) chopped onion

1 cup (150 g) chopped bell pepper

4 ounces (115 g) chopped green chiles

16 ounces (455 g) no-salt-added tomato sauce

2 cups (342 g) cooked pinto beans

$^1/_2$ teaspoon garlic powder

2 tablespoons taco seasoning

1 cup (235 ml) water

2 cups (240 g) grated Cheddar cheese

6 flour tortillas

In a large pot, brown beef, onion, and bell pepper. Add remaining ingredients except cheese and tortillas. Simmer 10 minutes. In a large casserole dish, alternately layer meat mixture, cheese, and tortillas, beginning with meat and ending with cheese. Bake at 350°F (180°C, gas mark 4) for 30 minutes.

Yield: 6 servings

Per serving: 280 g water; 583 calories (40% from fat, 27% from protein, 33% from carb); 35 g protein; 22 g total fat; 12 g saturated fat; 7 g monounsaturated fat; 1 g polyunsaturated fat; 42 g carbohydrate; 9 g fiber; 6 g sugar; 494 mg phosphorus; 414 mg calcium; 5 mg iron; 688 mg sodium; 949 mg potassium; 1640 IU vitamin A; 114 mg vitamin E; 51 mg vitamin C; 98 mg cholesterol

Taco Casserole

Call it Mexican lasagna if you wish, but in this case corn tortillas substitute for the noodles, layered with beef and beans.

1 pound (455 g) ground beef

1 cup (160 g) chopped onion

1 cup (150 g) chopped green bell pepper

1 teaspoon minced garlic

8 ounces (225 g) no-salt-added tomato sauce

2 cups (480 g) no-salt-added canned tomatoes

1 tablespoon chili powder

$^1/_2$ teaspoon oregano

$^1/_2$ teaspoon cumin

12 corn tortillas

2 cups (512 g) no-salt-added kidney beans

$^3/_4$ cup (90 g) shredded Cheddar cheese

In a skillet over medium heat, sauté the ground beef, onion, bell pepper, and garlic until the beef is done. Drain off excess fat. Add tomato sauce, tomatoes, and spices. Simmer mixture for 2 minutes. Place a layer of 4 tortillas in the bottom of a 9 × 13-inch (23 × 33-cm) baking pan that has been sprayed with nonstick vegetable oil spray. Place a layer of the beef mixture over top, then 4 more tortillas, the beans, the final 4 tortillas, and the rest of the beef mixture. Bake at 350°F (180°C, gas mark 4) for 30 minutes. Sprinkle with cheese and return to oven until cheese has melted.

Yield: 6 servings

Per serving: 258 g water; 443 calories (33% from fat, 25% from protein, 42% from carb); 29 g protein; 17 g total

fat; 7 g saturated fat; 6 g monounsaturated fat; 1 g polyunsaturated fat; 47 g carbohydrate; 11 g fiber; 5 g sugar; 465 mg phosphorus; 285 mg calcium; 5 mg iron; 374 mg sodium; 884 mg potassium; 863 IU vitamin A; 43 mg vitamin E; 34 mg vitamin C; 63 mg cholesterol

Mexican Spaghetti Pie

A Mexican-flavored version of spaghetti pie. The kidney beans provide extra fiber as well as flavor.

12 ounces (342 g) whole wheat spaghetti

4 tablespoons (55 g) unsalted butter

$^1/_4$ cup (25 g) grated Parmesan cheese

4 eggs, beaten

$^1/_2$ cup (80 g) chopped onion

1 pound (455 g) ground beef

2 cups (200 g) cooked kidney beans, drained

2 cups (480 g) no-salt-added canned tomatoes

6 ounces (170 g) no-salt-added tomato paste

4 ounces (115 g) canned green chiles, chopped

2 tablespoons chili powder

1 teaspoon cumin

$^1/_2$ cup (60 g) shredded Monterey Jack cheese

Cook and drain spaghetti, and let cool slightly. Stir in butter, Parmesan cheese, and eggs. Spread into the bottom of a large baking dish coated with nonstick vegetable oil spray. Brown onion and ground beef. Stir in kidney beans, undrained tomatoes, and tomato paste. Add chopped green chiles, chili powder, and cumin. Simmer for 30 minutes. Pour meat mixture over pasta in baking dish. Top with the shredded

cheese. Bake in a 350°F (180°C, gas mark 4) oven for 30 to 40 minutes or until brown.

Yield: 8 servings

Per serving: 152 g water; 607 calories (27% from fat, 25% from protein, 48% from carb); 36 g protein; 17 g total fat; 8 g saturated fat; 5 g monounsaturated fat; 2 g polyunsaturated fat; 68 g carbohydrate; 17 g fiber; 6 g sugar; 530 mg phosphorus; 236 mg calcium; 9 mg iron; 232 mg sodium; 1332 mg potassium; 1345 IU vitamin A; 106 mg vitamin E; 14 mg vitamin C; 183 mg cholesterol

Tip: If you like things spicier, add some red pepper flakes along with the other spices.

Chili Casserole

A Mexican meal in one pan. This is a fairly mild version, but you could increase the chili powder or add a chopped jalapeño to either the chili or the cornbread if you wanted to make it spicier.

1 pound (455 g) extra-lean ground beef (93% lean)

$^1/_2$ cup (80 g) onion, chopped

$^1/_2$ cup (75 g) red bell pepper, chopped

2 cups (450 g) no-salt-added kidney beans

2 cups (360 g) tomatoes, chopped and drained

1 cup (164 g) frozen corn

1 tablespoon (7.5 g) chili powder

1 teaspoon (2.5 g) cumin

$^1/_2$ teaspoon (1.5 g) garlic powder

$^1/_2$ cup (60 g) flour

$^1/_2$ cup (70 g) yellow cornmeal

2 tablespoons (26 g) sugar

1$^1/_2$ teaspoons (7 g) baking powder

1 cup (235 ml) skim milk

1 egg

1 tablespoon (15 ml) olive oil

Preheat oven to 425°F (220°C, or gas mark 7). Brown beef with onions and red bell pepper until beef is no longer pink. Add beans, tomatoes, corn, chili powder, cumin, and garlic powder and simmer for 5 minutes. In a large bowl, stir together flour, cornmeal, sugar, and baking powder. In a medium bowl, combine milk, egg, and oil and pour into flour mixture, stirring until just moistened. Spread beef mixture in a greased 8x8 baking dish. Spread cornmeal mixture over top. Bake for 10 to 12 minutes, or until cornbread is done.

Yield: 4 servings

Per serving: 669 calories (20% from fat, 28% from protein, 52% from carbohydrate); 39 g protein; 13 g total fat; 4 g saturated fat; 6 g monounsaturated fat; 2 g polyunsaturated fat; 74 g carbohydrate; 13 g fiber; 10 g sugar; 506 mg phosphorus; 288 mg calcium; 8 mg iron; 357 mg sodium; 1147 mg potassium; 1838 IU vitamin A; 38 mg ATE vitamin E; 49 mg vitamin C; 130 mg cholesterol; 340 g water

Enchilada Bake

An easy casserole dish with the taste of enchiladas.

1 pound (455 g) extra-lean ground beef (93% lean)

1/4 cup (40 g) onion, chopped

4 eggs

8 ounces (225 g) no-salt-added tomato sauce

2/3 cup (160 ml) fat-free evaporated milk

2 tablespoons (5 g) taco seasoning

1/4 cup (34 g) ripe olives, sliced

1 cup (28 g) corn chips

3/4 cup (90 g) low fat Cheddar cheese, shredded

Preheat oven to 350°F (180°C, or gas mark 4). In a skillet, cook beef and onion until meat is brown and onion is soft. Drain. Spread in the bottom of a 9-inch (23-cm) square baking dish that has been coated with nonstick vegetable oil spray. Beat together eggs, tomato sauce, milk, and taco seasoning. Pour over meat. Sprinkle with olives. Top with corn chips. Bake for 25 minutes, or until set in the center. Sprinkle cheese on top and return to oven just until cheese melts, about 3 minutes.

Yield: 6 servings

Per serving: 339 calories (38% from fat, 41% from protein, 22% from carbohydrate); 27 g protein; 11 g total fat; 3 g saturated fat; 4 g monounsaturated fat; 2 g polyunsaturated fat; 14 g carbohydrate; 1 g fiber; 6 g sugar; 322 mg phosphorus; 206 mg calcium; 3 mg iron; 455 mg sodium; 521 mg potassium; 586 IU vitamin A; 44 mg ATE vitamin E; 6 mg vitamin C; 197 mg cholesterol; 160 g water

Chiles Rellenos Casserole

Canned chile peppers are easy to find and convenient. You can also make this using fresh peppers if you have large mild chiles like ancho or poblano peppers available. If you're using fresh peppers, blanch for 30 to 60 seconds in boiling water before using.

2 cups (240 g) whole chile peppers

1 cup (115 g) low fat Cheddar cheese

$^1/_4$ cup (25 g) scallions, sliced

2 eggs

$^1/_2$ cup (120 ml) skim milk

$^1/_4$ cup (32 g) flour

$^3/_4$ cup (170 g) salsa

1 cup (115 g) part-skim mozzarella

Preheat oven to 325°F (170°C, or gas mark 3). Split chile peppers lengthwise and remove seeds and pith. Spread chiles in a single layer in a 9 × 13-inch (23 × 33-cm) baking dish sprayed with nonstick vegetable oil spray. Sprinkle Cheddar cheese and scallions over chiles. In a bowl, beat eggs, milk, and flour together until smooth. Pour over chiles and cheese. Bake for 50 minutes, or until a knife inserted in custard comes out clean. Meanwhile, mix salsa with the mozzarella cheese. Sprinkle over casserole and return to oven for 10 minutes or until cheese melts. Let stand for 5 minutes before serving.

Yield: 4 servings

Per serving: 227 calories (33% from fat, 39% from protein, 29% from carbohydrate); 22 g protein; 8 g total fat; 5 g saturated fat; 2 g monounsaturated fat; 1 g polyunsaturated fat; 16 g carbohydrate; 2 g fiber; 4 g sugar; 404 mg phosphorus; 445 mg calcium; 2 mg iron; 483 mg sodium; 405 mg potassium; 860 IU vitamin A; 74 mg ATE vitamin E; 62 mg vitamin C; 126 mg cholesterol; 210 g water

Mexican Lasagna

Lasagna with a southwestern twist.

$^3/_4$ pound (340 g) lasagna noodles

$^1/_2$ cup (80 g) onion, chopped

$^1/_2$ cup (75 g) red bell pepper, chopped

$^1/_2$ cup (82 g) frozen corn kernels, thawed

$^1/_2$ teaspoon (1.5 g) chopped garlic

2 cups (450 g) canned black beans, rinsed and drained

2 cups (460 g) refried beans

$2^3/_4$ cups (645 ml) no-salt-added tomato sauce

$^1/_2$ cup (115 g) salsa

$^1/_2$ cup (30 g) chopped fresh cilantro, divided

$1^1/_2$ cups (340 g) fat-free cottage cheese

1 cup (250 g) low fat ricotta cheese

$^1/_4$ cup (58 g) fat-free sour cream

1 cup (115 g) low fat Monterey Jack cheese, shredded

$^1/_4$ cup (50 g) black olives, sliced

Preheat oven to 350°F (180°C, or gas mark 4). Bring a large pot of lightly salted water to a boil. Add pasta and cook for 8 to 10 minutes or until al dente. Drain. Coat a large skillet with nonstick vegetable oil spray and place over medium heat. Sauté onion, red bell pepper, corn, and garlic until tender. Stir in black beans, refried beans, tomato sauce, salsa, and $^1/_4$ cup (15 g) cilantro. Cook until heated through and slightly thickened; set aside. In a large bowl, combine cottage cheese, ricotta, sour cream, Monterey Jack cheese, and remaining $^1/_4$ cup (15 g) chopped cilantro; set aside. Coat a 9 × 13-inch (23 × 33-cm) casserole dish with nonstick vegetable oil spray.

Arrange 3 of the cooked lasagna noodles in the bottom of the dish; cutting to fit if necessary. Spread with one-third of the bean mixture, then one-third of the cheese mixture. Repeat layers twice more. Cover and bake for 45 minutes. Garnish with sliced black olives.

Yield: 8 servings

Per serving: 438 calories (13% from fat, 25% from protein, 62% from carbohydrate); 27 g protein; 6 g total fat; 3 g saturated fat; 2 g monounsaturated fat; 1 g polyunsaturated fat; 66 g carbohydrate; 10 g fiber; 7 g sugar; 349 mg phosphorus; 243 mg calcium; 5 mg iron; 638 mg sodium; 914 mg potassium; 1041 IU vitamin A; 53 mg ATE vitamin E; 30 mg vitamin C; 22 mg cholesterol; 270 g water

Tip: This can be frozen unbaked and kept for up to a month. Simply thaw in refrigerator overnight and bake as directed. It tastes even better reheated the second day!

South-of-the-Border Pie

A slightly different take on Mexican food, you can use this rice and egg casserole either as a side dish or a meatless main dish.

1 tablespoon (15 ml) olive oil

1 cup (160 g) onion, chopped

1 teaspoon (2.6 g) chili powder

1 teaspoon (2.5 g) cumin

$1/2$ teaspoon (1.5 g) garlic powder

2 cups (450 g) canned kidney beans, drained

$1^1/2$ cups cooked brown rice

1 cup low fat Cheddar cheese, shredded

$^3/_4$ cup (180 ml) skim milk

2 eggs

Chopped green bell pepper and salsa for garnish (optional)

Preheat oven to 350°F (180°C, or gas mark 4). Heat oil in saucepan and cook onion. Stir in chili powder, cumin, and garlic powder and cook for 1 minute. Cool. Stir in beans, rice, cheese, milk, and eggs. Spray a 10-inch (25-cm) glass pie plate with nonstick vegetable oil spray. Add rice mixture. Bake uncovered for 30 minutes, or until center is just set. Let stand for 10 minutes. Garnish with chopped green pepper and serve with salsa, if desired.

Yield: 6 servings

Per serving: 477 calories (12% from fat, 23% from protein, 65% from carbohydrate); 28 g protein; 7 g total fat; 2 g saturated fat; 3 g monounsaturated fat; 1 g polyunsaturated fat; 78 g carbohydrate; 18 g fiber; 3 g sugar; 582 mg phosphorus; 255 mg calcium; 7 mg iron; 214 mg sodium; 1060 mg potassium; 312 IU vitamin A; 32 mg ATE vitamin E; 5 mg vitamin C; 145 mg cholesterol; 95 g water

Nacho Chicken Casserole

This is one of those easy throw-together-with-what-you-have-on-hand recipes. But it's the kind of thing that frequently comes up in those "We haven't had that in a while" conversations.

$1^1/2$ cups (84 g) unsalted tortilla chips, crushed

2 cups (220 g) cooked chicken breast, diced

1 cup (235 ml) low sodium cream of mushroom soup

8 ounces (225 g) fat-free sour cream

$^{1}/_{2}$ cup (58 g) low fat Cheddar cheese shredded

Preheat oven to 350°F (180°C, or gas mark 4). Line bottom of 1$^{1}/_{2}$-quart (1.4-L) casserole dish with crushed tortilla chips. Mix remaining ingredients, except cheese, and cover chips. Top with cheese. Bake for 15 minutes, or until cheese is bubbly.

Yield: 2 servings

Per serving: 602 calories (27% from fat, 49% from protein, 24% from carbohydrate); 58 g protein; 14 g total fat; 4 g saturated fat; 5 g monounsaturated fat; 4 g polyunsaturated fat; 28 g carbohydrate; 2 g fiber; 3 g sugar; 690 mg phosphorus; 326 mg calcium; 3 mg iron; 425 mg sodium; 1038 mg potassium; 544 IU vitamin A; 144 mg ATE vitamin E; 1 mg vitamin C; 174 mg cholesterol; 313 g water

Taco Quiche

A Mexican-flavored quiche. Baking it without a crust reduces the fat content to less than half of what it would be if you bought a pre-made piecrust.

$^{1}/_{2}$ pound (225 g) extra-lean ground beef (93% lean)

2 tablespoons (5.3 g) taco seasoning

$^{1}/_{2}$ cup (120 ml) water

$^{1}/_{2}$ cup (60 g) low fat Monterey Jack cheese, shredded

2 ounces (55 g) green chiles, seeded and diced

3 eggs

1 cup (235 ml) fat-free evaporated milk

Preheat oven to 375°F (190°C, or gas mark 5). Brown beef in skillet. Drain. Stir in taco seasoning mix and water, cover, and simmer until thickened. Cool 10 minutes. Add cheese and chiles and mix well. Spoon into 9-inch (23-cm) pie pan that has been sprayed with nonstick vegetable oil spray. Combine eggs and milk. Mix until smooth. Pour over meat mixture. Bake for 40 to 45 minutes, or until custard is set. Allow pie to stand 5 minutes before serving.

Yield: 6 servings

Per serving: 173 calories (30% from fat, 51% from protein, 19% from carbohydrate); 17 g protein; 4 g total fat; 2 g saturated fat; 2 g monounsaturated fat; 1 g polyunsaturated fat; 6 g carbohydrate; 0 g fiber; 5 g sugar; 229 mg phosphorus; 193 mg calcium; 2 mg iron; 321 mg sodium; 271 mg potassium; 451 IU vitamin A; 57 mg ATE vitamin E; 4 mg vitamin C; 130 mg cholesterol; 119 g water

Southwestern Beans

Quick and tasty bean dish with a little bit of a kick to it.

$^{1}/_{4}$ cup (36 g) poblano chiles, roasted and peeled

$^{1}/_{2}$ pound (225 g) chorizo, bulk

1 cup (100 g) green beans, sliced

1 cup (180 g) chopped tomato

2 cans (16 ounces each) pinto beans

Heat the oven to 350°F (180°C, gas mark 4). Cook and stir the chiles and chorizo together until the chorizo is done. Drain off excess fat. Mix the chorizo mixture and remaining ingredients in an ungreased 2-quart (2-L) casserole dish. Drain one can of pinto beans and leave one undrained. Bake uncovered until hot and bubbly. Serve.

Yield: 4 servings

Per serving: 85 g water; 275 calories (72% from fat, 21% from protein, 7% from carb); 15 g protein; 22 g total fat; 8 g saturated fat; 10 g monounsaturated fat; 2 g polyunsaturated fat; 5 g carbohydrate; 2 g fiber; 2 g sugar; 107 mg phosphorus; 20 mg calcium; 1 mg iron; 705 mg sodium; 391 mg potassium; 526 IU vitamin A; 0 mg vitamin E; 16 mg vitamin C; 50 mg cholesterol

Mexican-Style Beans

This recipe gives you beans similar to the canned "Mexi-beans." You can use it in recipes that call for them, as a starter for chili, or the way we had them for lunch, just spooned over rice with a little dollop of salsa on top.

8 ounces (225 g) dried kidney beans

6 cups (1.4 L) water

2 tablespoons (30 ml) vinegar

$^1/_2$ teaspoon (1.5 g) garlic powder

1 teaspoon (3 g) onion powder

1 tablespoon (7.5 g) chili powder

Rinse the beans and place in a large pot with the water. Bring to a boil and cook 2 minutes. Remove from heat and let stand for an hour. Return to heat; add vinegar, garlic powder, onion powder, and chili powder and simmer until beans are tender, 1 to 1$^1/_2$ hours. Add water or low sodium chicken broth if the beans get too dry.

Yield: 4 servings

Per serving: 199 calories (3% from fat, 27% from protein, 70% from carbohydrate); 14 g protein; 1 g total fat; 0 g saturated fat; 0 g monounsaturated fat; 0 g polyunsaturated fat; 36 g carbohydrate; 15 g fiber; 2 g sugar; 240 mg phosphorus; 100 mg calcium; 5 mg iron; 44 mg sodium; 851 mg potassium; 556 IU vitamin A; 0 mg ATE vitamin E; 4 mg vitamin C; 0 mg cholesterol; 368 g water

Mexican Topped Potatoes

Hot topped potatoes with a Mexican accent. Sure to be a hit with young people as well as adults.

2 baking potatoes

$^1/_2$ cup (115 g) low-fat cottage cheese

1 cup (171 g) cooked pinto beans, drained

$^1/_2$ cup (130 g) salsa

$^1/_4$ cup (25 g) chopped scallions

$^1/_2$ cup (50 g) black olives

$^1/_3$ cup (50 g) sliced red bell pepper

$^1/_2$ cup (58 g) shredded Cheddar cheese

Bake potatoes. Slit open. Loosen pulp with fork. Spoon over each potato: cottage cheese, beans, salsa, scallions, olives, bell pepper, and shredded cheese. Return to microwave or oven to reheat and melt cheese.

Yield: 2 servings

Per serving: 523 g water; 657 calories (22% from fat, 20% from protein, 58% from carb); 33 g protein; 17 g total

fat; 8 g saturated fat; 6 g monounsaturated fat; 1 g polyunsaturated fat; 98 g carbohydrate; 19 g fiber; 7 g sugar; 622 mg phosphorus; 418 mg calcium; 7 mg iron; 791 mg sodium; 2295 mg potassium; 1609 IU vitamin A; 97 mg vitamin E; 109 mg vitamin C; 39 mg cholesterol

Mexican Rice

A family favorite. A quick and flavorful use for leftover rice.

1 cup (220 g) cooked brown rice

2 tablespoons (28 ml) olive oil

$^1/_2$ cup (80 g) chopped onion

$^1/_4$ pound (113 g) shredded Cheddar cheese

1 jalapeño pepper, chopped

Brown rice in oil. Add remaining ingredients. Cover and simmer until heated through and cheese is melted.

Yield: 4 servings

Per serving: 67 g water; 237 calories (63% from fat, 14% from protein, 23% from carb); 9 g protein; 17 g total fat; 7 g saturated fat; 8 g monounsaturated fat; 1 g polyunsaturated fat; 14 g carbohydrate; 1 g fiber; 1 g sugar; 192 mg phosphorus; 214 mg calcium; 1 mg iron; 179 mg sodium; 86 mg potassium; 312 IU vitamin A; 73 mg vitamin E; 3 mg vitamin C; 30 mg cholesterol

Mexican Zucchini Oven Fries

These make a great alternative to French fries with a burger or other grilled meat.

2 medium zucchini

1 tablespoon (3 g) dried oregano

1 tablespoon (7 g) cumin

Preheat oven to 500°F (250°C, or gas mark 10). Cut zucchini in $^1/_4$ × 3-inch (0.6 × 7.5-cm) sticks, like French fries. Arrange zucchini on a nonstick baking sheet. Spray zucchini with nonstick vegetable oil spray. Combine oregano and cumin and sprinkle over the zucchini fries. Bake for 15 to 18 minutes. Serve hot with low sodium taco sauce or salsa for dipping.

Yield: 4 servings

Per serving: 18 calories (21% from fat, 20% from protein, 59% from carbohydrate); 1 g protein; 1 g total fat; 0 g saturated fat; 0 g monounsaturated fat; 0 g polyunsaturated fat; 3 g carbohydrate; 1 g fiber; 1 g sugar; 33 mg phosphorus; 35 mg calcium; 2 mg iron; 9 mg sodium; 202 mg potassium; 195 IU vitamin A; 0 mg ATE vitamin E; 11 mg vitamin C; 0 mg cholesterol; 59 g water

Mexican Noodles

This was kind of a throw-together that worked well. It makes a nice alternative to rice.

12 ounces (340 g) noodles

$^1/_4$ cup (24 g) dry cheese sauce mix

1 cup (235 ml) skim milk

$^1/_2$ teaspoon (1.3 g) cumin

$^1/_2$ teaspoon (1.5 g) onion powder

$^1/_4$ teaspoon (0.8 g) garlic powder

$^1/_2$ cup (115 g) salsa

Cook noodles according to package directions. Combine sauce mix, milk, cumin, onion powder, and garlic powder in a jar with a tight-fitting lid. Shake well until sauce mix is dissolved. Cook and stir until thickened and bubbly. Stir in noodles and salsa.

Yield: 6 servings

Per serving: 116 calories (16% from fat, 15% from protein, 69% from carbohydrate); 5 g protein; 2 g total fat; 1 g saturated fat; 1 g monounsaturated fat; 0 g polyunsaturated fat; 20 g carbohydrate; 3 g fiber; 1 g sugar; 121 mg phosphorus; 99 mg calcium; 0 mg iron; 204 mg sodium; 177 mg potassium; 242 IU vitamin A; 42 mg ATE vitamin E; 1 mg vitamin C; 5 mg cholesterol; 102 g water

Peas and Rice

Black-eyed peas are a southern tradition for New Year's Day. The more you eat on that day, the more prosperous you will be in the coming year. This pea recipe is easy to make and makes a hearty vegetarian meal or a great side dish with pork.

1 cup (250 g) dried black-eyed peas

4 cups (946 ml) water

3 teaspoons (6 g) low sodium chicken bouillon

$^1/_2$ teaspoon (1.5 g) crushed garlic

1 tablespoon (4 g) cilantro

1 tablespoon (4 g) fresh parsley

$^1/_2$ teaspoon (1 g) black pepper

$^1/_2$ cup (80 g) onion, chopped

2 cups (360 g) canned no-salt-added tomatoes

1 cup (195 g) uncooked rice

Combine black-eyed peas and water in large saucepan; add bouillon and garlic. Bring black-eyed pea mixture to a boil; reduce heat and stir in cilantro, parsley, and pepper. Cover and simmer for 15 minutes. Stir in onion and tomatoes. Cover and simmer for 15 minutes, or until black-eyed peas are almost soft. Stir in rice; cover. Cook for 20 minutes, or until rice and black-eyed peas are tender. Remove from heat and let stand.

Yield: 4 servings

Per serving: 231 calories (6% from fat, 21% from protein, 73% from carbohydrate); 13 g protein; 1 g total fat; 0 g saturated fat; 0 g monounsaturated fat; 1 g polyunsaturated fat; 44 g carbohydrate; 6 g fiber; 4 g sugar; 238 mg phosphorus; 99 mg calcium; 6 mg iron; 70 mg sodium; 873 mg potassium; 288 IU vitamin A; 0 mg ATE vitamin E; 15 mg vitamin C; 0 mg cholesterol; 401 g water

Mexican Beef Salad

A kind of taco salad without the tortillas, this makes a great light dinner for a hot day.

1 pound (455 g) ground beef, extra lean

$^1/_2$ cup (80 g) chopped onion

1 tablespoon chili powder

2 teaspoons oregano

$^1/_2$ teaspoon cumin

1 cup (100 g) cooked kidney beans, drained and rinsed

1 pound (455 g) chickpeas, drained and rinsed

1 cup (180 g) diced tomato

2 cups (110 g) iceberg lettuce

$^1/_2$ cup (58 g) shredded Cheddar cheese

Cook ground beef and onion in a skillet over medium-high heat until beef is no longer pink, 10 to 12 minutes. Drain. Stir in chili powder, oregano, and cumin. Cook for 1 minute. Mix in beans, chickpeas, and tomato. Portion lettuce onto serving plates. Top with shredded cheese. Then top with beef mixture.

Yield: 4 servings

Per serving: 263 g water; 601 calories (42% from fat, 27% from protein, 31% from carb); 41 g protein; 28 g total fat; 12 g saturated fat; 11 g monounsaturated fat; 3 g polyunsaturated fat; 47 g carbohydrate; 15 g fiber; 8 g sugar; 525 mg phosphorus; 242 mg calcium; 8 mg iron; 213 mg sodium; 1071 mg potassium; 1284 IU vitamin A; 43 mg vitamin E; 11 mg vitamin C; 96 mg cholesterol

Taco Salad

A meal on a plate. And you couldn't ask for more flavor.

1 pound (455 g) ground beef

1 tablespoon taco seasoning

2 cups (110 g) shredded lettuce

6 ounces (170 g) corn chips

2 cups (504 g) refried beans

1 cup (180 g) chopped tomato

$^1/_2$ cup (80 g) chopped onion

$^1/_2$ cup (75 g) chopped green bell pepper

$^1/_2$ cup (115 g) sour cream

$^1/_2$ cup (130 g) salsa

Brown the ground beef with the taco seasoning. Drain. Layer lettuce, chips, beef, beans, tomato, onion, and pepper. Top with sour cream and salsa.

Yield: 4 servings

Per serving: 318 g water; 523 calories (39% from fat, 25% from protein, 36% from carb); 33 g protein; 23 g total fat; 10 g saturated fat; 9 g monounsaturated fat; 2 g polyunsaturated fat; 48 g carbohydrate; 11 g fiber; 4 g sugar; 438 mg phosphorus; 183 mg calcium; 5 mg iron; 538 mg sodium; 1006 mg potassium; 842 IU vitamin A; 50 mg vitamin E; 31 mg vitamin C; 92 mg cholesterol

Mexican Bean Salad

A Mexican version of three bean salad, flavored with chili powder but without another dressing. Serve as is as a side dish or as a salad drizzled with Italian or other dressing.

1 cup (160 g) sliced red onion

$^1/_4$ cup (60 ml) water

1 tablespoon chili powder

1 cup (100 g) cooked green beans

1 cup (172 g) cooked black beans

1 cup (100 g) cooked kidney beans

1 cup (182 g) cooked navy beans

$^1/_2$ cup (82 g) frozen corn, thawed

2 tablespoons chopped cilantro

Place the onion in a saucepan with the water. Cook gently until the onion is soft and separated into rings, 4 to 5 minutes. Add the chili powder and stir until well mixed. Remove from heat. Combine all of the remaining ingredients in a large bowl and toss to mix well. Cover and chill for 1 to 2 hours to allow flavors to blend.

Yield: 6 servings

Per serving: 88 g water; 289 calories (4% from fat, 24% from protein, 73% from carb); 18 g protein; 1 g total fat; 0 g saturated fat; 0 g monounsaturated fat; 1 g polyunsaturated fat; 54 g carbohydrate; 17 g fiber; 4 g sugar; 333 mg phosphorus; 120 mg calcium; 6 mg iron; 26 mg sodium; 1070 mg potassium; 559 IU vitamin A; 0 mg vitamin E; 9 mg vitamin C; 0 mg cholesterol

Mexican Bean and Avocado Salad

A simple and tasty South-of-the-border bean salad. Cook dry beans according to package directions or drain canned beans.

2 cups (450 g) cooked kidney beans

2 cups (450 g) cooked garbanzo beans

1 cup (180 g) tomatoes, chopped

$^3/_4$ cup (105 g) cucumber, peeled and chopped

2 tablespoons (20 g) onion, diced

$^1/_2$ cup (115 g) avocado, mashed

$^1/_2$ cup (115 g) plain fat-free yogurt

$^1/_4$ teaspoon (0.8 g) minced garlic

$^1/_2$ teaspoon (1.3 g) cumin

4 cups (80 g) lettuce, shredded

In a large bowl, toss together the kidney beans, garbanzo beans, tomatoes, cucumber, and onion. In a small bowl, mix the avocado, yogurt, garlic, and cumin. Stir the avocado mixture into the bean mixture and chill. Serve on top of shredded lettuce.

Yield: 8 servings

Per serving: 172 calories (17% from fat, 19% from protein, 64% from carbohydrate); 9 g protein; 3 g total fat; 0 g saturated fat; 2 g monounsaturated fat; 1 g polyunsaturated fat; 29 g carbohydrate; 7 g fiber; 2 g sugar; 164 mg phosphorus; 75 mg calcium; 3 mg iron; 303 mg sodium; 506 mg potassium; 346 IU vitamin A; 0 mg ATE vitamin E; 11 mg vitamin C; 0 mg cholesterol; 159 g water

Mexican Bean and Corn Salad

A fairly simple salad, but full of flavor and loaded with fiber, providing 13 grams.

1 cup (164 g) cooked corn

1$^1/_2$ cups (150 g) cooked kidney beans

2 cups (110 g) shredded lettuce

$^1/_4$ cup (25 g) sliced black olives

2 tablespoons (18 g) chopped green chiles

$^1/_2$ cup (60 g) shredded Monterey Jack cheese

$^1/_2$ tablespoon tomato paste

2 tablespoons (28 ml) cider vinegar

6 tablespoons (90 ml) olive oil

$^1/_2$ teaspoon chili powder

Combine first 6 ingredients. Mix remaining ingredients thoroughly; add to salad.

Yield: 6 servings

Per serving: 67 g water; 349 calories (45% from fat, 16% from protein, 39% from carb); 15 g protein; 18 g total fat; 4 g saturated fat; 11 g monounsaturated fat; 2 g polyunsaturated fat; 35 g carbohydrate; 13 g fiber; 3 g sugar; 259 mg phosphorus; 161 mg calcium; 4 mg iron;

148 mg sodium; 755 mg potassium; 315 IU vitamin A; 21 mg vitamin E; 5 mg vitamin C; 10 mg cholesterol

Southwestern Vegetable Stew

This stew evokes not just the flavor of Mexico, but also that of the southwestern Native American tribes with the use of squash and corn. Delicious with cornbread.

$^3/_4$ cup (120 g) chopped onion

$^1/_2$ teaspoon finely chopped garlic

2 tablespoons (28 ml) vegetable oil

1 cup (150 g) red bell pepper, cut into strips

$^1/_2$ cup (72 g) poblano chiles, seeded and cut into strips

1 jalapeño pepper, seeded and chopped

1 cup (140 g) cubed acorn squash

4 cups (950 ml) low-sodium chicken broth

$^1/_2$ teaspoon black pepper

$^1/_2$ teaspoon ground coriander

1 cup (113 g) thinly sliced zucchini

1 cup (113 g) thinly sliced yellow squash

10 ounces (280 g) frozen corn

2 cups (342 g) cooked pinto beans, drained

Cook and stir onion and garlic in oil in 4-quart (4-L) Dutch oven over medium heat until onion is tender. Stir in bell pepper, poblano, and jalapeño. Cook 15 minutes. Stir in squash, broth, black pepper, and coriander. Heat to boiling; reduce heat. Cover and simmer until squash is tender, about 15 minutes. Stir in remaining ingredients. Cook uncovered, stirring occasionally, until zucchini is tender, about 10 minutes.

Yield: 6 servings

Per serving: 336 g water; 220 calories (24% from fat, 19% from protein, 57% from carb); 11 g protein; 6 g total fat; 1 g saturated fat; 2 g monounsaturated fat; 3 g polyunsaturated fat; 34 g carbohydrate; 8 g fiber; 5 g sugar; 199 mg phosphorus; 58 mg calcium;2 mg iron; 57 mg sodium; 759 mg potassium; 1001 IU vitamin A; 0 mg vitamin E; 54 mg vitamin C; 0 mg cholesterol

Mexican Bean and Barley Soup

Not quite chili and not quite bean soup, but definitely good. Cornbread is my personal choice of accompaniment.

$^1/_2$ cup (97 g) dried pinto beans

$^1/_2$ cup (125 g) dried kidney beans

$^1/_2$ cup (104 g) dried navy beans

$^1/_2$ cup (97 g) dried black beans

8 cups (1.9 L) water

$^1/_2$ cup (100 g) pearl barley

1 cup (160 g) chopped onion

2 bay leaves

2 teaspoons chili powder

2 teaspoons cumin

1 teaspoon oregano

$^1/_2$ teaspoon garlic powder

Rinse and pick over beans. Put into a 4- to 5-quart (4- to 5-L) heavy pot and cover with water. Let sit overnight. Drain. Add the water. Add barley, onion, and spices. Bring to a boil. Reduce heat to low. Cover and simmer for 2 hours, stirring occasionally, or until beans are tender, but still firm. Uncover. Increase heat to medium-low and boil, gently stirring occasionally, 45 to 60 minutes, until soup is slightly thickened. Discard bay leaves.

Yield: 6 servings

Per serving: 363 g water; 220 calories (5% from fat, 21% from protein, 74% from carb); 12 g protein; 1 g total fat; 0 g saturated fat; 0 g monounsaturated fat; 1 g polyunsaturated fat; 42 g carbohydrate; 13 g fiber; 2 g sugar; 229 mg phosphorus; 90 mg calcium;4 mg iron; 27 mg sodium; 679 mg potassium; 272 IU vitamin A; 0 mg vitamin E; 4 mg vitamin C; 0 mg cholesterol

Mexican Chicken Soup

Southwestern flavor without the heat.

1 pound (455 g) boneless chicken breasts cut in 1-inch (2.5-cm) cubes

1 cup (160 g) onion, chopped

4 cups (720 g) canned no-salt-added tomatoes

2 cups (470 ml) low sodium chicken broth

4 ounces (115 g) chopped chiles

1 teaspoon (1 g) dried oregano

1 teaspoon (2.5 g) cumin

1 cup (165 g) frozen corn, thawed

$^1/_2$ cup (75 g) green bell pepper, chopped

6 corn tortillas, cut in 1-inch (2.5-cm) strips

Mix first 7 ingredients (through cumin) in a slow cooker. Cover and cook on low for 7 to 8 hours. Turn

to high and stir in corn and green peppers. Cook 30 minutes, or until vegetables are tender. Preheat oven to 450°F (180°C, or gas mark 4). Place tortilla strips on baking sheets coated with nonstick vegetable oil spray. Bake for 6 minutes, or until crisp, but not brown. Spoon soup into bowls, top with tortilla strips.

Yield: 6 servings

Per serving: 208 calories (10% from fat, 42% from protein, 48% from carbohydrate); 23 g protein; 2 g total fat; 1 g saturated fat; 1 g monounsaturated fat; 1 g polyunsaturated fat; 26 g carbohydrate; 4 g fiber; 7 g sugar; 297 mg phosphorus; 94 mg calcium; 3 mg iron; 107 mg sodium; 771 mg potassium; 489 IU vitamin A; 5 mg ATE vitamin E; 75 mg vitamin C; 44 mg cholesterol; 366 g water

Tip: For a little added flavor, sprinkle with fresh cilantro.

Mexican Chicken Stew

A stew full of chicken and chunky vegetables, flavored with Mexican spices. Cooked while you are gone in the slow cooker, it gives the house a nice aroma to come home to.

$^1/_2$ cup (80 g) onion, coarsely chopped

2 boneless chicken breasts cut in 1-inch (2.5-cm) cubes

$^1/_2$ cup (75 g) green bell pepper, coarsely chopped

2 cups (225 g) zucchini, thickly sliced

1$^1/_2$ cups (270 g) plum tomatoes, chopped

$^1/_2$ cup (82 g) frozen corn, thawed

2 cups (470 ml) low sodium chicken broth

1 tablespoon (7.5 g) chili powder

$^1/_2$ tablespoon (3.5 g) cumin

1 tablespoon (3 g) dried oregano

¹/₂ teaspoon (1.5 g) garlic powder

Place onion in the bottom of a slow cooker. Cover with chicken and then green bell pepper, zucchini, tomatoes, and corn. Combine broth, chili powder, cumin, oregano, and garlic powder and pour over chicken. Cook on low 8 to 10 hours or on high 4 to 5 hours.

Yield: 4 servings

Per serving: 119 calories (14% from fat, 41% from protein, 45% from carbohydrate); 13 g protein; 2 g total fat; 0 g saturated fat; 1 g monounsaturated fat; 1 g polyunsaturated fat; 15 g carbohydrate; 4 g fiber; 5 g sugar; 176 mg phosphorus; 55 mg calcium; 2 mg iron; 91 mg sodium; 646 mg potassium; 1284 IU vitamin A; 2 mg ATE vitamin E; 37 mg vitamin C; 21 mg cholesterol; 305 g water

Tip: If you want a more substantial meal, you can serve this over rice.

Mexican Bean Soup

I created this recipe one weekend when I was looking for a fairly large pot of some kind of soup to use for lunches during the week. My original idea was chili, but I had lots of navy beans and no kidney or pinto ones, so this is what we came up with. This is a vegetarian version, but you could add some chicken to it if you're the kind who has to have meat. Chipotle peppers are dried, smoked jalapeños. In this recipe, I left the pepper whole so I could take it out at the end. If you can't find them in large markets near you, you could use fresh jalapeños. This makes a moderately spicy soup, but you can also adjust the heat to your desire by using more or less chipotle pepper.

1¹/₂ cups (375 g) dried navy beans

6 cups (1.4 L) water

¹/₂ chipotle pepper

¹/₂ cup (80 g) onion, chopped

¹/₂ teaspoon (1.5 g) garlic powder

1¹/₂ teaspoons (3.8 g) cumin

2 cups (360 g) canned no-salt-added tomatoes

6 ounces (170 g) frozen corn, thawed

8 ounces (225 g) orzo, or other small pasta

Soak beans in water overnight or bring to boil, boil for 1 minute, and let stand 1 hour. Add chipotle pepper, onion, garlic powder, and cumin and simmer for 1 to 1¹/₂ hours, or until beans are almost tender. Add tomatoes, corn, and pasta and cook until pasta and beans are done. Remove chipotle pepper before serving.

Yield: 8 servings

Per serving: 197 calories (4% from fat, 17% from protein, 78% from carbohydrate); 9 g protein; 1 g total fat; 0 g saturated fat; 0 g monounsaturated fat; 0 g polyunsaturated fat; 40 g carbohydrate; 5 g fiber; 3 g sugar; 151 mg phosphorus; 60 mg calcium; 3 mg iron; 237 mg sodium; 399 mg potassium; 293 IU vitamin A; 0 mg ATE vitamin E; 7 mg vitamin C; 0 mg cholesterol; 297 g water

Caribbean Turkey Soup

This makes a flavorful soup that is also a good way to use up leftover holiday turkey.

1¹/₂ pounds (680 g) turkey breast, cut into bite-sized pieces

1 teaspoon (2.5 g) paprika

1 cup (160 g) onion, coarsely chopped

$^1/_2$ cup (75 g) green bell pepper, coarsely chopped

$^1/_2$ teaspoon (1.5 g) finely chopped garlic

1 cup (100 g) celery, coarsely chopped

$^1/_2$ cup (35 g) mushrooms, sliced

2 cups (360 g) canned no-salt-added tomatoes

1 cup (235 ml) low sodium chicken broth

1 cup (134 g) frozen peas, thawed

$^1/_4$ teaspoon (0.5 g) black pepper

$^1/_4$ teaspoon (0.3 g) dried thyme

2 medium potatoes, peeled and chopped

1 tablespoon (0.4 g) dried parsley

$^1/_4$ teaspoon (0.3 g) dried oregano

In a large skillet or saucepan, combine turkey and paprika. Cook over medium heat, about 5 minutes. Remove turkey and set aside. Place onions, green bell pepper, garlic, celery, and mushrooms in skillet. Cook, stirring, about 4 minutes. Add remaining ingredients; mix well. Add turkey; cook, covered, over low heat about 40 minutes.

Yield: 6 servings

Per serving: 277 calories (8% from fat, 47% from protein, 45% from carbohydrate); 33 g protein; 3 g total fat; 1 g saturated fat; 0 g monounsaturated fat; 1 g polyunsaturated fat; 31 g carbohydrate; 6 g fiber; 6 g sugar; 379 mg phosphorus; 77 mg calcium; 4 mg iron; 203 mg sodium; 1274 mg potassium; 1044 IU vitamin A; 0 mg ATE vitamin E; 34 mg vitamin C; 68 mg cholesterol; 376 g water

Caribbean Fish Stew

This is a fairly spicy stew if you use the habanero pepper. I use a jalapeño instead, which still gives you some heat, but in moderation.

$^1/_2$ cup (65 g) carrot, sliced

1 cup (160 g) onion, sliced

2 tablespoons (28 g) grated fresh ginger

$^1/_2$ teaspoon (1.5 g) minced garlic

$^1/_2$ teaspoon (1 g) ground cloves

$^1/_2$ teaspoon (1 g) ground allspice

$^1/_2$ teaspoon (1 g) cardamom

$^1/_2$ teaspoon (1.1 g) turmeric

2 teaspoons (4 g) ground coriander

4 cups (360 g) canned no-salt-added tomatoes

12 ounces (355 ml) beer

1 habanero or jalapeño pepper, finely diced

2 medium potatoes, diced

1 pound tilapia (455 g) fillets, cut into 2-inch (5-cm) pieces

1 tablespoon (4 g) cilantro, chopped

$^1/_2$ cup (120 ml) lime juice

In a Dutch oven, sauté the carrot and onion until slightly soft, then add the ginger and garlic. When the vegetables are soft, add the cloves, allspice, cardamom, turmeric, and coriander and sauté about 1 minute longer. Add the tomatoes and beer and bring to a boil. Add the habanero pepper. Reduce the heat and let simmer for 20 minutes, then add the potatoes. When the potatoes are tender, add the fish. Cook another 5 minutes. Then add the cilantro and lime juice. Stir and serve.

Yield: 4 servings

Per serving: 395 calories (9% from fat, 32% from protein, 59% from carbohydrate); 31 g protein; 4 g total fat; 1 g saturated fat; 1 g monounsaturated fat; 1 g polyunsaturated fat; 56 g carbohydrate; 8 g fiber; 11 g sugar; 454 mg phosphorus; 181 mg calcium; 6 mg iron; 131 mg sodium; 2078 mg potassium; 3282 IU vitamin A; 53 mg ATE vitamin E; 59 mg vitamin C; 36 mg cholesterol; 589 g water

Tortillas

Newsletter subscriber Carla sent me this easy recipe for making flour tortillas. I have to admit they turned out well, and it wasn't nearly as difficult as I'd anticipated. I was afraid that it would be difficult to roll them thin enough, but it was actually easy to get them the way you find them at restaurants that hand make tortillas.

2 cups (250 g) flour

1 teaspoon (4.6 g) baking powder

1 tablespoon (14 g) unsalted butter

$^1/_2$ cup (120 ml) warm water

In a mixing bowl stir together flour and baking powder. Cut in butter until mixture resembles cornmeal. Add warm water and mix until dough can be gathered into a ball, adding more water if needed 1 tablespoon (15 ml) at a time. Let dough rest for 15 minutes. Divide dough into 12 portions; shape into balls. On a lightly floured surface roll each ball to a 7-inch (17.5-cm) round. Trim uneven edges to make a round tortilla. Cook in an ungreased skillet over medium heat (375°F, or 190°C) in an electric skillet) about $1^1/_2$ minutes per side, or until lightly browned.

Yield: 12 servings

Per serving: 84 calories (12% from fat, 10% from protein, 77% from carbohydrate); 2 g protein; 1 g total fat; 0 g saturated fat; 1 g monounsaturated fat; 0 g polyunsaturated fat; 16 g carbohydrate; 1 g fiber; 0 g sugar; 31 mg phosphorus; 24 mg calcium; 1 mg iron; 52 mg sodium; 24 mg potassium; 50 IU vitamin A; 11 mg ATE vitamin E; 0 mg vitamin C; 5 mg cholesterol; 13 g water

Whole Wheat Tortillas

It's easier than you think to make your own tortillas. For a long while I was afraid that I wouldn't be able to roll them thinly enough. Then I realized it doesn't matter. The ones real Mexican restaurants make on site are a lot thicker than the ones you get from the grocer's refrigerator case.

1 cup (120 g) whole wheat flour

$^1/_4$ teaspoon baking powder

$^1/_4$ teaspoon salt

$1^1/_2$ teaspoons (8 ml) oil

$^1/_4$ cup (60 ml) cold water

In bowl of food processor, combine flour, baking powder, and salt. Turn food processor on high and add oil. Add water gradually until mixture cleans sides of bowl and forms ball in center of bowl. Let the machine knead the dough for 2 minutes. Remove dough and divide into 4 parts. Let rest 10 minutes. Roll very thin on flour-covered board. Bake on lightly oiled or sprayed griddle. Turn when little bubbles appear and bake other side.

Yield: 4 servings

Per serving: 18 g water; 117 calories (16% from fat, 13% from protein, 70% from carb); 4 g protein; 2 g total fat; 0 g saturated fat; 1 g monounsaturated fat; 1 g polyunsaturated fat; 22 g carbohydrate; 4 g fiber; 0 g sugar; 110 mg phosphorus; 28 mg calcium; 1 mg iron; 180 mg sodium; 122 mg potassium; 3 IU vitamin A; 0 mg vitamin E; 0 mg vitamin C; 0 mg cholesterol

16

Cajun

We don't have a huge number of recipes in this chapter like some of the recent ones, but they are all favorites. There's more sausage recipes, this time for a substitute for garlicky, spicy andouille. There are some traditional Creole recipes. And then there are the Cajun ones that just couldn't be left out, such as gumbo, etouffee, jambalaya, and red beans and rice. Enough for several Mardi Gras celebrations.

Hot Creole Turkey Sausage

These are moderately spicy sausages. You can vary the heat by adjusting the amount of cayenne pepper.

1 jalapeño, stems and seed removed, chopped

$^1/_2$ teaspoon (0.9 g) cayenne pepper

1$^1/_2$ pounds (680 g) ground turkey

$^1/_2$ cup (80 g) onion, finely chopped

$^1/_2$ teaspoon (1.5 g) minced garlic

$^1/_2$ teaspoon (1 g) freshly ground black pepper

1 tablespoon (4 g) fresh parsley, minced

$^1/_4$ teaspoon (1.5 g) salt

$^1/_4$ teaspoon (0.3 g) dried thyme

1 bay leaf, crumbled

$^1/_8$ teaspoon allspice

$^1/_8$ teaspoon mace

Combine all ingredients and mix well (running the mixture through a grinder helps to ensure thorough mixing). Stuff casings and form into links or make into patties as desired. Refrigerate up to 3 days for flavors to blend. Sausages may be grilled, pan-fried, or oven-cooked.

Yield: 8 servings

Per serving: 151 calories (27% from fat, 70% from protein, 4% from carbohydrate); 25 g protein; 4 g total fat; 1 g saturated fat; 1 g monounsaturated fat; 1 g polyunsaturated fat; 1 g carbohydrate; 0 g fiber; 1 g sugar; 186 mg phosphorus; 26 mg calcium; 2 mg iron; 134 mg sodium; 280 mg potassium; 102 IU vitamin A; 0 mg ATE vitamin E; 2 mg vitamin C; 65 mg cholesterol; 66 g water

Tip: These are good for breakfast as well as a dinner meat and are a great addition to classic Cajun recipes such as jambalaya and gumbo.

Mild Cajun Turkey Sausage

This is a recipe for an andouille-type sausage. Not as hot as some Cajun sausages, this lower-fat version can be browned and crumbled into various dishes to give them that little extra bit of Cajun flavor.

1 pound (455 g) ground turkey

2 teaspoons (6 g) minced garlic

$^1/_4$ teaspoon (0.5 g) black pepper

$^1/_4$ teaspoon (0.5 g) cayenne pepper

1 teaspoon (5 ml) liquid smoke

$^1/_4$ teaspoon (0.6 g) paprika

$^1/_8$ teaspoon dried thyme

$^1/_8$ teaspoon dried sage

Mix spices thoroughly into turkey and grill, pan-fry, or bake as desired.

Yield: 8 servings

Per serving: 98 calories (27% from fat, 71% from protein, 2% from carbohydrate); 17 g protein; 3 g total fat; 1 g saturated fat; 1 g monounsaturated fat; 1 g polyunsaturated fat; 0 g carbohydrate; 0 g fiber; 0 g sugar; 122 mg phosphorus; 16 mg calcium; 1 mg iron; 40 mg sodium; 176 mg potassium; 62 IU vitamin A; 0 mg ATE vitamin E; 0 mg vitamin C; 43 mg cholesterol; 37 g water

Creole Sauce

This is perfect served with grilled chicken breasts or fish.

1 tablespoon (15 ml) olive oil

2 cups (320 g) onion, chopped

1 cup (150 g) yellow bell pepper, chopped

$^1/_2$ cup (60 g) celery, chopped

1 teaspoon (3 g) garlic, minced

4 cups (720 g) canned no-salt-added tomatoes, drained

1 cup (235 ml) low sodium chicken broth

1 teaspoon (0.8 g) fresh thyme

Heat oil in a heavy saucepan and cook onions, bell pepper, celery, and garlic over moderately low heat, stirring occasionally, until celery is softened. Add tomatoes, broth, and thyme and simmer sauce for 25 minutes, or until most of the liquid is evaporated.

Yield: 12 servings

Per serving: 43 calories (27% from fat, 13% from protein, 60% from carbohydrate); 2 g protein; 1 g total fat; 0 g saturated fat; 1 g monounsaturated fat; 0 g polyunsaturated fat; 7 g carbohydrate; 1 g fiber; 3 g sugar; 34 mg phosphorus; 36 mg calcium; 1 mg iron; 21 mg sodium; 252 mg potassium; 147 IU vitamin A; 0 mg ATE vitamin E; 38 mg vitamin C; 0 mg cholesterol; 137 g water

Tip: Sauce may be prepared 1 day ahead and kept chilled and covered, then reheated for serving.

Cajun Grilled Chicken

Nice Cajun flavor off the grill. Serve with rice and a steamed vegetable.

4 boneless chicken breasts

5 teaspoons (10 g) Cajun blackening spice mix

Cut slashes into the chicken $^1/_2$-inch (1.3-cm) deep to allow spices to penetrate the meat. Rub the spices into the chicken. Cook on a medium grill for about 25 minutes, or until done.

Yield: 4 servings

Per serving: 78 calories (11% from fat, 89% from protein, 0% from carbohydrate); 16 g protein; 1 g total fat; 0 g saturated fat; 0 g monounsaturated fat; 0 g polyunsaturated fat; 0 g carbohydrate; 0 g fiber; 0 g sugar; 139 mg phosphorus; 8 mg calcium; 1 mg iron; 46 mg sodium; 181 mg potassium; 15 IU vitamin A; 4 mg ATE vitamin E; 1 mg vitamin C; 41 mg cholesterol; 53 g water

Creole Chicken

This is a typical Creole recipe, with chicken cooked in a tomato-based sauce. It's good over rice or pasta.

$^1/_2$ cup (80 g) onion, chopped

1 cup (150 g) green bell pepper, chopped

2 cups (360 g) tomatoes, chopped

$^1/_2$ teaspoon (1.5 g) garlic powder

1 teaspoon (1 g) dried thyme

2 bay leaves

2 tablespoons (0.8 g) dried parsley

¹/₄ teaspoon (0.5 g) black pepper

¹/₈ teaspoon (0.3 g) cayenne pepper

2 boneless chicken breasts, cubed

In a heavy saucepan over high heat, cook the onion and green bell pepper, stirring, until they begin to color. Add the remaining ingredients. Cover and simmer for 10 to 15 minutes, or until chicken is cooked through.

Yield: 4 servings

Per serving: 73 calories (10% from fat, 50% from protein, 40% from carbohydrate); 10 g protein; 1 g total fat; 0 g saturated fat; 0 g monounsaturated fat; 0 g polyunsaturated fat; 8 g carbohydrate; 2 g fiber; 2 g sugar; 104 mg phosphorus; 24 mg calcium; 1 mg iron; 33 mg sodium; 369 mg potassium; 801 IU vitamin A; 2 mg ATE vitamin E; 54 mg vitamin C; 21 mg cholesterol; 151 g water

Chicken Creole with Mango

This recipe is a little more work than some, but it produces a very flavorful chicken. The fruit gives it that island character.

4 boneless chicken breasts

¹/₂ cup (120 ml) orange juice

¹/₄ cup (60 ml) lemon juice

1 teaspoon (3 g) minced garlic

¹/₄ teaspoon (0.5 g) black pepper

4 cups (946 ml) water

1 cup (150 g) green bell pepper, chopped

¹/₂ cup (65 g) carrots, sliced

1 cup (150 g) red bell pepper, chopped

1 cup (160 g) onion, cut in ¹/₂-inch (1.3-cm) slices

3 tablespoons (45 ml) cider vinegar

2 tablespoons (32 g) no-salt-added tomato paste

2 tablespoons (30 g) sugar

2 tablespoons (16 g) cornstarch

2 tablespoons (30 ml) water

2 mangoes, peeled, pitted and cut into ¹/₂-inch (1.3-cm) pieces

Combine chicken, orange juice, lemon juice, garlic, and black pepper in large bowl. Cover and let stand, turning occasionally, for 1 hour. Transfer chicken mixture to large saucepan; add water and green bell pepper. Heat to a boil, then reduce heat and simmer, covered, for 20 minutes, or until chicken is almost tender; remove chicken and pat dry. Meanwhile, skim grease from cooking liquid; add carrots, red bell pepper, onion, vinegar, tomato paste, and sugar. Dissolve cornstarch in water and stir into cooking liquid. Heat until mixture thickens and bubbles for 2 minutes; reduce heat. Add mangoes. Transfer chicken to platter. Spoon sauce over chicken.

Yield: 4 servings

Per serving: 283 calories (15% from fat, 26% from protein, 59% from carbohydrate); 19 g protein; 5 g total fat; 1 g saturated fat; 1 g monounsaturated fat; 2 g polyunsaturated fat; 43 g carbohydrate; 5 g fiber; 28 g sugar; 199 mg phosphorus; 56 mg calcium; 1 mg iron; 80 mg sodium; 772 mg potassium; 4954 IU vitamin A; 4 mg ATE vitamin E; 130 mg vitamin C; 41 mg cholesterol; 559 g water

Chicken Étouffée

One of the classic Cajun dishes, along with gumbo and jambalaya. Étouffée is meat served in a brown, tomato-flavored sauce. It's typically served over rice.

2 tablespoons (28 g) unsalted butter

1 cup (160 g) onion, chopped

1 tablespoon (8 g) flour

1 pound (455 g) boneless chicken breasts

$^3/_4$ cup (180 ml) water

2 tablespoons (30 ml) lemon juice

2 tablespoons (32 g) no-salt-added tomato paste

$^1/_4$ teaspoon (0.5 g) cayenne pepper

2 tablespoons (13 g) scallions, sliced

1 tablespoon (0.4 g) dried parsley

In a saucepan with a tight-fitting lid, melt butter, add onion, and cook over medium heat until tender. Stir in the flour, blend well. Add chicken, water, lemon, tomato paste, and cayenne pepper. Cook over low heat for 15 minutes, adding more water if necessary. Add scallions and parsley. Serve over steamed rice.

Yield: 4 servings

Per serving: 208 calories (31% from fat, 53% from protein, 15% from carbohydrate); 27 g protein; 7 g total fat; 5 g saturated fat; 2 g monounsaturated fat; 0 g polyunsaturated fat; 8 g carbohydrate; 1 g fiber; 3 g sugar; 249 mg phosphorus; 35 mg calcium; 1 mg iron; 147 mg sodium; 465 mg potassium; 607 IU vitamin A; 75 mg ATE vitamin E; 12 mg vitamin C; 76 mg cholesterol; 183 g water

Chicken Gumbo

Gumbo is *the* classic Cajun recipe, and this is one of my favorite recipes. Despite being low in sodium and fat, it has an excellent flavor that brings back memories of little restaurants just off Bourbon Street. Filé powder, or powdered sassafras leaves, is frequently used in Cajun cooking and acts as a flavoring and thickening agent.

2 pounds (905 g) boneless chicken breast

2 tablespoons (6 g) minced garlic

$^1/_4$ cup (60 ml) olive oil

1 cup (150 g) red bell peppers, chopped

1 cup (160 g) onion, chopped

$^1/_3$ cup (40 g) flour

2 cups (360 g) canned no-salt-added tomatoes

$^1/_2$ cup (90 g) frozen okra, thawed

$^1/_4$ teaspoon (1.3 ml) hot pepper sauce

1 tablespoon filé powder

Cook chicken with 5 cups (1.2 L) water and garlic until tender. Cut chicken into bite-sized pieces. Skim any fat off cooking liquid. Heat the oil in a skillet over medium heat and brown the red bell pepper and onions. Add the flour and brown. Gradually stir in some of the cooking liquid to make a roux (to desired thickness). Add tomatoes, cover and simmer for 30 minutes, adding more cooking liquid if needed. Add chicken and okra. Simmer for a few minutes. Season with hot pepper sauce. Add gumbo filé powder and stir until blended (it has a tendency to lump).

Yield: 8 servings

Per serving: 232 calories (33% from fat, 49% from protein, 18% from carbohydrate); 28 g protein; 8 g total fat; 1 g saturated fat; 5 g monounsaturated fat; 1 g

polyunsaturated fat; 11 g carbohydrate; 2 g fiber; 3 g sugar; 257 mg phosphorus; 47 mg calcium; 2 mg iron; 85 mg sodium; 504 mg potassium; 703 IU vitamin A; 7 mg ATE vitamin E; 34 mg vitamin C; 66 mg cholesterol; 184 g water

Cajun Chicken Kabobs

The yogurt, while not traditionally a Cajun ingredient, helps to keep the chicken moist and limit the spiciness.

1 pound (455 g) boneless chicken breast halves, cubed

5$^1/_2$ ounces (155 g) plain fat-free yogurt

1 tablespoon (9.6 g) Cajun seasoning

2 teaspoons (4 g) ground coriander

$^1/_2$ teaspoon (2.5 ml) lemon juice

1 cup (150 g) red bell pepper, diced

8 ounces (225 g) pineapple chunks

Preheat grill or broiler. Place the chicken in a bowl. Mix the yogurt, Cajun seasoning, coriander, and lemon juice together and stir into the chicken. Refrigerate for 10 to 15 minutes. Thread onto 4 large skewers, alternating with the red bell pepper and pineapple pieces. Place on the grill or under the broiler and cook for 10 to 15 minutes, turning occasionally, basting with any remaining marinade.

Yield: 4 servings

Per serving: 176 calories (9% from fat, 67% from protein, 24% from carbohydrate); 29 g protein; 2 g total fat; 0 g saturated fat; 0 g monounsaturated fat; 0 g polyunsaturated fat; 10 g carbohydrate; 1 g fiber; 9 g

sugar; 297 mg phosphorus; 105 mg calcium; 1 mg iron; 106 mg sodium; 557 mg potassium; 1233 IU vitamin A; 8 mg ATE vitamin E; 57 mg vitamin C; 67 mg cholesterol; 207 g water

Tip: We usually serve this over rice, but it's also good as part of a main dish salad.

Creole Chicken Spaghetti

This is a creamy, spicy dish that is typical of Creole cooking, which relies more heavily on the French influence than Cajun cooking does.

2 quarts (1.9 L) water

1 cup (160 g) onion, chopped, divided

1 cup (150 g) green bell pepper, chopped, divided

$^1/_2$ cup (50 g) celery, sliced, divided

$^1/_2$ teaspoon (1 g) black pepper

$^1/_2$ teaspoon (0.9 g) cayenne pepper

1 teaspoon (2.4 g) Cajun seasoning

1 pound (455 g) boneless chicken breast

2 tablespoons (30 ml) olive oil

1 cup (70 g) mushrooms, sliced

10.5-ounce (295-g) can low sodium cream of mushroom soup

$^1/_2$ cup (60 g) low fat Monterey Jack cheese, shredded

12 ounces (340 g) angel hair pasta

Bring water to a boil. Add $^1/_2$ cup (80 g) onion, $^1/_2$ cup (75 g) green pepper, and $^1/_4$ cup (25 g) celery. Stir in black pepper, cayenne pepper, and Cajun seasoning. Add boneless chicken breast and boil for 30 minutes, or until chicken is done. Strain and save cooking liquid. While chicken is cooking, heat olive oil in a skillet and sauté remaining bell pepper, onion, and celery until soft. When vegetables are almost done, add mushrooms and sauté until tender. Add cream of mushroom soup. Add cheese to vegetable mixture and stir until melted. Add 1 cup (235 ml) of reserved cooking liquid. Season vegetable mixture to taste with additional cayenne pepper and Cajun seasoning, if desired. Cut chicken into 1-inch (2.5-cm) cubes and add to mixture. Boil angel hair pasta in remaining cooking liquid according to package directions. Combine pasta with chicken sauce.

Yield: 4 servings

Per serving: 390 calories (30% from fat, 35% from protein, 35% from carbohydrate); 35 g protein; 13 g total fat; 3 g saturated fat; 6 g monounsaturated fat; 3 g polyunsaturated fat; 34 g carbohydrate; 6 g fiber; 5 g sugar; 420 mg phosphorus; 130 mg calcium; 2 mg iron; 218 mg sodium; 582 mg potassium; 413 IU vitamin A; 22 mg ATE vitamin E; 36 mg vitamin C; 70 mg cholesterol; 792 g water

Chicken with Okra

This makes a gumbo-like dish, almost a soup. It's best served over rice.

1 tablespoon (15 ml) olive oil

1 pound (455 g) boneless chicken breasts

1 cup (160 g) onion, coarsely chopped

1 cup (150 g) green bell peppers, coarsely chopped

$^1/_2$ cup (60 g) celery, sliced

$^1/_2$ teaspoon (1.5 g) minced garlic

$^2/_3$ pounds (305 g) okra, sliced

2 cups (360 g) tomatoes, chopped

$^1/_4$ cup (15 g) fresh parsley, chopped

$^1/_2$ teaspoon (1.3 g) paprika

1 bay leaf

$^1/_2$ cup (120 ml) low sodium chicken broth

$^1/_4$ cup (60 ml) white wine

$^1/_4$ teaspoon (1 ml) hot pepper sauce

Heat oil in a nonstick Dutch oven over medium heat. Add chicken and cook, stirring occasionally, for 10 minutes, or until brown on all sides. Remove chicken from pan. Add onion, green bell pepper, celery, and garlic; stir and cook for 5 minutes. Add okra and cook, stirring, for 5 minutes more. Stir in tomatoes, parsley, paprika, and bay leaf. Return chicken to Dutch oven and spoon vegetable mixture over top. In a small bowl, mix together chicken broth, wine and hot pepper sauce, pour over all. Cover, reduce heat to low, and cook for 30 minutes, or until chicken is done.

Yield: 4 servings

Per serving: 236 calories (21% from fat, 52% from protein, 27% from carbohydrate); 30 g protein; 5 g total fat; 1 g saturated fat; 3 g monounsaturated fat; 1 g polyunsaturated fat; 16 g carbohydrate; 5 g fiber; 4 g sugar; 322 mg phosphorus; 106 mg calcium; 2 mg iron; 174 mg sodium; 905 mg potassium; 1439 IU vitamin A; 7 mg ATE vitamin E; 75 mg vitamin C; 66 mg cholesterol; 351 g water

Slow Cooker Chicken Jambalaya

I'm a big fan of jambalaya and similar rice dishes. This is an easy way to make it, simple in preparation. And there's something very nice about coming home to a house that smells of Cajun cooking.

1 pound (455 g) boneless chicken breast

$^1/_2$ pound (225 g) Mild Cajun Turkey Sausage (see recipe page 348)

4 cups (720 g) canned no-salt-added tomatoes

$^1/_2$ cup (80 g) onion, chopped

$^1/_2$ cup (75 g) green pepper, chopped

1 cup (235 ml) low sodium chicken broth

$^1/_2$ cup (120 ml) white wine

2 teaspoons (2 g) dried oregano

2 teaspoons (0.2 g) dried parsley

2 teaspoons (5 g) Cajun seasoning

1 teaspoon (1.8 g) cayenne pepper

2 cups (330 g) cooked rice

Cut up chicken and crumble sausage. Add to slow cooker along with onion and green pepper. Add remaining ingredients, except rice. Cook on low for 6 to 8 hours. Half an hour before eating, add cooked rice; heat through.

Yield: 6 servings

Per serving: 202 calories (8% from fat, 45% from protein, 47% from carbohydrate); 21 g protein; 2 g total fat; 0 g saturated fat; 0 g monounsaturated fat; 0 g polyunsaturated fat; 22 g carbohydrate; 3 g fiber; 4 g sugar; 227 mg phosphorus; 79 mg calcium; 3 mg iron; 85 mg sodium; 607 mg potassium; 430 IU vitamin A; 5 mg ATE vitamin E; 27 mg vitamin C; 44 mg cholesterol; 312 g water

Chicken Jambalaya

I love a good jambalaya, and I have to admit stirring up quick and dirty jambalaya-ish dishes for many a Saturday lunch. This one is a little more effort, but it's worth it in my opinion.

1 pound (455 g) boneless chicken breast

4 cups (946 ml) water

2 cups (320 g) onion, chopped

$^1/_2$ cup (60 g) celery

3 tablespoons (30 g) garlic, minced

1 tablespoon (15 ml) olive oil

$^1/_2$ pound (225 g) Mild Cajun Turkey Sausage (see recipe page 348)

$^1/_2$ cup (75 g) green bell peppers

$^1/_4$ cup (25 g) scallions

2 cups (360 g) canned no-salt-added tomatoes, undrained

2 tablespoons (30 ml) Worcestershire sauce

$^1/_4$ teaspoon (0.3 g) dried thyme

$^1/_4$ teaspoon (0.5 g) cayenne pepper

2 cups (370 g) long-grain rice

In a large saucepan, combine the chicken breast, the water, half the chopped onion, half the chopped celery, and one-third of the garlic. Bring to a simmer over medium-high heat. Reduce the heat to medium-low and cook, partially covered, for 20 to 25 minutes, or until the chicken juices run clear when pierced with a fork. Remove the chicken breasts from the cooking liquid. In a sieve set over a large bowl, drain and reserve the cooking liquid, discarding the solids. You should have about 4 cups (946 ml) of liquid; add water, if necessary. Chop the breast meat coarsely and set it aside. Heat the oil in a 5-quart (4.7-L) Dutch oven. Add the sausage and cook over medium heat, stirring often, for 5 minutes, or until lightly browned. Then stir in the reserved cooking liquid; the remaining, onion, celery, and garlic; the green bell peppers; scallions; tomatoes with their juice; Worcestershire sauce; thyme; and cayenne pepper. Bring to a simmer, breaking up the tomatoes with a spoon. Stir in the rice and return to a simmer. Cook over medium-low heat, tightly covered, until the rice has absorbed all the liquid, about 25 minutes. Remove the Dutch oven from the heat, stir in the reserved chicken, cover, and let stand for 5 minutes.

Yield: 6 servings

Per serving: 439 calories (15% from fat, 27% from protein, 58% from carbohydrate); 29 g protein; 7 g total fat; 2 g saturated fat; 3 g monounsaturated fat; 1 g polyunsaturated fat; 63 g carbohydrate; 3 g fiber; 6 g sugar; 338 mg phosphorus; 92 mg calcium; 8 mg iron; 235 mg sodium; 682 mg potassium; 328 IU vitamin A; 21 mg ATE vitamin E; 45 mg vitamin C; 64 mg cholesterol; 397 g water

Blackened Salmon

Salmon blackened the Cajun way. This is one of the spicier recipes in this book. You can reduce the amount of cayenne pepper to suit your taste buds.

2 tablespoons (14 g) paprika

1 tablespoon (5 g) cayenne pepper

1 tablespoon (9 g) onion powder

$^1/_2$ teaspoon (1 g) white pepper

$^1/_2$ teaspoon (1 g) black pepper

$^1/_4$ teaspoon (0.3 g) dried thyme

$^1/_4$ teaspoon (0.2 g) dried basil

$^1/_4$ teaspoon (0.3 g) dried oregano

1 pound (455 g) salmon fillets

2 tablespoons (30 ml) olive oil

In a small bowl, mix paprika, cayenne pepper, onion powder, white pepper, black pepper, thyme, basil, and oregano. Brush salmon fillets on both sides with oil, and sprinkle evenly with the cayenne pepper mixture. Drizzle one side of each fillet with half the remaining oil. In a large, heavy skillet over high heat, cook salmon, oiled side down, for 2 to 5 minutes, or until blackened. Turn fillets, drizzle with remaining oil, and continue cooking until blackened and fish flakes easily with a fork.

Yield: 4 servings

Per serving: 289 calories (61% from fat, 32% from protein, 6% from carbohydrate); 23 g protein; 20 g total fat; 4 g saturated fat; 9 g monounsaturated fat; 6 g polyunsaturated fat; 5 g carbohydrate; 2 g fiber; 1 g sugar; 287 mg phosphorus; 33 mg calcium; 2 mg iron; 70 mg sodium; 541 mg potassium; 2439 IU vitamin A; 17 mg ATE vitamin E; 8 mg vitamin C; 67 mg cholesterol; 79 g water

Cajun Snapper

Somewhat spicy grilled snapper fillets. We prefer this with plain brown rice to help balance the more intense flavor of the fish.

2 pounds (910 g) snapper fillet

1 teaspoon (5 ml) hot pepper sauce

2 tablespoons (6 g) dried dill

$^1/_4$ cup (25 g) scallions, chopped

$^1/_4$ cup (38 g) green bell pepper, chopped

$^1/_4$ cup (38 g) red bell pepper, chopped

1 teaspoon (2.6 g) filé powder

1 cup (235 ml) sauterne wine

Lay snapper fillets in a pan that you have sprayed liberally with nonstick vegetable oil spray. Mix remaining ingredients together and pour over the fish. Cover the pan and marinate for 2 to 6 hours. Broil fish in oven or grill to desired doneness.

Yield: 6 servings

Per serving: 191 calories (12% from fat, 81% from protein, 7% from carbohydrate); 31 g protein; 2 g total fat; 0 g saturated fat; 0 g monounsaturated fat; 1 g polyunsaturated fat; 3 g carbohydrate; 0 g fiber; 1 g sugar; 317 mg phosphorus; 74 mg calcium; 1 mg iron; 107 mg sodium; 729 mg potassium; 483 IU vitamin A; 45 mg ATE vitamin E; 17 mg vitamin C; 56 mg cholesterol; 166 g water

Creole-Style Catfish

A simple, Creole-style recipe.

1 tablespoon (15 ml) olive oil

1 cup (160 g) onion, chopped

$^1/_2$ cup (50 g) celery, chopped

$^1/_2$ cup (75 g) green bell pepper, chopped

1 clove garlic, minced

2 cups (360 g) canned no-salt-added tomatoes

1 lemon, sliced

1 tablespoon (15 ml) Worcestershire sauce

1 tablespoon (7 g) paprika

1 bay leaf

$^1/_4$ teaspoon (0.3 g) dried thyme

$^1/_4$ teaspoon (1 ml) hot pepper sauce

2 pounds (905 g) catfish fillets

Heat the oil in a large skillet over medium heat. Add the onion, celery, green pepper, and garlic. Cook until soft. Add tomatoes and their liquid. Break the tomatoes with a spoon. Add lemon slices, Worcestershire sauce, paprika, bay leaf, thyme, and hot pepper sauce. Cook, stirring occasionally, for 15 minutes, or until the sauce is slightly thickened. Press fish pieces down into sauce and spoon some of the sauce over the top of the fish. Cover the pan and simmer gently for 10 minutes, or until the fish flakes easily with a fork. Serve over hot cooked rice.

Yield: 6 servings

Per serving: 260 calories (49% from fat, 38% from protein, 13% from carbohydrate); 25 g protein; 14 g total fat; 3 g saturated fat; 7 g monounsaturated fat; 3 g polyunsaturated fat; 9 g carbohydrate; 2 g fiber; 4 g sugar; 341 mg phosphorus; 55 mg calcium; 2 mg iron; 125 mg sodium; 746 mg potassium; 870 IU vitamin A; 23 mg ATE vitamin E; 31 mg vitamin C; 71 mg cholesterol; 242 g water

Tip: You can substitute any other white fish for the catfish.

Black-Eyed Pea Gumbo

Looking for a chili alternative? This could fit the bill. It has great flavor and is a lot lower in fat.

1 pound (455 g) black-eyed peas

1 tablespoon (15 ml) olive oil

1 cup (160 g) onion, chopped

$^1/_2$ cup (75 g) green bell pepper, chopped

$^1/_2$ cup (60 g) celery, chopped

2 cups (470 ml) low sodium chicken broth

1 cup (190 g) brown rice

2 cups (360 g) canned no-salt-added tomatoes

4 ounces (112 g) canned jalapeño, diced

$^1/_2$ teaspoon (1.5 g) minced garlic

Cook black-eyed peas according to package directions. Drain. Heat the olive oil in a large saucepan over medium heat and cook the onion, green bell pepper, and celery until tender. Add the chicken broth, rice, cooked black-eyed peas, tomatoes, jalapeño, and garlic. Bring to a boil, reduce heat to low, and simmer 45 minutes, or until rice is tender. Add water if soup is too thick.

Yield: 8 servings

Per serving: 210 calories (14% from fat, 16% from protein, 70% from carbohydrate); 9 g protein; 3 g total fat; 1 g saturated fat; 2 g monounsaturated fat; 1 g polyunsaturated fat; 38 g carbohydrate; 6 g fiber; 6 g sugar; 188 mg phosphorus; 51 mg calcium; 3 mg iron; 273 mg sodium; 519 mg potassium; 417 IU vitamin A; 0 mg ATE vitamin E; 18 mg vitamin C; 0 mg cholesterol; 199 g water

Hopping John Soup

This soup has a flavor of Hopping John, which is usually made as a skillet dish. The greens add an additional layer of flavor. This would make a good New Year's Day lunch, since you are supposed to eat black-eyed peas then for good luck.

$^1/_2$ cup (125 g) dried black-eyed peas

1 cup (235 ml) water

3 cups (710 ml) low sodium chicken broth

$^1/_4$ teaspoon (0.3 g) red pepper flakes

$^1/_2$ teaspoon (1.5 g) minced garlic

$^1/_4$ cup (50 g) uncooked rice

$^1/_2$ cup (80 g) onion, chopped

$^1/_2$ cup (75 g) green bell pepper, chopped

$^1/_4$ teaspoon (0.5 g) black pepper

1 teaspoon (2 g) celery seed

1 cup (235 ml) low sodium vegetable juice, such as V8

2 cubes low sodium chicken bouillon

2 cups (72 g) collard greens, chopped

Bring black-eyed peas, water, and broth to a boil in a large saucepan or Dutch oven. Boil uncovered for 2 minutes; remove from heat. Cover and let stand for 1 hour. Do not drain. Stir in red pepper flakes and garlic. Heat to a boil, then reduce heat, cover, and simmer for 1 to 1$^1/_2$ hours, or until black-eyed peas are tender. (Do not boil or peas will burst.) Stir in rice, onions, green bell pepper, black pepper, celery seed, vegetable juice, and bouillon cubes. Cover and simmer for 25 minutes, stirring occasionally. Cut stems out of the center of the collard green leaves. Slice and chop in small strips. Stir in collard greens and simmer until heated through.

Per serving: 109 calories (14% from fat, 25% from protein, 61% from carbohydrate); 7 g protein; 2 g total fat; 0 g saturated fat; 1 g monounsaturated fat; 0 g polyunsaturated fat; 18 g carbohydrate; 3 g fiber; 5 g sugar; 114 mg phosphorus; 69 mg calcium; 2 mg iron; 152 mg sodium; 466 mg potassium; 2244 IU vitamin A; 0 mg ATE vitamin E; 41 mg vitamin C; 0 mg cholesterol; 362 g water

Creole Beans

A taste of New Orleans, great with blackened chicken or fish.

$^1/_4$ cup (25 g) sliced celery

$^1/_4$ cup (40 g) coarsely chopped onion

$^1/_4$ cup (38 g) chopped green bell pepper

1 teaspoon unsalted butter

2 cups (480 g) no-salt-added canned tomatoes

$^1/_8$ teaspoon garlic powder

$^1/_8$ teaspoon black pepper

$1^1/_4$ cups (228 g) cooked navy beans

Cook celery, onion, and bell pepper in butter until tender—about 5 minutes. Break up large pieces of tomatoes. Add tomatoes and seasonings to cooked vegetables. Bring to a boil. Add beans and return to a boil. Reduce heat, cover, and simmer gently until flavors are blended and liquid is reduced—about 30 minutes. Stir occasionally to prevent sticking.

Yield: 2 servings

Per serving: 347 g water; 231 calories (11% from fat, 19% from protein, 70% from carb); 12 g protein; 3 g total fat; 1 g saturated fat; 1 g monounsaturated fat; 1 g polyunsaturated fat; 42 g carbohydrate; 15 g fiber; 8 g sugar; 223 mg phosphorus; 165 mg calcium; 5 mg iron; 43 mg sodium; 991 mg potassium; 472 IU vitamin A; 16 mg vitamin E; 39 mg vitamin C; 5 mg cholesterol

Cajun Red Beans and Rice

I've always been a fan of red beans and rice, although most of the packaged ones leave a lot to be desired from a healthy cooking standpoint. So I began experimenting. This is my favorite so far, producing a nice "gravy" with just enough heat, without being overpowering, and just slightly sweet. Feel free to vary the amount of spices to suit your idea of how hot they should be.

1 pound (455 g) dried kidney beans

6 cups (1.4 L) water

2 teaspoons (10 ml) hot pepper sauce

$^1/_2$ teaspoon (3 ml) Worcestershire sauce

2 tablespoons (30 ml) oil

$^3/_4$ cup (112 g) green bell pepper, chopped

1 cup (100 g) scallions, chopped

1 cup (160 g) onions, chopped

$^1/_2$ teaspoon (1.5 g) minced garlic

2 teaspoons (10 g) brown sugar

$^1/_4$ cup (30 g) flour

$^1/_2$ teaspoon (1 g) black pepper

$^1/_2$ teaspoon (1.2 g) Cajun seasoning

Place beans in a large pot and cover with water. Add hot pepper sauce and Worcestershire and allow to soak overnight. Heat oil in a large skillet over medium-high heat and sauté the green bell pepper, scallions, and onions until onions are soft. Add garlic, brown sugar, and flour. Stir constantly over medium heat for 5 to 6 minutes, or until browned. Add to pot with beans. Cook over low heat for 2 to 3 hours, or until beans are soft and mixture is thickened. Stir occasionally, adding water as needed. Add pepper and Cajun seasoning to suit your taste. Serve with rice.

Yield: 8 servings

Per serving: 136 calories (24% from fat, 17% from protein, 59% from carbohydrate); 6 g protein; 4 g total fat; 1 g saturated fat; 1 g monounsaturated fat; 2 g polyunsaturated fat; 21 g carbohydrate; 5 g fiber; 3 g sugar; 99 mg phosphorus; 39 mg calcium; 2 mg iron; 155 mg sodium; 333 mg potassium; 197 IU vitamin A; 0 mg ATE vitamin E; 16 mg vitamin C; 0 mg cholesterol; 259 g water

Cajun Rice

Just a little spicy, enough to give you that Cajun flavor. If you like more heat, add a little more hot pepper sauce. This makes quite a lot, which is good for me because I take the leftovers to work for lunch. You could halve the quantities if you want less.

2 tablespoons (30 ml) olive oil

$^1/_2$ cup (80 g) onion, chopped

$^1/_2$ cup (75 g) green bell pepper, chopped

$^1/_2$ cup (50 g) scallions, chopped

$^1/_2$ teaspoon (1.5 g) garlic, crushed

1 cup (70 g) mushrooms, sliced

2 cups (360 g) canned no-salt-added tomatoes

$^1/_4$ cup (35 g) chopped green chiles

1 teaspoon (2.4 g) Cajun seasoning

$^1/_4$ cup (15 g) chopped fresh cilantro

$^1/_8$ teaspoon hot pepper sauce

4 cups (660 g) cooked brown rice

Heat oil in a large skillet over medium-high heat and sauté the onion, green bell pepper, scallions, garlic, and mushrooms for 5 to 10 minutes, or until soft. Add the remaining ingredients except rice and mix well. Stir in the cooked rice, heat through, and serve.

Yield: 8 servings

Per serving: 394 calories (14% from fat, 9% from protein, 77% from carbohydrate); 8 g protein; 6 g total fat; 1 g saturated fat; 3 g monounsaturated fat; 1 g polyunsaturated fat; 76 g carbohydrate; 5 g fiber; 3 g sugar; 336 mg phosphorus; 51 mg calcium; 2 mg iron; 35 mg sodium; 408 mg potassium; 262 IU vitamin A; 0 mg ATE vitamin E; 17 mg vitamin C; 0 mg cholesterol; 103 g water

Okra Pilaf

A Cajun version of rice pilaf, with okra and tomatoes added. This makes a great side dish with blackened fish.

2 cups (200 g) okra, thinly sliced

2 slices low sodium bacon, diced

1 cup (150 g) green bell pepper, chopped

1 cup (160 g) onion, chopped

1 cup (195 g) uncooked rice

2 cups (470 ml) low sodium chicken broth

2 cups (360 g) canned no-salt-added tomatoes

In a large skillet, sauté okra and bacon until lightly browned. Add green bell peppers and onions; continue cooking until vegetables are crisp-tender. Add rice and chicken broth. Bring to a boil, stir once, cover, reduce heat and simmer for 20 minutes, or until rice is tender and liquid is absorbed. Add tomatoes; heat through and fluff with a fork.

Yield: 4 servings

Per serving: 149 calories (16% from fat, 19% from protein, 64% from carbohydrate); 8 g protein; 3 g total fat; 1 g saturated fat; 1 g monounsaturated fat; 0 g polyunsaturated fat; 26 g carbohydrate; 4 g fiber; 6 g sugar; 152 mg phosphorus; 103 mg calcium; 3 mg iron; 100 mg sodium; 649 mg potassium; 468 IU vitamin A; 0 mg ATE vitamin E; 55 mg vitamin C; 4 mg cholesterol; 372 g water

17

Salads

Salads are a natural choice for heart healthy eating. Whether it be the simplest vegetable salad or something more elaborate, they are full of nutritious vegetables, are naturally low in fat, and often contain significant amounts of fiber. We have some of those simple salads here, but also a lot of others including fruit salads, marinated vegetables, molds, dinner salads, and LOTS of salads featuring fiber-rich beans and other legumes.

Broccoli and Tomato Salad

As pretty as it is tasty, this salad is great with a piece of grilled meat or an egg dish like quiche.

1 pound (455 g) broccoli

1/4 pound (115 g) mushrooms

3/4 cup (75 g) olives, drained

8 ounces (225 g) cherry tomatoes

Dressing

1/3 cup (80 ml) olive oil

1 tablespoon (15 ml) white wine vinegar

1 tablespoon (15 ml) lemon juice

2 tablespoons chopped fresh parsley

1/4 cup (25 g) minced scallions

1/4 teaspoon minced garlic

1/4 teaspoon black pepper, fresh ground

Trim florets from broccoli, you should have about 1 quart (1 L). Reserve stems for another use. Drop broccoli florets into boiling water for 1 minute or just until they turn bright green; drain. Trim mushroom stems to 1/2 inch (1 cm). Combine broccoli, mushrooms, olives, and cherry tomatoes in bowl. Measure oil, vinegar, lemon juice, parsley, scallions, garlic, and pepper into small bowl. Whisk until blended. Pour dressing over vegetable mixture. Turn gently to coat vegetables. Cover and refrigerate 3 hours or more until ready to serve.

Yield: 4 servings

Per serving: 162 g water; 249 calories (72% from fat, 7% from protein, 20% from carb); 5 g protein; 21 g total fat; 3 g saturated fat; 15 g monounsaturated fat; 2 g polyunsaturated fat; 13 g carbohydrate; 5 g fiber; 3 g sugar; 104 mg phosphorus; 88 mg calcium; 2 mg iron; 261 mg sodium; 603 mg potassium; 1351 IU vitamin A; 0 mg vitamin E; 117 mg vitamin C; 0 mg cholesterol

Tip: This is a colorful salad to serve in a glass bowl.

Broccoli Cauliflower Salad

Simple salad that is good with grilled meat or any of a number of other meals.

1 pound (455 g) broccoli, cut in florets

1 pound (455 g) cauliflower, cut in florets

1 cup (160 g) thinly sliced red onion

1/2 cup (115 g) mayonnaise

1/4 cup (60 ml) vinegar

1/4 cup (50 g) sugar

1/4 cup (60 ml) salad oil

3 tablespoons (45 ml) mustard

Mix broccoli and cauliflower florets. Add onion and combine other ingredients. Pour over vegetables. Refrigerate 2 hours before serving.

Yield: 6 servings

Per serving: 174 g water; 307 calories (69% from fat, 6% from protein, 25% from carb); 4 g protein; 24 g total fat; 4 g saturated fat; 10 g monounsaturated fat; 9 g polyunsaturated fat; 20 g carbohydrate; 4 g fiber; 13 g sugar; 88 mg phosphorus; 63 mg calcium; 1 mg iron; 143 mg sodium; 413 mg potassium; 538 IU vitamin A; 15 mg vitamin E; 103 mg vitamin C; 7 mg cholesterol

Confetti Salad

Colorful, tasty, and good for you—what more could you ask? This makes a lot of salad, so you might want to cut the amounts in half, which is easier if you use frozen vegetables.

1 cup (150 g) peas

1 cup (164 g) white corn

2 cups (328 g) chickpeas

4 ounces (115 g) pimento, cut in strips

1 cup (150 g) green bell pepper, cut in strips

1 cup (100 g) green beans

1 cup (130 g) sliced carrot

1 cup (100 g) sliced celery

$1/4$ cup (25 g) sliced scallions

$1/2$ teaspoon black pepper, fresh ground

1 teaspoon celery seed

Dressing

$3/4$ cup (180 ml) vinegar

1 cup (200 g) sugar

$1/2$ cup (120 ml) olive oil

Drain liquid from any canned vegetables. Layer vegetables in bowl. Sprinkle with pepper and celery seed. To make the dressing, heat vinegar and sugar until sugar dissolves. Add oil. Cool slightly, pour over vegetables. Stir gently. Cover tightly. Marinate at least a day before serving.

Yield: 15 servings

Per serving: 89 g water; 185 calories (37% from fat, 6% from protein, 57% from carb); 3 g protein; 8 g total fat; 1 g saturated fat; 5 g monounsaturated fat; 1 g polyunsaturated fat; 27 g carbohydrate; 3 g fiber; 15 g sugar; 58 mg phosphorus; 28 mg calcium; 1 mg iron; 171 mg sodium; 195 mg potassium; 2002 IU vitamin A; 0 mg vitamin E; 19 mg vitamin C; 0 mg cholesterol

Corn Salad

Slightly sweet from the apple and very crunchy, this salad is great with barbecued meats.

1 cup (150 g) diced green bell pepper

1 avocado, cubed

1 cup (150 g) chopped apple

2 cups (328 g) corn, cooked and cooled

1 teaspoon Dijon mustard

1 tablespoon (15 ml) red wine vinegar

3 tablespoons (45 ml) olive oil

Place pepper, avocado, apple, and corn in salad bowl. Stir to mix. Combine remaining ingredients and pour over salad, tossing lightly.

Yield: 4 servings

Per serving: 151 g water; 234 calories (56% from fat, 5% from protein, 38% from carb); 3 g protein; 16 g total fat; 2 g saturated fat; 11 g monounsaturated fat; 2 g polyunsaturated fat; 24 g carbohydrate; 5 g fiber; 6 g sugar; 77 mg phosphorus; 14 mg calcium; 1 mg iron; 23 mg sodium; 386 mg potassium; 201 IU vitamin A; 0 mg vitamin E; 37 mg vitamin C; 0 mg cholesterol

Tip: For a Mexican salad, omit the apple and add a teaspoon of ground cumin to the dressing.

Pea Salad

Quick, how many kinds of peas can you name? This salad probably contains all of them.

1 cup (164 g) cooked chickpeas, drained and rinsed

1 cup (172 g) cooked black-eyed peas, drained

1 cup (130 g) frozen peas, cooked and cooled

$^1/_2$ cup (80 g) finely chopped onion

$^3/_4$ cup (114 g) finely chopped green bell pepper

$^1/_2$ cup (100 g) sugar

$^1/_3$ cup (78 ml) cider vinegar

$^1/_2$ cup (120 ml) olive oil

$^1/_4$ teaspoon black pepper

In a shallow container stir together all ingredients. Cover tightly and chill.

Yield: 6 servings

Per serving: 98 g water; 339 calories (50% from fat, 8% from protein, 43% from carb); 7 g protein; 19 g total fat; 3 g saturated fat; 13 g monounsaturated fat; 2 g polyunsaturated fat; 37 g carbohydrate; 6 g fiber; 22 g sugar; 113 mg phosphorus; 33 mg calcium; 2 mg iron; 92 mg sodium; 293 mg potassium; 662 IU vitamin A; 0 mg vitamin E; 20 mg vitamin C; 0 mg cholesterol 7

Tip: May be served on lettuce and garnished with cherry tomatoes or pimento and sliced cucumbers.

Curried Broccoli and Tomato Salad

A nice change of pace, with the broccoli and curry flavors adding an unusual twist.

$^1/_2$ pound (225 g) broccoli florets

1 cup (230 g) fat-free sour cream

$^1/_4$ cup (60 ml) skim milk

$^1/_2$ teaspoon (1 g) curry powder

$^1/_4$ teaspoon (0.8 g) dry mustard

$2^1/_2$ cups (50 g) lettuce

3 cups (540 g) tomatoes, cut in wedges

Steam broccoli for 5 minutes, or until crisp-tender. Drain and cool. Combine sour cream, milk, curry powder, and mustard. Pour over broccoli and refrigerate for 2 to 3 hours. To serve, divide lettuce between plates and arrange tomatoes and broccoli on top.

Yield: 5 servings

Per serving: 108 calories (8% from fat, 27% from protein, 65% from carbohydrate); 4 g protein; 1 g total fat; 0 g saturated fat; 0 g monounsaturated fat; 0 g polyunsaturated fat; 10 g carbohydrate; 1 g fiber; 1 g sugar; 119 mg phosphorus; 102 mg calcium; 1 mg iron; 51 mg sodium; 486 mg potassium; 2307 IU vitamin A; 56 mg ATE vitamin E; 67 mg vitamin C; 19 mg cholesterol; 209 g water

Fiesta Salad

A simple but flavorful main-dish salad. Good for those warmer spring evenings.

2 tablespoons (28 ml) olive oil

2 tablespoons (28 ml) lime juice

1 tablespoon (15 ml) lemon juice

$1/4$ teaspoon garlic powder

$1/2$ teaspoon cumin

$1/4$ teaspoon oregano

1 boneless chicken breast

4 cups (220 g) Romaine lettuce

16 cherry tomatoes

1 avocado, peeled and sliced

$1/4$ cup (27 g) shredded Swiss cheese

$1/2$ cup (36 g) crumbled tortilla chips

2 tablespoons (30 g) fat-free sour cream

$1/4$ cup (65 g) salsa

Combine first 6 ingredients in a resealable plastic bag. Add chicken breast and marinate at least 2 hours, turning occasionally. Grill or sauté chicken breast until no longer pink. Cut into $1/2$-inch-thick (1-cm) slices. Divide lettuce between two plates. Top with tomatoes, avocado, and chicken. Sprinkle with cheese and tortilla chips. Combine sour cream and salsa and pour over.

Yield: 2 servings

Per serving: 236 g water; 457 calories (55% from fat, 16% from protein, 28% from carb); 19 g protein; 28 g total fat; 4 g saturated fat; 18 g monounsaturated fat; 4 g polyunsaturated fat; 32 g carbohydrate; 10 g fiber; 3 g sugar; 315 mg phosphorus; 268 mg calcium; 3 mg iron; 263 mg sodium; 1187 mg potassium; 6614 IU vitamin A; 24 mg vitamin E; 64 mg vitamin C; 33 mg cholesterol

Grilled Vegetable Orzo Salad

We made this to have with a grilled chicken breast, thinking we might as well put the rest of the grill to use while it was on. The leftovers provided lunch for several days.

1 cup (124 g) zucchini, cut into 1-inch (2.5-cm) cubes

$1/2$ cup (75 g) red bell pepper, cut into 1-inch (2.5-cm) cubes

$1/2$ cup (75 g) yellow bell pepper, cut into 1-inch (2.5-cm) cubes

1 cup (160 g) red onion, cut into 1-inch (2.5-cm) cubes

$1/2$ teaspoon (1.5 g) minced garlic

3 tablespoons (45 ml) olive oil, divided

1 teaspoon (2 g) freshly ground black pepper, divided

8 ounces (225 g) orzo

$1/3$ cup (80 ml) lemon juice

$1/4$ cup (35 g) pine nuts, toasted

Prepare the grill. Toss zucchini, bell peppers, onion, and garlic with 1 tablespoon (15 ml) olive oil and $1/2$ teaspoon (1 g) pepper in a large bowl. Transfer to a grill basket. Grill for 15 to 20 minutes, or until browned, stirring occasionally. Meanwhile, cook the orzo according to package directions. Drain and transfer to a large serving bowl. Add the roasted vegetables to the pasta. Combine the lemon juice and remaining olive oil and pepper and pour on the pasta and vegetables. Let cool to room temperature. Stir in the pine nuts.

Yield: 8 servings

Per serving: 201 calories (37% from fat, 10% from protein, 53% from carbohydrate); 5 g protein; 9 g total fat; 1 g saturated fat; 5 g monounsaturated fat; 2 g polyunsaturated fat; 27 g carbohydrate; 2 g fiber; 3 g sugar; 99 mg phosphorus; 19 mg calcium; 2 mg iron; 5 mg sodium; 244 mg potassium; 373 IU vitamin A; 0 mg ATE vitamin E; 63 mg vitamin C; 0 mg cholesterol; 75 g water

Marinated Cauliflower Salad

Yes, it says cauliflower salad, but this dish also gets a nice fiber boost from tomatoes, carrots, and artichokes.

2 cups (200 g) cauliflower, cut into florets

1 cup (300 g) artichoke hearts, drained and quartered

12 cherry tomatoes, halved

$^1/_2$ cup (65 g) thinly sliced carrot

$^1/_2$ cup (80 g) red onion, peeled, sliced, separated into rings

1 cup (130 g) frozen peas, thawed and drained

2 tablespoons (16 g) sesame seeds, toasted

$^1/_2$ cup (120 ml) Italian dressing

Combine vegetables and sesame seeds in large container. Stir in dressing. Cover and refrigerate several hours.

Yield: 6 servings

Per serving: 116 g water; 143 calories (49% from fat, 11% from protein, 39% from carb); 4 g protein; 8 g total fat; 1 g saturated fat; 2 g monounsaturated fat; 4 g polyunsaturated fat; 15 g carbohydrate; 5 g fiber; 5 g sugar; 94 mg phosphorus; 75 mg calcium; 2 mg iron; 440 mg sodium; 338 mg potassium; 2624 IU vitamin A; 0 mg vitamin E; 30 mg vitamin C; 0 mg cholesterol

Marinated Mediterranean Vegetables

This is a great salad with just a piece of meat, or as the main dish with a little chicken or seafood added.

$^1/_2$ cup (120 ml) olive oil

$^1/_4$ cup (60 ml) red wine vinegar

1 tablespoon (15 ml) light corn syrup

1 teaspoon dried basil

$^1/_2$ teaspoon black pepper

$^1/_2$ cup (35 g) sliced mushrooms

$^3/_4$ pound (340 g) fresh asparagus, slightly cooked, cut into 2-inch (5-cm) pieces

1 cup (164 g) cooked chickpeas, drained

$^1/_4$ cup (25 g) sliced black olives

$^1/_4$ cup (25 g) sliced green olives

10 ounces (280 g) artichoke hearts, cooked

1 cup (160 g) thinly sliced red onion

Combine first 5 ingredients. Add to all vegetables in nonaluminum bowl. Marinate at least 1 hour or overnight. Drain and serve on lettuce leaves.

Yield: 4 servings

Per serving: 255 g water; 419 calories (62% from fat, 7% from protein, 30% from carb); 8 g protein; 30 g total fat; 4 g saturated fat; 21 g monounsaturated fat; 4 g polyunsaturated fat; 33 g carbohydrate; 9 g fiber; 5 g sugar; 164 mg phosphorus; 85 mg calcium; 4 mg iron; 372 mg sodium; 565 mg potassium; 859 IU vitamin A; 0 mg vitamin E; 14 mg vitamin C; 0 mg cholesterol

Marinated Vegetable Salad

I really like marinated vegetables, especially in the summer when you can just add them to some lettuce to make a refreshing and filling salad.

$^1/_2$ cup (56 g) sliced zucchini

$^1/_2$ cup (56 g) sliced yellow squash

$^1/_2$ cup (36 g) broccoli florets

$^1/_2$ cup (50 g) cauliflower florets

$^1/_4$ cup (33 g) sliced carrot

$^1/_4$ cup (40 g) thinly sliced red onion

15 cherry tomatoes, halved

4 ounces (115 g) mushrooms, sliced

Marinade

1 cup (235 ml) olive oil

$^1/_2$ cup (120 ml) red wine vinegar

$^1/_4$ cup (60 ml) lemon juice

1 teaspoon oregano

1 teaspoon dry mustard

1 teaspoon minced onion

$^1/_2$ teaspoon pressed garlic

Mix vegetables in a bowl. Combine marinade ingredients and pour over vegetables. Refrigerate for several hours or overnight.

Yield: 8 servings

Per serving: 71 g water; 265 calories (91% from fat, 2% from protein, 7% from carb); 1 g protein; 27 g total fat; 4 g saturated fat; 20 g monounsaturated fat; 3 g polyunsaturated fat; 5 g carbohydrate; 2 g fiber; 1 g sugar; 29 mg phosphorus; 16 mg calcium; 1 mg iron; 10 mg sodium; 228 mg potassium; 1046 IU vitamin A; 0 mg vitamin E; 21 mg vitamin C; 0 mg cholesterol

Marinated Zucchini Salad

This is a nice summer salad that can help to use up those extra zucchini when the garden is producing more than you can eat.

2 cups (220 g) thinly sliced zucchini

$^1/_2$ cup (35 g) thinly sliced mushrooms

1 cup (300 g) artichoke hearts, drained and sliced

1 can bamboo shoots, drained

$^1/_2$ cup (120 ml) Italian dressing

Mix all but dressing together in a large bowl. Pour dressing over ingredients and stir to mix. Marinate several hours or overnight.

Yield: 4 servings

Per serving: 181 g water; 129 calories (57% from fat, 10% from protein, 32% from carb); 4 g protein; 9 g total fat; 1 g saturated fat; 2 g monounsaturated fat; 4 g polyunsaturated fat; 11 g carbohydrate; 4 g fiber; 5 g sugar; 76 mg phosphorus; 26 mg calcium; 1 mg iron; 520 mg sodium; 368 mg potassium; 212 IU vitamin A; 0 mg vitamin E; 14 mg vitamin C; 0 mg cholesterol

Roasted Corn Salad

I know this one sounds a little strange, but it turns out really well. It has a sort of Mexican flavor to it and would be good with just about any kind of grilled meat.

4 ears corn
$^1/_4$ cup (38 g) red bell pepper, chopped
$^1/_4$ cup (40 g) onion, chopped
2 tablespoons (30 ml) honey
$^1/_4$ cup (60 ml) lime juice
1 tablespoon (4 g) fresh coriander
$^1/_4$ teaspoon (0.6 g) cumin

Husk and clean corn. Wrap in aluminum foil. Grill over medium heat until tender, turning often. Cut corn from cobs. Stir in pepper and onion. Mix together remaining ingredients. Pour over vegetables. Stir to mix. Refrigerate at least 2 hours or overnight before serving.

Yield: 4 servings

Per serving: 101 calories (3% from fat, 8% from protein, 89% from carbohydrate); 2 g protein; 0 g total fat; 0 g saturated fat; 0 g monounsaturated fat; 0 g polyunsaturated fat; 26 g carbohydrate; 2 g fiber; 12 g sugar; 51 mg phosphorus; 15 mg calcium; 1 mg iron; 6 mg sodium; 184 mg potassium; 329 IU vitamin A; 0 mg ATE vitamin E; 22 mg vitamin C; 0 mg cholesterol; 88 g water

Spinach and Toasted Walnut Salad

Simple two-ingredient salad. Raspberry-walnut vinaigrette dressing (such as Wish-Bone brand) goes perfectly with this.

$^1/_4$ cup (30 g) chopped walnuts
1 pound (455 g) fresh spinach, deveined and torn into bite-size pieces

Place walnuts in preheated 350°F (180°C, gas mark 4) oven for 8 to 10 minutes. Watch carefully, as they do burn easily. Set aside. Place 1 cup spinach on each of 4 chilled plates and spoon 1 tablespoon raspberry-walnut vinaigrette dressing (such as Wish-Bone) over the top. Top each with 1 tablespoon toasted walnuts.

Yield: 4 servings

Per serving: 101 g water; 85 calories (47% from fat, 26% from protein, 27% from carb); 6 g protein; 5 g total fat; 0 g saturated fat; 1 g monounsaturated fat; 3 g polyunsaturated fat; 7 g carbohydrate; 5 g fiber; 1 g sugar; 97 mg phosphorus; 178 mg calcium; 2 mg iron; 110 mg sodium; 383 mg potassium; 13680 IU vitamin A; 0 mg vitamin E; 3 mg vitamin C; 0 mg cholesterol

Spinach Salad

This different kind of salad recipe comes from one of my wife's co-workers. It is a request for every luncheon and get-together they have, and it's easy to understand why. We made a main dish out of it by topping it with some grilled boneless chicken breast that had been marinating in extra dressing.

For Salad:

$^1/_2$ pound (225 g) spinach

$^1/_2$ pound (225 g) strawberries, hulled and halved

$^1/_4$ cup (40 g) red onion, sliced

$^1/_2$ cup (50 g) cucumber, sliced

$^1/_3$ cup (30 g) almonds, sliced

For Dressing:

1 lemon

2 tablespoons (30 ml) white wine vinegar

1 tablespoon (15 ml) olive oil

$^1/_3$ cup (68 g) sugar

Combine salad ingredients. Zest the lemon and squeeze juice into a small bowl. Mix juice with other dressing ingredients. Toss salad and dressing just before serving.

Yield: 6 servings

Per serving: 142 calories (39% from fat, 10% from protein, 51% from carbohydrate); 4 g protein; 7 g total fat; 1 g saturated fat; 4 g monounsaturated fat; 1 g polyunsaturated fat; 20 g carbohydrate; 3 g fiber; 14 g sugar; 73 mg phosphorus; 87 mg calcium; 1 mg iron; 40 mg sodium; 267 mg potassium; 4576 IU vitamin A; 0 mg ATE vitamin E; 29 mg vitamin C; 0 mg cholesterol; 96 g water

Spinach and Artichoke Salad

An easy salad with lots of flavor from an unusual combination of ingredients. And that's not even to mention the fact that it contains almost half your daily target of fiber.

$^1/_4$ cup (60 ml) lemon juice

1 teaspoon sugar

$^1/_2$ teaspoon minced garlic

$^1/_4$ teaspoon black pepper

4 cups (120 g) fresh spinach, cleaned and torn

$^1/_2$ cup (50 g) chopped scallions

1 avocado, cubed

14 ounces (397 g) artichoke hearts, drained and halved

Combine first 4 ingredients to make dressing. Toss with remaining ingredients.

Yield: 4 servings

Per serving: 305 g water; 175 calories (29% from fat, 22% from protein, 49% from carb); 12 g protein; 7 g total fat; 1 g saturated fat; 3 g monounsaturated fat; 1 g polyunsaturated fat; 25 g carbohydrate; 14 g fiber; 4 g sugar; 180 mg phosphorus; 327 mg calcium; 5 mg iron; 242 mg sodium; 1064 mg potassium; 23256 IU vitamin A; 0 mg vitamin E; 22 mg vitamin C; 0 mg cholesterol

Molded Vegetable Salad

This molded salad is another of those traditional family recipes. This one is seen most often at Easter, along with ham, turkey, and potato salad.

6 ounces (170 g) lemon gelatin

2 cups (475 ml) boiling water

$2^1/_4$ cups (535 ml) cold water, divided

1 tablespoon unflavored gelatin

1 cup (180 g) chopped tomato

$^1/_2$ cup (75 g) chopped green bell pepper

$^1/_2$ cup (80 g) chopped onion

$^1/_2$ cup (60 g) sliced cucumber

$^1/_2$ cup (65 g) sliced carrot

1 cup (70 g) shredded cabbage

$^1/_4$ cup (60 ml) cider vinegar

Prepare lemon gelatin according to package directions using 2 cups each boiling and cold water. Dissolve 1 tablespoon unflavored gelatin in $^1/_4$ cup (60 ml) cold water. Let stand 5 minutes. Add this to the lemon gelatin mixture. Refrigerate until consistency of unbeaten egg whites or soft custard. Combine the remaining ingredients. Stir into chilled gelatin and pour into a 7-cup well-oiled mold or bowl. Chill at least 8 hours in refrigerator until firm.

Yield: 8 servings

Per serving: 191 g water; 140 calories (1% from fat, 9% from protein, 91% from carb); 3 g protein; 0 g total fat; 0 g saturated fat; 0 g monounsaturated fat; 0 g polyunsaturated fat; 33 g carbohydrate; 1 g fiber; 29 g sugar; 62 mg phosphorus; 18 mg calcium; 0 mg iron; 163 mg sodium; 135 mg potassium; 1513 IU vitamin A; 0 mg vitamin E; 18 mg vitamin C; 0 mg cholesterol

Coleslaw

This makes a fairly sour slaw, which is just fine with me, especially if you are planning to put it on barbecue sandwiches. You could add more sugar or a little honey if you like it sweeter.

2 cups (140 g) cabbage, shredded

$^1/_3$ cup (40 g) carrot, shredded

$^1/_4$ cup (56 g) low fat mayonnaise

$^1/_4$ cup (60 g) fat-free sour cream

2 tablespoons (30 ml) vinegar

2 tablespoons (26 g) sugar

$^1/_4$ teaspoon (0.5 g) celery seed

$^1/_4$ teaspoon (0.8 g) onion powder

Stir dressing ingredients together. Pour over cabbage and carrot and stir to mix.

Yield: 6 servings

Per serving: 75 calories (46% from fat, 5% from protein, 49% from carbohydrate); 1 g protein; 3 g total fat; 1 g saturated fat; 0 g monounsaturated fat; 0 g polyunsaturated fat; 8 g carbohydrate; 1 g fiber; 6 g sugar; 27 mg phosphorus; 28 mg calcium; 0 mg iron; 95 mg sodium; 97 mg potassium; 1281 IU vitamin A; 10 mg ATE vitamin E; 11 mg vitamin C; 7 mg cholesterol; 52 g water

Island Slaw

A sweet and spicy version of coleslaw to go with your grilled meats.

2 cups (140 g) shredded cabbage

$^1/_2$ cup (55 g) shredded carrot

$^1/_2$ cup (36 g) shredded broccoli

$^1/_4$ cup (50 g) sugar

3 tablespoons (45 ml) white wine vinegar

2 tablespoons (28 ml) olive oil

1 teaspoon vanilla extract

1 teaspoon black pepper

$^1/_4$ teaspoon ground ginger

$^1/_8$ teaspoon cayenne pepper

Mix vegetables in a large bowl. Combine remaining ingredients; stir until well blended. Just before serving, pour over cabbage mixture; toss gently.

Yield: 4 servings

Per serving: 79 g water; 137 calories (45% from fat, 4% from protein, 51% from carb); 1 g protein; 7 g total fat; 1 g saturated fat; 5 g monounsaturated fat; 1 g polyunsaturated fat; 18 g carbohydrate; 2 g fiber; 14 g sugar; 27 mg phosphorus; 33 mg calcium; 1 mg iron; 21 mg sodium; 189 mg potassium; 3016 IU vitamin A; 0 mg vitamin E; 28 mg vitamin C; 0 mg cholesterol

Mexican Coleslaw

Coleslaw with a little hint of Mexican flavor. Great with grilled meats.

$^1/_2$ cup (35 g) shredded red cabbage

$^1/_4$ teaspoon cumin

1 cup (70 g) shredded green cabbage

$^1/_4$ cup (28 g) pared, grated carrot

$^1/_4$ teaspoon black pepper, fresh ground

$^1/_4$ cup (60 g) plain fat-free yogurt

2 tablespoons (28 ml) lime juice

Combine all ingredients in a medium mixing bowl. Serve at once or refrigerate and serve cold.

Yield: 3 servings

Per serving: 77 g water; 31 calories (4% from fat, 22% from protein, 73% from carb); 2 g protein; 0 g total fat; 0 g saturated fat; 0 g monounsaturated fat; 0 g polyunsaturated fat; 6 g carbohydrate; 2 g fiber; 4 g sugar; 50 mg phosphorus; 66 mg calcium; 0 mg iron; 33 mg sodium; 188 mg potassium; 1997 IU vitamin A; 0 mg vitamin E; 23 mg vitamin C; 0 mg cholesterol

Reduced-Fat Potato Salad

Time for a little picnic stuff. Feel free to vary the vegetables to whatever suits you best.

6 medium potatoes

$^1/_2$ cup (115 g) low fat mayonnaise

$^1/_4$ cup (60 g) fat-free sour cream

2 teaspoons (6 g) dry mustard

1 teaspoon (3 g) onion powder

2 tablespoons (30 ml) honey

$^1/_2$ teaspoon (1 g) black pepper

1 tablespoon (0.4 g) dried parsley

$^1/_2$ teaspoon (1 g) celery seed

$^1/_4$ teaspoon (0.3 g) dried dill

$^1/_4$ cup (37 g) green bell pepper, chopped

$^1/_4$ cup (25 g) celery, sliced

$^1/_2$ cup (65 g) carrot, sliced

Boil potatoes until done. Rinse in cold water and allow to cool. Mix together mayonnaise, sour cream, mustard, onion powder, honey, black pepper, parsley, celery seed, and dill. Pour over potatoes and stir to coat. Fold in green bell pepper, celery, and carrot.

Yield: 6 servings

Per serving: 371 calories (18% from fat, 8% from protein, 74% from carbohydrate); 8 g protein; 7 g total fat; 1 g saturated fat; 0 g monounsaturated fat; 0 g

polyunsaturated fat; 69 g carbohydrate; 7 g fiber; 11 g sugar; 256 mg phosphorus; 63 mg calcium; 3 mg iron; 198 mg sodium; 1778 mg potassium; 1993 IU vitamin A; 10 mg ATE vitamin E; 39 mg vitamin C; 11 mg cholesterol; 339 g water

Tip: Recipes often say to boil the potatoes whole, then peel and chop them, but I find I get better results by cutting them into smaller pieces first. Unless you have very small potatoes to boil whole, the outside will be mushy before the inside is done.

Garbanzo and Pasta Salad

Garbanzo beans can be purchased dried or canned. If using dried beans, cook according to package directions. For canned beans, be sure to drain and rinse them before using.

4 ounces (115 g) pasta

2 cups (480 g) cooked garbanzo beans

$^1/_2$ cup (75 g) red bell pepper, chopped

$^1/_3$ cup (33 g) celery, sliced

$^1/_3$ cup (43 g) carrot, sliced

$^1/_4$ cup (25 g) scallions, chopped

3 tablespoons (45 ml) balsamic vinegar

2 tablespoons (28 g) low fat mayonnaise

2 teaspoons (10 g) mustard

$^1/_2$ teaspoon (1 g) black pepper

$^1/_4$ teaspoon (0.2 g) dried Italian seasoning

4 cups (80 g) leaf lettuce, torn into bite-sized pieces

Cook pasta according to directions, omitting salt. Drain and rinse well under cold water until pasta is cool; drain well. Combine pasta, garbanzo beans, red bell pepper, celery, carrot, and scallions in medium bowl. Whisk together vinegar, mayonnaise, mustard, black pepper, and Italian seasoning in small bowl until blended. Pour over salad; toss to coat evenly. Cover and refrigerate up to 8 hours. Arrange lettuce on individual plates. Spoon salad over lettuce.

Yield: 8 servings

Per serving: 150 calories (16% from fat, 15% from protein, 69% from carbohydrate); 6 g protein; 3 g total fat; 0 g saturated fat; 0 g monounsaturated fat; 1 g polyunsaturated fat; 26 g carbohydrate; 4 g fiber; 1 g sugar; 103 mg phosphorus; 39 mg calcium; 1 mg iron; 226 mg sodium; 239 mg potassium; 2589 IU vitamin A; 2 mg ATE vitamin E; 18 mg vitamin C; 13 mg cholesterol; 87 g water

Tip: This recipe can also be used as a vegetarian main dish, yielding 4 servings.

Tomato Pasta Salad

A cool and pleasing side dish with a simple dressing.

2 cups (300 g) dried pasta

1 cup (230 g) fat-free sour cream

$^1/_4$ cup (60 ml) skim milk

1 tablespoon (4 g) fresh dill

1 tablespoon (15 ml) vinegar

$^1/_2$ teaspoon (1 g) black pepper

2 cups (270 g) cucumber, chopped

2 cups (360 g) tomatoes, chopped

Cook pasta in boiling salted water until al dente. Drain and rinse in cold water. Transfer cooked pasta to a large serving bowl. In a separate bowl, mix together sour cream, milk, dill, vinegar, and pepper. Set dressing aside. Mix cucumbers and tomatoes into the pasta. Pour dressing over pasta mixture and toss thoroughly to combine. Cover, and refrigerate at least 1 hour and preferably overnight. Stir just before serving.

Yield: 8 servings

Per serving: 91 calories (9% from fat, 19% from protein, 72% from carbohydrate); 3 g protein; 1 g total fat; 0 g saturated fat; 0 g monounsaturated fat; 0 g polyunsaturated fat; 11 g carbohydrate; 1 g fiber; 1 g sugar; 76 mg phosphorus; 57 mg calcium; 1 mg iron; 23 mg sodium; 211 mg potassium; 409 IU vitamin A; 35 mg ATE vitamin E; 11 mg vitamin C; 19 mg cholesterol; 92 g water

Whole Wheat Pasta Salad

An updated version of pasta salad, with more fiber and great taste.

8 ounces (225 g) whole wheat pasta

$^{1}/_{2}$ cup (30 g) finely chopped fresh parsley

$^{1}/_{4}$ cup (25 g) halved cherry scallions

$^{1}/_{2}$ cup (90 g) diced tomato, peeled and seeded

$^{1}/_{4}$ cup (38 g) chopped green bell pepper

$^{1}/_{4}$ cup (60 ml) lemon juice

$^{1}/_{4}$ cup (60 ml) olive oil

$^{1}/_{2}$ teaspoon black pepper, fresh ground

Cook pasta in boiling water until tender. Drain and rinse under cold water. Drain thoroughly. Turn pasta into large bowl. Stir in parsley, scallions, tomato, and bell pepper. In separate bowl, mix lemon juice, oil, and black pepper. Pour over pasta mixture, mixing well. Cover and chill. To serve, garnish with lettuce leaves and tomato wedges or lemon and lime slices if desired.

Yield: 4 servings

Per serving: 57 g water; 331 calories (37% from fat, 10% from protein, 53% from carb); 9 g protein; 14 g total fat; 2 g saturated fat; 10 g monounsaturated fat; 2 g polyunsaturated fat; 46 g carbohydrate; 6 g fiber; 1 g sugar; 161 mg phosphorus; 43 mg calcium; 3 mg iron; 11 mg sodium; 264 mg potassium; 887 IU vitamin A; 0 mg vitamin E; 28 mg vitamin C; 0 mg cholesterol

Grapefruit, Avocado, and Spinach Salad

This is a great salad. I like to make a double batch of the dressing and use half to marinate boneless chicken breasts to grill as an accompaniment.

1$^{1}/_{2}$ pounds (680 g) fresh spinach

3 red grapefruit

2 avocados

$^{1}/_{4}$ cup (60 ml) orange juice

2 tablespoons (30 ml) lemon juice

1 teaspoon sugar

2 tablespoons (28 ml) white wine vinegar

$^{1}/_{2}$ cup (120 ml) olive oil

Remove stems from spinach. Wash spinach thoroughly and dry. Tear leaves into bite-size pieces.

Wrap gently in paper towels and refrigerate in plastic bags until ready to toss salad. Peel and section grapefruit. Slice avocados into quarters, then cut each slice into 2-inch (5-cm) chunks. Combine remaining ingredients for dressing. At serving time, toss spinach with dressing. Add grapefruit and avocados and gently toss again, or arrange grapefruit and avocado slices on bed of dressed spinach on individual serving plates. Pass additional dressing, if desired.

Yield: 6 servings

Per serving: 240 g water; 422 calories (52% from fat, 7% from protein, 41% from carb); 8 g protein; 26 g total fat; 4 g saturated fat; 18 g monounsaturated fat; 3 g polyunsaturated fat; 45 g carbohydrate; 10 g fiber; 2 g sugar; 138 mg phosphorus; 43 mg calcium; 2 mg iron; 8 mg sodium; 465 mg potassium; 397 IU vitamin A; 0 mg vitamin E; 55 mg vitamin C; 0 mg cholesterol

Cabbage Fruit Salad

A great dish for fall when cabbage and apples are in season. It features a sweet creamy dressing.

2 cups (140 g) raw, shredded cabbage

1 medium apple, diced and unpeeled

1 tablespoon (15 ml) lemon juice

$^1/_2$ cup (75 g) raisins

$^1/_4$ cup (60 ml) pineapple juice

$1^1/_2$ teaspoons lemon juice

1 tablespoon sugar

$^1/_2$ cup (115 g) sour cream

Prepare cabbage and apple. Use lemon juice to wet apple to prevent darkening. Toss cabbage, raisins, and apple. Mix fruit juices and sugar. Add sour cream, stir until smooth; add to salad and chill.

Yield: 4 servings

Per serving: 102 g water; 169 calories (31% from fat, 5% from protein, 64% from carb); 2 g protein; 6 g total fat; 4 g saturated fat; 2 g monounsaturated fat; 0 g polyunsaturated fat; 29 g carbohydrate; 2 g fiber; 20 g sugar; 58 mg phosphorus; 64 mg calcium; 1 mg iron; 24 mg sodium; 338 mg potassium; 244 IU vitamin A; 50 mg vitamin E; 24 mg vitamin C; 13 mg cholesterol

Cranberry Walnut Mold

This mold always reminds me of fall, with its cranberries and apples.

1 cup ground (110 g) cranberries

1 cup (245 g) ground apples

1 cup (200 g) sugar

3 ounces (85 g) lemon gelatin

1 cup (235 ml) hot water

1 cup (235 ml) pineapple juice

$^1/_2$ cup (75 g) seedless green grapes, cut up

$^1/_4$ cup (30 g) chopped walnuts

Combine cranberries, apples, and sugar. Dissolve gelatin in hot water. Add juice, chill. Add cranberry mixture, grapes, and nuts. Put in mold and congeal.

Yield: 6 servings

Per serving: 101 g water; 314 calories (9% from fat, 3% from protein, 87% from carb); 3 g protein; 3 g total fat;

0 g saturated fat; 1 g monounsaturated fat; 2 g
polyunsaturated fat; 73 g carbohydrate; 2 g fiber; 66 g
sugar; 54 mg phosphorus; 15 mg calcium; 0 mg iron;
69 mg sodium; 123 mg potassium; 19 IU vitamin A; 0 mg
vitamin E; 5 mg vitamin C; 0 mg cholesterol

Orange Avocado Salad

Fresh and citrusy with a sesame/poppyseed dressing, this
salad would dress up any meal. Particularly good with
chicken or fish.

2 tablespoons (40 g) honey

1 tablespoon sesame seeds

1 teaspoon poppyseeds

$^1/_4$ teaspoon onion powder

2 tablespoons (28 ml) vegetable oil

2 tablespoons (28 ml) cider vinegar

$^1/_4$ teaspoon Worcestershire sauce

4 cups (220 g) lettuce, torn into bite-size pieces

2 oranges, separated into sections

1 avocado, diced

Combine first 4 ingredients in blender until well
blended. With blender running, add oil, vinegar, and
Worcestershire sauce in a slow, steady stream. Blend
until thickened. Toss lettuce, oranges, and avocado.
Drizzle with dressing.

Yield: 4 servings

Per serving: 183 g water; 209 calories (51% from fat,
4% from protein, 45% from carb); 2 g protein; 13 g total
fat; 2 g saturated fat; 5 g monounsaturated fat; 5 g
polyunsaturated fat; 25 g carbohydrate; 5 g fiber; 19 g

sugar; 54 mg phosphorus; 67 mg calcium; 1 mg iron;
14 mg sodium; 461 mg potassium; 621 IU vitamin A; 0 mg
vitamin E; 55 mg vitamin C; 0 mg cholesterol

Overnight Layered Fruit Salad

This makes a great presentation if you layer it in a glass
trifle bowl. But more importantly, it tastes good.

2 cups (110 g) shredded iceberg lettuce

2 Golden Delicious apples

2 oranges

2 cups (300 g) seedless green grapes

$^1/_3$ cup (75 g) mayonnaise

$^1/_3$ cup (77 g) sour cream

1 cup (115 g) shredded Cheddar cheese

Spread lettuce on bottom of 2-quart (2-L) serving
dish. Core and quarter apples; slice thinly and layer
over lettuce. Peel and section oranges; squeeze a
teaspoon or so of orange juice onto the apples.
Arrange sectioned orange on top of apple slices.
Layer grapes. Combine mayonnaise and sour cream
in small bowl; spread over grapes. Sprinkle shredded
cheese over all. Cover dish tightly with plastic wrap.
Refrigerate overnight.

Yield: 6 servings

Per serving: 159 g water; 268 calories (61% from fat,
10% from protein, 29% from carb); 7 g protein; 19 g total
fat; 7 g saturated fat; 5 g monounsaturated fat; 6 g
polyunsaturated fat; 20 g carbohydrate; 3 g fiber; 16 g
sugar; 150 mg phosphorus; 210 mg calcium; 0 mg iron;
215 mg sodium; 285 mg potassium; 611 IU vitamin A;
80 mg vitamin E; 36 mg vitamin C; 33 mg cholesterol

Raspberry-Cranberry Mold

Pineapple and cranberry in a raspberry base . . . almost all my favorite fruits.

6 ounces (170 g) raspberry gelatin

2 cups (310 g) crushed pineapple with syrup, drained

16 ounces (455 g) whole berry cranberry sauce, undrained

1 cup (120 g) halved walnuts

Dissolve gelatin in 4 cups (950 ml) boiling water; add drained pineapple and the undrained cranberry sauce; mix well. Chill until partially set, then add walnuts and pour into 9 × 13-inch (23 × 33-cm) dish or mold. Chill until set.

Yield: 10 servings

Per serving: 71 g water; 237 calories (27% from fat, 7% from protein, 66% from carb); 5 g protein; 8 g total fat; 0 g saturated fat; 2 g monounsaturated fat; 4 g polyunsaturated fat; 41 g carbohydrate; 2 g fiber; 38 g sugar; 94 mg phosphorus; 17 mg calcium; 1 mg iron; 93 mg sodium; 131 mg potassium; 43 IU vitamin A; 0 mg vitamin E; 5 mg vitamin C; 0 mg cholesterol

Spinach and Orange Section Salad

A great salad, this could easily be made a full meal by adding some chicken or shrimp.

1 pound (455 g) spinach, washed, trimmed, drained

1/2 pound (35 g) sliced cleaned mushrooms

5 ounces (140 g) water chestnuts, drained, rinsed

4 oranges, peeled, sectioned

2 tablespoons (28 ml) orange juice

1 tablespoon (15 ml) Dick's Reduced Sodium Soy Sauce (see recipe page 25)

1/4 teaspoon dry mustard

1/8 teaspoon black pepper, fresh ground

Tear spinach into bite-size pieces. Toss with mushrooms, water chestnuts, and orange sections. Combine remaining ingredients in jar with tight-fitting lid. Shake well. Before serving, pour over spinach mixture; toss lightly.

Yield: 8 servings

Per serving: 174 g water; 88 calories (5% from fat, 18% from protein, 78% from carb); 4 g protein; 1 g total fat; 0 g saturated fat; 0 g monounsaturated fat; 0 g polyunsaturated fat; 19 g carbohydrate; 5 g fiber; 10 g sugar; 79 mg phosphorus; 127 mg calcium; 1 mg iron; 55 mg sodium; 543 mg potassium; 7049 IU vitamin A; 0 mg vitamin E; 53 mg vitamin C; 0 mg cholesterol

Black Bean Salad

This is a main-dish salad, with black beans and smoked turkey. If you don't have any smoked turkey, regular leftover turkey breast will do just as well. This salad has a lot of flavor, and the curry powder adds color. I use a fat-free vinaigrette dressing and don't miss the oil at all.

3/4 cup (188 g) dried black beans

3/4 cup (188 g) dried black-eyed peas

1 cup (160 g) onion, chopped

2 cups (225 g) smoked turkey breast

1 cup (235 ml) low fat Italian salad dressing

1 cup (100 g) scallions, chopped

1¹/₃ cups (200 g) red bell pepper, chopped

1¹/₄ cups (205 g) frozen corn, thawed

¹/₄ cup (15 g) cilantro, chopped

2 teaspoons (4 g) curry powder

¹/₂ teaspoon (0.6 g) red pepper flakes

Place beans and peas in separate saucepans. Cover with water. Add half of the onion to each. Bring to a boil and boil for 1 minute. Remove from heat, cover, and let stand for 1 hour. Add additional water to saucepans if needed. Divide turkey between pans. Simmer one hour or until beans are tender. Drain. Combine beans, black-eyed peas, and turkey in a large bowl. Pour Italian dressing over while hot. Add scallions, red bell pepper, corn, cilantro, curry powder, and red pepper flakes. Toss to mix. Cover and refrigerate overnight or serve warm.

Yield: 8 servings

Per serving: 161 calories (19% from fat, 36% from protein, 45% from carbohydrate); 15 g protein; 4 g total fat; 1 g saturated fat; 1 g monounsaturated fat; 1 g polyunsaturated fat; 19 g carbohydrate; 4 g fiber; 5 g sugar; 156 mg phosphorus; 37 mg calcium; 2 mg iron; 439 mg sodium; 421 mg potassium; 1059 IU vitamin A; 0 mg ATE vitamin E; 37 mg vitamin C; 26 mg cholesterol; 143 g water

Bean and Artichoke Salad

A tasty variation on three bean salad. Serve over lettuce or as a side dish.

¹/₂ cup (50 g) green beans, cooked

¹/₂ cup (50 g) yellow beans, cooked

¹/₂ cup (50 g) cooked kidney beans

1 jar (6 ounces) artichoke hearts

¹/₄ cup (48 g) chopped pimento

¹/₄ cup (60 ml) Italian dressing

Cook and drain beans. Chop artichoke hearts. Save the juice. Combine beans, hearts, and pimento. Add dressing to the juice of the hearts and pour over mixture. Refrigerate at least 2 hours or overnight.

Yield: 4 servings

Per serving: 99 g water; 158 calories (25% from fat, 19% from protein, 56% from carb); 8 g protein; 5 g total fat; 1 g saturated fat; 1 g monounsaturated fat; 2 g polyunsaturated fat; 23 g carbohydrate; 10 g fiber; 3 g sugar; 144 mg phosphorus; 57 mg calcium; 3 mg iron; 284 mg sodium; 565 mg potassium; 532 IU vitamin A; 0 mg vitamin E; 19 mg vitamin C; 0 mg cholesterol

Black-Eyed Pea Salad

A great-tasting salad with Mediterranean flavor. You could make a whole meal of it by increasing the portion and adding a little cooked chicken.

2 cups (344 g) cooked black-eyed peas, drained

¹/₄ cup (40 g) chopped red onion

¹/₄ cup (38 g) chopped green bell pepper

3 ounces (85 g) feta cheese

¹/₂ cup (55 g) sun-dried tomatoes, oil packed

¹/₄ cup (60 ml) balsamic vinegar

1 tablespoon (15 ml) Dijon mustard

1 tablespoon (20 g) honey

In a medium bowl, mix the peas, onion, bell pepper, and feta. In a separate bowl, combine the sun-dried tomatoes, vinegar, mustard, and honey. Drizzle over the salad and gently toss to coat. Refrigerate 1 hour before serving

Yield: 4 servings

Per serving: 111 g water; 225 calories (28% from fat, 20% from protein, 52% from carb); 11 g protein; 7 g total fat; 4 g saturated fat; 2 g monounsaturated fat; 1 g polyunsaturated fat; 30 g carbohydrate; 7 g fiber; 10 g sugar; 205 mg phosphorus; 138 mg calcium; 2 mg iron; 322 mg sodium; 597 mg potassium; 368 IU vitamin A; 27 mg vitamin E; 25 mg vitamin C; 19 mg cholesterol

Black-Eyed Pea and Rice Salad

A nice side salad of rice and black-eyed peas. Perfect accompaniment to meat grilled with Caribbean spices.

3 cups (660 g) cooked brown rice

1¹/₂ cups (258 g) cooked black-eyed peas

1 tablespoon (15 ml) Dijon mustard

¹/₂ teaspoon black pepper, fresh ground

¹/₄ cup (60 ml) red wine vinegar

¹/₄ cup (60 ml) olive oil

¹/₂ cup (80 g) sliced red onion

¹/₂ teaspoon minced garlic

¹/₂ cup (55 g) grated carrot

¹/₄ cup chopped fresh parsley

Cook the rice and the peas in advance. Whisk the mustard, pepper, and vinegar until dissolved. Drizzle in the oil while whisking. Toss the black-eyed peas and the rice with the vinaigrette. Mix in the onion, garlic, carrot, and parsley. Serve over Romaine or Boston lettuce if desired.

Yield: 8 servings

Per serving: 56 g water; 371 calories (22% from fat, 9% from protein, 69% from carb); 9 g protein; 9 g total fat; 1 g saturated fat; 6 g monounsaturated fat; 2 g polyunsaturated fat; 64 g carbohydrate; 5 g fiber; 3 g sugar; 280 mg phosphorus; 32 mg calcium; 2 mg iron; 37 mg sodium; 335 mg potassium; 2043 IU vitamin A; 0 mg vitamin E; 2 mg vitamin C; 0 mg cholesterol

Tip: Can be prepared a day ahead and stored in the refrigerator. Allow it to come to room temperature before serving.

Chickpea and Vegetable Salad

A nice combination of salad ingredients set off by a fresh homemade dressing. Serve over lettuce leaves.

2 cups (328 g) cooked chickpeas

1 cup (150 g) green bell pepper, cut in strips

$^1/_4$ cup (40 g) chopped onion

1 cup (180 g) tomato, cut in thin wedges, or 12 cherry tomatoes

2 tablespoons chopped fresh parsley

Dressing

1 tablespoon (15 ml) lemon juice

2 tablespoons (28 ml) olive oil

3 tablespoons (45 ml) water

$^1/_8$ teaspoon cayenne pepper

$^1/_4$ cup (60 ml) rice vinegar

2 teaspoons fresh basil

$^1/_2$ teaspoon dry mustard

Place chickpeas in a nonmetal bowl. Combine dressing ingredients, pour over them, and marinate in the refrigerator for an hour or two. Add rest of ingredients, toss well, and serve.

Yield: 4 servings

Per serving: 158 g water; 220 calories (36% from fat, 14% from protein, 49% from carb); 8 g protein; 9 g total fat; 1 g saturated fat; 5 g monounsaturated fat; 2 g polyunsaturated fat; 28 g carbohydrate; 8 g fiber; 5 g sugar; 161 mg phosphorus; 60 mg calcium; 3 mg iron; 13 mg sodium; 442 mg potassium; 607 IU vitamin A; 0 mg vitamin E; 46 mg vitamin C; 0 mg cholesterol

Broccoli, Navy Bean, and Cashew Salad

A main dish or side salad that will fill you up as well as satisfy your taste buds.

1 cup (71 g) broccoli

$^1/_2$ cup (91 g) cooked navy beans

$^1/_2$ cup (120 ml) Italian dressing

4 cups (220 g) iceberg lettuce

$^1/_4$ cup (35 g) cashews

$^1/_4$ cup (60 g) plain fat-free yogurt

Steam broccoli until tender but still crunchy and combine with navy beans. Marinade in Italian dressing; chill overnight. Wash and dry lettuce and tear into bite-size pieces. Drain beans and broccoli; add them to lettuce. Add cashews and yogurt just before serving.

Yield: 4 servings

Per serving: 123 g water; 249 calories (45% from fat, 13% from protein, 42% from carb); 9 g protein; 13 g total fat; 2 g saturated fat; 4 g monounsaturated fat; 5 g polyunsaturated fat; 27 g carbohydrate; 6 g fiber; 7 g sugar; 204 mg phosphorus; 98 mg calcium; 3 mg iron; 515 mg sodium; 584 mg potassium; 517 IU vitamin A; 0 mg vitamin E; 23 mg vitamin C; 0 mg cholesterol

Four Bean Salad

If three bean salad is good, why not go it one better?

10 ounces (280 g) green beans

10 ounces (280 g) yellow beans

2 cups (320 g) chickpeas

2 cups (200 g) kidney beans

$^1/_2$ cup (75 g) chopped green bell pepper

$^1/_2$ cup (80 g) chopped onion

1 cup (200 g) sugar

1 cup (235 ml) cider vinegar

³/₄ cup (180 ml) vegetable oil

¹/₂ teaspoon black pepper

If beans are frozen, cook until crisp-tender; if canned, drain. Combine with the bell pepper and onion; set aside. Combine remaining ingredients; pour over vegetables, mixing well. Cover and marinate in the refrigerator for 24 hours, stirring occasionally.

Yield: 8 servings

Per serving: 145 g water; 351 calories (43% from fat, 8% from protein, 50% from carb); 7 g protein; 17 g total fat; 2 g saturated fat; 5 g monounsaturated fat; 9 g polyunsaturated fat; 44 g carbohydrate; 8 g fiber; 21 g sugar; 119 mg phosphorus; 64 mg calcium; 2 mg iron; 150 mg sodium; 392 mg potassium; 271 IU vitamin A; 0 mg vitamin E; 18 mg vitamin C; 0 mg cholesterol

Tip: This will keep for up to a week in the refrigerator.

Marinated Bean and Corn Salad

Mexican-flavored salad. This makes a big batch, but it keeps well in the refrigerator. I like it just as is for a quick lunch to take to work.

1 cup (100 g) cooked kidney beans

1 cup (171 g) cooked pinto beans

1 cup (164 g) cooked chickpeas

1 cup (172 g) cooked black beans

10 ounces (280 g) frozen corn, thawed

¹/₂ cup (80 g) chopped onion

¹/₄ cup chopped fresh parsley

¹/₂ cup (50 g) thinly sliced celery

¹/₃ cup (80 ml) olive oil

¹/₄ cup (60 ml) red wine vinegar

¹/₂ teaspoon minced garlic

¹/₄ teaspoon chili powder

¹/₄ teaspoon cumin

¹/₄ teaspoon red pepper flakes

Drain beans; put into large bowl. Add corn, onion, and parsley; toss to mix. Mix remaining ingredients in small bowl. Pour over bean and corn mixture; toss to coat. Refrigerate covered overnight. Taste and adjust seasonings. Serve at room temperature.

Yield: 8 servings

Per serving: 104 g water; 291 calories (30% from fat, 16% from protein, 54% from carb); 12 g protein; 10 g total fat; 1 g saturated fat; 7 g monounsaturated fat; 1 g polyunsaturated fat; 40 g carbohydrate; 10 g fiber; 2 g sugar; 214 mg phosphorus; 68 mg calcium; 3 mg iron; 104 mg sodium; 658 mg potassium; 244 IU vitamin A; 0 mg vitamin E; 8 mg vitamin C; 0 mg cholesterol

Pinto Bean and Wild Rice Salad

This salad offers a variety of options on the basic recipe. Feel free to substitute other greens like endive or radicchio, brown rice for the wild, and other beans for the pintos. It will still be healthy and delicious.

³/₄ cup (145 g) dried pinto beans

1¹/₂ cups (83 g) lettuce

1¹/₂ cups (247 g) cooked wild rice

¹/₂ cup (120 ml) olive oil

3 tablespoons (45 ml) red wine vinegar

2 tablespoons chopped fresh chives

$^1/_2$ teaspoon minced garlic

$^1/_4$ teaspoon black pepper

Soak the beans overnight in water to cover. Drain the beans, rinse them under cold running water, and place them in a saucepan with fresh water to cover. Bring to a boil over high heat, then reduce the heat and simmer several hours until the beans are soft and the skins begin to split. Add water when necessary to keep the beans from drying, and stir occasionally to prevent them from burning and sticking. Remove from the heat, drain, and allow to cool. In a bowl, toss together the lettuce, beans, and rice. Cover and chill in the refrigerator at least 30 minutes. In a blender, combine the oil, vinegar, chives, garlic, and pepper. Blend until the chives and garlic are finely pureed. Pour the dressing over the salad just before serving.

Yield: 6 servings

Per serving: 42 g water; 337 calories (49% from fat, 9% from protein, 42% from carb); 8 g protein; 19 g total fat; 3 g saturated fat; 13 g monounsaturated fat; 2 g polyunsaturated fat; 36 g carbohydrate; 5 g fiber; 1 g sugar; 210 mg phosphorus; 24 mg calcium; 1 mg iron; 6 mg sodium; 298 mg potassium; 142 IU vitamin A; 0 mg vitamin E; 1 mg vitamin C; 0 mg cholesterol

Tip: You may use canned beans that have been rinsed and drained in place of the cooked dried beans.

Spinach and Black-Eyed Pea Salad

A tasty salad of marinated black-eyed peas over spinach.

$^1/_2$ pound (225 g) black-eyed peas

1 cup (160 g) chopped onion

$^1/_2$ teaspoon minced garlic

4 cups (950 ml) water

14 ounces (400 g) artichoke hearts

1 tablespoon (15 ml) Dijon mustard

1 tablespoon (15 ml) Worcestershire sauce

$^1/_2$ pound (225 g) spinach leaves

4 slices bacon, cooked and crumbled

Sort and wash peas; place in a Dutch oven with next 3 ingredients. Bring to a boil; reduce heat, and simmer 40 minutes or until peas are tender. Drain. Keep peas warm. Drain artichoke hearts, reserving marinade. Chop artichoke hearts and add to black-eyed peas. Combine reserved marinade, mustard, and Worcestershire; pour over peas and toss gently. Arrange spinach leaves on individual salad plates; spoon salad onto spinach. Sprinkle with crumbled bacon and serve warm.

Yield: 6 servings

Per serving: 302 g water; 132 calories (20% from fat, 25% from protein, 56% from carb); 9 g protein; 3 g total fat; 1 g saturated fat; 1 g monounsaturated fat; 1 g polyunsaturated fat; 20 g carbohydrate; 7 g fiber; 4 g sugar; 147 mg phosphorus; 73 mg calcium; 3 mg iron; 249 mg sodium; 622 mg potassium; 3688 IU vitamin A; 1 mg vitamin E; 21 mg vitamin C; 6 mg cholesterol

Chicken Main-Dish Salad

A meal-on-a-plate type. This makes a good hot weather dinner when you don't really feel like doing much cooking.

For Dressing:

6 tablespoons (90 ml) olive oil

$1/4$ teaspoon (0.8 g) minced garlic

1 tablespoon (15 ml) lemon juice

2 tablespoons (30 ml) red wine vinegar

$1/2$ teaspoon (2.5 ml) Worcestershire sauce

For Salad:

1 pound (455 g) boneless chicken breasts

12 ounces (340 g) Romaine lettuce

1 cup (30 g) croutons

$1/4$ cup (25 g) Parmesan cheese, grated

$1/4$ teaspoon (0.5 g) freshly ground black pepper

Combine dressing ingredients in a jar with a tight-fitting lid and shake well. Place half of the dressing in a resealable plastic bag with chicken breasts and marinate several hours. Remove chicken and discard dressing. Grill chicken until done and slice into strips. Place lettuce on plates and top with chicken. Add croutons, sprinkle with cheese and pepper. Serve with remaining dressing.

Yield: 4 servings

Per serving: 290 calories (44% from fat, 43% from protein, 13% from carbohydrate); 31 g protein; 14 g total fat; 3 g saturated fat; 8 g monounsaturated fat; 2 g polyunsaturated fat; 9 g carbohydrate; 2 g fiber; 1 g sugar; 304 mg phosphorus; 117 mg calcium; 2 mg iron; 235 mg sodium; 531 mg potassium; 4992 IU vitamin A; 14 mg ATE vitamin E; 25 mg vitamin C; 71 mg cholesterol; 178 g water

Pepper Steak Salad

Although this doesn't actually contain any soy sauce, the flavor is definitely Asian.

For Marinade/Dressing:

$1/4$ cup (60 ml) balsamic vinegar

2 tablespoons (30 ml) sesame oil

$1/2$ teaspoon (0.9 g) ground ginger

1 tablespoon (13 g) sugar

$1/4$ teaspoon (0.8 g) minced garlic

1 ounce (28 g) sesame seeds

4 ounces (115 g) leftover roast beef

For Salad:

$1/2$ pound (225 g) lettuce, shredded

4 ounces (115 g) snow peas

$1/2$ cup (65 g) carrots, sliced

1 cup (70 g) cabbage, shredded

4 ounces (115 g) mushrooms, sliced

$1/2$ cup (75 g) red bell pepper, sliced

4 ounces (115 g) mung bean sprouts

To make the marinade/dressing: Combine vinegar, sesame oil, ginger, sugar, garlic, and sesame seeds. Pour into a resealable plastic bag. Slice beef and add to marinade in bag for 1 to 2 hours. Drain, reserving liquid.

To make the salad: Toss salad ingredients, top with beef slices. Spoon remaining dressing over.

Yield: 4 servings

Per serving: 216 calories (51% from fat, 23% from protein, 26% from carbohydrate); 13 g protein; 13 g total fat; 2 g saturated fat; 5 g monounsaturated fat; 5 g polyunsaturated fat; 15 g carbohydrate; 5 g fiber; 8 g sugar; 184 mg phosphorus; 121 mg calcium; 3 mg iron; 38 mg sodium; 491 mg potassium; 3932 IU vitamin A; 0 mg ATE vitamin E; 54 mg vitamin C; 25 mg cholesterol; 217 g water

Avocado and Crabmeat Salad

This is another of those "fancy" salads that are good when you have guests. But go ahead and treat yourself even if there is no one but family. This makes enough that it could be a whole meal in itself.

1 cup (230 g) fat-free sour cream

4 tablespoons (64 g) low-fat mayonnaise

1 teaspoon Worcestershire sauce

1 avocado

1 cup asparagus, cut in 1-inch (2.5-cm) pieces

$^{1}/_{4}$ cup (25 g) sliced black olives

1 pound (455 g) crabmeat

1 can artichoke hearts, quartered

Combine sour cream, mayonnaise, and Worcestershire to make sauce. Peel and coarsely chop avocado. Combine asparagus, black olives, crabmeat, artichoke, and avocado. Pour sauce over salad and mix.

Yield: 8 servings

Per serving: 130 g water; 172 calories (42% from fat, 38% from protein, 20% from carb); 14 g protein; 7 g total fat; 1 g saturated fat; 2 g monounsaturated fat; 1 g polyunsaturated fat; 7 g carbohydrate; 3 g fiber; 1 g sugar; 229 mg phosphorus; 82 mg calcium; 1 mg iron; 740 mg sodium; 396 mg potassium; 361 IU vitamin A; 35 mg vitamin E; 10 mg vitamin C; 44 mg cholesterol

Tip: Serve on lettuce garnished with cherry tomatoes.

Niçoise Salad

A main-dish salad that lets diners choose their ingredients from a central platter. The ingredients are typical of the type of salad served in Nice, France.

1 ounce (28 g) anchovies, minced

2 teaspoons Dijon mustard

3 tablespoons (45 ml) red wine vinegar

$^{1}/_{4}$ cup (60 ml) olive oil

4 cups (20 g) butter lettuce

1 can tuna, drained

2 eggs, hard cooked, halved

1 large tomato, cut into wedges

2 medium potatoes, peeled, cooked, and sliced

$^{1}/_{2}$ cup (50 g) green beans, cooked, drained, and cooled

$^{1}/_{2}$ cup (75 g) sliced and slivered green bell pepper

$^{1}/_{2}$ cup (80 g) red onion, cut in rounds

$^{1}/_{2}$ cup (50 g) black olives, drained

$^{1}/_{2}$ cup (35 g) thinly sliced mushrooms

14 ounces (400 g) artichoke hearts, drained

$^{1}/_{2}$ cup (17 g) alfalfa sprouts

Combine first 4 ingredients to make dressing. Line a platter with butter lettuce. Place tuna in center.

Arrange rest of ingredients in groups around tuna. Either serve as a salad or stuff pita bread halves with any ingredients from platter. Drizzle with dressing.

Yield: 4 servings

Per serving: 465 g water; 459 calories (40% from fat, 21% from protein, 39% from carb); 25 g protein; 21 g total fat; 4 g saturated fat; 13 g monounsaturated fat; 3 g polyunsaturated fat; 47 g carbohydrate; 11 g fiber; 6 g sugar; 394 mg phosphorus; 130 mg calcium; 5 mg iron; 568 mg sodium; 1630 mg potassium; 2695 IU vitamin A; 42 mg vitamin E; 47 mg vitamin C; 143 mg cholesterol

White Bean and Tuna Salad

This makes a great luncheon salad. It can also be a main dish in somewhat larger portions.

2 cups (200 g) cooked cannellini beans, drained and rinsed

13 ounces (368 g) tuna, drained

1 cup (180 g) seeded, diced tomato

$^1/_2$ cup (80 g) chopped red onion

2 tablespoons (30 ml) lemon juice

3 teaspoons (15 ml) Dijon mustard

$^1/_3$ cup (80 ml) olive oil

$^1/_4$ cup chopped fresh basil

Combine beans, tuna, tomato, and onion in large bowl. Combine lemon juice and mustard in small bowl. Gradually whisk in olive oil. Add to salad. Mix in basil.

Yield: 4 servings

Per serving: 192 g water; 406 calories (47% from fat, 29% from protein, 24% from carb); 30 g protein; 21 g total fat; 3 g saturated fat; 14 g monounsaturated fat; 3 g polyunsaturated fat; 24 g carbohydrate; 8 g fiber; 2 g sugar; 375 mg phosphorus; 129 mg calcium; 4 mg iron; 303 mg sodium; 769 mg potassium; 530 IU vitamin A; 6 mg vitamin E; 12 mg vitamin C; 39 mg cholesterol

Tip: Cannellini beans are large white beans like kidney beans. If you can't find them, you can substitute navy or pea beans.

Tofu Salad

Fresh Asian-style vegetables and tofu along with an Asian dressing give this main-dish salad a different kind of flavor.

For Salad:

$^1/_2$ pound (225 g) lettuce, shredded

4 ounces (115 g) snow peas

$^1/_2$ cup (65 g) carrot, shredded

1 cup (70 g) cabbage, shredded

$^1/_2$ cup (35 g) mushrooms, sliced

$^1/_2$ cup (75 g) red bell pepper, sliced

4 ounces (115 g) mung bean sprouts

$^1/_2$ cup (90 g) tomato, sliced

12 ounces (340 g) tofu, drained and cubed

For Dressing:

1 tablespoon (15 ml) rice vinegar

2 tablespoons (30 ml) sesame oil

3 tablespoons (45 ml) Dick's Reduced Sodium Soy Sauce (see recipe page 25)

2 cloves garlic, crushed

1 tablespoon (8 g) sesame seeds

$^1/_2$ teaspoon (0.9 g) ground ginger

To make the salad: Toss salad ingredients.

To make the dressing: Combine dressing ingredients and spoon dressing over salad.

Yield: 6 servings

Per serving: 111 calories (19% from fat, 7% from protein, 75% from carbohydrate); 5 g protein; 6 g total fat; 1 g saturated fat; 2 g monounsaturated fat; 4 g polyunsaturated fat; 57 g carbohydrate; 3 g fiber; 5 g sugar; 92 mg phosphorus; 55 mg calcium; 1 mg iron; 72 mg sodium; 365 mg potassium; 2728 IU vitamin A; 0 mg ATE vitamin E; 38 mg vitamin C; 0 mg cholesterol; 185 g water

18

Side Dishes

This chapter contains mostly vegetable side dishes. The starchier ones are in the next chapter. As such, everything I said in the notes about the salad chapter applies here too. These are the kind of things that you can't eat too much of, and the variety here should give you a great start. As a little added bonus the chapter ends with a couple of recipes for stuffing and a number of recipes for baked beans and other healthy legume side dishes.

Stuffed Tomatoes

Tomatoes stuffed with a rice/cheese/veggie mix make a nice side dish for just about any kind of meat.

6 medium tomatoes

2 tablespoons (28 ml) olive oil

$^1/_3$ cup (33 g) chopped celery

2 tablespoons (20 g) chopped onion

2 cups (440 g) cooked brown rice

$^1/_4$ cup (25 g) grated Parmesan cheese

1 tablespoon chopped fresh parsley

1 teaspoon basil

$^1/_8$ teaspoon black pepper

$^1/_8$ teaspoon garlic powder

Cut thin slice from top of each tomato. Set tops aside. Scoop out center of tomatoes; chop pulp, and set aside. Place shells upside down on paper towels to drain. Lightly oil 9-inch (23-cm) pie plate or round baking dish. Place tomatoes in dish. Cover with aluminum foil. Preheat oven to 350°F (180°C, gas mark 4). Heat oil in medium saucepan. Add celery and onion. Sauté over moderate heat until celery is tender. Remove from heat. Add reserved tomato pulp, rice, cheese, parsley, basil, pepper, and garlic powder; mix well. Fill tomato shells with rice mixture. Replace tomato tops, if desired. Bake at 350°F (180°C, gas mark 4), 30 to 45 minutes or until tomatoes are tender.

Yield: 6 servings

Per serving: 197 g water; 164 calories (36% from fat, 11% from protein, 53% from carb); 5 g protein; 7 g total fat;
2 g saturated fat; 4 g monounsaturated fat; 1 g polyunsaturated fat; 23 g carbohydrate; 3 g fiber; 1 g sugar; 124 mg phosphorus; 67 mg calcium; 1 mg iron; 86 mg sodium; 392 mg potassium; 1036 IU vitamin A; 5 mg vitamin E; 40 mg vitamin C; 4 mg cholesterol

Tip: Use one lightly oiled custard cup for each tomato instead of pie plate or baking dish, if desired.

Avocado-Stuffed Tomatoes

Particularly good as an appetizer or side dish for a Mexican meal.

4 tomatoes

1 avocado

$^1/_4$ teaspoon lemon juice

$^1/_2$ teaspoon chili powder

$^1/_4$ cup (38 g) chopped green bell pepper

1 teaspoon parsley

$^1/_4$ teaspoon coriander

Cut tops off tomatoes and scoop out insides. Save insides for another dish. Mash avocado and mix with the rest of the ingredients. Stuff into the tomato shells.

Yield: 4 servings

Per serving: 174 g water; 91 calories (51% from fat, 8% from protein, 41% from carb); 2 g protein; 6 g total fat; 1 g saturated fat; 3 g monounsaturated fat; 1 g polyunsaturated fat; 11 g carbohydrate; 4 g fiber; 0 g sugar; 57 mg phosphorus; 15 mg calcium; 1 mg iron; 20 mg sodium; 529 mg potassium; 1134 IU vitamin A; 0 mg vitamin E; 50 mg vitamin C; 0 mg cholesterol

Scalloped Tomatoes

My mother used to make scalloped tomatoes, but for some reason we never did. We recently rediscovered them, and they are now a regular treat on our table.

2 tablespoons (30 ml) olive oil

$^1/_2$ cup (80 g) onion, chopped

2 slices bread, coarsely crumbled

3 cups (540 g) tomatoes, sliced

Preheat oven to 350°F (180°C, or gas mark 4). Heat oil in a skillet and cook onion until softened. Add bread crumbs and stir to coat. Layer half the tomatoes in a 1-quart (946-ml) casserole dish. Top with half the crumb mixture. Repeat layers. Bake for 30 minutes.

Yield: 6 servings

Per serving: 88 calories (50% from fat, 8% from protein, 42% from carbohydrate); 2 g protein; 5 g total fat; 1 g saturated fat; 3 g monounsaturated fat; 1 g polyunsaturated fat; 10 g carbohydrate; 2 g fiber; 2 g sugar; 41 mg phosphorus; 17 mg calcium; 1 mg iron; 59 mg sodium; 207 mg potassium; 464 IU vitamin A; 0 mg ATE vitamin E; 20 mg vitamin C; 0 mg cholesterol; 86 g water

Roasted Italian Vegetables

This is the perfect side dish with an Italian meat like the chicken breasts in Chapter 13.

2 tablespoons (30 ml) olive oil

$^1/_2$ teaspoon (1.5 g) minced garlic

$^1/_2$ teaspoon (0.4 g) dried basil

$^1/_2$ teaspoon (0.5 g) dried oregano

$^1/_2$ cup (80 g) onion, sliced into wedges

$^1/_2$ cup (75 g) green bell pepper, cut in 1-inch (2.5-cm) pieces

$^1/_4$ cup (45 g) plum tomato halves

$^1/_2$ cup (56 g) zucchini, cut in 1-inch (2.5-cm) slices

$^1/_2$ cup (35 g) mushrooms, cut in half

Preheat oven to 400°F (200°C, or gas mark 6). Combine oil, garlic, basil, and oregano in a resealable plastic bag. Add onion, green bell pepper, tomatoes, zucchini, and mushrooms and shake to coat evenly. Coat a 9 x 13-inch (23 x 33-cm) roasting pan with nonstick vegetable oil spray. Place the vegetables in a single layer in the pan. Roast for 20 minutes, or until crisp.

Yield: 4 servings

Per serving: 79 calories (75% from fat, 5% from protein, 20% from carbohydrate); 1 g protein; 7 g total fat; 1 g saturated fat; 5 g monounsaturated fat; 1 g polyunsaturated fat; 4 g carbohydrate; 1 g fiber; 2 g sugar; 26 mg phosphorus; 15 mg calcium; 0 mg iron; 4 mg sodium; 159 mg potassium; 195 IU vitamin A; 0 mg ATE vitamin E; 21 mg vitamin C; 0 mg cholesterol; 67 g water

Green Beans with Caramelized Pearl Onions

This makes a nice alternative to the usual green bean casserole. It's easier to make and lower in sodium, and the sweet flavor goes well with many different meals.

2 pounds (910 g) fresh green beans

1 pound (455 g) pearl onions

$1/3$ cup (75 g) unsalted butter

$1/2$ cup (115 g) brown sugar

Arrange beans in a steamer basket over boiling water. Cover and steam 15 minutes; set aside. Place onions in boiling water for 3 minutes. Drain and rinse with cold water. Cut off root ends of onions and peel. Arrange onions in steamer basket over boiling water. Cover and steam 5 minutes. Set onions aside. Melt butter in a heavy skillet over medium heat. Add sugar, and cook, stirring constantly, until bubbly. Add onions; cook 3 minutes, stirring constantly. Add beans and cook, stirring constantly, until thoroughly heated.

Yield: 8 servings

Per serving: 155 g water; 177 calories (37% from fat, 6% from protein, 57% from carb); 3 g protein; 8 g total fat; 1 g saturated fat; 3 g monounsaturated fat; 2 g polyunsaturated fat; 27 g carbohydrate; 5 g fiber; 17 g sugar; 64 mg phosphorus; 68 mg calcium; 2 mg iron; 15 mg sodium; 370 mg potassium; 1120 IU vitamin A; 72 mg vitamin E; 23 mg vitamin C; 0 mg cholesterol

Tip: If you don't have a steamer, you can boil the vegetables.

Sesame Green Beans

These beans are a perfect side dish. They taste great and are low in fat and calories and high in fiber. What more could you ask?

1 teaspoon sesame seeds

1 pound (455 g) green beans, thawed if frozen

$1/2$ cup (120 ml) low-sodium chicken broth

2 teaspoons (10 ml) lemon juice

Toast sesame seeds in a heavy nonstick skillet over medium heat, about 3 minutes, shaking pan constantly until seeds are browned and have popped. Add green beans and broth. Cover skillet and cook 7 to 8 minutes or until green beans are tender and liquid is evaporated. Remove from heat. Stir in lemon juice before serving.

Yield: 4 servings

Per serving: 134 g water; 45 calories (12% from fat, 21% from protein, 67% from carb); 3 g protein; 1 g total fat; 0 g saturated fat; 0 g monounsaturated fat; 0 g polyunsaturated fat; 9 g carbohydrate; 4 g fiber; 2 g sugar; 57 mg phosphorus; 51 mg calcium; 1 mg iron; 16 mg sodium; 269 mg potassium; 783 IU vitamin A; 0 mg vitamin E; 20 mg vitamin C; 0 mg cholesterol

Spicy Limas

This recipe comes from a newsletter subscriber, who provided options for baking or cooking in the slow cooker. It's great as a stand-alone dish serving about 8 people or served over brown rice, whole grain pasta, or vegetable pasta.

2 cups (404 g) dried lima beans

4 cups (940 ml) water

2 teaspoons Mrs. Dash extra spicy

$1/2$ teaspoon crushed garlic

1 cup (160 g) chopped onion

$1/2$ cup (75 g) chopped green bell pepper

2 cups (480 g) no-salt-added canned tomatoes

1 tablespoon (20 g) honey

1 teaspoon basil

$^1/_4$ cup thyme

Cook dried lima beans according to package directions. Mix all ingredients except lima beans together. Carefully stir in lima beans. Place in 2- to 4-quart (2- to 4-L) covered baking dish. Cover and bake at 350°F (180°C, gas mark 4) for $1^1/_2$ hours, or until liquid is absorbed and vegetables are tender. Slow cooker option: Soak lima beans 6 to 8 hours in enough water to cover sufficiently and drain. Cook beans in covered slow cooker on low overnight (6 to 8 hours) and drain. Mix all other ingredients into slow cooker, cover, and cook on high for 1 hour or until vegetables are tender. Carefully stir in lima beans. Cook on low until liquid is absorbed.

Yield: 8 servings

Per serving: 206 g water; 183 calories (3% from fat, 22% from protein, 76% from carb); 10 g protein; 1 g total fat; 0 g saturated fat; 0 g monounsaturated fat; 0 g polyunsaturated fat; 36 g carbohydrate; 10 g fiber; 8 g sugar; 194 mg phosphorus; 94 mg calcium; 6 mg iron; 21 mg sodium; 944 mg potassium; 170 IU vitamin A; 0 mg vitamin E; 15 mg vitamin C; 0 mg cholesterol

Green Beans and Tomatoes

A different twist on green beans. Good with grilled meat.

$^1/_2$ pound (225 g) green beans

1 tablespoon (15 ml) olive oil

$^1/_4$ cup (38 g) red bell pepper, chopped

$^1/_4$ cup (40 g) onion, chopped

1 cup (180 g) tomatoes, chopped

$^1/_2$ teaspoon (0.4 g) dried basil

$^1/_2$ teaspoon (0.6 g) dried rosemary

Cook green beans in boiling water until tender. Drain and set aside. In a skillet, heat oil and sauté red bell pepper and onion until soft. Add tomatoes, basil, and rosemary. Stir in green beans and heat through.

Yield: 4 servings

Per serving: 62 calories (48% from fat, 9% from protein, 43% from carbohydrate); 2 g protein; 4 g total fat; 1 g saturated fat; 2 g monounsaturated fat; 0 g polyunsaturated fat; 7 g carbohydrate; 3 g fiber; 2 g sugar; 36 mg phosphorus; 28 mg calcium; 1 mg iron; 8 mg sodium; 239 mg potassium; 925 IU vitamin A; 0 mg ATE vitamin E; 32 mg vitamin C; 0 mg cholesterol; 104 g water

Bean Salad

This makes a fairly traditional three-bean salad. You can use either low sodium canned kidney beans or cook dried beans ahead of time.

$^1/_2$ cup (120 ml) cider vinegar

$^1/_4$ cup (50 g) sugar

$^1/_4$ cup (60 ml) oil

$^1/_4$ teaspoon (0.8 g) garlic powder

$^1/_4$ teaspoon (0.5 g) black pepper

12 ounces (340 g) frozen green beans, thawed

12 ounces (340 g) frozen yellow (wax) beans, thawed

1 cup (225 g) cooked kidney beans

$^1/_4$ cup (40 g) onion, diced

$^1/_4$ cup (37 g) green bell peppers, diced

Combine vinegar, sugar, oil, garlic powder, and black pepper in a saucepan. Heat until sugar melts. In a skillet, cook green, yellow, and kidney beans with onions and peppers until just tender. Combine vinegar mixture and vegetables and stir to mix. Refrigerate overnight.

Yield: 6 servings

Per serving: 194 calories (42% from fat, 9% from protein, 49% from carbohydrate); 5 g protein; 9 g total fat; 1 g saturated fat; 3 g monounsaturated fat; 5 g polyunsaturated fat; 24 g carbohydrate; 6 g fiber; 10 g sugar; 90 mg phosphorus; 54 mg calcium; 2 mg iron; 79 mg sodium; 394 mg potassium; 476 IU vitamin A; 0 mg ATE vitamin E; 24 mg vitamin C; 0 mg cholesterol; 153 g water

Tip: This will keep in the refrigerator for up to a week, but it probably won't last that long.

Vegetable-Stuffed Peppers

This dish could become a main dish with the addition of some ground turkey or cheese for protein. As it is, it makes a nice-looking, as well as tasty, side dish. The vegetable mixture, basically succotash in a pepper, can also be served alone.

2 green bell peppers

1 tablespoon (15 ml) olive oil

$^1/_4$ cup (40 g) onion, chopped

6 ounces (170 g) frozen corn, thawed

2 cups (360 g) canned no-salt-added tomatoes, drained

6 ounces (170 g) frozen lima beans, thawed

$^1/_4$ teaspoon (0.8 g) garlic powder

$^1/_2$ teaspoon (0.4 g) dried basil

$^1/_2$ cup (60 g) bread crumbs

Preheat oven to 350°F (180°C, or gas mark 4). Cut the green bell peppers in half lengthwise. Remove the tops and discard the seeds. Heat enough water in a saucepan to cover the peppers and boil for 3 to 5 minutes, or until just beginning to get soft. Drain. In a large skillet, heat olive oil and cook onion until soft, but not brown. Stir in corn, tomatoes, lima beans, garlic powder, and basil. Mix well. Place peppers in an 8 x 8-inch (20 x 20-cm) baking dish. Fill with vegetable mixture. Sprinkle bread crumbs on top. Bake for 20 minutes.

Yield: 4 servings

Per serving: 202 calories (20% from fat, 14% from protein, 66% from carbohydrate); 8 g protein; 5 g total fat; 1 g saturated fat; 3 g monounsaturated fat; 1 g polyunsaturated fat; 36 g carbohydrate; 7 g fiber; 8 g sugar; 136 mg phosphorus; 87 mg calcium; 3 mg iron; 132 mg sodium; 639 mg potassium; 497 IU vitamin A; 0 mg ATE vitamin E; 76 mg vitamin C; 0 mg cholesterol; 256 g water

Vegetable Bake

We were getting a little tired of the same old plain vegetables, so I threw together something a little different to have with roast beef.

12 ounces (340 g) frozen winter vegetable mix

6 ounces (170 g) Brussels sprouts

1 cup (235 ml) skim milk

$^1/_2$ cup (115 g) fat-free sour cream

2 tablespoons (16 g) cornstarch

4 ounces (115 g) water chestnuts

2 ounces (55 g) low fat Cheddar cheese, shredded

Preheat oven to 350°F (180°C, or gas mark 4). Cook winter vegetable mix and Brussels sprouts according to package directions. Mix milk, sour cream, and cornstarch until blended. Cook and stir until bubbly and thickened. Stir in vegetables and water chestnuts. Sprinkle with cheese. Place in 9 x 13-inch (23 x 33-cm) baking dish and bake for 10 minutes, or until cheese is melted.

Yield: 6 servings

Per serving: 120 calories (9% from fat, 29% from protein, 62% from carbohydrate); 7 g protein; 1 g total fat; 1 g saturated fat; 0 g monounsaturated fat; 0 g polyunsaturated fat; 16 g carbohydrate; 4 g fiber; 2 g sugar; 158 mg phosphorus; 141 mg calcium; 1 mg iron; 113 mg sodium; 312 mg potassium; 2778 IU vitamin A; 51 mg ATE vitamin E; 23 mg vitamin C; 11 mg cholesterol; 131 g water

Zucchini Cakes

These are a light, flavorful way to use up some of that extra zucchini when the garden is really producing.

4 cups (500 g) zucchini, grated

2 eggs

$^1/_4$ teaspoon (0.8 g) minced garlic

1 tablespoon (0.4 g) dried parsley

1 tablespoon (5 g) lemon zest

1 cup (115 g) bread crumbs

$^1/_4$ cup (60 ml) olive oil

Stir together zucchini, eggs, garlic, parsley, lemon zest, and bread crumbs. Divide into 6 balls. Heat half of the oil in a large skillet. Shape 3 balls into patties about $^1/_2$-inch (1.3-cm) thick. Fry until the bottom is golden, then turn and fry the other side. Repeat with remaining balls and oil.

Yield: 6 servings

Per serving: 182 calories (52% from fat, 13% from protein, 35% from carbohydrate); 6 g protein; 11 g total fat; 2 g saturated fat; 7 g monounsaturated fat; 2 g polyunsaturated fat; 16 g carbohydrate; 2 g fiber; 3 g sugar; 87 mg phosphorus; 59 mg calcium; 2mg iron; 178 mg sodium; 227 mg potassium; 294 IU vitamin A; 0 mg ATE vitamin E; 16 mg vitamin C; 70 mg cholesterol; 98 g water

Zucchini Squares

Another quiche-like dish, featuring shredded zucchini. Cut into smaller squares, this makes a great appetizer.

2 tablespoons (30 ml) olive oil

1 cup (160 g) onion, chopped

1 teaspoon (3 g) minced garlic

$^1/_4$ cup (15 g) fresh parsley, minced

$^1/_2$ cup (35 g) mushrooms, sliced

6 cups (745 g) zucchini, shredded

6 eggs

$^1/_2$ cup (60 g) low fat sharp Cheddar cheese, grated

1 cup (100 g) Parmesan cheese, grated

1 teaspoon (0.6 g) dried marjoram

$^1/_2$ cup (60 g) bread crumbs, toasted

Preheat oven to 350°F (180°C, or gas mark 4). Heat oil in a large skillet and sauté onion, garlic, parsley, and mushrooms. Add zucchini and sauté until barely softened. Mix eggs, cheeses, and marjoram. Add zucchini mixture to mixing bowl. Mix well and pour into a 9 x 13-inch (23 x 33-cm) glass baking dish that has been coated with nonstick vegetable oil spray. Sprinkle with bread crumbs. Bake for 30 to 40 minutes, or until a knife inserted near the center comes out clean. Allow to cool and cut into 2-inch (5-cm) squares to serve.

Yield: 6 servings

Per serving: 214 calories (52% from fat, 27% from protein, 21% from carbohydrate); 15 g protein; 12 g total fat; 4 g saturated fat; 5 g monounsaturated fat; 1 g polyunsaturated fat; 11g carbohydrate; 2 g fiber; 3 g sugar; 271 mg phosphorus; 231 mg calcium; 0 mg iron; 314 mg sodium; 292 mg potassium; 635 IU vitamin A; 80 mg ATE vitamin E; 20 mg vitamin C; 197 mg cholesterol; 153 g water

Zucchini Casserole

Another use for excess zucchini that I seem to have late each summer. This side dish goes well with chicken or fish.

3 cups (339 g) thinly sliced zucchini

1 cup (160 g) finely chopped red onion

2 tablespoons (28 ml) olive oil

4 ounces (115 g) chopped green chiles

6 tablespoons (45 g) whole wheat flour

$^1/_4$ cup chopped fresh parsley

$^1/_4$ teaspoon black pepper

3 cups (450 g) grated Monterey Jack cheese

2 eggs, lightly beaten

2 cups (450 g) cottage cheese

1 cup (100 g) grated Parmesan cheese

Sauté zucchini and onion in oil and place in large casserole dish. Cover with chiles, flour, parsley, and pepper. Sprinkle Monterey Jack cheese on top. Mix eggs and cottage cheese in bowl and spoon evenly over top of casserole. Sprinkle with Parmesan cheese. Bake at 350°F (180°C, gas mark 4) for 35 minutes.

Yield: 8 servings

Per serving: 140 g water; 358 calories (59% from fat, 30% from protein, 11% from carb); 27 g protein; 24 g total fat; 13 g saturated fat; 8 g monounsaturated fat; 1 g polyunsaturated fat; 10 g carbohydrate; 2 g fiber; 3 g sugar; 421 mg phosphorus; 548 mg calcium; 2 mg iron; 544 mg sodium; 287 mg potassium; 785 IU vitamin A; 132 mg vitamin E; 17 mg vitamin C; 117 mg cholesterol

Corn and Zucchini Bake

Something a little different in a vegetable side dish, with corn and zucchini contributing to a cheese-flavored custard.

3 cups (340 g) zucchini, sliced

1 tablespoon (15 ml) olive oil

$^1/_4$ cup (40 g) onion, chopped

10 ounces (280 g) frozen corn, thawed

1 cup (110 g) low fat Swiss cheese, shredded

2 eggs

$^1/_4$ cup (30 g) bread crumbs

2 tablespoons (13 g) Parmesan cheese, grated

Preheat oven to 350°F (180°C, or gas mark 4). Cook zucchini in boiling water until soft. Drain and mash with fork. Heat oil in a small skillet and sauté onion until soft. Combine zucchini, onion, corn, Swiss cheese, and eggs. Pour into a 1-quart (946 ml) casserole dish coated with nonstick vegetable oil spray. Combine bread crumbs and Parmesan, sprinkle over top. Place casserole dish on a baking sheet and bake, uncovered, for 40 minutes, or until a knife inserted near the center comes out clean.

Yield: 6 servings

Per serving: 154 calories (29% from fat, 31% from protein, 40% from carbohydrate); 12 g protein; 5 g total fat; 2 g saturated fat; 2 g monounsaturated fat; 1 g polyunsaturated fat; 16 g carbohydrate; 2 g fiber; 4 g sugar; 233 mg phosphorus; 267 mg calcium; 1 mg iron; 168 mg sodium; 247 mg potassium; 243 IU vitamin A; 11 mg ATE vitamin E; 12 mg vitamin C; 80 mg cholesterol; 132 g water

Cheesy Squash Bake

This is a great way to use extra yellow squash from the garden. It makes a good summer meal with just a simple piece of grilled chicken.

6 cups (680 g) yellow squash, sliced

1 cup (230 g) fat-free sour cream

2 eggs

2 tablespoons (16 g) flour

1 cup (115 g) low fat Cheddar cheese, shredded

$^1/_3$ cup (38 g) bread crumbs

Preheat oven to 350°F (180°C, or gas mark 4). Slice squash and cook in boiling water until tender. Combine sour cream, eggs, and flour. In a 9 x 13-inch (23 x 33-cm) baking dish coated with nonstick vegetable oil spray, layer half the squash, half the egg mixture, and half the cheese. Repeat layers. Sprinkle bread crumbs on top. Bake for 20 to 25 minutes, or until set.

Yield: 8 servings

Per serving: 121 calories (21% from fat, 38% from protein, 41% from carbohydrate); 9 g protein; 2 g total fat; 1 g saturated fat; 1 g monounsaturated fat; 0 g polyunsaturated fat; 9 g carbohydrate; 1 g fiber; 2 g sugar; 169 mg phosphorus; 129 mg calcium; 1 mg iron; 176 mg sodium; 335 mg potassium; 373 IU vitamin A; 40 mg ATE vitamin E; 15 mg vitamin C; 65 mg cholesterol; 128 g water

Scalloped Zucchini

Another of those old-time sort of recipes. We sometimes make a meal of this by adding 1 pound (455 g) of browned ground turkey to the mixture.

4 cups (500 g) zucchini, chopped

$^1/_2$ cup (80 g) onion, chopped

2 tablespoons (30 ml) olive oil

$^1/_2$ cup (50 g) Parmesan cheese, grated

$^1/_2$ cup (50 g) cracker crumbs

2 eggs

Preheat oven to 350°F (180°C, or gas mark 4). Cook zucchini in boiling water until nearly done. Drain, reserving $\frac{1}{2}$ cup (120 ml) of liquid, and chop coarsely. Heat oil in a skillet and cook onion until soft. Stir all ingredients together and pour into a $1\frac{1}{2}$-quart (1.4-L) baking dish coated with nonstick vegetable oil spray. Bake for 40 minutes, or until set.

Yield: 8 servings

Per serving: 111 calories (49% from fat, 21% from protein, 29% from carbohydrate); 6 g protein; 6 g total fat; 2 g saturated fat; 3 g monounsaturated fat; 1 g polyunsaturated fat; 8 g carbohydrate; 1 g fiber; 2 g sugar; 102 mg phosphorus; 102 mg calcium; 1 mg iron; 179 mg sodium; 150 mg potassium; 208 IU vitamin A; 7 mg ATE vitamin E; 11 mg vitamin C; 56 mg cholesterol; 82 g water

Summer Squash Casserole

A good way to use up extra zucchini or yellow squash from the garden. I take whatever leftover ends of homemade bread there are, grind them into bread crumbs, and store them in the freezer for just this kind of recipe.

4 zucchini or yellow squash, sliced

1 cup (160 g) sliced onion

1 tablespoon unsalted butter, melted

$\frac{1}{4}$ cup (60 g) sour cream

$\frac{1}{8}$ teaspoon paprika

2 tablespoons chopped chives

2 cups (230 g) whole wheat bread crumbs

Cook squash and onion until almost tender. Stir together butter, sour cream, paprika, and chives. Add

drained squash. Place in $1\frac{1}{2}$-quart (1.5-L) baking dish sprayed with nonstick vegetable oil spray. Top with bread crumbs. Bake at 350°F (180°C, gas mark 4) for 20 minutes.

Yield: 6 servings

Per serving: 34 g water; 191 calories (28% from fat, 11% from protein, 61% from carb); 5 g protein; 6 g total fat; 3 g saturated fat; 1 g monounsaturated fat; 1 g polyunsaturated fat; 29 g carbohydrate; 2 g fiber; 3 g sugar; 77 mg phosphorus; 85 mg calcium; 2 mg iron; 56 mg sodium; 128 mg potassium; 191 IU vitamin A; 33 mg vitamin E; 3 mg vitamin C; 9 mg cholesterol

Cheese-Sauced Cauliflower

The sight of a whole head of cauliflower is an impressive display for what is usually considered a lowly vegetable.

1 medium head of cauliflower

2 tablespoons (16 g) flour

$\frac{1}{8}$ teaspoon (0.3 g) white pepper

2 tablespoons (30 ml) olive oil

1 cup (235 ml) skim milk

$\frac{3}{4}$ cup (90 g) low fat Cheddar cheese, shredded

1 teaspoon (5 g) mustard

Bring 1 cup (235 ml) of water to boil in a saucepan large enough to hold the cauliflower head. Add the cauliflower to the pan, cover, and cook for 20 minutes, or until tender. Transfer to a serving plate. Blend flour and pepper into oil in a saucepan. Stir in milk. Cook and stir until thickened. Stir in cheese and mustard, and heat until cheese melts. Pour over cauliflower.

Yield: 6 servings

Per serving: 124 calories (44% from fat, 25% from protein, 30% from carbohydrate); 8 g protein; 6 g total fat; 1 g saturated fat; 4 g monounsaturated fat; 1 g polyunsaturated fat; 10 g carbohydrate; 3 g fiber; 3 g sugar; 168 mg phosphorus; 148 mg calcium; 1 mg iron; 144 mg sodium; 266 mg potassium; 133 IU vitamin A; 35 mg ATE vitamin E; 55 mg vitamin C; 4 mg cholesterol; 163 g water

Broccoli Casserole

A delightful way to make broccoli something a little different.

6 cups (420 g) broccoli florets

10 ounces (280 g) low sodium cream of mushroom soup

$^1/_4$ cup (60 g) low fat mayonnaise

$^1/_4$ cup (30 g) low fat Cheddar cheese

1 tablespoon (15 ml) lemon juice

$^1/_3$ cup (33 g) cracker crumbs

Preheat oven to 350°F (180°C, or gas mark 4). Cook broccoli in boiling water for 10 to 15 minutes, or until soft. Pour into a 1$^1/_2$–quart (1.4-L) casserole dish coated with nonstick vegetable oil spray. Combine remaining ingredients except cracker crumbs. Pour over broccoli. Top with crumbs. Bake, uncovered, for 35 minutes.

Yield: 6 servings

Per serving: 112 calories (39% from fat, 17% from protein, 45% from carbohydrate); 5 g protein; 5 g total fat; 1 g saturated fat; 0 g monounsaturated fat; 1 g polyunsaturated fat; 13 g carbohydrate; 1 g fiber; 2 g sugar; 113 mg phosphorus; 75 mg calcium; 1 mg iron; 203 mg sodium; 431 mg potassium; 2164 IU vitamin A; 4 mg ATE vitamin E; 67 mg vitamin C; 6 mg cholesterol; 117 g water

Mock Spaghetti

This makes a nice meat-free meal with just a salad for accompaniment. I've found that microwaving a spaghetti squash seems to work out better than baking it. It stays soft and juicy and takes less than half the time.

1 medium spaghetti squash

2 cups (360 g) canned diced tomatoes, no-salt-added

2 cups (140 g) mushrooms, sliced

$^1/_2$ cup (65 g) carrot, grated

$^1/_2$ cup (75 g) green bell pepper, chopped

$^1/_2$ cup (67 g) frozen peas, thawed

1 tablespoon (2.1 g) Italian seasoning

$^1/_2$ tablespoon (5 g) garlic powder

$^1/_4$ cup (60 ml) red wine

4 ounces (115 g) part-skim mozzarella, shredded

Pierce squash to center in several places. Microwave on high for 20 minutes, turning several times during cooking if microwave does not have a turntable. Slice in half lengthwise. When cool enough to handle, remove seeds and shred squash into strands with a fork. Place tomatoes, mushrooms, carrot, green bell pepper, peas, Italian seasoning, garlic powder, and red wine in a heavy saucepan and bring to a boil. Reduce heat, cover, and simmer for 15 to 20 minutes, or until vegetables are tender and sauce is thickened. Serve sauce over squash. Sprinkle with cheese.

Yield: 4 servings

Per serving: 171 calories (30% from fat, 25% from protein, 45% from carbohydrate); 11 g protein; 6 g total fat; 3 g saturated fat; 1 g monounsaturated fat; 1 g polyunsaturated fat; 19 g carbohydrate; 3 g fiber; 3 g sugar; 228 mg phosphorus; 275 mg calcium; 2 mg iron; 278 mg sodium; 570 mg potassium; 3881 IU vitamin A; 35 mg ATE vitamin E; 41 mg vitamin C; 18 mg cholesterol; 270 g water

Creamed Spinach

Creamed spinach is one of those dishes that kids tend to hate. Then they grow up and realize how good it really is.

3 tablespoons (24 g) flour

2 cups (470 ml) skim milk

$^1/_2$ cup (40 g) Parmesan cheese, shredded

1 tablespoon (15 ml) olive oil

$^1/_2$ cup (80 g) onion, finely chopped

$^1/_2$ teaspoon (1.5 g) minced garlic

12 ounces (340 g) frozen chopped spinach, thawed and squeezed dry

Shake flour and milk together in a jar with a tight-fitting lid until flour is dissolved. Pour into a saucepan, cook over medium heat and stir until thickened. Add Parmesan and stir until melted. In another pot, heat the oil and sauté the onion and garlic; add spinach. Cook for 10 minutes, or until

spinach is hot and onion is translucent. Add sauce and mix thoroughly.

Yield: 4 servings

Per serving: 191 calories (35% from fat, 28% from protein, 37% from carbohydrate); 14 g protein; 8 g total fat; 3 g saturated fat; 4 g monounsaturated fat; 1 g polyunsaturated fat; 18 g carbohydrate; 4 g fiber; 1 g sugar; 284 mg phosphorus; 451 mg calcium; 2 mg iron; 347 mg sodium; 533 mg potassium; 10563 IU vitamin A; 90 mg ATE vitamin E; 5 mg vitamin C; 13 mg cholesterol; 207 g water

Greens

A traditional, long-cooked southern vegetable. None of this crisp-tender stuff for these people. Red pepper flakes are optional, depending on how hot you like your food.

2 pounds (905 g) collard greens or kale

3 slices low sodium bacon

$^1/_4$ cup (40 g) onion, chopped

$^1/_2$ teaspoon (1.5 g) black pepper

1 tablespoon (13 g) sugar

Rinse greens thoroughly. Cut off stems and chop coarsely. Brown bacon in the bottom of a stew pot or Dutch oven. Remove. Place greens, onion, pepper, and sugar in the pot. Add enough water to cover. Cover and cook for 45 minutes to 1 hour, or until tender. Drain. Crumble bacon over.

Yield: 6 servings

Per serving: 78 calories (24% from fat, 24% from protein, 52% from carbohydrate); 5 g protein; 2 g total fat; 1 g saturated fat; 1 g monounsaturated fat; 0 g

polyunsaturated fat; 11 g carbohydrate; 6 g fiber; 3 g sugar; 39 mg phosphorus; 222 mg calcium; 0 mg iron; 72 mg sodium; 290 mg potassium; 10084 IU vitamin A; 0 mg ATE vitamin E; 54 mg vitamin C; 4 mg cholesterol; 143 g water

Southern-Style Greens

This makes a perfect accompaniment to grilled or smoked pork. The spices and honey make it more special than just boiled greens.

2 pounds (905 g) kale or collard greens

$^1/_2$ cup (80 g) onion, chopped

$^1/_2$ cup (75 g) red bell pepper, chopped

$^1/_2$ cup (75 g) green bell pepper, chopped

$^1/_2$ cup (120 ml) cider vinegar

1 tablespoon (15 ml) honey

$^1/_2$ teaspoon (1.5 g) garlic powder

$^1/_2$ teaspoon (1.5 g) freshly ground black pepper

1 teaspoon (5 ml) hot pepper sauce

Combine all ingredients in a large pot with 4 cups (946 ml) water. Bring to a boil, cover, reduce heat, and simmer for $1^1/_2$ hours.

Yield: 6 servings

Per serving: 103 calories (9% from fat, 19% from protein, 72% from carbohydrate); 5 g protein; 1 g total fat; 0 g saturated fat; 0 g monounsaturated fat; 1 g polyunsaturated fat; 21 g carbohydrate; 4 g fiber; 4 g sugar; 97 mg phosphorus; 212 mg calcium; 3 mg iron; 73 mg sodium; 765 mg potassium; 23697 IU vitamin A; 0 mg ATE vitamin E; 208 mg vitamin C; 0 mg cholesterol; 183 g water

Amish-Style Red Cabbage

Sweet and sour red cabbage recipe from Amish country, where sweets and sours are a part of life.

$^1/_4$ cup (60 g) brown sugar, packed

$^1/_4$ cup (60 ml) cider vinegar

$^1/_2$ teaspoon (1 g) caraway seed

$^1/_8$ teaspoon (0.2 g) red pepper flakes

$^1/_4$ cup (60 ml) water

4 cups (280 g) red cabbage, shredded

2 cups (300 g) apple, cubed

Combine first 5 ingredients (through water) in a saucepan and heat until sugar is dissolved. Stir in cabbage and apple. Cook about 15 minutes for crisp cabbage or longer for softer cabbage.

Yield: 5 servings

Per serving: 88 calories (2% from fat, 5% from protein, 93% from carbohydrate); 1 g protein; 0 g total fat; 0 g saturated fat; 0 g monounsaturated fat; 0 g polyunsaturated fat; 22 g carbohydrate; 2 g fiber; 18 g sugar; 31 mg phosphorus; 46 mg calcium; 1 mg iron; 25 mg sodium; 263 mg potassium; 815 IU vitamin A; 0 mg ATE vitamin E; 42 mg vitamin C; 0 mg cholesterol; 126 g water

Corn Relish

This makes a nice addition to salads as well as being useful just as a relish. It will keep for at least a week in the refrigerator.

10 ounces (280 g) frozen corn

$^1/_2$ cup (100 g) sugar

1 tablespoon (8 g) cornstarch

$^1/_2$ cup (120 ml) cider vinegar

$^1/_3$ cup (80 ml) water

2 tablespoons (15 g) celery, finely chopped

2 tablespoons (19 g) green bell pepper, finely chopped

2 tablespoons (20 g) onion, finely chopped

2 tablespoons (24 g) pimentos, chopped

1 teaspoon (2.2 g) turmeric

$^1/_2$ teaspoon (1.5 g) dry mustard

Cook corn according to package directions; set aside. In saucepan combine sugar and cornstarch. Stir in vinegar and water. Add corn and remaining ingredients. Cook and stir until thickened and bubbly. Cover and refrigerate.

Yield: 8 servings

Per serving: 90 calories (5% from fat, 6% from protein, 90% from carbohydrate); 1 g protein; 1 g total fat; 0 g saturated fat; 0 g monounsaturated fat; 0 g polyunsaturated fat; 21 g carbohydrate; 1 g fiber; 14 g sugar; 36 mg phosphorus; 5 mg calcium; 0 mg iron; 8 mg sodium; 132 mg potassium; 170 IU vitamin A; 0 mg ATE vitamin E; 7 mg vitamin C; 0 mg cholesterol; 60 g water

Brussels Sprouts with Tarragon Mustard Butter

This recipe came from my daughter. She's a Brussels sprouts fan who wishes we had them more often, so she went searching online for recipes. This is a variation of one she found, and it's a winner.

1 pound (455 g) Brussels sprouts

$^1/_2$ cup (120 ml) water

4 tablespoons (55 g) unsalted butter

2 tablespoons (28 ml) Dijon mustard

1 teaspoon dried tarragon

$^1/_4$ teaspoon black pepper

Cook the Brussels sprouts in the water in a covered saucepan just until a knife tip inserted in the center meets no resistance. Drain. Melt butter in a skillet over medium heat. Whisk in mustard until smooth. Stir in the tarragon. Cook until bubbly, about 30 seconds. Stir in sprouts, stirring to coat evenly. Continue cooking just until heated through. Sprinkle with pepper.

Yield: 4 servings

Per serving: 137 g water; 155 calories (65% from fat, 11% from protein, 24% from carb); 5 g protein; 12 g total fat; 7 g saturated fat; 3 g monounsaturated fat; 1 g polyunsaturated fat; 10 g carbohydrate; 5 g fiber; 2 g sugar; 76 mg phosphorus; 40 mg calcium; 1 mg iron; 105 mg sodium; 349 mg potassium; 1417 IU vitamin A; 95 mg vitamin E; 52 mg vitamin C; 31 mg cholesterol

Creamed Celery and Peas

Another recipe with a different-than-usual combination of ingredients.

$^1/_3$ cup (78 ml) water

2 cups (200 g) sliced celery

10 ounces (280 g) frozen peas

$^1/_2$ cup (115 g) sour cream

$^1/_2$ teaspoon rosemary

$^1/_8$ teaspoon garlic powder

$^1/_4$ cup (27 g) slivered almonds

In a saucepan, bring water to boil. Add celery, cover, and cook for 8 minutes. Add peas; return to boil. Cover and cook 3 minutes more. Drain. Combine sour cream and spices; mix well. Place vegetables in a serving bowl. Top with sour cream mixture. Sprinkle with almonds.

Yield: 6 servings

Per serving: 101 g water; 266 calories (60% from fat, 16% from protein, 24% from carb); 11 g protein; 17 g total fat; 1 g saturated fat; 11 g monounsaturated fat; 4 g polyunsaturated fat; 15 g carbohydrate; 7 g fiber; 5 g sugar; 232 mg phosphorus; 120 mg calcium; 2 mg iron; 198 mg sodium; 427 mg potassium; 1223 IU vitamin A; 20 mg vitamin E; 6 mg vitamin C; 8 mg cholesterol

Grilled Eggplant

If you are grilling almost any kind of meat, sprinkle it with Italian seasoning and grill this eggplant at the same time to accompany it.

1 eggplant

$^1/_3$ cup (80 ml) olive oil

$^1/_2$ teaspoon garlic powder

$^1/_2$ teaspoon Italian seasoning

$^1/_8$ teaspoon black pepper

Peel the eggplant and then cut into $^3/_4$-inch (2-cm) slices. Combine oil, garlic, and Italian seasoning; stir well. Brush eggplant slices with oil mixture, and sprinkle with pepper. Place eggplant about 3 to 4 inches (10 cm) from coals. Grill over medium coals 10 minutes or until tender, turning and basting occasionally.

Yield: 6 servings

Per serving: 71 g water; 125 calories (84% from fat, 3% from protein, 14% from carb); 1 g protein; 12 g total fat; 2 g saturated fat; 9 g monounsaturated fat; 1 g polyunsaturated fat; 5 g carbohydrate; 3 g fiber; 2 g sugar; 20 mg phosphorus; 8 mg calcium; 0 mg iron; 2 mg sodium; 180 mg potassium; 28 IU vitamin A; 0 mg vitamin E; 2 mg vitamin C; 0 mg cholesterol

Grilled Vegetable Stacks

Serve these as a side dish or add a portobello mushroom at the bottom of the stack to turn them into a vegetarian main dish.

$^1/_2$ teaspoon minced garlic

$^1/_4$ cup (60 ml) balsamic vinegar

$^1/_4$ cup (60 ml) olive oil

1 teaspoon basil

4 slices eggplant

1 cup (180 g) sliced tomato

4 slices red onion

1 cup (113 g) sliced zucchini

4 ounces (115 g) Swiss cheese

Combine garlic, vinegar, oil, and basil. In a large resealable plastic bag or bowl, pour marinade over all vegetables except tomato. Let sit for about 30 minutes. Remove vegetables from marinade and grill for 10 to 15 minutes or until browned and tender. To assemble stacks, layer eggplant, tomato, cheese, onion slices, and zucchini. Insert a metal or wooden skewer through the center of each stack from top to bottom. Return to grill for about 5 minutes or until cheese is melted. Carefully transfer stacks to serving plate and pull out skewers.

Yield: 4 servings

Per serving: 546 g water; 308 calories (44% from fat, 17% from protein, 40% from carb); 14 g protein; 16 g total fat; 3 g saturated fat; 10 g monounsaturated fat; 2 g polyunsaturated fat; 33 g carbohydrate; 17 g fiber; 14 g sugar; 318 mg phosphorus; 334 mg calcium; 2 mg iron; 90 mg sodium; 1317 mg potassium; 556 IU vitamin A; 11 mg vitamin E; 23 mg vitamin C; 10 mg cholesterol

Harvest Vegetable Curry

A flavorful curry containing a variety of vegetables. Feel free to substitute, depending on availability and your taste.

1 cup (130 g) sliced carrot

2 cups (280 g) cubed butternut squash

2 cups (142 g) broccoli florets

1 cup (150 g) red bell pepper, cut in strips

1 cup (113 g) zucchini, cut in wedges

1 cup (160 g) red onion, quartered

1 cup (164 g) cooked chickpeas, drained

1 tablespoon (15 ml) olive oil

1 tablespoon curry powder

2 tablespoons minced gingerroot

1 teaspoon cumin

1 teaspoon minced garlic

$1/4$ teaspoon red pepper flakes

$1/4$ cup (60 ml) low-sodium chicken broth

2 tablespoons (30 ml) lemon juice

3 cups (660 g) cooked brown rice

2 tablespoons chopped fresh cilantro

Steam carrot and squash for 5 minutes. Add broccoli, bell pepper, zucchini, and red onion and steam for 5 minutes. Add chickpeas; steam for 3 to 5 minutes or until all vegetables are tender-crisp. Meanwhile, in a small saucepan, heat oil over medium heat and cook curry powder, gingerroot, cumin, garlic, and red pepper flakes, stirring often, for 2 minutes. Add broth and lemon juice and simmer uncovered for 2 minutes. Toss vegetables with sauce. Serve over hot rice or couscous. Sprinkle with cilantro.

Yield: 6 servings

Per serving: 201 g water; 477 calories (11% from fat, 10% from protein, 79% from carb); 12 g protein; 6 g total fat; 1 g saturated fat; 3 g monounsaturated fat; 2 g polyunsaturated fat; 96 g carbohydrate; 8 g fiber; 6 g sugar; 415 mg phosphorus; 97 mg calcium; 3 mg iron; 158 mg sodium; 784 mg potassium; 10191 IU vitamin A; 0 mg vitamin E; 75 mg vitamin C; 0 mg cholesterol

Roasted Vegetables

A simple but tasty way to cook vegetables.

3 potatoes, cubed

3 turnips, cubed

1 cup (130 g) carrot, sliced 1 inch (2.5 cm) long

$^1/_2$ cup (75 g) green bell pepper, cut in chunks

$^1/_2$ cup (75 g) red bell pepper, cut in chunks

4 ounces (115 g) mushrooms

$^1/_2$ teaspoon onion powder

$^1/_4$ teaspoon garlic powder

$^1/_2$ teaspoon thyme

Place vegetables in a single layer in a roasting pan. Spray with nonstick olive oil spray. Sprinkle with spices. Roast at 350°F (180°C, gas mark 4) until done, about 30 minutes, turning once.

Yield: 6 servings

Per serving: 239 g water; 158 calories (3% from fat, 12% from protein, 86% from carb); 5 g protein; 0 g total fat; 0 g saturated fat; 0 g monounsaturated fat; 0 g polyunsaturated fat; 36 g carbohydrate; 5 g fiber; 5 g sugar; 152 mg phosphorus; 40 mg calcium; 2 mg iron; 50 mg sodium; 1082 mg potassium; 4037 IU vitamin A; 0 mg vitamin E; 50 mg vitamin C; 0 mg cholesterol

Potato and Carrot Bake

Looking for a different side dish for beef? Instead of boiled potatoes and carrots, try this.

6 potatoes, peeled, finely grated

1 cup (110 g) peeled, finely grated carrot

1 cup (160 g) finely chopped onion

3 eggs, beaten

6 tablespoons (45 g) whole wheat flour

2 tablespoons chopped parsley

$^1/_2$ teaspoon black pepper, fresh ground

1 teaspoon paprika

Preheat oven to 375°F (190°C, gas mark 5). In a large bowl, blend potato, carrot, and onion. Stir in eggs until well mixed. Stir in flour, parsley, and black pepper. Pour into a 9 x 13-inch (23 x 33-cm) pan coated with nonstick vegetable oil spray, filling to the top (it will shrink), and sprinkle with paprika. Bake 1 hour or until browned.

Yield: 8 servings

Per serving: 273 g water; 259 calories (9% from fat, 14% from protein, 77% from carb); 9 g protein; 3 g total fat; 1 g saturated fat; 1 g monounsaturated fat; 1 g polyunsaturated fat; 52 g carbohydrate; 6 g fiber; 5 g sugar; 242 mg phosphorus; 53 mg calcium; 3 mg iron; 59 mg sodium; 1404 mg potassium; 3043 IU vitamin A; 29 mg vitamin E; 28 mg vitamin C; 89 mg cholesterol

Spinach Casserole

Sort of an onion-flavored version of creamed spinach. Good with steak or chicken.

20 ounces (560 g) frozen spinach, cooked and drained

$^1/_2$ packet onion soup mix

8 ounces (225 g) sour cream

1 teaspoon lemon juice

$^1/_2$ cup (58 g) shredded Cheddar cheese

Combine all ingredients except cheese in casserole dish coated with nonstick vegetable oil spray. Top with cheese. Bake at 325°F (170°C, gas mark 3) for 20 to 30 minutes.

Yield: 4 servings

Per serving: 179 g water; 191 calories (57% from fat, 22% from protein, 21% from carb); 12 g protein; 13 g total fat; 8 g saturated fat; 4 g monounsaturated fat; 1 g polyunsaturated fat; 11 g carbohydrate; 5 g fiber; 1 g sugar; 209 mg phosphorus; 397 mg calcium; 3 mg iron; 339 mg sodium; 519 mg potassium; 17473 IU vitamin A; 99 mg vitamin E; 4 mg vitamin C; 39 mg cholesterol

Mixed Vegetable Casserole

Creamy, nice vegetable bake, good with fish or chicken.

10 ounces (280 g) frozen lima beans

10 ounces (280 g) frozen peas

10 ounces (280 g) frozen green beans

$^1/_2$ cup (80 g) diced onion

1 tablespoon (15 ml) olive oil

$^1/_2$ cup (115 g) mayonnaise

$^1/_2$ cup (115 g) sour cream

$^1/_4$ cup (25 g) grated Parmesan cheese

Cook frozen vegetables according to package directions. Drain vegetables. Sauté onion in oil until tender. Stir in mayonnaise and sour cream. Fold in

vegetables. Put in 2-quart (2-L) casserole dish coated with nonstick vegetable oil spray. Top with Parmesan cheese. Cook 20 minutes at 350°F (180°C, gas mark 4).

Yield: 6 servings

Per serving: 146 g water; 303 calories (60% from fat, 12% from protein, 29% from carb); 9 g protein; 21 g total fat; 5 g saturated fat; 6 g monounsaturated fat; 8 g polyunsaturated fat; 22 g carbohydrate; 7 g fiber; 4 g sugar; 172 mg phosphorus; 116 mg calcium; 2 mg iron; 346 mg sodium; 429 mg potassium; 1542 IU vitamin A; 40 mg vitamin E; 16 mg vitamin C; 19 mg cholesterol

Spinach Artichoke Casserole

This can be used as an appetizer spread on crackers or bread or as a side dish with a meal.

1 can artichoke hearts

30 ounces (840 g) frozen spinach, drained and squeezed

8 ounces (225 g) fat-free cream cheese, softened

6 tablespoons (90 ml) skim milk

2 tablespoons (28 g) mayonnaise

$^1/_4$ teaspoon black pepper

$^1/_3$ cup (33 g) grated Parmesan cheese

Spray 2-quart (2-L) ovenproof bowl with nonstick vegetable oil spray. Put artichoke hearts in bowl and then spinach. Mix cream cheese, milk, mayonnaise, and pepper. Pour over spinach and press spinach into the liquid. Sprinkle Parmesan cheese on top and bake at 375°F (190°C, gas mark 5) for 40 minutes.

Yield: 6 servings

Per serving: 200 g water; 214 calories (35% from fat, 31% from protein, 34% from carb); 14 g protein; 7 g total fat; 2 g saturated fat; 2 g monounsaturated fat; 3 g polyunsaturated fat; 15 g carbohydrate; 7 g fiber; 1 g sugar; 210 mg phosphorus; 352 mg calcium; 4 mg iron; 391 mg sodium; 634 mg potassium; 17488 IU vitamin A; 88 mg vitamin E; 5 mg vitamin C; 28 mg cholesterol

Vegetable Medley

A good way to come up with a veggie side dish on those days when the garden didn't yield enough of any one thing. Feel free to use your imagination (and refrigerator veggie drawer contents) when deciding what ingredients to use.

$^1/_2$ pound (225 g) green beans

1 cup (180 g) chopped tomato

1 cup (113 g) cubed zucchini

$^1/_4$ teaspoon garlic powder

1 teaspoon basil

Wash, trim, and cook beans until almost tender. Drain. Return to pan with other ingredients and cook to desired doneness.

Yield: 4 servings

Per serving: 116 g water; 30 calories (5% from fat, 20% from protein, 75% from carb); 2 g protein; 0 g total fat; 0 g saturated fat; 0 g monounsaturated fat; 0 g polyunsaturated fat; 7 g carbohydrate; 3 g fiber; 2 g sugar; 44 mg phosphorus; 33 mg calcium; 1 mg iron; 8 mg sodium; 296 mg potassium; 780 IU vitamin A; 0 mg vitamin E; 19 mg vitamin C; 0 mg cholesterol

Cranberry Yam Bake

Here's a nice combination of traditional holiday flavors, but good any time of year.

3 cups (330 g) sliced sweet potatoes

$^1/_2$ cup (60 g) whole wheat pastry flour

$^1/_2$ cup (115 g) brown sugar

$^1/_2$ cup (40 g) quick-cooking oats

$^1/_2$ teaspoon cinnamon

$^1/_3$ cup (75 g) unsalted butter

2 cups (200 g) cranberries

2 tablespoons (26 g) sugar

Peel sweet potatoes, slice, and cook until soft. Drain. Combine flour, brown sugar, oats, and cinnamon. Cut in butter until crumbly. Sprinkle cranberries with sugar. In a 2-quart (2-L) casserole dish coated with nonstick vegetable oil spray, layer half the potatoes, half the cranberries, and half the crumbs. Repeat the layers. Bake at 250°F (120°C, gas mark $^1/_2$) for 35 minutes.

Yield: 8 servings

Per serving: 126 g water; 301 calories (25% from fat, 6% from protein, 69% from carb); 5 g protein; 9 g total fat; 2 g saturated fat; 4 g monounsaturated fat; 3 g polyunsaturated fat; 54 g carbohydrate; 6 g fiber; 25 g sugar; 124 mg phosphorus; 58 mg calcium; 2 mg iron; 40 mg sodium; 429 mg potassium; 19714 IU vitamin A; 72 mg vitamin E; 19 mg vitamin C; 0 mg cholesterol

Stuffed Oranges

This is a great side dish to have with pork. I can see it for something like Thanksgiving dinner, maybe with a few of the required mini marshmallows on top.

6 yams

4 oranges

$^1/_2$ cup (112 g) unsalted butter, melted

$^1/_2$ cup (115 g) brown sugar

$^1/_4$ teaspoon nutmeg

$^1/_4$ teaspoon cinnamon

$^1/_2$ cup (75 g) raisins

1 ounce (28 ml) Grand Marnier

$^1/_2$ cup (55 g) chopped pecans

Bake yams at 350°F (180°C, gas mark 4) until tender. Cut oranges in half, scoop out pulp, and chop half of it. Peel yams, put in mixing bowl with chopped orange pulp, melted butter, sugar, nutmeg, cinnamon, raisins, and Grand Marnier. Mix well and stuff orange halves. Sprinkle top with pecans. Bake in a 350°F (180°C, gas mark 4) oven, 20 minutes.

Yield: 8 servings

Per serving: 133 g water; 367 calories (40% from fat, 3% from protein, 57% from carb); 3 g protein; 17 g total fat; 8 g saturated fat; 6 g monounsaturated fat; 2 g polyunsaturated fat; 54 g carbohydrate; 6 g fiber; 30 g sugar; 82 mg phosphorus; 72 mg calcium; 1 mg iron; 14 mg sodium; 779 mg potassium; 648 IU vitamin A; 95 mg vitamin E; 58 mg vitamin C; 30 mg cholesterol

Butternut Squash Bake

A sweet and different way to serve winter squash. This is good with pork, chicken, or fish.

$^3/_4$ cup (94 g) flour

$^3/_4$ cup (170 g) brown sugar

2 teaspoons (4.6 g) cinnamon

1 teaspoon (1.9 g) ground allspice

$^1/_4$ cup (55 g) unsalted butter

1 butternut squash

1 cup (235 ml) maple syrup

$^1/_2$ cup (50 g) pecans, chopped

Preheat oven to 350°F (180°C, or gas mark 4). In a bowl, combine flour, sugar, cinnamon, and allspice. Cut in butter until crumbly. Peel squash and cut into $^1/_2$-inch (1.3-cm) thick slices, removing seeds. Place half of squash in a greased 8 x 8-inch (20 x 20-cm) baking dish. Sprinkle with half of the flour mixture. Repeat layers. Drizzle with maple syrup. Sprinkle pecans on top. Cover with foil. Bake for 1 hour. Remove foil. Bake for 10 minutes more.

Yield: 10 servings

Per serving: 285 calories (26% from fat, 3% from protein, 71% from carbohydrate); 2 g protein; 9 g total fat; 6 g saturated fat; 2 g monounsaturated fat; 0 g polyunsaturated fat; 53 g carbohydrate; 2 g fiber; 37 g sugar; 51 mg phosphorus; 78 mg calcium; 2 mg iron; 61 mg sodium; 362 mg potassium; 6198 IU vitamin A; 55 mg ATE vitamin E; 12 mg vitamin C; 10 mg cholesterol; 61 g water

Sweet Potatoes, Squash, and Apples

This makes a great side dish with pork.

2 cups (266 g) sweet potatoes, cut in 1-inch (2.5-cm) cubes

2 cups (280 g) butternut squash, cut in 1-inch (2.5-cm) cubes

1 cup (150 g) apple, peeled and sliced

1/4 cup (60 ml) apple juice concentrate

1/2 teaspoon (1.2 g) cinnamon

Cook sweet potatoes and squash in water until almost soft. Drain, return to pan. Add apple and juice concentrate. Cook until apple is tender. Sprinkle with cinnamon.

Yield: 6 servings

Per serving: 113 calories (2% from fat, 7% from protein, 91% from carbohydrate); 2 g protein; 0 g total fat; 0 g saturated fat; 0 g monounsaturated fat; 0 g polyunsaturated fat; 27 g carbohydrate; 4 g fiber; 9 g sugar; 53 mg phosphorus; 55 mg calcium; 1 mg iron; 31 mg sodium; 433 mg potassium; 22177 IU vitamin A; 0 mg ATE vitamin E;25 mg vitamin C; 0 mg cholesterol; 144 g water

Spicy Sweet Potatoes

A slightly spicy, different way to serve sweet potatoes.

2 sweet potatoes, peeled and cubed

1 teaspoon (5 ml) canola oil

1/4 cup (38 g) red bell pepper, chopped

1/4 cup (40 g) onion, chopped

1/4 cup (60 g) brown sugar

1/4 cup (60 ml) orange juice

2 teaspoons (10 ml) lime juice

1 1/2 teaspoons (3 g) jerk seasoning

Cook sweet potatoes in boiling water until just tender. Drain well. Heat oil in large skillet. Add sweet potatoes, red bell peppers, and onions to pan and mix well. Cook until vegetables caramelize. Combine brown sugar, orange and lime juices, and jerk seasoning in a small bowl. Add juice mixture to pan with vegetables and cook over medium heat to reduce liquid until syrupy.

Yield: 4 servings

Per serving: 133 calories (9% from fat, 4% from protein, 87% from carbohydrate); 1 g protein; 1 g total fat; 0 g saturated fat; 1 g monounsaturated fat; 0 g polyunsaturated fat; 30 g carbohydrate; 2 g fiber; 18 g sugar; 35 mg phosphorus; 37 mg calcium; 1 mg iron; 27 mg sodium; 288 mg potassium; 12189 IU vitamin A; 0 mg ATE vitamin E; 28 mg vitamin C; 0 mg cholesterol; 94 g water

Better Than Stove Top

Do-it-yourself stuffing that beats the boxed stuff in both taste and nutrition.

1/2 cup (80 g) chopped onion

1/4 cup (25 g) sliced celery

$^1/_4$ cup (55 g) unsalted butter, divided

1 tablespoon parsley flakes

$^1/_2$ teaspoon black pepper, fresh ground

$^1/_2$ teaspoon sage

$^1/_2$ teaspoon thyme

1 cup (235 ml) low-sodium chicken broth

2 cups (230 g) whole wheat bread crumbs

In a saucepan, sauté onion and celery in 1 tablespoon butter until tender. Stir in remaining ingredients, except bread crumbs, and simmer for 5 minutes. Add bread crumbs, cover, turn off heat, and allow to sit for 8 to 10 minutes.

Yield: 4 servings

Per serving: 88 g water; 336 calories (39% from fat, 11% from protein, 50% from carb); 9 g protein; 15 g total fat; 8 g saturated fat; 4 g monounsaturated fat; 2 g polyunsaturated fat; 42 g carbohydrate; 3 g fiber; 4 g sugar; 120 mg phosphorus; 122 mg calcium; 3 mg iron; 102 mg sodium; 225 mg potassium; 431 IU vitamin A; 95 mg vitamin E; 2 mg vitamin C; 31 mg cholesterol

Sausage Stuffing

A little different kind of stuffing, with sausage and cheese providing a flavor boost.

1 pound (455 g) whole wheat bread, day old

$^1/_2$ cup (120 ml) skim milk

10 ounces (280 g) frozen spinach

1 pound (455 g) turkey breakfast sausage (see Chapter 5)

1 cup (160 g) diced onion

1 cup (70 g) sliced mushrooms

1 teaspoon crushed garlic

1 tablespoon unsalted butter

1 cup (115 g) shredded Monterey Jack cheese

3 egg yolks

Discard ends of bread and tear remaining loaf into pieces; place in a bowl. Pour just enough milk over bread to cover; soak for 5 minutes. Strain out milk, squeeze bread dry, and set aside. Cook spinach per directions on package, cool, squeeze dry, and set aside. In a skillet, fry sausage, crumbling as you cook it. Drain grease; set aside. Sauté onion, mushrooms, and garlic in butter until onion becomes translucent. Add spinach and sausage to onion and garlic, mix well; set aside to cool. Combine bread and spinach mixture with cheese. Add egg yolks. Combine all ingredients into a 12 x 9 x 4-inch (30 x 23 x 10-cm) casserole dish coated with nonstick vegetable oil spray. Bake covered in 350°F (180°C, gas mark 4) oven for 35 to 45 minutes, or until heated through.

Yield: 8 servings

Per serving: 140 g water; 483 calories (38% from fat, 25% from protein, 37% from carb); 23 g protein; 29 g total fat; 12 g saturated fat; 12 g monounsaturated fat; 4 g polyunsaturated fat; 33 g carbohydrate; 4 g fiber; 5 g sugar; 327 mg phosphorus; 306 mg calcium; 4 mg iron; 229 mg sodium; 480 mg potassium; 4603 IU vitamin A; 86 mg vitamin E; 4 mg vitamin C; 141 mg cholesterol

Stuffing

Almost everyone has different herbs and additives they like in their stuffing. Feel free to change the seasonings with such ingredients as thyme and basil. You can also add other things like mushrooms, chopped turkey giblets, etc., if this is something you would normally do. The longer you let the bread cubes dry out before making the stuffing, the more broth you will need.

1 pound (455 g) whole wheat bread, cubed or crumbled

2 cups (475 ml) low-sodium chicken broth

1 cup (160 g) chopped onion

$1/2$ cup (50 g) chopped celery

2 teaspoons tarragon

1 teaspoon sage

1 teaspoon poultry seasoning

$1^1/2$ teaspoons black pepper

Combine all ingredients and toss lightly. Place in a 9 x 13-inch (23 x 33-cm) baking dish coated with nonstick vegetable oil spray. Bake at 350°F (180°C, gas mark 4) until heated through, about 30 minutes.

Yield: 12 servings

Per serving: 68 g water; 114 calories (13% from fat, 18% from protein, 69% from carb); 5 g protein; 2 g total fat; 0 g saturated fat; 0 g monounsaturated fat; 1 g polyunsaturated fat; 20 g carbohydrate; 2 g fiber; 3 g sugar; 77 mg phosphorus; 64 mg calcium; 2 mg iron; 213 mg sodium; 142 mg potassium; 31 IU vitamin A; 0 mg vitamin E; 1 mg vitamin C; 0 mg cholesterol

Barbecued Baked Beans

This recipe starts with canned pork and beans, then expands on it to give it that homemade taste.

4 slices low-sodium bacon, diced

1 cup (160 g) chopped onion

$1/3$ cup (67 g) sugar

$1/3$ cup (75 g) packed brown sugar

$1/4$ cup (60 ml) ketchup

$1/4$ cup (60 ml) barbecue sauce

1 tablespoon (15 ml) mustard

$1/2$ teaspoon black pepper

$1/2$ teaspoon chili powder

16 ounces (455 g) pork and beans, undrained

16 ounces (455 g) kidney beans, rinsed and drained

16 ounces (455 g) great northern beans, rinsed and drained

In a large skillet, cook bacon and onion until meat is done and onion is tender. Drain any fat. Combine all remaining ingredients except beans. Add to meat mixture; mix well. Stir in beans. Place in a $2^1/2$-quart (2.5-L) casserole dish coated with nonstick vegetable oil spray. Bake, covered, at 350°F (180°C, gas mark 4) for 1 hour or until heated through.

Yield: 8 servings

Per serving: 147 g water; 317 calories (8% from fat, 17% from protein, 74% from carb); 14 g protein; 3 g total fat; 1 g saturated fat; 1 g monounsaturated fat; 0 g polyunsaturated fat; 61 g carbohydrate; 12 g fiber; 23 g sugar; 248 mg phosphorus; 113 mg calcium; 4 mg iron; 446 mg sodium; 731 mg potassium; 127 IU vitamin A; 0 mg vitamin E; 6 mg vitamin C; 8 mg cholesterol

Brown Beans

A fairly traditional baked bean recipe, flavored with bacon and sweetened with both molasses and brown sugar.

$2^1/_2$ cups (483 g) dried pinto beans

4 ounces (115 g) bacon, cut up

1 cup (160 g) chopped onion

$1/_2$ teaspoon minced garlic

$1/_8$ teaspoon black pepper

2 tablespoons (40 g) molasses

1 teaspoon Worcestershire sauce

$1/_2$ cup (120 ml) ketchup

1 tablespoon (15 ml) vinegar

$1/_2$ cup (115 g) brown sugar

$1/_8$ teaspoon dry mustard

$1^1/_2$ tablespoons cornstarch

$1^1/_4$ cups (295 ml) cold water

Presoak beans in water to cover overnight. Bring to boiling; cover and simmer until tender. Drain. Mix remaining ingredients. Add mixture to cooked beans. Bake about 45 minutes.

Yield: 6 servings

Per serving: 139 g water; 333 calories (22% from fat, 17% from protein, 61% from carb); 14 g protein; 8 g total fat; 3 g saturated fat; 4 g monounsaturated fat; 1 g polyunsaturated fat; 52 g carbohydrate; 7 g fiber; 27 g sugar; 228 mg phosphorus; 77 mg calcium; 3 mg iron; 462 mg sodium; 710 mg potassium; 195 IU vitamin A; 2 mg vitamin E; 7 mg vitamin C; 21 mg cholesterol

Cowboy Pinto Beans

Simply spiced, but good with a lot of different meals.

4 cups (950 ml) water

2 cups (386 g) dried pinto beans

$1/_2$ cup (80 g) chopped onion

1 teaspoon cumin

$1/_2$ teaspoon crushed garlic

$1/_4$ cup (60 ml) olive oil

1 slice low-sodium bacon, cut into 1-inch pieces

Mix the water, beans, and onion in a 4-quart (4-L) Dutch oven. Cover and heat to boiling. Boil 2 minutes and remove from the heat; let stand for 1 hour. Add just enough water to the beans to cover. Stir in the remaining ingredients and heat to boiling. Cover and reduce the heat. Boil gently, stirring occasionally, until the beans are very tender, about 2 hours (add water during the cooking time if necessary); drain the beans.

Yield: 6 servings

Per serving: 177 g water; 317 calories (29% from fat, 18% from protein, 52% from carb); 14 g protein; 10 g total fat; 2 g saturated fat; 7 g monounsaturated fat; 1 g polyunsaturated fat; 42 g carbohydrate; 10 g fiber; 2 g sugar; 277 mg phosphorus; 84 mg calcium; 4 mg iron; 28 mg sodium; 932 mg potassium; 5 IU vitamin A; 0 mg vitamin E; 5 mg vitamin C; 1 mg cholesterol

New England Baked Beans

Traditional New England–style baked beans, sweetened with maple syrup and slow cooked.

1 pound (455 g) navy beans

6 cups (1.4 L) water

2 slices bacon, cut in 1-inch (2.5-cm) cubes

1 cup (160 g) chopped onion

$^2/_3$ cup (160 ml) maple syrup

3 tablespoons (60 g) molasses

Mix all ingredients in a bean pot or ovenproof casserole dish. Bake at 275°F (140°C, gas mark 1) for 5 hours.

Yield: 6 servings

Per serving: 327 g water; 235 calories (6% from fat, 12% from protein, 83% from carb); 7 g protein; 2 g total fat; 0 g saturated fat; 1 g monounsaturated fat; 0 g polyunsaturated fat; 50 g carbohydrate; 4 g fiber; 29 g sugar; 127 mg phosphorus; 95 mg calcium; 2 mg iron; 416 mg sodium; 501 mg potassium; 2 IU vitamin A; 0 mg vitamin E; 3 mg vitamin C; 3 mg cholesterol

Rancher Beans

Just the sort of thing you'd want for dinner after a day riding fences on the ranch—something hot, spicy, and filling.

8 slices bacon

2 jalapeño peppers, seeded and chopped

$^1/_2$ teaspoon chopped garlic

1 cup (160 g) chopped onion

$^1/_4$ cup (60 ml) beer

1 tablespoon (15 ml) red wine vinegar

4 cups (684 g) cooked pinto beans, drained

6 ounces (170 g) no-salt-added tomato paste

Heat the oven to 375°F (190°C, gas mark 5). Cook the bacon in a skillet until crisp, then stir in the jalapeños, garlic, and onion. Cook and stir until the onion is tender, then drain the excess fat. Mix the bacon mixture and remaining ingredients in a 2-quart (2-L) casserole dish coated with nonstick vegetable oil spray. Bake uncovered, stirring once, until the beans are hot and bubbly, about 45 minutes.

Yield: 6 servings

Per serving: 134 g water; 261 calories (18% from fat, 24% from protein, 58% from carb); 16 g protein; 5 g total fat; 2 g saturated fat; 2 g monounsaturated fat; 1 g polyunsaturated fat; 39 g carbohydrate; 12 g fiber; 5 g sugar; 259 mg phosphorus; 71 mg calcium; 3 mg iron; 278 mg sodium; 898 mg potassium; 474 IU vitamin A; 1 mg vitamin E; 11 mg vitamin C; 12 mg cholesterol

Refried Beans

This makes a big batch of refried beans. The use of the slow cooker makes it easy to prepare. They freeze very nicely, so you can pack some away for the next time. The flavor is fairly traditional (despite the rather untraditional coffee in the ingredients) and not too spicy at all.

1 pound (455 g) pinto beans

4 cups (940 ml) water

1 cup (235 ml) coffee

1 teaspoon minced garlic

1 cup (160 g) diced onion

1 tablespoon cumin

2 teaspoons chili powder

1$\frac{1}{2}$ teaspoons oregano

Rinse beans and place in a large bowl covered with water overnight. Drain and place in slow cooker along with remaining ingredients. Stir well, cover, and cook 8 to 10 hours or until beans are tender. Use a potato masher or large spoon to mash the beans until desired consistency.

Yield: 12 servings

Per serving: 114 g water; 121 calories (4% from fat, 24% from protein, 72% from carb); 7 g protein; 1 g total fat; 0 g saturated fat; 0 g monounsaturated fat; 0 g polyunsaturated fat; 22 g carbohydrate; 5 g fiber; 1 g sugar; 141 mg phosphorus; 50 mg calcium; 2 mg iron; 12 mg sodium; 502 mg potassium; 139 IU vitamin A; 0 mg vitamin E; 3 mg vitamin C; 0 mg cholesterol

Cowgirl Beans

I'm not quite sure why I decided these were cowgirl, rather than cowboy, beans, but whatever you call them they are good. The tomatoes add a little different texture and taste than typical baked beans, and the jalapeños add a little heat.

1$\frac{1}{4}$ cups (241 g) dried pinto beans

6$\frac{1}{2}$ cups (1.5 L) water

$\frac{3}{4}$ cup (120 g) finely chopped onion, divided

1 tablespoon (15 ml) olive oil

2 teaspoons jalapeño pepper, seeded and chopped

$\frac{3}{4}$ cup (135 g) finely diced tomato

6 tablespoons chopped cilantro

Pick over the beans and wash them well. Put them in a kettle, add the water, bring to a boil, and simmer for 1 hour. Add half of the onion. Continue cooking uncovered 30 to 45 minutes longer. Heat the oil in a small skillet and add the remaining onion and the jalapeño. Cook briefly until the onion is wilted. Add the tomato and cilantro and cook, stirring, for 3 more minutes. Add the tomato mixture to the beans and continue to simmer, about 5 more minutes.

Yield: 6 servings

Per serving: 299 g water; 172 calories (15% from fat, 21% from protein, 64% from carb); 9 g protein; 3 g total fat; 0 g saturated fat; 2 g monounsaturated fat; 0 g polyunsaturated fat; 28 g carbohydrate; 7 g fiber; 2 g sugar; 177 mg phosphorus; 61 mg calcium; 2 mg iron; 17 mg sodium; 649 mg potassium; 298 IU vitamin A; 0 mg vitamin E; 10 mg vitamin C; 0 mg cholesterol

Baked Beans

A picnic's not a picnic without baked beans. These also freeze well, so you might want to make a double batch while you're at it.

$\frac{1}{2}$ pound (225 g) dried navy beans

4 cups (946 ml) water

1 cup (235 ml) chili sauce

$\frac{3}{4}$ cup (120 g) onion, chopped

2 tablespoons (30 ml) molasses

2 tablespoons (30 g) brown sugar

1 $1/2$ teaspoons (4.5 g) dry mustard

$1/4$ teaspoon (0.8 g) garlic powder

1 cup (235 ml) water

Place beans and 4 cups (946 ml) water in a large saucepan. Bring to a boil and cook for 1 minute. Remove from heat and let stand for 1 hour, then return to heat and simmer for 1 hour, or until almost done. Drain. Mix beans with remaining ingredients. Place in a 1 $1/2$ quart (1.4 L) baking dish. Cover and bake for 4 hours at 300°F. Add water if needed during cooking.

Yield: 6 servings

Per serving: 107 calories (4% from fat, 13% from protein, 83% from carbohydrate); 4 g protein; 0 g total fat; 0 g saturated fat; 0 g monounsaturated fat; 0 g polyunsaturated fat; 23 g carbohydrate; 3 g fiber; 12 g sugar; 60 mg phosphorus; 56 mg calcium; 1 mg iron; 454 mg sodium; 262 mg potassium; 670 IU vitamin A; 0 mg ATE vitamin E; 9 mg vitamin C; 0 mg cholesterol; 280 g water

Black Beans

These beans are best served over rice. Feel free to increase the pepper sauce if you like things spicy—the lunch I had with the leftovers when I added more hot sauce and cumin was even better than the original meal.

1 cup (250 g) dried black beans

4 cups (946 ml) water

1 tablespoon (15 ml) olive oil

1 cup (160 g) onion, chopped

1 tablespoon (10 g) minced garlic

$1/2$ cup (75 g) red bell pepper, diced

$1/4$ cup (60 ml) vinegar

$1/8$ teaspoon (0.6 ml) hot pepper sauce

1 teaspoon (2.5 g) cumin

$1/4$ cup (15 g) fresh cilantro, chopped

Soak beans in water overnight. Cook over medium heat for 1 $1/2$ hours, or until tender. Heat the oil in a large skillet and sauté the onion until tender. Add the garlic and red bell pepper and sauté an additional 2 minutes. Add the drained beans, vinegar, hot pepper sauce, and cumin. Bring to a boil and simmer 5 minutes. Stir in the cilantro. Serve over rice.

Yield: 4 servings

Per serving: 114 calories (29% from fat, 16% from protein, 55% from carbohydrate); 5 g protein; 4 g total fat; 1 g saturated fat; 2 g monounsaturated fat; 0 g polyunsaturated fat; 16 g carbohydrate; 5 g fiber; 3 g sugar; 83 mg phosphorus; 36 mg calcium; 1 mg iron; 14 mg sodium; 287 mg potassium; 765 IU vitamin A; 0 mg ATE vitamin E; 28 mg vitamin C; 0 mg cholesterol; 335 g water

Bean Patties

A tasty side dish made from leftover beans. Great with a pork chop and some greens.

1 $1/2$ cups (256 g) cooked pinto beans, drained

1 cup (160 g) finely chopped onion

$1/2$ cup (120 ml) fat-free evaporated milk

$1/2$ cup (62 g) flour

2 tablespoons (28 ml) olive oil

Mash pinto beans. Add onion and milk. Add enough flour to make patties. Heat oil in a heavy skillet.

Spoon bean mixture into skillet, flattening into a pattie. Fry until brown, turning once.

Yield: 4 servings

Per serving: 103 g water; 249 calories (26% from fat, 16% from protein, 57% from carb); 10 g protein; 7 g total fat; 1 g saturated fat; 5 g monounsaturated fat; 1 g polyunsaturated fat; 36 g carbohydrate; 7 g fiber; 6 g sugar; 185 mg phosphorus; 134 mg calcium; 2 mg iron; 39 mg sodium; 461 mg potassium; 127 IU vitamin A; 38 mg vitamin E; 4 mg vitamin C; 1 mg cholesterol

Tip: You can substitute any other kind of leftover beans you have for the pinto beans.

New Year's Day Black-Eyed Pea Salad

This has become a traditional New Year's Day dish in our house. It's a way to get the black-eyed peas for luck that still goes with the roast beef dinner that we always have. Even children will usually eat a little of this, ensuring luck for the year.

1 teaspoon Dijon mustard

1 1/2 teaspoons (8 ml) cider vinegar

1 1/2 teaspoons (8 ml) olive oil

2 cups (344 g) cooked black-eyed peas

10 ounces (280 g) frozen corn, thawed

1/2 cup (75 g) finely chopped red bell pepper

1/4 cup (40 g) finely chopped red onion

In a medium container, whisk the mustard, vinegar, and oil. Add all the vegetables. Toss to combine.

Yield: 4 servings

Per serving: 139 g water; 198 calories (14% from fat, 19% from protein, 68% from carb); 10 g protein; 3 g total fat; 1 g saturated fat; 2 g monounsaturated fat; 1 g polyunsaturated fat; 36 g carbohydrate; 8 g fiber; 7 g sugar; 176 mg phosphorus; 25 mg calcium; 2 mg iron; 30 mg sodium; 567 mg potassium; 795 IU vitamin A; 0 mg vitamin E; 32 mg vitamin C; 0 mg cholesterol

Black-Eyed Pea Salad

This recipe comes to us from the South, with roots back to Africa.

1 1/2 cups (250 g) dried black-eyed peas, cooked and drained

1 cup (160 g) onion, minced

1/2 cup (75 g) green bell pepper, chopped

1/2 cup (75 g) red bell pepper, chopped

1 teaspoon (3 g) minced garlic

3 tablespoons (45 ml) red wine vinegar

2 tablespoons (30 ml) olive oil

1/2 teaspoon (0.5 g) dried thyme

Pour the drained black-eyed peas into a medium bowl and add the onion, green and red bell peppers, and garlic. In another bowl, combine the vinegar, olive oil, and thyme to form the marinade. Pour the marinade over the black-eyed pea mixture, cover with plastic wrap, and refrigerate overnight so that the flavors blend, stirring occasionally.

Yield: 4 servings

Per serving: 172 calories (37% from fat, 14% from protein, 48% from carbohydrate); 6 g protein; 7 g total fat; 1 g saturated fat; 5 g monounsaturated fat; 1 g polyunsaturated fat; 21 g carbohydrate; 6 g fiber; 6 g sugar; 100 mg phosphorus; 31 mg calcium; 2 mg iron; 7 mg sodium; 378 mg potassium; 705 IU vitamin A; 0 mg ATE vitamin E; 44 mg vitamin C; 0 mg cholesterol; 123 g water

Marinated Black-Eyed Peas

This particular marinated vegetable recipe is almost entirely black-eyed peas. It's become traditional in our family to serve this as part of a New Year's dinner salad so you get the black-eyed peas that you are supposed to eat that day for luck.

4 cups (688 g) cooked black-eyed peas, drained

$^1/_2$ cup (120 ml) olive oil

$^1/_3$ cup (78 ml) white wine vinegar

$^1/_4$ cup (40 g) chopped onion

1 teaspoon garlic powder

$^1/_8$ teaspoon black pepper

$^1/_4$ teaspoon Tabasco sauce

Combine all ingredients in a large bowl, stirring well. Cover and marinate in refrigerator 3 days. Before serving, garnish with rings of onion and pepper, if desired.

Yield: 6 servings

Per serving: 94 g water; 316 calories (53% from fat, 12% from protein, 35% from carb); 10 g protein; 19 g total fat; 3 g saturated fat; 13 g monounsaturated fat; 2 g

polyunsaturated fat; 28 g carbohydrate; 7 g fiber; 6 g sugar; 143 mg phosphorus; 29 mg calcium; 3 mg iron; 8 mg sodium; 451 mg potassium; 88 IU vitamin A; 0 mg vitamin E; 4 mg vitamin C; 0 mg cholesterol

Black-Eyed Peas and Lentils

This makes a great side dish for chicken or pork. It tastes great, and it's a great choice for a day when you need a fiber boost, with 10 grams.

$^1/_2$ pound (225 g) black-eyed peas

$^1/_2$ pound (225 g) lentils

1 cup (160 g) chopped onion

2 cups (480 g) no-salt-added canned tomatoes

$^1/_4$ teaspoon black pepper

$^1/_2$ teaspoon basil

Soak peas and lentils overnight or for several hours. Combine all ingredients in large pot, and cover with water. Cook for approximately 1 hour, seasoning to taste.

Yield: 4 servings

Per serving: 226 g water; 178 calories (4% from fat, 24% from protein, 72% from carb); 11 g protein; 1 g total fat; 0 g saturated fat; 0 g monounsaturated fat; 0 g polyunsaturated fat; 34 g carbohydrate; 10 g fiber; 8 g sugar; 206 mg phosphorus; 73 mg calcium; 4 mg iron; 21 mg sodium; 711 mg potassium; 197 IU vitamin A; 0 mg vitamin E; 17 mg vitamin C; 0 mg cholesterol

Dal

A traditional Indian food, made with lentils or split peas.

1 cup (192 g) lentils

4 cups (950 ml) low-sodium chicken broth

2 tablespoons (16 g) grated gingerroot

$^1/_4$ teaspoon turmeric

$^1/_8$ teaspoon cardamom

$^1/_4$ teaspoon cayenne pepper

$^1/_2$ teaspoon cumin

2 tablespoons fresh cilantro

Rinse the lentils and combine them in a medium-size saucepan with the broth. Bring the broth to a boil, then lower the heat and simmer for 1 hour. Add spices, continue to cook briefly, and serve with fresh, whole wheat flatbread.

Yield: 2 servings

Per serving: 537 g water; 201 calories (15% from fat, 35% from protein, 51% from carb); 19 g protein; 4 g total fat; 1 g saturated fat; 1 g monounsaturated fat; 1 g polyunsaturated fat; 27 g carbohydrate; 8 g fiber; 3 g sugar; 330 mg phosphorus; 47 mg calcium; 5 mg iron; 149 mg sodium; 840 mg potassium; 282 IU vitamin A; 0 mg vitamin E; 3 mg vitamin C; 0 mg cholesterol

Dal with Tomato and Onion

Another version of dal, this one with added vegetables.

2 cups (384 g) lentils

1 cup (160 g) chopped onion

$^1/_2$ cup (90 g) chopped tomato

1 tablespoon grated gingerroot

1 teaspoon coriander

$^3/_4$ teaspoon garam masala

2 tablespoons chopped fresh cilantro

Wash and pick through dry lentils. Soak for 2 hours. Drain water. Put lentils in a saucepan and add water to cover plus 1 inch (2.5 cm). Bring to a boil. Boil vigorously for 5 minutes. Drain water and rinse well. Add fresh water to lentils to cover plus 2 inches (5 cm). Bring to a boil and reduce to a simmer. Simmer until tender, about 30 minutes. While cooking, check constantly to make sure there is enough water to cover. If not, add some. Stir in remaining ingredients during last 30 minutes of cooking.

Yield: 4 servings

Per serving: 125 g water; 136 calories (3% from fat, 27% from protein, 70% from carb); 10 g protein; 0 g total fat; 0 g saturated fat; 0 g monounsaturated fat; 0 g polyunsaturated fat; 25 g carbohydrate; 9 g fiber; 4 g sugar; 196 mg phosphorus; 33 mg calcium; 4 mg iron; 6 mg sodium; 488 mg potassium; 261 IU vitamin A; 0 mg vitamin E; 8 mg vitamin C; 0 mg cholesterol

Chickpea Loaf

This makes a nice, and different, sort of side dish. It also has plenty of protein and other good things to be used as a vegetarian main dish.

$^3/_4$ cup (90 g) whole wheat bread crumbs

$^1/_4$ cup (25 g) oat bran

1 egg white

$^1/_2$ cup (80 g) finely chopped onion

$^1/_2$ cup (55 g) grated carrot

$^1/_4$ cup (25 g) finely chopped celery

2 cups (328 g) chickpeas, cooked and mashed

$^1/_4$ teaspoon thyme

$^1/_2$ teaspoon savory

1 teaspoon basil

2 tablespoons chopped fresh parsley

Combine the bread crumbs and oat bran. Add the egg white and mix. Add the other ingredients. Put the mixture in a loaf pan or casserole dish, nonstick or sprayed with nonstick vegetable oil spray. Bake for 1 hour at 350°F (180°C, gas mark 4).

Yield: 6 servings

Per serving: 88 g water; 170 calories (9% from fat, 16% from protein, 74% from carb); 7 g protein; 2 g total fat; 0 g saturated fat; 0 g monounsaturated fat; 1 g polyunsaturated fat; 32 g carbohydrate; 5 g fiber; 2 g sugar; 115 mg phosphorus; 68 mg calcium; 3 mg iron; 286 mg sodium; 257 mg potassium; 1968 IU vitamin A; 6 mg vitamin E; 7 mg vitamin C; 0 mg cholesterol

Pasta with Chickpeas

There was a time when eating pasta with beans just seemed strange to me. But no more. If it still does to you, this might be a good recipe to start with to overcome that.

3 cups (492 g) cooked chickpeas

1 cup (160 g) chopped onion

$^1/_2$ teaspoon oregano

$^1/_2$ teaspoon garlic powder

$^1/_4$ teaspoon black pepper, fresh ground

2 cups (480 g) no-salt-added canned tomatoes, chopped

$^1/_2$ teaspoon sugar

$^1/_4$ cup (60 ml) dry red wine

3 cups (420 g) cooked whole wheat pasta

Combine the chickpeas and their liquid in a large saucepan with the onion, oregano, garlic powder, and pepper. Cook over medium heat for 10 minutes. Add the tomatoes, sugar, and wine. Bring to a boil; cover, reduce heat, and simmer for 30 minutes. Add the cooked pasta and stir well. Serve in soup bowls.

Yield: 6 servings

Per serving: 195 g water; 361 calories (5% from fat, 16% from protein, 79% from carb); 15 g protein; 2 g total fat; 0 g saturated fat; 0 g monounsaturated fat; 1 g polyunsaturated fat; 73 g carbohydrate; 11 g fiber; 4 g sugar; 270 mg phosphorus; 93 mg calcium; 4 mg iron; 375 mg sodium; 526 mg potassium; 129 IU vitamin A; 0 mg vitamin E; 14 mg vitamin C; 0 mg cholesterol

Chickpea Salad

Something a little different, based on chickpeas. Serve as a side dish or over lettuce as a salad.

14 ounces (397 g) artichoke hearts

$^1/_4$ cup (60 ml) lemon juice

$^1/_2$ teaspoon black pepper

$^1/_2$ teaspoon minced garlic

2 cups (328 g) canned chickpeas, drained

16 cherry tomatoes, halved

3 eggs, hard cooked, cut in wedges

Drain artichoke hearts and reserve liquid. Make a dressing by combining artichoke liquid, lemon juice, pepper, and garlic. Set aside. In a bowl, place 6 chopped artichoke hearts, the chickpeas, and the tomatoes. Pour the dressing over the mixture and refrigerate. Let marinate 6 to 12 hours. Before serving, top with chopped egg.

Yield: 4 servings

Per serving: 215 g water; 267 calories (20% from fat, 21% from protein, 59% from carb); 15 g protein; 6 g total fat; 2 g saturated fat; 2 g monounsaturated fat; 1 g polyunsaturated fat; 41 g carbohydrate; 11 g fiber; 2 g sugar; 251 mg phosphorus; 88 mg calcium; 3 mg iron; 471 mg sodium; 699 mg potassium; 823 IU vitamin A; 58 mg vitamin E; 30 mg vitamin C; 178 mg cholesterol

Lentils

This recipe can be used as a side dish or as the center of a meatless meal. And it provides a large serving of fiber while being low in fat.

1 cup (192 g) dried lentils

1 tablespoon (15 ml) olive oil

$^1/_2$ cup (80 g) onion, chopped

3 cups (710 ml) water

Soak the lentils using the traditional overnight method or the quick soak method on the bag. Heat oil in a skillet and sauté onions until just soft.

Combine lentils, onions, and water in a pan and bring to a boil over high heat. Reduce to low heat, cover, and cook for 30 minutes. Drain and serve

Yield: 2 servings

Per serving: 191 calories (33% from fat, 19% from protein, 48% from carbohydrate); 9 g protein; 7 g total fat; 1 g saturated fat; 5 g monounsaturated fat; 1 g polyunsaturated fat; 24 g carbohydrate; 9 g fiber; 3 g sugar; 190 mg phosphorus; 39 mg calcium; 3 mg iron; 14 mg sodium; 427 mg potassium; 9 IU vitamin A; 0 mg ATE vitamin E; 4 mg vitamin C; 0 mg cholesterol; 459 g water

Curried Chickpeas

This makes a great side dish with grilled chicken (try the Indian Chicken recipe in Chapter 6).

1 tablespoon (15 ml) olive oil

1 tablespoon (11 g) mustard seeds

dash red pepper flakes

$^1/_2$ cup (80 g) shallot, minced

4 cups (960 g) cooked chickpeas

$^1/_2$ teaspoon (1.1 g) turmeric

$^1/_2$ teaspoon (1.3 g) cumin

$^1/_4$ teaspoon (0.5 g) ground ginger

$^1/_4$ cup (15 g) fresh cilantro

Heat oil in a large saucepan and fry mustard seeds until they begin to pop. Add red pepper flakes and shallots and sauté until shallots are soft. Add chickpeas, turmeric, cumin, ginger, and enough water to prevent sticking. Simmer for 15 minutes, then sprinkle with cilantro.

Yield: 6 servings

Per serving: 220 calories (23% from fat, 19% from protein, 59% from carbohydrate); 11 g protein; 6 g total fat; 1 g saturated fat; 3 g monounsaturated fat; 2 g polyunsaturated fat; 33 g carbohydrate; 9 g fiber; 5 g sugar; 210 mg phosphorus; 72 mg calcium; 4 mg iron; 11 mg sodium; 394 mg potassium; 309 IU vitamin A; 0 mg ATE vitamin E; 3 mg vitamin C; 0 mg cholesterol; 78 g water

Yield: 6 servings

Per serving: 80 g water; 149 calories (47% from fat, 21% from protein, 32% from carb); 8 g protein; 8 g total fat; 5 g saturated fat; 2 g monounsaturated fat; 1 g polyunsaturated fat; 12 g carbohydrate; 3 g fiber; 1 g sugar; 163 mg phosphorus; 183 mg calcium; 1 mg iron; 261 mg sodium; 223 mg potassium; 2587 IU vitamin A; 57 mg vitamin E; 15 mg vitamin C; 23 mg cholesterol

Chickpea and Vegetable Casserole

Simple casserole of chickpeas and veggies that would be good with any meat.

8 ounces (225 g) dried chickpeas

$1/2$ cup (65 g) diced carrot

$1/2$ cup (50 g) diced scallions

1 cup (180 g) diced tomato

$1/4$ cup (38 g) diced green bell pepper

$1/2$ tablespoon vegetable seasoning

$1/2$ tablespoon paprika

1 cup (115 g) shredded Cheddar cheese

Soak beans overnight with three times as much water. The next morning rinse the beans, place in a pot with twice as much water, cover, and bring to a boil. Reduce to simmer and simmer for about 35 minutes. Dice carrot into chunks and steam for 15 minutes. Dice other vegetables and mix with chickpeas and seasonings. Place in well-buttered casserole dish, cover, and bake at 325°F (170°C, gas mark 3) for 35 minutes. After 25 minutes put a layer of cheese on top.

19

Potatoes, Pasta, Rice, and Other Grains

Another favorite food type of mine. I love almost any kind of potatoes and there are a number of recipes here. But beyond that there are some areas where I've made some changes in recent years, discovering that whole grain versions of pasta, rice and other grains were not only better for you, but, surprise, they tasted better than the old, more highly processed ones I used to eat. So now I almost always eat whole grain pasta and brown rice and we've added more barley, bulgur, and other whole grains. I'm sure they are better for me, but I'm really eating them because I like them better.

Garlic Fried Potatoes

A nice flavorful side dish to use with a simple grilled piece of meat.

1 pound (455 g) red potatoes, cubed

1 cup (235 ml) low-sodium chicken broth

1 tablespoon (15 ml) olive oil

$^3/_4$ teaspoon crushed garlic

Wash potatoes and cut into $^1/_2$-inch (1-cm) cubes; do not peel. Heat chicken broth in a nonstick skillet just large enough to hold the potatoes in 1 layer. Add potatoes, cover, and simmer 5 minutes. Chicken broth will evaporate. Add olive oil and garlic. Toss for 5 minutes over medium heat. Add black pepper to taste.

Yield: 4 servings

Per serving: 112 g water; 265 calories (13% from fat, 9% from protein, 78% from carb); 6 g protein; 4 g total fat; 1 g saturated fat; 3 g monounsaturated fat; 0 g polyunsaturated fat; 53 g carbohydrate; 9 g fiber; 2 g sugar; 133 mg phosphorus; 42 mg calcium; 8 mg iron; 42 mg sodium; 704 mg potassium; 11 IU vitamin A; 0 mg vitamin E; 15 mg vitamin C; 0 mg cholesterol

Spicy Oven-Baked French Fries

Southwestern flavors blend with spicy mustard for a zippy alternative to deep-fried fries. Feel free to increase the cayenne, red pepper, and chili powder if you like them spicier. You won't want to let the ketchup bottle near the table!

3 tablespoons (45 ml) olive oil

2 tablespoons (28 ml) lime juice

$^1/_2$ teaspoon minced garlic

$^1/_2$ teaspoon red pepper flakes

$^1/_4$ teaspoon cayenne pepper

1 teaspoon chili powder

2 tablespoons (28 ml) Dijon mustard

$^1/_2$ teaspoon black pepper

4 potatoes, peeled and cut into $^1/_4$-inch-thick (0.5-cm) fries

Preheat the oven to 400°F (200°C, gas mark 6). In a large bowl, stir together the olive oil, lime juice, garlic, red pepper flakes, cayenne pepper, chili powder, mustard, and pepper. Add the potato slices and stir until evenly coated. Arrange fries in a single layer on a large baking sheet. Bake for 20 minutes in the preheated oven. Then turn the fries over and continue to bake for 10 to 15 more minutes, until crispy and browned.

Yield: 6 servings

Per serving: 164 g water; 239 calories (27% from fat, 6% from protein, 67% from carb); 4 g protein; 7 g total fat; 1 g saturated fat; 5 g monounsaturated fat; 1 g polyunsaturated fat; 41 g carbohydrate; 4 g fiber; 2 g sugar; 88 mg phosphorus; 22 mg calcium; 1 mg iron; 71 mg sodium; 684 mg potassium; 228 IU vitamin A; 0 mg vitamin E; 17 mg vitamin C; 0 mg cholesterol

Home Fried Potatoes

This is a traditional breakfast kind of dish, but also works just as well as a side dish at dinner.

4 potatoes

1 cup (160 g) chopped onion

4 tablespoons (55 g) unsalted butter

$^1/_2$ teaspoon black pepper, fresh ground

Boil potatoes until almost done through. Drain. Coarsely chop potatoes and onion. Melt butter in a heavy skillet. Add potatoes and onion. Grind pepper over. Fry until browned, turning frequently.

Yield: 4 servings

Per serving: 270 g water; 376 calories (28% from fat, 6% from protein, 66% from carb); 6 g protein; 12 g total fat; 7 g saturated fat; 3 g monounsaturated fat; 1 g polyunsaturated fat; 64 g carbohydrate; 6 g fiber; 4 g sugar; 135 mg phosphorus; 38 mg calcium; 1 mg iron; 18 mg sodium; 1048 mg potassium; 365 IU vitamin A; 95 mg vitamin E; 25 mg vitamin C; 31 mg cholesterol

Potato Dumplings

Try these with sauerbraten or just plain grilled pork chops.

4 potatoes

1 egg, beaten

3 tablespoons (24 g) cornstarch

1 cup (115 g) whole wheat bread crumbs

$^1/_4$ teaspoon black pepper

$^1/_4$ cup (31 g) flour

Peel potatoes and boil in salted water until soft. Drain and mash smoothly. Blend in egg, cornstarch, bread crumbs, and pepper. Mix thoroughly and shape into dumplings. You may need to add flour to make

dumplings hold together. Roll each dumpling in flour and drop into rapidly boiling water. Cover and cook for about 15 or 20 minutes.

Yield: 6 servings

Per serving: 163 g water; 271 calories (7% from fat, 10% from protein, 83% from carb); 7 g protein; 2 g total fat; 1 g saturated fat; 1 g monounsaturated fat; 1 g polyunsaturated fat; 57 g carbohydrate; 4 g fiber; 3 g sugar; 128 mg phosphorus; 54 mg calcium; 2 mg iron; 48 mg sodium; 703 mg potassium; 51 IU vitamin A; 13 mg vitamin E; 15 mg vitamin C; 39 mg cholesterol

Potato and Vegetable Hash

Adding vegetables makes hash-browned potatoes a more complete side dish, but they are good for breakfast this way too. Depending on the meal, a number of different herbs can be added. We sprinkled them with a little garlic powder and basil just before turning.

2 potatoes, shredded

$^1/_2$ cup (80 g) shredded onion

$^1/_4$ cup (38 g) shredded red bell pepper

$^1/_4$ cup (38 g) shredded green bell pepper

$^1/_4$ cup (28 g) shredded zucchini

$^1/_3$ cup (60 g) finely chopped tomato

2 tablespoons (28 ml) olive oil

Shred all vegetables except tomato. Mix together. Heat oil in a large skillet. Add vegetables and spread to an even layer. Cook until lightly browned. Turn over and add chopped tomato on top. Cover and cook until tender. Cut in wedges to serve.

Yield: 6 servings

Per serving: 114 g water; 136 calories (30% from fat, 6% from protein, 64% from carb); 2 g protein; 5 g total fat; 1 g saturated fat; 3 g monounsaturated fat; 1 g polyunsaturated fat; 22 g carbohydrate; 2 g fiber; 2 g sugar; 51 mg phosphorus; 14 mg calcium; 0 mg iron; 7 mg sodium; 404 mg potassium; 300 IU vitamin A; 0 mg vitamin E; 23 mg vitamin C; 0 mg cholesterol

Grilled Potatoes

This makes a very tasty variation on baked potatoes when you grill a steak or chops. It can also be cooked in the oven those days when you aren't firing up the grill.

4 potatoes

1 onion, sliced

Scrub potatoes and make 2 or 3 crosswise slices almost through. Place an onion slice in each cut. Wrap potatoes in heavy-duty foil and grill for 30 to 45 minutes, or until done.

Yield: 4 servings

Per serving: 274 calories (2% from fat, 10% from protein, 88% from carbohydrate); 7 g protein; 1 g total fat; 0 g saturated fat; 0 g monounsaturated fat; 0 g polyunsaturated fat; 62 g carbohydrate; 7 g fiber; 5 g sugar; 237 mg phosphorus; 46 mg calcium; 3 mg iron; 24 mg sodium; 1737 mg potassium; 27 IU vitamin A; 0 mg ATE vitamin E; 35 mg vitamin C; 0 mg cholesterol; 334 g water

Baked Fried Potatoes

Instead of French fries, make these baked fries. The texture and taste is similar to the frozen steak fries in the supermarket.

4 large potatoes

1 tablespoon (15 ml) olive oil

Preheat oven to 400°F (200°C, or gas mark 6). Scrub potatoes. Cut each in half lengthwise. Cut each half into 4 spears. Place potatoes in a large pot of boiling water, bring water back to a boil, and boil for 3 minutes. Drain in a colander. Coat a cooking sheet with nonstick vegetable oil spray. Mix the olive oil and potatoes in bowl and toss to coat. Bake for 15 minutes, or until tender. Drain on paper towels.

Yield: 4 servings

Per serving: 288 calories (12% from fat, 9% from protein, 79% from carbohydrate); 7 g protein; 4 g total fat; 1 g saturated fat; 2 g monounsaturated fat; 1 g polyunsaturated fat; 59 g carbohydrate; 6 g fiber; 4 g sugar; 225 mg phosphorus; 37 mg calcium; 3 mg iron; 22 mg sodium; 1679 mg potassium; 26 IU vitamin A; 0 mg ATE vitamin E; 32 mg vitamin C; 0 mg cholesterol; 299 g water

Tip: You can vary these with any combination of herbs and spices that appeal to you. Just toss them with the potatoes after coating them in the oil.

Fat-Free Mashed Potatoes

These make a flavorful addition to any meal, spicing up a piece of plain grilled meat.

4 medium red potatoes

$1/2$ teaspoon (1.5 g) roasted garlic

2 tablespoons (30 g) fat-free cream cheese

$1/4$ cup (60 ml) skim milk

1 teaspoon (1 g) chives

1 tablespoon (4 g) fresh parsley, chopped.

Cube the potatoes (you may peel them or leave unpeeled). Place in a saucepan of water, bring to a boil, and simmer until potatoes are soft, but not mushy. Drain very well. Place potatoes in a large mixing bowl; add garlic, cream cheese, and milk. Beat mixture until it reaches desired consistency, adding more milk if needed, then add the chives and parsley and mix well.

Yield: 4 servings

Per serving: 139 calories (2% from fat, 12% from protein, 86% from carbohydrate); 4 g protein; 0 g total fat; 0 g saturated fat; 0 g monounsaturated fat; 0 g polyunsaturated fat; 28 g carbohydrate; 5 g fiber; 1 g sugar; 88 mg phosphorus; 52 mg calcium; 4 mg iron; 44 mg sodium; 380 mg potassium; 178 IU vitamin A; 23 mg ATE vitamin E; 10 mg vitamin C; 5 mg cholesterol; 47 g water

Tip: If you don't want to roast your own garlic, you can find jars of it in the fresh vegetable sections of many large grocery stores.

Potato Pie

This is a great side dish—sort of a cross between scalloped potatoes and macaroni and cheese.

2 large potatoes, peeled and shredded

6 ounces (170 g) shredded low fat Cheddar cheese, divided

$1/2$ cup (120 ml) skim milk

$1/2$ cup (80 g) onion, chopped

$1/2$ teaspoon (1 g) black pepper

4 eggs

Preheat oven to 350°F (180°C, or gas mark 4). Spray a 9-inch (23-cm) pie plate with nonstick vegetable oil spray. Mix potatoes and $1/2$ cup (58 g) cheese. Press into bottom and up sides of prepared pie plate. Stir onion, pepper, remaining cheese, and eggs together. Pour into crust. Bake for 45 to 50 minutes, or until a knife inserted near the center comes out clean. Let stand 5 minutes before serving.

Yield: 6 servings

Per serving: 184 calories (18% from fat, 33% from protein, 49% from carbohydrate); 15 g protein; 4 g total fat; 2 g saturated fat; 1 g monounsaturated fat; 1 g polyunsaturated fat; 23 g carbohydrate; 2 g fiber; 2 g sugar; 290 mg phosphorus; 185 mg calcium; 2 mg iron; 268 mg sodium; 675 mg potassium; 260 IU vitamin A; 30 mg ATE vitamin E; 12 mg vitamin C; 147 mg cholesterol; 182 g water

Baked Potato Casserole

This is a casserole version of hot-topped potatoes. It makes a nice presentation and allows everyone to take exactly how much they want.

6 large potatoes

6 slices low sodium bacon, cooked, drained, and crumbled

1 cup (115 g) low fat Cheddar cheese, shredded

2 cups (300 g) frozen broccoli, thawed

$^1/_4$ cup (25 g) scallions, sliced

Preheat oven to 350°F (180°C, or gas mark 4). Boil, bake, or microwave the potatoes until tender. Cut potatoes in half, leaving the skins on, and arrange in a large casserole dish. Press down with a fork. Spread bacon bits over potatoes. Boil or steam broccoli, chop, and add to top of casserole. Spread grated cheese over top. Bake for 20 to 25 minutes or until hot and cheese is melted. Garnish with scallions.

Yield: 6 servings

Per serving: 351 calories (14% from fat, 18% from protein, 68% from carbohydrate); 16 g protein; 6 g total fat; 2 g saturated fat; 2 g monounsaturated fat; 1 g polyunsaturated fat; 62 g carbohydrate; 7 g fiber; 4 g sugar; 396 mg phosphorus; 146 mg calcium; 3 mg iron; 250 mg sodium; 1846 mg potassium; 305 IU vitamin A; 14 mg ATE vitamin E; 60 mg vitamin C; 13 mg cholesterol; 344 g water

Slow Cooker Scalloped Potatoes

Another one of those classic comfort foods. In this version, I simplify the preparation by using the slow cooker to create tender, creamy potatoes.

2 cups (470 ml) water

1 teaspoon (3 g) cream of tartar

5 medium potatoes, thinly sliced

$^1/_4$ cup (30 g) all-purpose flour

$^1/_8$ teaspoon (0.3 g) freshly ground black pepper

$1^1/_2$ cups (355 ml) skim milk

1 cup (115 g) low fat Cheddar cheese, shredded

Combine water and cream of tartar in large bowl. Stir. Add potatoes and stir well. This will help keep potatoes from darkening. Drain. Pour potatoes into a slow cooker. Stir flour and pepper together in a saucepan. Whisk in milk gradually until no lumps remain. Heat and stir until boiling and thickened. Stir in cheese to melt. Pour over potatoes in cooker. Cover. Cook on low for 6 to 8 hours.

Yield: 6 servings

Per serving: 305 calories (6% from fat, 19% from protein, 75% from carbohydrate); 14 g protein; 2 g total fat; 1 g saturated fat; 1 g monounsaturated fat; 0 g polyunsaturated fat; 57 g carbohydrate; 5 g fiber; 4 g sugar; 360 mg phosphorus; 205 mg calcium; 2 mg iron; 204 mg sodium; 1573 mg potassium; 195 IU vitamin A; 51 mg ATE vitamin E; 32 mg vitamin C; 6 mg cholesterol; 339 g water

German Potato Bake

The flavor of German potato salad in a casserole. Great with pork or chicken.

6 slices low sodium bacon

2 tablespoons (16 g) flour

$1/4$ cup (60 ml) cider vinegar

2 cups (470 ml) low sodium chicken broth

2 tablespoons (30 g) brown sugar

$1/4$ cup (25 g) scallions, sliced diagonally

$1/4$ teaspoon (0.5 g) celery seed

6 medium potatoes, cooked and sliced

Preheat oven to 400°F (200°C, or gas mark 6). In a skillet, cook bacon until crisp; remove to a paper towel–lined plate to drain. Wipe out skillet. Shake flour and vinegar together in a jar with a tight-fitting lid until dissolved. Pour into skillet and add remaining ingredients except potatoes. Cook, stirring until thickened. In $1^{1}/_{2}$-quart (1.4-L) shallow baking dish arrange potatoes; pour broth mixture over the top. Bake for 30 minutes. Garnish with bacon.

Yield: 6 servings

Per serving: 345 calories (11% from fat, 13% from protein, 75% from carbohydrate); 12 g protein; 4 g total fat; 1 g saturated fat; 2 g monounsaturated fat; 1 g polyunsaturated fat; 67 g carbohydrate; 6 g fiber; 8 g sugar; 298 mg phosphorus; 51 mg calcium; 3 mg iron; 132 mg sodium; 1832 mg potassium; 70 IU vitamin A; 1 mg ATE vitamin E; 33 mg vitamin C; 9 mg cholesterol; 390 g water

Two-Tone Twice-Baked Potatoes

This is one of those ideas that make you wonder why you never thought of it before. We had it as part of our Christmas dinner, and everyone thought it was a great idea.

3 baking potatoes

3 sweet potatoes

$1/3$ cup (77 g) sour cream

3 tablespoons (45 ml) skim milk

4 tablespoons chives

Pierce potatoes with a fork. Bake at 400°F (200°C, gas mark 6) until tender, 60 to 70 minutes. Cut a slice off the top of each baking potato. Scoop out the pulp, leaving the skin intact. Place in a bowl and mix together with half the sour cream, milk, and chives. Repeat with the sweet potatoes. Place sweet potato mixture in one end of each potato skin and baking potato mixture in the other end. Bake at 350°F (180°C, gas mark 4) until heated through, about 10 to 15 minutes.

Yield: 6 servings

Per serving: 190 g water; 227 calories (12% from fat, 9% from protein, 79% from carb); 6 g protein; 3 g total fat; 2 g saturated fat; 1 g monounsaturated fat; 0 g polyunsaturated fat; 46 g carbohydrate; 5 g fiber; 6 g sugar; 149 mg phosphorus; 70 mg calcium; 2 mg iron; 47 mg sodium; 1012 mg potassium; 12084 IU vitamin A; 27 mg vitamin E; 25 mg vitamin C; 6 mg cholesterol

Twice-Baked Potatoes

With the addition of ground beef, these potatoes become a whole meal. The microwave also makes it a quick meal.

4 medium potatoes

8 ounces (225 g) ground beef, extra lean

1 cup (71 g) finely chopped broccoli florets

1 cup (235 ml) water

1 cup (115 g) shredded Cheddar cheese, divided

$^1/_2$ cup (115 g) sour cream

$^1/_4$ teaspoon black pepper, fresh ground

$^1/_4$ cup (25 g) sliced scallions

Pierce potatoes all over with a fork. Place in the microwave and cook, turning once or twice, until the potatoes are soft, about 10 minutes. Meanwhile, brown meat in a large skillet over medium-high heat, stirring often, about 3 minutes. Transfer to a large bowl. Increase heat to high, add broccoli and water to the skillet, cover, and cook until tender, 4 to 5 minutes. Drain the broccoli; add to the meat. Carefully cut off the top third of the cooked potatoes; reserve the tops for another use. Scoop the insides out into a medium bowl. Place the potato shells in a small baking dish. Add $^1/_2$ cup (58 g) Cheddar, sour cream, and pepper to the potato insides and mash with a fork or potato masher. Add scallions and the potato mixture to the broccoli and meat; stir to combine. Evenly divide the potato mixture among the potato shells and top with the remaining Cheddar cheese. Microwave on high until the filling is hot and the cheese is melted, 2 to 4 minutes.

Yield: 4 servings

Per serving: 452 g water; 572 calories (39% from fat, 19% from protein, 43% from carb); 27 g protein; 25 g total fat; 13 g saturated fat; 8 g monounsaturated fat; 1 g polyunsaturated fat; 62 g carbohydrate; 6 g fiber; 4 g sugar; 517 mg phosphorus; 326 mg calcium; 4 mg iron; 285 mg sodium; 1989 mg potassium; 1064 IU vitamin A; 115 mg vitamin E; 50 mg vitamin C; 86 mg cholesterol

Reduced-Fat Macaroni and Cheese

This isn't exactly the same as the boxes of macaroni and cheese. On the other hand, this recipe contains only 3 grams of saturated fat and has the nutritional advantage of having real cheese.

12 ounces (340 g) elbow macaroni

$^1/_2$ cup (120 ml) skim milk

1 cup (250 g) low fat ricotta cheese

$^1/_4$ cup (40 g) onion, diced

$^1/_4$ teaspoon (0.5 g) black pepper

1 cup (115 g) shredded low fat Cheddar cheese, divided

Preheat oven to 350°F (180°C, or gas mark 4). Cook macaroni according to package directions, omitting salt. Drain. In a food processor or blender combine milk, ricotta cheese, onion, and pepper. Process until smooth. Pour into a bowl and add macaroni and $^1/_4$ cup (30 g) Cheddar cheese. Mix well. Spray a 1-quart (946 ml) baking dish with nonstick vegetable oil spray. Pour in macaroni mixture and top with remaining cheese. Cover and bake for 30 minutes. Uncover and bake an additional 10 minutes.

Yield: 6 servings

Per serving: 316 calories (16% from fat, 24% from protein, 60% from carbohydrate); 18 g protein; 6 g total fat; 3 g saturated fat; 2 g monounsaturated fat; 0 g polyunsaturated fat; 47 g carbohydrate; 2 g fiber; 2 g sugar; 314 mg phosphorus; 246 mg calcium; 2 mg iron; 202 mg sodium; 240 mg potassium; 245 IU vitamin A; 69 mg ATE vitamin E; 1 mg vitamin C; 18 mg cholesterol; 74 g water

Pasta and Bean Salad

This is another salad that could be a full meal if you want. A simple dressing brings out the flavor of the vegetables.

3 tablespoons (45 ml) vinegar

$^1/_4$ cup (60 ml) light corn syrup

$^1/_4$ cup (60 ml) olive oil

10 ounces (280 g) frozen green beans

1 cup (100 g) chopped celery

1 cup (150 g) chopped green bell pepper

1 cup (160 g) thinly sliced red onion

1 cup (182 g) cooked navy beans

2 cups (280 g) cooked whole wheat pasta

In medium saucepan, stir together vinegar and corn syrup. Bring to full boil, remove from heat, and cool. Add oil. Cook frozen beans according to directions; drain; cool. In large bowl mix vegetables, navy beans, and pasta. Pour vinegar and oil mixture over vegetables. Refrigerate 24 hours, stirring occasionally.

Yield: 6 servings

Per serving: 123 g water; 394 calories (22% from fat, 13% from protein, 65% from carb); 13 g protein; 10 g total fat; 1 g saturated fat; 7 g monounsaturated fat; 2 g polyunsaturated fat; 67 g carbohydrate; 11 g fiber; 8 g sugar; 267 mg phosphorus; 100 mg calcium; 4 mg iron; 32 mg sodium; 717 mg potassium; 494 IU vitamin A; 0 mg vitamin E; 31 mg vitamin C; 0 mg cholesterol

Sweet Potato Fries

Try these instead of regular French fries. Sweet potatoes are lower in carbohydrates and are particularly rich in vitamin A. The egg coating that makes them nice and crisp can be used for regular potatoes too.

3 sweet potatoes

1 egg white

$^1/_4$ teaspoon (0.6 g) cinnamon

Preheat oven to 450°F (230°C, or gas mark 8). Cut potatoes into strips. In a bowl, beat together the egg white and cinnamon until frothy. Stir in potatoes and toss to coat well. Spread in a single layer on a baking sheet coated with nonstick vegetable oil spray. Bake for 20 to 25 minutes, or until crispy on the outside and soft inside.

Yield: 6 servings

Per serving: 62 calories (4% from fat, 11% from protein, 85% from carbohydrate); 2 g protein; 0 g total fat; 0 g saturated fat; 0 g monounsaturated fat; 0 g polyunsaturated fat; 13 g carbohydrate; 2 g fiber; 4 g sugar; 31 mg phosphorus; 24 mg calcium; 1 mg iron; 30 mg sodium; 191 mg potassium; 11903 IU vitamin A;

0 mg ATE vitamin E; 10 mg vitamin C; 0 mg cholesterol; 65 g water

Twice-Baked Sweet Potatoes

Sweet potatoes are almost always boiled. Take a tip from restaurants and bake them instead. A little sprinkle of brown sugar and cinnamon will help you forget about adding butter to them. They are an excellent source of vitamins A and C.

4 sweet potatoes

$1/4$ cup (60 g) brown sugar

1 teaspoon cinnamon

2 tablespoons (28 g) unsalted butter

Scrub potatoes and score the skin with a knife to allow the steam to escape. Bake at 375°F (190°C, gas mark 5) until done, about 45 minutes. Or microwave until tender, about 10 minutes. Scoop out centers and mix with remaining ingredients.

Yield: 4 servings

Per serving: 123 g water; 219 calories (24% from fat, 4% from protein, 72% from carb); 2 g protein; 6 g total fat; 4 g saturated fat; 1 g monounsaturated fat; 0 g polyunsaturated fat; 41 g carbohydrate; 4 g fiber; 22 g sugar; 53 mg phosphorus; 61 mg calcium; 2 mg iron; 47 mg sodium; 399 mg potassium; 23946 IU vitamin A; 48 mg vitamin E; 19 mg vitamin C; 15 mg cholesterol

Couscous with Peppers and Onions

For anyone not familiar with couscous, it's a very small Middle Eastern pasta. It can be used as a base for curries, tomato sauces, or any number of other things, or by itself as a side dish. This variation adds a few vegetables for flavor and color.

1 tablespoon (15 ml) olive oil

$1/4$ cup (40 g) onion, finely chopped

$1/4$ cup (38 g) red bell pepper, finely chopped

$1/4$ cup (25 g) celery, finely chopped

$1 1/2$ cups (355 ml) low sodium chicken broth

1 cup (175 g) dry couscous

Heat oil in a skillet and sauté onion, red bell pepper, and celery until tender. In a large saucepan, bring broth to a boil. Stir in couscous and sautéed vegetables. Cover and let stand 5 minutes. Fluff with a fork before serving.

Yield: 4 servings

Per serving: 214 calories (18% from fat, 14% from protein, 68% from carbohydrate); 8 g protein; 4 g total fat; 1 g saturated fat; 3 g monounsaturated fat; 1 g polyunsaturated fat; 36 g carbohydrate; 3 g fiber; 1 g sugar; 107 mg phosphorus; 20 mg calcium; 1 mg iron; 37 mg sodium; 200 mg potassium; 320 IU vitamin A; 0 mg ATE vitamin E; 13 mg vitamin C; 0 mg cholesterol; 114 g water

Moroccan Couscous

A delicious side dish with a Middle Eastern flavor. Serve with grilled chicken for a great meal.

1 cup (160 g) chopped onion

1 cup (130 g) sliced carrot

1 cup (100 g) sliced celery

1 cup (70 g) sliced mushrooms

$^1/_2$ cup (60 g) chopped walnuts

5 tablespoons (75 ml) olive oil, divided

2 cups (328 g) cooked chickpeas, drained

8 ounces (225 g) no-salt-added tomato sauce

$^1/_2$ cup (75 g) raisins

2 teaspoons curry powder

$^1/_4$ teaspoon cayenne pepper

1 teaspoon paprika

1$^1/_2$ cups (355 ml) water

1 cup (175 g) couscous

To make the vegetable mixture, in a large pan, brown onion, carrot, celery, mushrooms, and walnuts in 3 tablespoons olive oil. Add next 6 ingredients, bring to boil, cover, and simmer for 40 minutes. To make the couscous, boil the water with the remaining olive oil. Pour over couscous, stir, cover, and let stand for 5 minutes or until water is absorbed. Serve vegetables over steaming couscous.

Yield: 4 servings

Per serving: 335 g water; 676 calories (37% from fat, 11% from protein, 53% from carb); 18 g protein; 28 g total fat; 3 g saturated fat; 15 g monounsaturated fat; 8 g polyunsaturated fat; 92 g carbohydrate; 13 g fiber; 19 g sugar; 351 mg phosphorus; 116 mg calcium; 4 mg iron; 421 mg sodium; 1040 mg potassium; 6085 IU vitamin A; 0 mg vitamin E; 19 mg vitamin C; 0 mg cholesterol

Barley-Stuffed Green Peppers

You can either use these as a side dish with a simple piece of meat or make them a full meal by adding some ground beef or turkey to the mixture.

1 tablespoon (15 ml) olive oil

2 cups (140 g) chopped mushrooms

1 cup (160 g) chopped onion

1$^1/_2$ cups (235 g) cooked pearl barley

2 tablespoons chopped fresh parsley

$^1/_4$ teaspoon thyme

$^1/_4$ teaspoon black pepper

1 cup (115 g) shredded Monterey Jack cheese

4 green bell peppers

1 cup (245 g) no-salt-added tomato sauce

Preheat oven to 350°F (180°C, gas mark 4). Heat the oil in a large skillet. Add mushrooms and onion and cook, stirring until the onion is browned. Stir in the barley, parsley, thyme, and pepper. Stir in the cheese; set aside. Cut off the tops of the peppers; remove and discard the seeds. Spoon $^1/_4$ of the mixture into each pepper. Stand the peppers upright in a baking dish just large enough to accommodate them. Pour the sauce over the peppers. Bake 30 minutes or until the peppers are tender.

Yield: 4 servings

Per serving: 284 g water; 474 calories (28% from fat, 17% from protein, 55% from carb); 20 g protein; 16 g total fat; 7 g saturated fat; 6 g monounsaturated fat; 2 g polyunsaturated fat; 67 g carbohydrate; 17 g fiber; 9 g sugar; 421 mg phosphorus; 307 mg calcium; 4 mg iron;

201 mg sodium; 1008 mg potassium; 1193 IU vitamin A; 63 mg vitamin E; 134 mg vitamin C; 29 mg cholesterol

Tip: Vary the flavor by adding other spices or using spaghetti sauce.

Barley with Mushrooms

Barley by itself can be pretty plain, but mushrooms and other vegetables give this dish a great flavor boost.

1 tablespoon (15 ml) olive oil

$^1/_2$ cup (80 g) chopped onion

$^1/_2$ cup (65 g) finely chopped carrot

$^1/_2$ cup (75 g) chopped red bell pepper

$^1/_2$ teaspoon finely minced garlic

$^1/_2$ pound (225 g) coarsely sliced mushrooms

1 cup (200 g) pearl barley

$1^3/_4$ cups (410 ml) low-sodium beef broth, divided

2 tablespoons minced fresh parsley

3 tablespoons minced fresh dill

2 tablespoons (30 ml) fresh lemon juice

In a 10-inch (25-cm) sauté pan, heat oil over medium heat. Add onion, carrot, pepper, and garlic. Sauté for 3 minutes. Add mushrooms; sauté and toss for 3 minutes. Add barley and continue cooking until lightly browned, about 5 minutes. Add 1 cup (235 ml) of broth; cover and simmer over medium-low heat for 15 minutes. Add the remaining broth and continue simmering until the liquid is absorbed, about 10 minutes longer, stirring now and then. Stir in the parsley, dill, and lemon juice.

Yield: 4 servings

Per serving: 217 g water; 241 calories (18% from fat, 15% from protein, 67% from carb); 10 g protein; 5 g total fat; 1 g saturated fat; 3 g monounsaturated fat; 1 g polyunsaturated fat; 42 g carbohydrate; 10 g fiber; 4 g sugar; 215 mg phosphorus; 80 mg calcium; 4 mg iron; 88 mg sodium; 663 mg potassium; 3579 IU vitamin A; 0 mg vitamin E; 35 mg vitamin C; 0 mg cholesterol

Barley and Pine Nut Casserole

A simple but flavorful side dish with the additional crunch of pine nuts. Good with any grilled meat, especially ones with Italian seasoning.

1 cup (200 g) pearl barley

$^1/_2$ cup (70 g) pine nuts, divided

3 tablespoons (42 g) unsalted butter, divided

1 cup (160 g) chopped onion

$^1/_2$ cup (30 g) minced fresh parsley

$^1/_4$ cup (25 g) minced scallions

$^1/_4$ teaspoon black pepper, freshly ground

3 cups (355 ml) low-sodium chicken broth, heated to boiling

Preheat oven to 375°F (190°C, gas mark 5). Rinse and drain barley. Toast pine nuts in 1 tablespoon butter in a skillet. Remove nuts with slotted spoon and set aside. Add remaining butter to skillet with onion and barley, stir until toasted. Stir in nuts, parsley, scallions, and pepper. Spoon into a 1 $^1/_2$-quart (1.5-L) casserole dish. Pour hot broth over casserole and mix well. Bake uncovered for 1 hour and 15 minutes.

Yield: 6 servings

Per serving: 152 g water; 268 calories (48% from fat, 12% from protein, 41% from carb); 8 g protein; 15 g total fat; 5 g saturated fat; 4 monounsaturated fat; 5 g polyunsaturated fat; 29 g carbohydrate; 6 g fiber; 2 g sugar; 196 mg phosphorus; 35 mg calcium; 2 mg iron; 45 mg sodium; 390 mg potassium; 651 IU vitamin A; 48 mg vitamin E; 10 mg vitamin C; 15 mg cholesterol

Barley Casserole

This barley casserole is flavored with beef broth, making it a great choice to have with steak or roast beef.

$^1/_2$ cup (80 g) chopped onion

2 tablespoons (28 ml) olive oil

2 cups (400 g) pearl barley

6 cups (1.4 L) low-sodium beef broth

$^1/_4$ teaspoon black pepper

1 cup (235 ml) boiling water

Sauté onion in oil until transparent. Add barley and continue cooking until barley is lightly browned. Put in 2-quart (2-L) casserole dish that has been sprayed with nonstick vegetable oil spray. Just before baking, bring broth to a boil. Add broth, pepper, and water to barley and stir gently. Bake covered 1 hour or until barley is tender. Add more water or broth if necessary.

Yield: 8 servings

Per serving: 218 g water; 209 calories (20% from fat, 15% from protein, 65% from carb); 8 g protein; 5 g total fat;
1 g saturated fat; 3 g monounsaturated fat; 1 g

polyunsaturated fat; 35 g carbohydrate; 8 g fiber; 1 g sugar; 148 mg phosphorus; 29 mg calcium; 2 mg iron; 112 mg sodium; 320 mg potassium; 13 IU vitamin A; 0 mg vitamin E; 1 mg vitamin C; 0 mg cholesterol

Barley Mushroom Pilaf

A quick and easy way to give barley some extra flavor. We like this with chicken, but it would go with a number of meals.

2 teaspoons (10 ml) olive oil

$^1/_2$ cup (35 g) sliced mushrooms

1 cup (200 g) pearl barley

3 cups (710 ml) low-sodium chicken broth

2 tablespoons chopped scallions

$^1/_4$ teaspoon rosemary

2 tablespoons grated Parmesan cheese

Heat olive oil in saucepan; add mushrooms and sauté until limp. Add barley, broth, scallions, and rosemary. Bring to a boil. Reduce heat to low, cover, and cook 45 minutes or until barley is tender and liquid is absorbed. Sprinkle Parmesan cheese over pilaf and serve.

Yield: 4 servings

Per serving: 189 g water; 228 calories (20% from fat, 18% from protein, 62% from carb); 11 g protein; 5 g total fat; 1 g saturated fat; 3 g monounsaturated fat; 1 g polyunsaturated fat; 37 g carbohydrate; 8 g fiber; 1 g sugar; 207 mg phosphorus; 60 mg calcium; 2 mg iron; 108 mg sodium; 403 mg potassium; 56 IU vitamin A; 4 mg vitamin E; 1 mg vitamin C; 3 mg cholesterol

Barley Risotto

Not exactly like traditional risotto, but still a delightful side dish.

$^1/_2$ cup (100 g) pearl barley

1 teaspoon (5 ml) olive oil

3 tablespoons (21 g) minced carrot

3 tablespoons (30 g) minced onion

3 tablespoons (24 g) minced celery

1 teaspoon rosemary

1 bay leaf

$^1/_2$ teaspoon black pepper

$1^1/_2$ cups (355 ml) vegetable broth

Put barley in heavy skillet over low heat and toast. Shake pan frequently. When barley turns light brown and smells nutty, about 15 to 20 minutes, remove from skillet. Heat oil in skillet, add minced vegetables, and sauté for 3 minutes. Add barley and stir to coat grains. Add herbs and broth. Simmer, covered, until barley is tender and liquid is absorbed, about 35 minutes. Remove bay leaf.

Yield: 4 servings

Per serving: 108 g water; 138 calories (24% from fat, 11% from protein, 65% from carb); 4 g protein; 4 g total fat;
1 g saturated fat; 2 g monounsaturated fat; 1 g polyunsaturated fat; 23 g carbohydrate; 5 g fiber; 1 g sugar; 87 mg phosphorus; 27 mg calcium; 1 mg iron; 450 mg sodium; 187 mg potassium; 1041 IU vitamin A; 0 mg vitamin E; 3 mg vitamin C; 0 mg cholesterol

Barley Salad

A cool and crunchy salad. Serve over lettuce leaves with grilled meat for a summer treat.

$^1/_2$ cup (78 g) cooked pearl barley

$^1/_2$ cup (62 g) water chestnuts, drained and sliced

1 cup (100 g) chopped celery

$^1/_4$ cup (38 g) chopped green bell pepper

$^1/_3$ cup (58 g) pimentos

$^1/_4$ cup (40 g) chopped onion

1 cup (150 g) cubed ham

1 tablespoon Italian seasoning

$^1/_3$ cup (67 g) sugar

$^1/_4$ cup (60 ml) olive oil

$^1/_4$ cup (60 ml) red wine vinegar

Mix together barley, water chestnuts, celery, bell pepper, pimentos, onion, and ham. Cover and chill. In a screw-top jar, combine remaining ingredients. Cover and shake well. Pour over salad and stir to mix just before serving.

Yield: 4 servings

Per serving: 108 g water; 358 calories (43% from fat, 12% from protein, 45% from carb); 11 g protein; 17 g total fat; 3 g saturated fat; 11 g monounsaturated fat; 2 g polyunsaturated fat; 41 g carbohydrate; 6 g fiber; 19 g sugar; 164 mg phosphorus; 39 mg calcium; 2 mg iron; 404 mg sodium; 458 mg potassium; 630 IU vitamin A; 0 mg vitamin E; 24 mg vitamin C; 14 mg cholesterol

Tabbouleh

Tabbouleh is a Middle Eastern salad of bulgur wheat. The chickpeas are not traditional, but add a nice touch of flavor and up the fiber content.

4 cups (950 ml) water, boiling

1 1/2 cups (210 g) bulgur

3/4 cup (123 g) cooked chickpeas

1 1/2 cups (90 g) minced fresh parsley

3/4 cup (72 g) fresh mint

1/4 cup (25 g) chopped scallions

1 cup (180 g) chopped tomato

1/2 cup (120 ml) lemon juice

1/4 cup (60 ml) olive oil

1/2 teaspoon black pepper, to taste

Pour boiling water over bulgur. Let stand covered about 2 hours until light and fluffy. Remove excess water by shaking in a strainer and squeezing with hands. Combine cooked, squeezed bulgur, cooked beans, parsley, and mint (if fresh mint is not available, substitute more fresh parsley). Add scallions, tomato, lemon juice, olive oil, and pepper. Chill for at least 1 hour. May be used as a light meal or as salad.

Yield: 6 servings

Per serving: 236 g water; 234 calories (36% from fat, 10% from protein, 55% from carb); 6 g protein; 10 g total fat; 1 g saturated fat; 7 g monounsaturated fat; 1 g polyunsaturated fat; 34 g carbohydrate; 9 g fiber; 1 g sugar; 139 mg phosphorus; 70 mg calcium; 4 mg iron; 56 mg sodium; 392 mg potassium; 1932 IU vitamin A; 0 mg vitamin E; 38 mg vitamin C; 0 mg cholesterol

Bulgur Pilaf

A simple dish that can be used as a side dish similar to cooked rice.

2 tablespoons (28 ml) olive oil

1/2 cup (50 g) chopped celery

1 cup (160 g) chopped onion

1 cup (70 g) sliced mushrooms

1 cup (140 g) bulgur

1/2 teaspoon dried dill

1/4 teaspoon dried oregano

1/4 teaspoon black pepper, fresh ground

2 cups (475 ml) low-sodium chicken broth

Heat oil in a large skillet; add celery, onion, and mushrooms. Stir constantly until vegetables are tender. Add bulgur and cook until golden. Add seasonings and chicken broth. Cover and bring to a boil. Reduce heat and simmer 15 minutes.

Yield: 6 servings

Per serving: 122 g water; 148 calories (31% from fat, 13% from protein, 56% from carb); 5 g protein; 5 g total fat;
1 g saturated fat; 4 g monounsaturated fat; 1 g polyunsaturated fat; 22 g carbohydrate; 5 g fiber; 2 g sugar; 114 mg phosphorus; 24 mg calcium; 1 mg iron; 37 mg sodium; 267 mg potassium; 49 IU vitamin A; 0 mg vitamin E; 3 mg vitamin C; 0 mg cholesterol

Bulgur Wheat with Squash

Sometimes grain side dishes can be pretty plain. This one gets its flavor from butternut squash, and it turns out to be a winning combination.

1 1/2 tablespoons (21 g) unsalted butter

1/2 cup (80 g) chopped onion

1 cup (140 g) peeled and cubed butternut squash

1/2 cup (70 g) bulgur

2 whole cloves

2 cinnamon sticks

1 bay leaf

1 cup (235 ml) low-sodium chicken broth

Melt butter over medium heat. Add onion and squash. Cook until onion is soft. Add bulgur, cloves, cinnamon, and bay leaf. Stir until bulgur is brown. Stir in chicken broth. Cover and bring to a boil. Reduce heat and cook 15 minutes. Remove bay leaf and cinnamon sticks.

Yield: 4 servings

Per serving: 108 g water; 131 calories (32% from fat, 11% from protein, 57% from carb); 4 g protein; 5 g total fat; 3 g saturated fat; 1 g monounsaturated fat; 0 g polyunsaturated fat; 20 g carbohydrate; 4 g fiber; 2 g sugar; 89 mg phosphorus; 31 mg calcium; 1 mg iron; 24 mg sodium; 277 mg potassium; 3855 IU vitamin A; 36 mg vitamin E; 9 mg vitamin C; 11 mg cholesterol

Vegetable Bulgur Salad

Healthy salad full of the goodness of whole wheat and vegetables.

1 cup (70 g) bulgur

1 cup (235 ml) boiling water

1/2 cup (65 g) coarsely chopped carrot

1/2 cup (80 g) green sliced onion

1/2 cup (75 g) chopped green bell pepper

1/4 cup (25 g) sliced celery

1/4 cup (60 ml) lemon juice

1/3 cup (80 ml) olive oil

1/2 teaspoon pressed garlic

1 1/2 teaspoons basil

1/2 teaspoon dry mustard

1/2 teaspoon black pepper, fresh ground

Cover bulgur with boiling water and let stand 1 hour. Cool; then add vegetables. Mix remaining ingredients to make dressing. Add dressing, cover, and let stand 4 hours.

Yield: 4 servings

Per serving: 125 g water; 300 calories (53% from fat, 6% from protein, 40% from carb); 5 g protein; 19 g total fat; 3 g saturated fat; 13 g monounsaturated fat; 2 g polyunsaturated fat; 32 g carbohydrate; 8 g fiber; 2 g sugar; 124 mg phosphorus; 42 mg calcium; 1 mg iron; 27 mg sodium; 313 mg potassium; 2944 IU vitamin A; 0 mg vitamin E; 26 mg vitamin C; 0 mg cholesterol

Rice and Beans

An easy stovetop preparation for a tasty rice and bean dish. Use as a side dish or make it a whole meal.

1 cup (190 g) brown rice

2 cups (475 ml) water

1 cup (160 g) chopped onion

1 tablespoon (15 ml) olive oil

$^1/_2$ teaspoon crushed garlic

1 cup (180 g) diced tomato

1 cup (113 g) chopped zucchini

$^1/_2$ teaspoon oregano

2 cups (200 g) cooked kidney beans, drained (can be pink or black)

1 cup (115 g) shredded Cheddar cheese

In medium saucepan, combine rice and water. Bring to a boil; reduce heat, cover, and simmer 35 minutes. Sauté onion in oil in a large saucepan until tender. Stir in remaining ingredients except cheese. Heat to boiling, reduce heat, and simmer until vegetables are tender. Stir in rice and heat through. Serve with cheese sprinkled over.

Yield: 4 servings

Per serving: 325 g water; 356 calories (37% from fat, 21% from protein, 42% from carb); 19 g protein; 15 g total fat; 8 g saturated fat; 6 g monounsaturated fat; 1 g polyunsaturated fat; 38 g carbohydrate; 11 g fiber; 3 g sugar; 364 mg phosphorus; 323 mg calcium; 4 mg iron; 223 mg sodium; 651 mg potassium; 637 IU vitamin A; 85 mg vitamin E; 19 mg vitamin C; 35 mg cholesterol

Two Bean and Rice Salad

This makes a lot of salad, but it will keep well in the refrigerator for up to a week.

3 cups (495 g) cooked, chilled rice

2 cups (342 g) cooked pinto beans, rinsed and drained

2 cups (344 g) cooked black beans, rinsed and drained

10 ounces (280 g) frozen peas, thawed

1 cup (100 g) sliced celery

1 cup (160 g) chopped red onion

8 ounces (225 g) chopped green chiles, drained

$^1/_4$ cup chopped fresh cilantro

$^1/_3$ cup (78 ml) white wine vinegar

$^1/_4$ cup (60 ml) olive oil

2 tablespoons (30 ml) water

$^1/_2$ teaspoon garlic powder

$^1/_2$ teaspoon black pepper

In a $2^1/_2$-quart (2.5-L) covered container, combine cooked rice, pinto beans, black beans, peas, celery, onion, chiles, and cilantro. In screw-top jar, combine remaining ingredients. Cover and shake well to mix. Add dressing to rice mixture; toss gently to mix. Cover and chill several hours.

Yield: 10 servings

Per serving: 157 g water; 238 calories (23% from fat, 16% from protein, 61% from carb); 9 g protein; 6 g total fat; 1 g saturated fat; 4 g monounsaturated fat; 1 g polyunsaturated fat; 37 g carbohydrate; 9 g fiber; 2 g sugar; 162 mg phosphorus; 59 mg calcium; 3 mg iron; 193 mg sodium; 435 mg potassium; 743 IU vitamin A; 0 mg vitamin E; 13 mg vitamin C; 0 mg cholesterol

Wild Rice and Barley Salad

We like this as a side dish with grilled chicken. Serve over lettuce.

1 3/4 cups (410 ml) low-sodium chicken broth

1/2 cup (85 g) brown and wild rice mix

1/2 cup (100 g) pearl barley

3/4 cup (123 g) cooked chickpeas

1/3 cup (50 g) golden raisins

1/4 cup (25 g) sliced scallions

2 tablespoons (28 ml) red wine vinegar

1 1/2 teaspoons (8 ml) olive oil

1 teaspoon Dijon mustard

1/4 teaspoon black pepper

2 tablespoons chopped fresh basil

2 tablespoons (18 g) slivered almonds, toasted

Combine first 3 ingredients in a medium saucepan; bring to a boil. Cover, reduce heat, and simmer 40 minutes or until liquid is absorbed. Remove from heat and let stand, covered, 5 minutes. Spoon rice mixture into a medium bowl. Add chickpeas, raisins, and scallions. Combine vinegar and next 3 ingredients in a small bowl; stir with a whisk. Pour over rice mixture; toss well. Cover; chill 2 hours. Stir in basil and almonds.

Yield: 8 servings

Per serving: 76 g water; 156 calories (17% from fat, 15% from protein, 69% from carb); 6 g protein; 3 g total fat; 0 g saturated fat; 2 g monounsaturated fat; 1 g polyunsaturated fat; 28 g carbohydrate; 4 g fiber; 5 g sugar; 133 mg phosphorus; 39 mg calcium; 2 mg iron; 94 mg sodium; 276 mg potassium; 91 IU vitamin A; 0 mg vitamin E; 2 mg vitamin C; 0 mg cholesterol

Brown Rice Pilaf

When I make something like this, it makes me wonder why I don't cook brown rice more often. It has such a nice flavor and crunchy texture. And it's so simple.

2 cups (470 ml) low sodium chicken broth

1/2 cup (120 ml) water

1 cup (190 g) brown rice

2 tablespoons (20 g) minced onion

1/8 teaspoon (0.4 g) garlic powder

Place broth and water in a saucepan. Bring to boil. Add rice, onion, and garlic powder. Reduce heat, cover, and simmer for 45 minutes or until rice is done.

Yield: 4 servings

Per serving: 199 calories (9% from fat, 13% from protein, 78% from carbohydrate); 6 g protein; 2 g total fat; 0 g saturated fat; 1 g monounsaturated fat; 1 g polyunsaturated fat; 39 g carbohydrate; 2 g fiber; 1 g sugar; 198 mg phosphorus; 23 mg calcium; 1 mg iron; 41 mg sodium; 248 mg potassium; 1 IU vitamin A; 0 mg ATE vitamin E; 2 mg vitamin C; 0 mg cholesterol; 150 g water

Herbed Brown Rice

Flavored with dill and thyme, this is great with fish.

2 tablespoons (30 ml) olive oil

1 cup (160 g) onion, chopped

1/2 teaspoon (1.5 g) chopped garlic

1 cup (190 g) brown rice

2 1/2 cups (590 ml) water

2 teaspoons (2 g) dried dill

1/2 teaspoon (0.7 g) thyme

1/2 teaspoon (1 g) black pepper

In a medium pot, heat the oil. Add onions, garlic, and rice, and sauté for 5 minutes, stirring frequently. Add the water, dill, thyme, and pepper. Stir until well combined. Bring to a boil, then reduce heat and simmer, covered, for 40 minutes, or until the water is absorbed. After 30 minutes, check to see if there is a lot of water left in the pot; if so, remove the cover for the remainder of the cooking time. Let the cooked rice stand in the pot, covered, for 15 minutes.

Yield: 4 servings

Per serving: 250 calories (29% from fat, 7% from protein, 64% from carbohydrate); 4 g protein; 8 g total fat; 1 g saturated fat; 5 g monounsaturated fat; 1 g polyunsaturated fat; 40 g carbohydrate; 2 g fiber; 2 g sugar; 170 mg phosphorus; 38 mg calcium; 1 mg iron; 11 mg sodium; 186 mg potassium; 37 IU vitamin A; 0 mg ATE vitamin E; 3 mg vitamin C; 0 mg cholesterol; 188 g water

Brown Rice with Spinach

Baked brown rice and spinach, with just enough cheese to add a little extra flavor.

1 cup (190 g) brown rice

1 pound (455 g) fresh spinach

1 tablespoon (15 ml) olive oil

3/4 cup (120 g) onion, minced

1/4 teaspoon (0.8 g) minced garlic

1 teaspoon (1 g) dried thyme, chopped

1/4 cup (15 g) minced fresh parsley

1/4 cup (30 g) low fat Provolone cheese, shredded

3 eggs

Preheat oven to 350°F (180°C, or gas mark 4). Cook rice according to package directions until tender but still undercooked (about 30 minutes). Drain, rinse with cold water, drain again, and set aside. Wash spinach and remove stems. In a large skillet, cook the spinach in the water that clings to the leaves until the spinach is wilted. Remove from skillet, cool, and chop coarsely. In the same skillet, heat the oil and sauté the onion until softened. Add the garlic and thyme. Combine the rice, spinach, onion mixture, parsley, Provolone, and eggs. Coat a 1 1/2-quart (1.4 L) baking dish with nonstick vegetable oil spray and add the spinach mixture. Cover with foil and bake for 25 minutes. Remove foil and cook for 5 minutes more.

Yield: 4 servings

Per serving: 320 calories (23% from fat, 21% from protein, 57% from carbohydrate); 16 g protein; 8 g total fat; 2 g saturated fat; 4 g monounsaturated fat; 2 g polyunsaturated fat; 45 g carbohydrate; 7 g fiber; 3 g sugar; 320 mg phosphorus; 289 mg calcium; 5 mg iron; 272 mg sodium; 580 mg potassium; 14245 IU vitamin A; 19 mg ATE vitamin E; 10 mg vitamin C; 166 mg cholesterol; 178 g water

Risotto with Sun-Dried Tomatoes

Every once in a while, when I'm looking for something different, I decide that risotto is worth the effort. We had this one with fish topped with a sun-dried tomato mixture. In order to get the real Italian-type risotto, you need to buy short-grained rice, such as Arborio.

4 cups (946 ml) low sodium chicken broth

2 tablespoons (30 ml) olive oil

$1/_2$ cup (80 g) onion, chopped

$1/_2$ cup (75 g) yellow bell peppers, chopped

$1 1/_2$ cups (300 g) Arborio rice

$1/_2$ cup (120 ml) white wine

$1/_4$ cup (28 g) oil-packed sun-dried tomatoes, drained

Heat the broth in a large saucepan to almost boiling; reduce heat and keep hot. Sauté the onion and pepper in the olive oil in a large skillet or Dutch oven until softened. Add the rice and sauté until translucent, but not brown. Add the wine and simmer until liquid is almost completely absorbed. Add 1 cup (235 ml) of the broth and simmer until liquid is almost completely absorbed, stirring occasionally. Continue adding broth 1 cup (235 ml) at a time, stirring frequently and allowing it to cook until liquid is absorbed after each addition. After all broth is added, stir until rice is tender, about 20 minutes total cooking time. Stir in sun-dried tomatoes and simmer until heated through.

Yield: 4 servings

Per serving: 224 calories (40% from fat, 14% from protein, 46% from carbohydrate); 7 g protein; 9 g total fat; 2 g saturated fat; 6 g monounsaturated fat; 1 g polyunsaturated fat; 24 g carbohydrate; 1 g fiber; 2 g sugar; 131 mg phosphorus; 34 mg calcium; 2 mg iron; 94 mg sodium; 447 mg potassium; 135 IU vitamin A; 0 mg ATE vitamin E; 51 mg vitamin C; 0 mg cholesterol; 341 g water

Wild Rice and Fruit Pilaf

This sounds like a holiday sort of recipe, but it would be good any time of year.

2 cups (470 ml) low sodium chicken broth

1 cup (160 g) uncooked wild rice, rinsed

1 tablespoon (15 ml) olive oil

1 cup (160 g) onion, sliced in thin wedges

2 teaspoons (10 g) brown sugar, firmly packed

$1/_4$ cup (38 g) golden raisins

$1/_4$ cup (38 g) dried cranberries

$1/_4$ cup (60 ml) orange juice

1 teaspoon (1.7 g) orange peel

$1/_4$ teaspoon (0.5 g) white pepper

Combine chicken broth and wild rice in a medium saucepan; bring to a boil. Reduce heat, cover, and simmer for 40 minutes, or until rice is almost tender. Heat the oil in a small saucepan and sauté onion and brown sugar. Cook for 10 minutes, stirring occasionally, until onion is tender and lightly browned. Add cooked onions, raisins, cranberries, orange juice, orange peel, and pepper to rice mixture. Cover and simmer for 10 minutes, or until rice is tender.

Yield: 6 servings

Per serving: 186 calories (15% from fat, 13% from protein, 73% from carbohydrate); 6 g protein; 3 g total fat; 1 g saturated fat; 2 g monounsaturated fat; 1 g polyunsaturated fat; 36 g carbohydrate; 3 g fiber; 11 g sugar; 157 mg phosphorus; 22 mg calcium; 1 mg iron; 29 mg sodium; 301 mg potassium; 15 IU vitamin A; 0 mg ATE vitamin E; 6 mg vitamin C; 0 mg cholesterol; 114 g water

Brown Rice Fritters

Almost sweet enough to be a dessert, but also good as a side dish.

2 cups (440 g) cooked brown rice

3 eggs, beaten

$^1/_4$ teaspoon vanilla extract

$^1/_2$ teaspoon nutmeg

$^1/_4$ cup (50 g) sugar

6 tablespoons (48 g) flour

1 tablespoon baking powder

Combine rice, eggs, vanilla, nutmeg, and sugar and mix well. Sift dry ingredients together and stir into rice mixture. Drop by spoonfuls into hot deep fat (360°F) and fry until brown. Drain on absorbent paper, sprinkle with confectioners' sugar, and serve hot.

Yield: 6 servings

Per serving: 70 g water; 176 calories (18% from fat, 14% from protein, 68% from carb); 6 g protein; 4 g total fat; 1 g saturated fat; 1 g monounsaturated fat; 1 g polyunsaturated fat; 30 g carbohydrate; 1 g fiber; 9 g

sugar; 167 mg phosphorus; 158 mg calcium; 1 mg iron; 286 mg sodium; 75 mg potassium; 137 IU vitamin A; 39 mg vitamin E; 0 mg vitamin C; 118 mg cholesterol

Tomato Pilaf

A delicious side dish for any meal where you would normally have rice or noodles.

2 cups (480 g) no-salt-added canned tomatoes

2 teaspoons (10 ml) olive oil

$^1/_2$ cup (80 g) minced onion

1 cup (140 g) bulgur

$^1/_2$ cup (30 g) chopped fresh parsley

Drain tomatoes, reserving juice. Heat oil in a skillet and add onion. Sauté until tender. Add bulgur and brown for 1 minute until golden colored. Put in casserole dish. Add enough water to reserved tomato juice to make 2 cups (475 ml) liquid. Pour over wheat mixture along with parsley and tomatoes. Cover. Bake at 350°F (180°C, gas mark 4) for 45 minutes. Remove cover; stir and bake, uncovered, 5 minutes longer.

Yield: 4 servings

Per serving: 141 g water; 171 calories (14% from fat, 12% from protein, 73% from carb); 6 g protein; 3 g total fat; 0 g saturated fat; 2 g monounsaturated fat; 1 g polyunsaturated fat; 34 g carbohydrate; 8 g fiber; 4 g sugar; 138 mg phosphorus; 64 mg calcium; 3 mg iron; 27 mg sodium; 440 mg potassium; 776 IU vitamin A; 0 mg vitamin E; 23 mg vitamin C; 0 mg cholesterol

Rice and Cheese Casserole

Cheesy rice side dish that is a good use for leftover rice. And is good enough that you may want to make sure some is left over.

2 cups (440 g) cooked brown rice

1 cup (115 g) shredded Cheddar cheese

2 tablespoons (20 g) chopped onion

3 eggs, slightly beaten

Place rice in a 1$^1/_2$-quart (1.5-L) baking dish. Combine remaining ingredients and pour over rice. Bake in moderate oven for 25 minutes.

Yield: 4 servings

Per serving: 120 g water; 303 calories (48% from fat, 21% from protein, 31% from carb); 16 g protein; 16 g total fat; 8 g saturated fat; 5 g monounsaturated fat; 1 g polyunsaturated fat; 24 g carbohydrate; 2 g fiber; 1 g sugar; 332 mg phosphorus; 271 mg calcium; 1 mg iron; 269 mg sodium; 138 mg potassium; 535 IU vitamin A; 144 mg vitamin E; 0 mg vitamin C; 212 mg cholesterol

Southern Rice Pilaf

Rice with lots of good things added to it.

2 cups (380 g) brown rice

4 tablespoons (55 g) unsalted butter, melted

$^1/_2$ teaspoon cumin seeds

$^1/_4$ teaspoon cinnamon

2 whole cloves

1 cup (150 g) peas

3$^1/_2$ cups (830 ml) water

$^1/_2$ cup (80 g) finely sliced onion

$^1/_4$ cup (27 g) slivered almonds

$^1/_4$ cup (35 g) raisins

Wash rice, drain, and set aside for about 30 minutes. Put half the butter in a saucepan, add the cumin seeds, and heat. When cumin seeds turn slightly brown, add cinnamon and cloves and the peas. Fry for a minute and add the rice. Mix for another minute. Add the water, and after it starts to boil, cover and put on low heat and cook until done, about 35 to 45 minutes. To decorate, take half the remaining butter and fry the onion until lightly brown and sprinkle on top of rice. With the rest of the butter, fry slivered almonds and raisins until lightly brown and sprinkle on top of the onion and rice. Serve hot.

Yield: 4 servings

Per serving: 332 g water; 333 calories (45% from fat, 8% from protein, 47% from carb); 7 g protein; 17 g total fat; 8 g saturated fat; 6 g monounsaturated fat; 2 g polyunsaturated fat; 40 g carbohydrate; 6 g fiber; 10 g sugar; 180 mg phosphorus; 66 mg calcium; 2 mg iron; 144 mg sodium; 291 mg potassium; 1199 IU vitamin A; 95 mg vitamin E; 6 mg vitamin C; 31 mg cholesterol

Curried Rice Salad

Spiced rice dish that can be served either chilled or warm. The spices give a Middle Eastern or Indian sort of flavor.

1 cup (185 g) rice, long cooking

2 tablespoons (28 g) unsalted butter

1/2 cup (80 g) chopped onion

1/2 teaspoon minced garlic

1/2 teaspoon ginger

1/2 teaspoon cinnamon

1 bay leaf

1/4 teaspoon ground coriander

1/4 teaspoon ground black pepper

1/4 teaspoon turmeric

1/4 teaspoon ground cumin

1/8 teaspoon cayenne pepper

1/4 cup (35 g) golden raisins

1/4 cup (27 g) slivered almonds, toasted

1/2 cup (82 g) cooked chickpeas, drained

1/2 cup (75 g) fresh peas, or defrosted frozen peas

Place the rice in a colander and rinse under cold running water. Place the rinsed rice in a large bowl and cover with 2 cups (475 ml) of water. Let soak 30 minutes. Drain and reserve the water for cooking. In a large pot, heat the butter over medium-high heat. Add the onion and cook, stirring, for 3 minutes. Add the garlic and ginger, and cook, stirring, for 45 seconds. Add the cinnamon, bay leaf, coriander, pepper, turmeric, cumin, and cayenne, and cook, stirring, until fragrant, about 45 seconds. Add the rice and cook, stirring, for 2 minutes. Add the reserved soaking liquid and raisins, and bring to a boil. Reduce the heat to low, stir, cover, and simmer until the water is absorbed and the rice is tender, 20 minutes. Remove from the heat and let sit covered for 15 minutes. Fluff the rice with a fork and transfer to a large bowl. Combine with the remaining ingredients. Remove bay leaf. Serve warm or chilled.

Yield: 4 servings

Per serving: 54 g water; 368 calories (28% from fat, 10% from protein, 62% from carb); 9 g protein; 12 g total fat; 4 g saturated fat; 5 g monounsaturated fat; 2 g polyunsaturated fat; 58 g carbohydrate; 6 g fiber; 9 g sugar; 187 mg phosphorus; 82 mg calcium; 4 mg iron; 21 mg sodium; 355 mg potassium; 631 IU vitamin A; 48 mg vitamin E; 5 mg vitamin C; 15 mg cholesterol

Mediterranean Rice Salad

This is another one of those salads that I'm always glad makes a lot so I have some left over for lunch the next day.

2 1/2 cups (550 g) cooked, cooled brown rice

1/2 cup (50 g) chopped celery

1/2 cup (75 g) chopped green bell pepper

1/4 cup (48 g) chopped pimento

1/4 cup (25 g) chopped scallions

Dressing

6 ounces (170 g) artichoke hearts, undrained, chopped

1 cup (225 g) mayonnaise

1 teaspoon oregano

Mix ingredients well. Combine dressing ingredients, pour over rice mixture, and stir to blend.

Yield: 6 servings

Per serving: 120 g water; 374 calories (70% from fat, 4% from protein, 26% from carb); 4 g protein; 30 g total fat; 5 g saturated fat; 7 g monounsaturated fat; 16 g polyunsaturated fat; 24 g carbohydrate; 3 g fiber; 1 g sugar; 103 mg phosphorus; 31 mg calcium; 1 mg iron;

237 mg sodium; 193 mg potassium; 499 IU vitamin A; 29 mg vitamin E; 19 mg vitamin C; 14 mg cholesterol

Warm Rice Salad

This is a good side salad, but I also like it as a meal in itself, with maybe a little leftover chicken added on top.

1 tablespoon unsalted butter

$^1/_2$ cup (72 g) almonds

3 cups (355 ml) low-sodium chicken broth

$^1/_2$ cup (95 g) brown rice

$^1/_2$ cup (100 g) pearl barley

$^1/_2$ cup (75 g) raisins

2 tablespoons chopped fresh parsley

Vinaigrette

1 tablespoon (15 ml) red wine vinegar

$^1/_2$ teaspoon Dijon mustard

$^1/_8$ teaspoon black pepper

4 teaspoons (20 ml) olive oil

In pie plate, microwave butter until melted. Stir in almonds; microwave on high for 2 minutes or until browned, stirring often. Chop and set aside. In 8-cup casserole dish, microwave broth, rice, and barley at high for 8 minutes or until boiling; stir. Cover and microwave at medium (50%) for 45 minutes or until tender; stir in raisins. Let stand for 10 minutes. To make the vinaigrette: Combine vinegar, mustard, and pepper; whisk in oil. Stir into casserole; add parsley. Mound onto lettuce-lined plate; garnish with almonds.

Yield: 4 servings

Per serving: 203 g water; 371 calories (42% from fat, 12% from protein, 46% from carb); 12 g protein; 19 g total fat; 4 g saturated fat; 11 g monounsaturated fat; 3 g polyunsaturated fat; 45 g carbohydrate; 7 g fiber; 14 g sugar; 246 mg phosphorus; 71 mg calcium; 3 mg iron; 74 mg sodium; 563 mg potassium; 254 IU vitamin A; 24 mg vitamin E; 3 mg vitamin C; 8 mg cholesterol

20

Quick Breads

Quick breads are one of those things that can be really bad for your heart healthy diet, high in fat and sodium and mostly empty calories from white flour and white sugar. We've attacked that problem head on, creating a long list of healthy quick breads for you to choose from. There are biscuits, cornbread, coffee cakes, and more than 30 kinds of muffins. Most have both reduced fat and whole grains to make them healthier. As mentioned in Chapter 1 you could also easily make them lower in sodium by using a reduced sodium or sodium-free baking powder. For example, the biscuits in the first recipe that have 255 mg of sodium would have only 13 with sodium-free baking powder.

Reduced Fat Biscuits

This is a basic biscuit recipe, to which you could add other herbs and spices, a little low fat cheese, or whatever strikes your fancy. They can be made as drop biscuits as well as the rolled and cut version described below.

2 cups (250 g) flour

4 teaspoons (18.4 g) baking powder

2 teaspoons (8 g) sugar

$^1/_2$ teaspoon (1.5 g) cream of tartar

$^1/_4$ cup (56 g) unsalted butter

$^2/_3$ cup (160 ml) skim milk

Preheat oven to 450°F (230°C, or gas mark 8). Stir together flour, baking powder, sugar, and cream of tartar. Cut in butter until mixture resembles coarse crumbs. Add milk. Stir until just mixed. Knead gently on a floured surface a few times. Press to $^1/_2$-inch (1.3-cm) thickness. Cut out with a $2^1/_2$-inch (6.3-cm) biscuit cutter. Transfer to an ungreased baking sheet. Bake for 10 to 12 minutes, or until golden brown.

Yield: 10 servings

Per serving: 142 calories (30% from fat, 9% from protein, 60% from carbohydrate); 3 g protein; 5 g total fat; 4 g saturated fat; 1 g monounsaturated fat; 0 g polyunsaturated fat; 21 g carbohydrate; 1 g fiber; 1 g sugar; 89 mg phosphorus; 139 mg calcium; 1 mg iron; 255 mg sodium; 87 mg potassium; 273 IU vitamin A; 65 mg ATE vitamin E; 0 mg vitamin C; 10 mg cholesterol; 19 g water

Tip: If you don't have a biscuit cutter, you can use a drinking glass or just cut the dough into squares with a knife.

Whole Wheat Biscuits

A small variation of the standard biscuit recipe. I added a little dill to them when we had them with the Swedish Salmon Stew (see recipe page 230). You could also add a little cheese or other herbs and spices. If you don't have a biscuit cutter, you can use a drinking glass or just cut it into squares with a knife.

$1^1/_2$ cups (188 g) flour

$^1/_2$ cup (60 g) whole wheat flour

2 teaspoons (8 g) sugar

1 tablespoons (13.8 g) baking powder

$^1/_4$ cup (56 g) unsalted butter

$^2/_3$ cup (160 ml) skim milk

Preheat oven to 450°F (230°C, or gas mark 8). Stir together flours, sugar, and baking powder. Cut in butter until mixture resembles coarse crumbs. Add milk. Stir until just mixed. Knead gently on a floured surface a few times. Press to $^1/_2$-inch (1.3-cm) thickness. Cut out with a $2^1/_2$-inch (6.3-cm) biscuit cutter. Transfer to an ungreased baking sheet. Bake for 10 to 12 minutes, or until golden brown.

Yield: 10 servings

Per serving: 141 calories (30% from fat, 10% from protein, 60% from carbohydrate); 4 g protein; 5 g total fat; 4 g saturated fat; 1 g monounsaturated fat; 0 g polyunsaturated fat; 22 g carbohydrate; 1 g fiber; 1 g sugar; 153 mg phosphorus; 275 mg calcium; 2 mg iron; 498 mg sodium; 80 mg potassium; 274 IU vitamin A; 65 mg ATE vitamin E; 0 mg vitamin C; 10 mg cholesterol; 19 g water

Lower-Fat Restaurant-Style Biscuits

This recipe has the flakiness and the buttery flavor typical of biscuits served at fast food chicken restaurants, but without the fat and sodium.

2 cups (250 g) flour

1 tablespoon (13.8 g) baking powder

4 tablespoons (56 g) unsalted butter, divided

2 ounces (55 g) fat-free sour cream

1/2 cup (120 ml) club soda, at room temperature

Preheat oven to 375°F (190°C, or gas mark 5). Stir flour and baking powder together. Cut in 2 tablespoons (28 g) butter with a pastry blender or two knives until mixture resembles coarse crumbs. Mix sour cream and club soda into flour mixture. Turn out onto a lightly floured surface and knead lightly. Roll or pat to 1/2-inch (1.3-cm) thickness. Cut into 6 biscuits with a biscuit cutter or sharp knife. Place biscuits in an 8 × 8-inch (20 × 20-cm) baking dish sprayed with nonstick vegetable oil spray. Melt remaining butter and pour over the top. Bake for 20 to 25 minutes, or until golden brown.

Yield: 6 servings

Per serving: 232 calories (32% from fat, 9% from protein, 59% from carbohydrate); 5 g protein; 8 g total fat; 6 g saturated fat; 2 g monounsaturated fat; 0 g polyunsaturated fat; 33 g carbohydrate; 1 g fiber; 0 g sugar; 109 mg phosphorus; 158 mg calcium; 2 mg iron; 335 mg sodium; 66 mg potassium; 435 IU vitamin A; 101 mg ATE vitamin E; 0 mg vitamin C; 14 mg cholesterol; 34 g water

Lower-Fat Cornbread

Cornbread goes well with a lot of things. (It's also great reheated with a little honey or syrup for breakfast.) I've found here, like with a lot of recipes, that reducing the amount of fat called for doesn't really affect the end product at all.

1 cup (140 g) cornmeal

1 cup (125 g) flour

1/4 cup (50 g) sugar

1 tablespoon (13.8 g) baking powder

2 tablespoons (28 g) unsalted butter

1 cup (235 ml) skim milk

1 egg

Preheat oven to 425°F (220°C, or gas mark 7). Mix together cornmeal, flour, sugar, and baking powder. Cut in butter until mixture resembles coarse crumbs. Stir milk and egg together and add to dry ingredients, stirring until just mixed. Place in a 9-inch (23-cm) square pan sprayed with nonstick vegetable oil spray and bake for 20 to 25 minutes.

Yield: 12 servings

Per serving: 133 calories (17% from fat, 11% from protein, 73% from carbohydrate); 4 g protein; 2 g total fat; 1 g saturated fat; 0 g monounsaturated fat; 0 g polyunsaturated fat; 24 g carbohydrate; 1 g fiber; 4 g sugar; 81 mg phosphorus; 103 mg calcium; 1 mg iron; 165 mg sodium; 88 mg potassium; 189 IU vitamin A; 35 mg ATE vitamin E; 0 mg vitamin C; 35 mg cholesterol; 26 g water

Mexican-Style Cornbread

This goes well with any chili.

1 cup (140 g) cornmeal

1 cup (120 g) whole wheat pastry flour

3 tablespoons (41 g) baking powder

$^1/_4$ cup (55 g) unsalted butter

1 cup (235 ml) skim milk

1 egg

1 cup (164 g) frozen corn

1 can chopped jalapeño peppers

$^1/_2$ cup (58 g) shredded Cheddar cheese

Stir dry ingredients together. Cut in butter until mixture resembles coarse crumbs. Stir together milk and egg. Add to dry ingredients and stir until just mixed. Stir in remaining ingredients. Place in 8 × 8-inch (20 × 20-cm) baking dish coated with nonstick vegetable oil spray and bake at 425°F (220°C, gas mark 7) until done, about 20 minutes.

Yield: 9 servings

Per serving: 37 g water; 209 calories (37% from fat, 13% from protein, 50% from carb); 7 g protein; 9 g total fat; 5 g saturated fat; 2 g monounsaturated fat; 1 g polyunsaturated fat; 27 g carbohydrate; 2 g fiber; 0 g sugar; 242 mg phosphorus; 369 mg calcium; 2 mg iron; 561 mg sodium; 153 mg potassium; 375 IU vitamin A; 88 mg vitamin E; 1 mg vitamin C; 44 mg cholesterol

Corn Fritters

A fried bread typical of the New Orleans area. Similar to hush puppies, these can also be served as a side dish with fish or other traditional southern foods like black-eyed peas.

2 cups (240 g) whole wheat pastry flour

1 tablespoon baking powder

$^1/_4$ cup (50 g) sugar

2 eggs

1 cup (235 ml) skim milk

$^1/_4$ cup (55 g) unsalted butter, melted

1$^1/_2$ cups (246 g) frozen corn, thawed

Stir together flour, baking powder, and sugar. Combine eggs, milk, and butter. Fold in dry ingredients; add corn last. Drop by tablespoons into hot vegetable oil and deep-fry about 5 minutes or until golden brown. Sprinkle with confectioners' sugar or serve with syrup.

Yield: 6 servings

Per serving: 86 g water; 321 calories (28% from fat, 13% from protein, 59% from carb); 11 g protein; 11 g total fat; 6 g saturated fat; 3 g monounsaturated fat; 1 g polyunsaturated fat; 50 g carbohydrate; 6 g fiber; 10 g sugar; 308 mg phosphorus; 221 mg calcium; 2 mg iron; 299 mg sodium; 385 mg potassium; 514 IU vitamin A; 114 mg vitamin E; 3 mg vitamin C; 100 mg cholesterol

Pasta Fritters

A different sort of use for leftover pasta.

2 cups (280 g) leftover spaghetti

$^1/_4$ cup (25 g) chopped scallions

$^1/_2$ cup (56 g) shredded zucchini

$^1/_3$ cup (78 ml) canola oil

1 egg

1 cup (120 g) whole wheat pastry flour

$^1/_8$ teaspoon black pepper

1 cup (235 ml) water

About 35 minutes before serving, coarsely chop cooked spaghetti, chop scallions, and shred zucchini; set aside. In 12-inch (30-cm) skillet, over high heat, heat canola oil until very hot. Meanwhile prepare batter. In medium bowl, with wire whisk or fork, mix egg, flour, pepper, and water. Stir in spaghetti mixture. Drop mixture into hot oil in skillet by $^1/_4$ cups into 4 mounds about 2 inches (5 cm) apart. With pancake turner, flatten each to make 3-inch (7.5-cm) pancake. Cook fritters until golden brown on both sides; drain fritters on paper towels. Keep warm. Repeat with remaining mixture, adding more oil if needed.

Yield: 6 servings

Per serving: 92 g water; 254 calories (48% from fat, 10% from protein, 42% from carb); 6 g protein; 14 g total fat; 1 g saturated fat; 8 g monounsaturated fat; 4 g polyunsaturated fat; 28 g carbohydrate; 5 g fiber; 1 g sugar; 132 mg phosphorus; 24 mg calcium; 2 mg iron; 21 mg sodium; 152 mg potassium; 123 IU vitamin A; 15 mg vitamin E; 3 mg vitamin C; 35 mg cholesterol

Banana Pumpkin Muffins

These moist pumpkin muffins have a spiced brown sugar topping.

$^1/_2$ cup (112 g) pureed banana

$^1/_2$ cup (123 g) canned pumpkin

$^1/_2$ cup (100 g) sugar

$^1/_4$ cup (60 ml) skim milk

$^1/_4$ cup (60 ml) canola oil

1 egg

1$^3/_4$ cups (210 g) whole wheat pastry flour

2 teaspoons baking powder

1 teaspoon pumpkin pie spice

Topping:
$^1/_2$ cup (115 g) packed brown sugar

$^1/_2$ cup (40 g) rolled oats

$^1/_2$ teaspoon pumpkin pie spice

Mix pureed banana, pumpkin, sugar, milk, oil, and egg until well blended. Combine flour, baking powder, and pumpkin pie spice. Spoon into muffin tins coated with nonstick vegetable oil spray. Top each with 1 tablespoon of the sugar-spice mixture. Bake in preheated 375°F (190°C, gas mark 5) oven for 20 minutes or until toothpick inserted into muffin comes out clean.

Yield: 12 servings

Per serving: 19 g water; 195 calories (26% from fat, 7% from protein, 67% from carb); 4 g protein; 6 g total fat; 1 g saturated fat; 3 g monounsaturated fat; 2 g polyunsaturated fat; 34 g carbohydrate; 3 g fiber; 18 g

sugar; 112 mg phosphorus; 74 mg calcium; 1 mg iron; 96 mg sodium; 151 mg potassium; 1629 IU vitamin A; 11 mg vitamin E; 0 mg vitamin C; 18 mg cholesterol

Blueberry Oatmeal Muffins

Quick muffins with great blueberry taste.

3 cups (384 g) biscuit baking mix

$^1/_2$ cup (115 g) packed brown sugar

$^3/_4$ cup (60 g) quick-cooking oats

1 teaspoon cinnamon

2 eggs, well beaten

1$^1/_2$ cups (355 ml) skim milk

$^1/_4$ cup (55 g) unsalted butter, melted

2 cups (290 g) blueberries

Combine biscuit mix, brown sugar, oats, and cinnamon. Mix eggs, milk, and butter. Add dry ingredients all at once and stir until just blended; fold in blueberries. Spoon into muffin pans coated with nonstick vegetable oil spray, filling each cup two-thirds full. Bake in preheated 400°F (200°C, gas mark 6) oven for 15 to 20 minutes. Remove from pans and place on rack to cool.

Yield: 18 servings

Per serving: 40 g water; 167 calories (34% from fat, 9% from protein, 57% from carb); 4 g protein; 6 g total fat; 3 g saturated fat; 3 g monounsaturated fat; 1 g polyunsaturated fat; 24 g carbohydrate; 2 g fiber; 10 g sugar; 166 mg phosphorus; 77 mg calcium; 1 mg iron; 266 mg sodium; 124 mg potassium; 161 IU vitamin A; 43 mg vitamin E; 2 mg vitamin C; 34 mg cholesterol

Tip: To up the fiber even more, use the Reduced Fat Whole Wheat Baking Mix in Chapter 18.

Carrot Apple Muffins

These are one of my all-time favorite muffins—very moist and tasty. I like to make a batch on the weekend so I have them available for quick breakfasts during the week.

$^1/_2$ cup (75 g) raisins

2 cups (240 g) whole wheat pastry flour

1 cup (200 g) sugar

2 teaspoons baking soda

2 teaspoons cinnamon

$^3/_4$ cup (83 g) grated carrot

1 green apple, grated

$^1/_2$ cup (55 g) sliced almonds

$^1/_2$ cup (40 g) sweet shredded coconut

3 eggs

$^2/_3$ cup (160 ml) vegetable oil

2 teaspoons vanilla extract

Soak raisins in hot water to cover for 30 minutes; drain thoroughly. Preheat oven to 350°F (180°C, gas mark 4). Mix flour, sugar, baking soda, and cinnamon in bowl. Stir in raisins, carrot, apple, almonds, and coconut. Beat eggs with oil and vanilla to blend. Stir into flour mixture until just combined. Divide into muffin cups. Bake until golden brown and tested, 20 to 22 minutes. Cool 5 minutes before removing from pan.

Yield: 12 servings

Per serving: 31 g water; 343 calories (45% from fat, 7% from protein, 48% from carb); 6 g protein; 18 g total fat;

3 g saturated fat; 6 g monounsaturated fat; 8 g polyunsaturated fat; 42 g carbohydrate; 4 g fiber; 24 g sugar; 140 mg phosphorus; 39 mg calcium; 2 mg iron; 39 mg sodium; 244 mg potassium; 1420 IU vitamin A; 19 mg vitamin E; 1 mg vitamin C; 59 mg cholesterol

Peanut Butter Banana Muffins

A tasty way to use up leftover bananas.

2 cups (240 g) whole wheat pastry flour

$^1/_2$ cup (100 g) sugar

1 tablespoon baking powder

$^1/_2$ cup (130 g) crunchy peanut butter

2 tablespoons (28 g) unsalted butter

$^1/_2$ cup (120 ml) skim milk

2 eggs

1 cup (225 g) mashed banana

$^1/_2$ cup (73 g) chopped unsalted dry-roasted peanuts

Combine first 3 ingredients in a mixing bowl. Cut in peanut butter and butter until mixture resembles coarse crumbs. Add milk, eggs, banana, and peanuts and stir until just mixed. Fill muffin pans coated with nonstick vegetable oil spray two-thirds full. Bake at 400°F (200°C, gas mark 6) for 15 to 17 minutes.

Yield: 12 servings

Per serving: 33 g water; 251 calories (39% from fat, 13% from protein, 48% from carb); 9 g protein; 12 g total fat; 3 g saturated fat; 5 g monounsaturated fat; 3 g polyunsaturated fat; 32 g carbohydrate; 4 g fiber; 12 g sugar; 184 mg phosphorus; 104 mg calcium; 1 mg iron; 195 mg sodium; 300 mg potassium; 139 IU vitamin A; 35 mg vitamin E; 2 mg vitamin C; 45 mg cholesterol

Raspberry Almond Muffins

These are a real taste treat, with their hidden raspberry and almond surprise.

5 ounces (140 g) almond paste

$^1/_2$ cup (112 g) unsalted butter, room temperature

$^3/_4$ cup (150 g) sugar

2 eggs

1 teaspoon baking powder

$^1/_2$ teaspoon baking soda

1 teaspoon almond extract

2 cups (240 g) whole wheat pastry flour

1 cup (235 ml) buttermilk

$^1/_4$ cup (80 g) raspberry preserves

Heat oven to 350°F (180°C, gas mark 4). Line muffin pans with paper baking cups or spray with nonstick vegetable oil spray. Cut almond paste into 12 pieces and pat each piece into a round disk about 1 $^1/_2$ inches (4 cm) across. In a large bowl, beat butter until creamy. Beat in sugar until pale and fluffy. Beat in eggs, one at a time. Then mix in baking powder, baking soda, and almond extract. With a rubber spatula fold in 1 cup (120 g) of flour, then the buttermilk, and lastly the remaining flour until well blended. Spoon about 2 tablespoons of batter into each cup and smooth surface with your fingers. Top with a level teaspoon of raspberry preserves, then with a piece of almond paste. Top each muffin with another 2 tablespoons of batter. Bake 25 to 30 minutes or until lightly browned. Turn out onto a rack and let stand at least 10 minutes.

Yield: 12 servings

Per serving: 33 g water; 280 calories (39% from fat, 8% from protein, 53% from carb); 6 g protein; 12 g total fat; 6 g saturated fat; 5 g monounsaturated fat; 1 g polyunsaturated fat; 39 g carbohydrate; 3 g fiber; 21 g sugar; 148 mg phosphorus; 82 mg calcium; 1 mg iron; 80 mg sodium; 170 mg potassium; 289 IU vitamin A; 78 mg vitamin E; 1 mg vitamin C; 61 mg cholesterol

Cranberry–Oat Bran Muffins

Cranberry-orange flavor in a good-for-you muffin.

2 cups (200 g) cranberries

1 1/2 cups (150 g) oat bran

1 teaspoon orange peel

1 cup (200 g) sugar

1/3 cup (75 g) brown sugar

2 1/2 cups (300 g) whole wheat pastry flour

1 tablespoon baking powder

1/2 teaspoon allspice

1/4 cup (60 ml) canola oil

1/2 cup (120 ml) skim milk

2 eggs

1/2 cup (55 g) chopped pecans

Preheat oven to 350°F (180°C, gas mark 4). Chop cranberries and add to oat bran along with orange peel and both sugars. Combine flour, baking powder, and allspice. Combine oil, milk, and eggs. Add to flour mixture. Blend in nuts and cranberry mixture. Fill mini muffin pans and bake 10 to 12 minutes.

Yield: 12 servings

Per serving: 23 g water; 348 calories (24% from fat, 7% from protein, 69% from carb); 6 g protein; 10 g total fat; 1 g saturated fat; 5 g monounsaturated fat; 3 g polyunsaturated fat; 63 g carbohydrate; 5 g fiber; 37 g sugar; 186 mg phosphorus; 118 mg calcium; 3 mg iron; 166 mg sodium; 207 mg potassium; 127 IU vitamin A; 36 mg vitamin E; 1 mg vitamin C; 40 mg cholesterol

Strawberry-Rhubarb Muffins

These muffins taste like spring—that's really the only way to say it.

1 3/4 cups (210 g) whole wheat pastry flour

3/4 cup (150 g) sugar, divided

2 1/2 teaspoons baking powder

1 egg, lightly beaten

3/4 cup (175 ml) skim milk

1/3 cup (80 ml) canola oil

3/4 cup (80 g) minced rhubarb

1/2 cup (85 g) sliced strawberries

Heat oven to 400°F (200°C, gas mark 6). Mix flour, 1/2 cup (100 g) sugar, and the baking powder in large bowl. Combine egg, milk, and oil in small bowl; stir into flour mixture with fork just until moistened. Fold rhubarb and sliced strawberries into batter. Fill muffin tins coated with nonstick vegetable oil spray two-thirds full with batter. Sprinkle tops with remaining sugar. Bake until golden, 20 to 25 minutes. Remove from tins; cool on wire racks.

Yield: 12 servings

Per serving: 31 g water; 181 calories (34% from fat, 8% from protein, 58% from carb); 4 g protein; 7 g total fat; 1 g saturated fat; 4 g monounsaturated fat; 2 g polyunsaturated fat; 27 g carbohydrate; 2 g fiber; 13 g sugar; 109 mg phosphorus; 94 mg calcium; 1 mg iron; 120 mg sodium; 137 mg potassium; 69 IU vitamin A; 17 mg vitamin E; 5 mg vitamin C; 18 mg cholesterol

Per serving: 34 g water; 157 calories (41% from fat, 9% from protein, 50% from carb); 4 g protein; 7 g total fat; 1 g saturated fat; 4 g monounsaturated fat; 2 g polyunsaturated fat; 20 g carbohydrate; 3 g fiber; 6 g sugar; 122 mg phosphorus; 89 mg calcium; 1 mg iron; 120 mg sodium; 163 mg potassium; 71 IU vitamin A; 17 mg vitamin E; 5 mg vitamin C; 18 mg cholesterol

Whole Wheat Strawberry-Banana Muffins

These are a seasonal sort of thing, good with fresh strawberries.

1 $^1/_2$ cups (180 g) whole wheat pastry flour

$^1/_4$ cup (50 g) sugar

$^1/_4$ cup (28 g) wheat germ

2 $^1/_2$ teaspoons baking powder

$^1/_2$ teaspoon baking soda

1 egg

$^3/_4$ cup (175 ml) skim milk

$^1/_3$ cup (80 ml) canola oil

$^1/_2$ cup (112 g) mashed banana

$^1/_2$ cup (85 g) chopped strawberries

Stir together the dry ingredients. Mix together the rest of the ingredients and stir into dry, stirring until just moistened. Spoon into sprayed or paper-lined muffin tins. Bake at 350°F (180°C, gas mark 4) for 20 to 25 minutes, until done.

Yield: 12 servings

Bran Applesauce Muffins

Most people tend to think of bran muffins as something you need to force yourself to eat. These are not like that, but are moist and flavorful.

1 $^1/_4$ cups (150 g) whole wheat pastry flour

$^3/_4$ cup (30 g) bran flakes cereal, crushed

$^1/_2$ cup (100 g) sugar

1 teaspoon baking soda

1 teaspoon cinnamon

$^1/_2$ teaspoon nutmeg

1 cup (245 g) applesauce

$^1/_2$ cup (120 ml) canola oil

1 teaspoon vanilla extract

2 eggs

$^1/_2$ cup (75 g) raisins

1 tablespoon sugar

$^1/_2$ teaspoon cinnamon

Heat oven to 400°F (200°C, gas mark 6). Line 12 muffin cups with paper baking cups or spray with nonstick vegetable oil spray. Lightly spoon flour into measuring cup; level off. In large bowl, combine all ingredients except the sugar and cinnamon; mix well.

Spoon batter into prepared muffin cups, filling two-thirds full. In small bowl, combine the sugar and cinnamon; sprinkle over top of each muffin. Bake at 400°F (200°C, gas mark 6) for 15 to 20 minutes or until toothpick inserted in center comes out clean. Immediately remove from pan. Serve warm.

Yield: 12 servings

Per serving: 27 g water; 224 calories (41% from fat, 6% from protein, 53% from carb); 4 g protein; 11 g total fat; 1 g saturated fat; 6 g monounsaturated fat; 3 g polyunsaturated fat; 31 g carbohydrate; 3 g fiber; 17 g sugar; 87 mg phosphorus; 19 mg calcium; 1 mg iron; 44 mg sodium; 148 mg potassium; 185 IU vitamin A; 13 mg vitamin E; 2 mg vitamin C; 39 mg cholesterol

Oat Bran Muffins

So good you won't guess that they are good for you.

2¼ cups (225 g) oat bran

1 tablespoon baking powder

¼ cup (35 g) raisins

¼ cup (28 g) chopped pecans

2 eggs

2 tablespoons (28 ml) olive oil

¼ cup (85 g) honey

1¼ cups (295 ml) water

Preheat oven to 425°F (220°C, gas mark 7). Put dry ingredients, raisins, and pecans in mixing bowl. Beat eggs, olive oil, honey, and water lightly. Add this mixture to dry ingredients and stir until moistened. Line muffin pans with paper liners or spray with nonstick vegetable oil spray and fill about half full. Bake for 15 to 17 minutes.

Yield: 12 servings

Per serving: 34 g water; 113 calories (39% from fat, 9% from protein, 52% from carb); 3 g protein; 5 g total fat; 1 g saturated fat; 3 g monounsaturated fat; 1 g polyunsaturated fat; 16 g carbohydrate; 1 g fiber; 9 g sugar; 97 mg phosphorus; 93 mg calcium; 3 mg iron; 168 mg sodium; 89 mg potassium; 129 IU vitamin A; 38 mg vitamin E; 1 mg vitamin C; 39 mg cholesterol

Tip: Cover when cooled, as they dry quickly.

Orange Bran Muffins

Good moist bran muffins with just a hint of orange flavor.

2½ cups (300 g) whole wheat pastry flour

1 tablespoon baking soda

3 cups (177 g) raisin bran cereal

½ cup (100 g) sugar

1 teaspoon cinnamon

1½ tablespoons orange peel

2 cups (460 g) plain fat-free yogurt

2 eggs, beaten

½ cup (120 ml) canola oil

In large bowl, mix flour and baking soda. Add the cereal, sugar, cinnamon, and orange peel, mixing well. Briefly but thoroughly mix in yogurt, beaten eggs, and cooking oil. Spoon into muffin tins that have been lined with paper liners or sprayed with nonstick vegetable oil spray. Bake for 20 minutes in a 375°F (190°C, gas mark 5) oven.

Yield: 12 servings

Per serving: 46 g water; 283 calories (33% from fat, 11% from protein, 56% from carb); 8 g protein; 11 g total

fat; 2 g saturated fat; 3 g monounsaturated fat; 6 g polyunsaturated fat; 42 g carbohydrate; 5 g fiber; 17 g sugar; 233 mg phosphorus; 106 mg calcium; 2 mg iron; 136 mg sodium; 314 mg potassium; 183 IU vitamin A; 53 mg vitamin E; 2 mg vitamin C; 40 mg cholesterol

Oat Bran Raisin Muffins

Another healthy and tasty muffin treat, this one loaded with artery-cleaning oat bran cereal.

2$^1/_4$ cups (225 g) oat bran

$^1/_2$ cup (75 g) raisins

1 tablespoon (14 g) baking powder

$^1/_4$ cup (60 g) packed brown sugar

1$^1/_4$ cups (285 ml) skim milk

2 eggs

3 tablespoons (45 ml) canola oil

Preheat oven to 425°F (220°C, or gas mark 7). In a large bowl, combine oat bran, raisins, baking powder, and brown sugar. Combine milk, eggs, and oil. Stir into dry ingredients until just moistened. Coat 12 muffin cups with nonstick vegetable oil spray or line with paper liners. Spoon batter into prepared pan and bake for 15 minutes, or until done.

Yield: 12 servings

Per serving: 120 calories (31% from fat, 11% from protein, 57% from carbohydrate); 4 g protein; 4 g total fat; 0 g saturated fat; 2 g monounsaturated fat; 1 g polyunsaturated fat; 18 g carbohydrate; 1 g fiber; 10 g sugar; 119 mg phosphorus; 133 mg calcium; 3 mg iron; 189 mg sodium; 186 mg potassium; 172 IU vitamin A;

40 mg ATE vitamin E; 1 mg vitamin C; 36 mg cholesterol; 33 g water

Oat Bran Apple Muffins

I've always been fond of apple muffins, and the extra cholesterol-fighting benefit of oat bran in these makes them even more appealing.

$^3/_4$ cup (90 g) flour

$^3/_4$ cup (90 g) whole wheat flour

1$^1/_2$ teaspoons (3.5 g) cinnamon

1 teaspoon (4.6 g) baking powder

$^1/_2$ teaspoon (2.3 g) baking soda

1 cup (235 ml) buttermilk

$^1/_2$ cup (50 g) oat bran

$^1/_4$ cup (60 g) packed brown sugar

2 tablespoons (30 ml) canola oil

1 egg

1$^1/_2$ cups (225 g) apple, peeled, cored, and chopped

Preheat oven to 400°F (200°C, or gas mark 6). Coat twelve muffin cups with nonstick vegetable oil spray or line with paper liners. In a large bowl, combine flours, cinnamon, baking powder, and baking soda. In a medium bowl, beat buttermilk, oat bran, brown sugar, oil, and egg until blended. Stir buttermilk mixture into flour mixture just until combined. Fold in apples. Divide batter among muffin cups. Bake 18 to 20 minutes or until wooden pick inserted in centers comes out clean.

Yield: 12 servings

Per serving: 119 calories (22% from fat, 11% from protein, 67% from carbohydrate); 3 g protein; 3 g total fat; 0 g saturated fat; 2 g monounsaturated fat; 1 g polyunsaturated fat; 20 g carbohydrate; 2 g fiber; 7 g sugar; 80 mg phosphorus; 64 mg calcium; 2 mg iron; 133 mg sodium; 125 mg potassium; 49 IU vitamin A; 7 mg ATE vitamin E; 1 mg vitamin C; 17 mg cholesterol; 37 g water

Bran Muffins

Those who think bran muffins have to be dry, tasteless creations should try this recipe. While still providing a fiber boost, these muffins are moist and delicious.

1 $^1/_4$ cups (150 g) whole wheat flour

1 cup (100 g) wheat bran

$^1/_4$ cup (50 g) sugar

2 teaspoons (9.2 g) baking powder

1 cup (235 ml) skim milk

1 tablespoon (15 ml) canola oil

$^1/_4$ cup (60 ml) molasses

1 egg

$^1/_2$ teaspoon (1.2 g) cinnamon

$^1/_4$ teaspoon (0.6 g) nutmeg

1 tablespoon (5 g) orange zest

$^1/_2$ cup (65 g) carrot, grated

Preheat oven to 350°F (180°C, or gas mark 4). Coat 12 muffin cups with nonstick vegetable oil spray or line with paper liners. Mix first 4 ingredients. In a second bowl, mix remaining ingredients. Combine until just moistened. Spoon batter into prepared pan and bake for 20 to 22 minutes.

Yield: 12 servings

Per serving: 116 calories (13% from fat, 12% from protein, 74% from carbohydrate); 4 g protein; 2 g total fat; 0 g saturated fat; 1 g monounsaturated fat; 1 g polyunsaturated fat; 24 g carbohydrate; 4 g fiber; 8 g sugar; 143 mg phosphorus; 103 mg calcium; 2 mg iron; 110 mg sodium; 284 mg potassium; 961 IU vitamin A; 13 mg ATE vitamin E; 1 mg vitamin C; 17 mg cholesterol; 31 g water

Apple Muffins

Weekends are a good time to do a little breakfast baking. Not only do you have the time, but if your family is like mine, there are likely to be more people around to enjoy it. And the leftovers make a good grab-and-go breakfast for the first few days of the work week. These muffins are fat-free, owing to the substitution of applesauce for the usual oil.

1 $^1/_2$ cups (185 g) flour

$^1/_4$ cup (50 g) plus 2 teaspoons (25 g) sugar, divided

2 $^1/_2$ teaspoons (11.5 g) baking powder

1 teaspoon (2.3 g) cinnamon, divided

$^3/_4$ cup (180 ml) skim milk

1 egg

$^1/_3$ cup (80 ml) applesauce

1 cup (150 g) apple, peeled and chopped

Preheat oven to 400°F (200°C, or gas mark 6). In a large bowl, stir together flour, $^1/_4$ cup (50 g) sugar, baking powder, and $^1/_2$ teaspoon (1.2 g) cinnamon. Make a well in the center. Stir together milk, egg, applesauce, and apple. Add all at once to dry ingredients. Stir until just moistened. Spoon into greased or paper-lined muffin pans. Mix together remaining $^1/_2$ teaspoon (1.2 g) cinnamon and 2 teaspoons (25 g) sugar. Sprinkle over the tops of the muffins. Bake for 20 minutes.

Apple Butter Muffins

Sweet enough to eat without adding any toppings.

2 cups (250 g) flour

1 tablespoon (13.8 g) baking powder

2 tablespoons (25 g) sugar

5 tablespoons (70 g) unsalted butter

1 egg

$^1/_2$ cup (120 ml) skim milk

6 tablespoons (90 ml) apple butter, divided

2 tablespoons (30 g) brown sugar

1 tablespoon (8 g) flour

$^1/_4$ teaspoon (0.6 g) cinnamon

Preheat oven to 400°F (200°C, or gas mark 6). Combine flour, baking powder, and sugar in a mixing bowl. Cut in butter until mixture resembles coarse crumbs. Combine egg, milk, and 2 tablespoons (30 ml) of the apple butter. Stir until just moistened. Spoon into 12 paper-lined or greased muffin cups. Top each with 1 teaspoon (5 ml) of the apple butter. Combine brown sugar, flour, and cinnamon and sprinkle over the top. Bake for 20 to 25 minutes.

Yield: 12 servings

Apple Raisin Muffins

You could cook some apples to use for these muffins, but I happened to have a can of unsweetened apple pie filling on hand when I made them, and that is a lot easier.

$^1/_2$ cup (120 ml) water

$^1/_2$ cup (75 g) raisins

1 $^1/_2$ cups (180 g) flour

$^1/_4$ cup (50 g) sugar

2 $^1/_2$ teaspoons (11.5 g) baking powder

$^1/_2$ teaspoon (1.2 g) cinnamon

1 cup (260 g) unsweetened apple pie filling

1 egg

$^1/_4$ cup (60 ml) skim milk

Preheat oven to 400°F (200°C, or gas mark 6). Place raisins in water. Heat in microwave for 2 minutes. Allow to cool for 10 minutes. Stir together flour, sugar, baking powder, and cinnamon. Make a well in the center. Cut up the apples in the filling. Stir together apples, egg, milk, and cooled raisin mixture. Add all at once to dry ingredients. Stir until just moistened. Spoon into greased or paper-lined muffin pans. Bake for 20 minutes.

Yield: 12 servings

Per serving: 112 calories (4% from fat, 9% from protein, 87% from carbohydrate); 3 g protein; 0 g total fat; 0 g saturated fat; 0 g monounsaturated fat; 0 g polyunsaturated fat; 25 g carbohydrate; 1 g fiber; 11 g sugar; 58 mg phosphorus; 74 mg calcium; 1 mg iron; 116 mg sodium; 107 mg potassium; 38 IU vitamin A; 3 mg ATE vitamin E; 0 mg vitamin C; 17 mg cholesterol; 36 g water

Strawberry Muffins

A muffin with a flavor like strawberry shortcake. Less sweet than most muffins, with just enough cream cheese to give it a little flavor surprise. Baby food replaces the oil in this recipe, adding flavor and removing fat.

1$^3/_4$ cups (215 g) flour

2 tablespoons (25 g) sugar

3 teaspoons (13.8 g) baking powder

1 egg

$^3/_4$ cup (180 ml) skim milk

$^1/_3$ cup (80 g) baby food bananas

6 ounces (170 g) frozen strawberries, thawed and drained

6 tablespoons (90 g) fat-free cream cheese

Preheat oven to 400°F (200°C, or gas mark 6). Stir together flour, sugar, and baking powder. Combine egg, milk, and baby food bananas. Stir into dry ingredients, mixing until just moistened. Stir in strawberries. Spoon two-thirds of the batter into the bottom of paper-lined or greased muffin cups. Place $^1/_2$ tablespoon (7.5 g) cream cheese in each cup. Divide remaining batter evenly among muffin cups. Bake for 20 to 25 minutes, or until done.

Yield: 12 servings

Per serving: 112 calories (5% from fat, 16% from protein, 79% from carbohydrate); 4 g protein; 1 g total fat; 0 g saturated fat; 0 g monounsaturated fat; 0 g polyunsaturated fat; 20 g carbohydrate; 1 g fiber; 3 g sugar; 83 mg phosphorus; 106 mg calcium; 1 mg iron; 164 mg sodium; 106 mg potassium; 106 IU vitamin A; 23 mg ATE vitamin E; 10 mg vitamin C; 22 mg cholesterol; 43 g water

Fresh Berry Muffins

Sweet muffins with a real berry flavor.

2 cups (250 g) flour

2 teaspoons (9.6 g) baking powder

2 tablespoons (25 g) sugar

1 egg

2 tablespoons (28 g) unsalted butter, melted

1 cup (235 ml) skim milk

$^1/_2$ cup (85 g) strawberries, sliced

Preheat oven to 350°F (180°C, or gas mark 4). Stir together the flour, baking powder, and sugar. In a medium bowl, mix together the remaining ingredients and stir into the dry ingredients, stirring until just moistened. Spoon into greased or paper-lined muffin cups. Bake for 20 to 25 minutes, or until done.

Yield: 12 servings

Per serving: 116 calories (18% from fat, 13% from protein, 69% from carbohydrate); 4 g protein; 2 g total fat; 2 g saturated fat; 0 g monounsaturated fat; 0 g polyunsaturated fat; 20 g carbohydrate; 1 g fiber; 2 g sugar; 70 mg phosphorus; 82 mg calcium; 1 mg iron; 103 mg sodium;

87 mg potassium; 145 IU vitamin A; 31 mg ATE vitamin E; 4 mg vitamin C; 23 mg cholesterol; 31 g water

Blueberry Muffins

These are a real breakfast treat. And you won't even notice that they are fat-free.

1 1/2 cups (180 g) flour

6 tablespoons (75 g) sugar, divided

2 1/2 teaspoons (11.5 g) baking powder

1 teaspoon (2.3 g) cinnamon, divided

1 egg

3/4 cup (180 ml) skim milk

1/3 cup (80 ml) applesauce

1/2 cup (73 g) blueberries

Preheat oven to 400°F (200°C, or gas mark 6). Stir together flour, 4 tablespoons (50 g) sugar, baking powder, and 1/2 teaspoon (1.2 g) cinnamon. Make a well in the center. Stir together milk, egg, and applesauce. Add all at once to dry ingredients. Stir until just moistened. Stir in blueberries. Spoon into greased or paper-lined muffin cups. Mix together remaining cinnamon and sugar. Sprinkle over the tops of the muffins. Bake for 20 minutes.

Yield: 12 servings

Per serving: 99 calories (4% from fat, 12% from protein, 85% from carbohydrate); 3 g protein; 0 g total fat; 0 g saturated fat; 0 g monounsaturated fat; 0 g polyunsaturated fat; 21 g carbohydrate; 1 g fiber; 8 g sugar; 63 mg phosphorus; 86 mg calcium; 1 mg iron; 120 mg sodium; 73 mg potassium; 56 IU vitamin A; 9 mg ATE vitamin E; 1 mg vitamin C; 17 mg cholesterol; 31 g water

Cranberry Orange Muffins

Easy to make and a good, healthy way to start the day.

1 3/4 cups (215 g) flour

1/4 cup (50 g) sugar

2 1/2 tablespoons (7 g) baking powder

1 egg

1/4 cup (60 ml) orange juice

2 tablespoons (30 ml) canola oil

1/4 cup (60 ml) applesauce

1/2 cup (75 g) dried cranberries

Preheat oven to 400°F (200°C, or gas mark 6). Stir together flour, sugar, and baking powder. Combine egg, orange juice, oil, and applesauce. Add all at once to dry ingredients. Stir until just mixed. Fold in cranberries. Fill 12 greased or paper-lined muffin cups. Bake for 20 to 25 minutes.

Yield: 12 servings

Per serving: 129 calories (19% from fat, 8% from protein, 73% from carbohydrate); 3 g protein; 3 g total fat; 0 g saturated fat; 1 g monounsaturated fat; 1 g polyunsaturated fat; 24 g carbohydrate; 1 g fiber; 8 g sugar; 90 mg phosphorus; 176 mg calcium; 1 mg iron; 315 mg sodium; 53 mg potassium; 24 IU vitamin A; 0 mg ATE vitamin E; 2 mg vitamin C; 17 mg cholesterol; 17 g water

Cranberry Sauce Muffins

A good use for leftover cranberry sauce, and great-tasting too.

1 1/2 cups (180 g) flour

1/2 cup (100 g) sugar

2 teaspoons (9.2 g) baking powder

1/2 teaspoon (1.2 g) cinnamon

1/2 teaspoon (0.9 g) ground ginger

1/2 cup (120 ml) applesauce

1 egg

1/2 cup (140 g) whole berry cranberry sauce

1/2 cup (120 ml) orange juice

Preheat oven to 400°F (200°C, or gas mark 6). Stir together flour, sugar, baking powder, cinnamon, and ginger. Combine applesauce, egg, cranberry sauce, and orange juice. Add to dry ingredients and stir until just mixed. Spoon into greased or paper-lined muffin cups. Bake for 19 to 20 minutes.

Yield: 12 servings

Per serving: 121 calories (3% from fat, 8% from protein, 89% from carbohydrate); 2 g protein; 0 g total fat; 0 g saturated fat; 0 g monounsaturated fat; 0 g polyunsaturated fat; 27 g carbohydrate; 1 g fiber; 14 g sugar; 43 mg phosphorus; 53 mg calcium; 1 mg iron; 95 mg sodium; 66 mg potassium; 35 IU vitamin A; 0 mg ATE vitamin E; 4 mg vitamin C; 17 mg cholesterol; 31 g water

Leftover Cranberry Muffins

One more use for your leftover cranberry sauce, this one paired with oats and whole wheat flour for extra nutrition.

1 cup quick cooking oats

3/4 cup skim milk

1 1/2 cups whole wheat pastry flour

1 tablespoon baking powder

1/4 cup brown sugar

1 cup whole berry cranberry sauce

1 egg

1 teaspoon vanilla

1/4 cup walnuts, chopped

Combine oats and milk and set aside for 15 minutes. Combine flour, baking powder, and sugar and stir to mix well. Add the oat mixture and the remaining ingredients, stirring until just moistened. Coat muffin pan with non-stick cooking spray and fill 3/4 full with batter. Bake at 350°F for 18 minutes or until done.

Yield: 12 servings

Per serving: 161 calories (16% from fat, 11% from protein, 73% from carb); 5 g protein; 3 g total fat; 0 g saturated fat; 1 g monounsaturated fat; 2 g polyunsaturated fat; 30 g carb; 3 g fiber; 13 g sugar; 145 mg phosphorus; 108 mg calcium; 148 mg sodium; 151 mg potassium; 71 IU vitamin A; 17 mg vitamin E; 1 mg vitamin C; 18 mg cholesterol

Peach Muffins

A good way to start a cold Saturday morning . . . or a warm one. This recipe uses a trick I read somewhere for reducing fat in baked goods. Instead of the usual suggestion to replace the oil with applesauce, here we use peach baby food, which adds to the peach flavor of the muffins.

For muffins:

1 cup (125 g) flour

$^1/_2$ cup (40 g) oatmeal

$^1/_4$ cup (50 g) sugar

$2^1/_2$ teaspoons (11.5 g) baking powder

1 egg

$^3/_4$ cup (180 ml) skim milk

$^1/_3$ cup (80 g) baby food peaches

$^1/_2$ cup (100 g) peaches, diced

$^1/_2$ teaspoon (2.5 ml) almond extract

For topping:

2 tablespoons (25 g) sugar

$^1/_2$ teaspoon (1.2 g) cinnamon

To make the muffins: Preheat oven to 400°F (200°C, or gas mark 6). Stir together the flour, oatmeal, sugar, and baking powder. Make a well in the center. Stir together egg, milk, and baby food. Add all at once to dry ingredients. Stir until just moistened. Stir in peaches and almond extract. Spoon into greased or paper-lined muffin cups.

To make the topping: Mix together sugar and cinnamon. Sprinkle over the tops of the muffins. Bake for 20 minutes.

Yield: 12 servings

Per serving: 106 calories (7% from fat, 13% from protein, 80% from carbohydrate); 3 g protein; 1 g total fat; 0 g saturated fat; 0 g monounsaturated fat; 0 g polyunsaturated fat; 21 g carbohydrate; 1 g fiber; 8 g sugar; 92 mg phosphorus; 88 mg calcium; 1 mg iron; 121 mg sodium; 109 mg potassium; 83 IU vitamin A; 9 mg ATE vitamin E; 3 mg vitamin C; 17 mg cholesterol; 32 g water

Tropical Muffins

For those mornings when you are trying to escape the last cold, wet days of winter, these muffins make it a little easier to picture Hawaii.

$1^3/_4$ cups (215 g) flour

$^1/_4$ cup (60 g) brown sugar

$2^1/_2$ teaspoons (11.5 g) baking powder

1 egg

$^3/_4$ cup (180 ml) skim milk

$^1/_3$ cup (80 ml) applesauce

6 ounces (170 g) crushed pineapple with syrup, drained

$^1/_4$ cup (18 g) flaked dried coconut

Preheat oven to 400°F (200°C, or gas mark 6). In a medium bowl, stir together flour, brown sugar, and baking powder. Combine egg, milk, and applesauce and add to dry ingredients. Stir until just mixed. Stir in pineapple and coconut. Spoon into muffin cups lined with paper or coated with nonstick vegetable oil spray. Bake for 20 to 25 minutes.

Yield: 12 servings

Per serving: 112 calories (7% from fat, 11% from protein, 81% from carbohydrate); 3 g protein; 1 g total fat; 1 g saturated fat; 0 g monounsaturated fat; 0 g polyunsaturated fat; 23 g carbohydrate; 1 g fiber; 7 g

sugar; 68 mg phosphorus; 90 mg calcium; 1 mg iron; 123 mg sodium; 106 mg potassium; 57 IU vitamin A; 9 mg ATE vitamin E; 1 mg vitamin C; 17 mg cholesterol; 39 g water

Whole Wheat Banana Muffins

Another fresh muffin idea, this time with a way to get rid of those overripe bananas.

1 egg

$^3/_4$ cup (180 ml) skim milk

$^1/_3$ cup (80 ml) applesauce

$^1/_2$ cup (115 g) banana, mashed

1 cup (125 g) flour

$^1/_2$ cup (60 g) whole wheat flour

$^1/_4$ cup (28 g) wheat germ

$2^1/_2$ teaspoons (11.5 g) baking powder

$^1/_4$ teaspoon (0.6 g) cinnamon

Preheat oven to 375°F (190°C, or gas mark 5). Combine egg, milk, applesauce, and banana. Stir together remaining ingredients. Add milk mixture and stir until just combined. Spoon into 12 lined or greased muffin cups. Bake for 20 to 25 minutes.

Yield: 12 servings

Per serving: 86 calories (7% from fat, 17% from protein, 76% from carbohydrate); 4 g protein; 1 g total fat; 0 g saturated fat; 0 g monounsaturated fat; 0 g polyunsaturated fat; 17 g carbohydrate; 2 g fiber; 2 g sugar; 103 mg phosphorus; 87 mg calcium; 1 mg iron; 121 mg sodium; 138 mg potassium; 61 IU vitamin A; 9 mg ATE vitamin E; 1 mg vitamin C; 17 mg cholesterol; 33 g water

Date Muffins

I've always been fond of muffins for breakfast. And the good news is that there are lots of nice, healthy recipes for them. Like these whole wheat date muffins, for example.

1 cup (125 g) whole wheat flour

1 cup (125 g) flour

2 tablespoons (25 g) sugar

4 teaspoons (18.4 g) baking powder

1 egg

1 cup (235 ml) skim milk

2 tablespoons (30 ml) canola oil

$^1/_2$ cup (55 g) dates, chopped

Preheat oven to 400°F (200°C, or gas mark 6). Combine flours, sugar, and baking powder. Combine egg, milk, and oil; mix well and add dates. Add to dry ingredients, stirring only until flour mixture is moistened. Fill greased muffin pans and bake for 20 to 25 minutes, or until a wooden pick inserted in the center comes out clean.

Yield: 12 servings

Per serving: 135 calories (18% from fat, 12% from protein, 70% from carbohydrate); 4 g protein; 3 g total fat; 0 g saturated fat; 1 g monounsaturated fat; 1 g polyunsaturated fat; 24 g carbohydrate; 2 g fiber; 7 g sugar; 113 mg phosphorus; 130 mg calcium; 1 mg iron; 185 mg sodium; 155 mg potassium; 62 IU vitamin A; 13 mg ATE vitamin E; 0 mg vitamin C; 17 mg cholesterol; 27 g water

Graham Cracker Muffins

These are very popular around our house. The graham crackers give them flavor as well as whole-grain goodness.

2 cups (168 g) graham crackers, crushed

$^1/_4$ cup (50 g) sugar

2 teaspoons (9.2 g) baking powder

1 cup (235 ml) skim milk

1 egg, slightly beaten

2 tablespoons (30 ml) honey

Preheat oven to 400°F (200°C, or gas mark 6). Grease 12 muffin cups or line with paper muffin liners. In a large bowl, combine cracker crumbs, sugar, and baking powder. Stir in milk, egg, and honey; mixing just until moistened. Spoon batter into prepared muffin cups. Bake for 15 to 18 minutes, or until a wooden pick inserted in the center comes out clean. Let stand for 5 minutes.

Yield: 12 servings

Per serving: 99 calories (15% from fat, 10% from protein, 76% from carbohydrate); 2 g protein; 2 g total fat; 0 g saturated fat; 1 g monounsaturated fat; 1 g polyunsaturated fat; 19 g carbohydrate; 0 g fiber; 11 g sugar; 61 mg phosphorus; 81 mg calcium; 1 mg iron; 187 mg sodium; 76 mg potassium; 61 IU vitamin A; 13 mg ATE vitamin E; 0 mg vitamin C; 17 mg cholesterol; 24 g water

Chocolate Muffins

Something for those days when you're looking for a sweeter breakfast.

2 cups (250 g) flour

$^3/_4$ cup (150 g) sugar

$2^1/_2$ teaspoons (11.5 g) baking powder

2 tablespoons (11 g) instant coffee granules

1 cup (235 ml) warm skim milk

$^1/_2$ cup (120 ml) applesauce

1 egg

1 teaspoon (5 ml) vanilla

$^3/_4$ cup (170 g) miniature chocolate chips

Preheat oven to 375°F (190°C, or gas mark 5). In a bowl, combine flour, sugar, and baking powder. In another bowl, stir coffee into milk until dissolved. Add applesauce, egg, and vanilla and mix well. Stir into dry ingredients until just moistened. Stir in chocolate chips. Fill greased or paper-lined muffin pans two-thirds full. Bake for 17 to 20 minutes, or until muffins are done.

Yield: 12 servings

Per serving: 201 calories (16% from fat, 9% from protein, 75% from carbohydrate); 4 g protein; 4 g total fat; 2 g saturated fat; 1 g monounsaturated fat; 0 g polyunsaturated fat; 38 g carbohydrate; 1 g fiber; 19 g sugar; 97 mg phosphorus; 112 mg calcium; 1 mg iron; 132 mg sodium; 140 mg potassium; 82 IU vitamin A; 18 mg ATE vitamin E; 0 mg vitamin C; 20 mg cholesterol; 35 g water

Streusel Muffins

These muffins are relatively low fat as well as low sodium, and they taste like old-fashioned coffee cake.

For Streusel:

$^1/_2$ cup (115 g) brown sugar

2 tablespoons (16 g) flour

2 teaspoons (4.6 g) cinnamon

For Muffins:

$1^1/_2$ cups (188 g) flour

$^1/_2$ cup (100 g) sugar

2 teaspoons (9.6 g) baking powder

$^1/_4$ cup (56 g) unsalted butter

$^1/_2$ cup (120 ml) skim milk

1 egg

To make the streusel: Stir together brown sugar, flour, and cinnamon. Set aside.

To make the muffins: Preheat oven to 375°F (190°C, or gas mark 5). Stir together flour, sugar, and baking powder. Cut in butter until mixture resembles coarse crumbs. Combine milk and egg. Add to dry ingredients and stir until just mixed. Divide half the batter evenly among 12 greased or paper-lined muffin cups. Sprinkle with half the streusel topping. Top with remaining batter and then remaining streusel topping. Bake for 20 to 25 minutes.

Yield: 12 servings

Per serving: 172 calories (21% from fat, 7% from protein, 72% from carbohydrate); 3 g protein; 4 g total fat; 4 g saturated fat; 0 g monounsaturated fat; 0 g polyunsaturated fat; 31 g carbohydrate; 1 g fiber; 17 g sugar; 58 mg phosphorus; 81 mg calcium; 1 mg iron; 142 mg sodium; 92 mg potassium; 241 IU vitamin A; 52 mg ATE vitamin E; 0 mg vitamin C; 23 mg cholesterol; 16 g water

Good-for-You Muffins

These are my all-time favorite muffins, just packed with things that are good for you, as well as good-tasting.

$^1/_2$ cup (80 g) raisins

2 cups (250 g) flour

1 cup (200 g) sugar

2 teaspoons (9.2 g) baking soda

2 teaspoons (4.6 g) cinnamon

$^3/_4$ cup (98 g) carrot, grated

1 green apple, grated

$^1/_2$ cup (60 g) sliced almonds

$^1/_2$ cup (35 g) shredded coconut

3 eggs

$^2/_3$ cup (160 ml) applesauce

2 teaspoons (10 ml) vanilla

Soak raisins in enough hot water to cover for 30 minutes; drain thoroughly. Preheat oven to 350°F (180°C, or gas mark 4). Mix flour, sugar, baking soda, and cinnamon in bowl. Stir in raisins, carrots, apple, almonds, and coconut. Beat egg with applesauce and vanilla to blend. Stir into flour mixture until just combined. Divide batter evenly among 12 greased or paper-lined muffin cups. Bake for 20 to 22 minutes, or until golden brown and a wooden pick inserted in the center comes out clean. Cool 5 minutes before removing from pan.

Yield: 12 servings

Per serving: 241 calories (18% from fat, 9% from protein, 73% from carbohydrate); 6 g protein; 5 g total fat; 1 g saturated fat; 2 g monounsaturated fat; 1 g polyunsaturated fat; 45 g carbohydrate; 2 g fiber; 24 g sugar; 86 mg phosphorus; 37 mg calcium; 2 mg iron; 247 mg sodium; 226 mg potassium; 1411 IU vitamin A; 0 mg ATE vitamin E; 1 mg vitamin C; 52 mg cholesterol; 46 g water

Cinnamon Honey Scones

These are sort of a free-form scone, rather than the more traditional wedges. Serve warm with honey and butter to bring out the flavor of the scones even more.

1$^3/_4$ cups (220 g) whole wheat pastry flour

1$^1/_2$ teaspoons baking powder

$^1/_4$ teaspoon cinnamon

6 tablespoons (85 g) unsalted butter, softened

1 tablespoon (20 g) honey

$^1/_2$ cup (120 ml) skim milk

1 egg

Preheat oven to 450°F (230°C, gas mark 8). Line baking sheet with aluminum foil. In a bowl, mix the flour, baking powder, and cinnamon with a wooden spoon. Work butter into mixture by hand until mixture is yellow. Add honey and milk, then egg. Stir with wooden spoon until thoroughly mixed. Scoop spoonful of dough and drop onto baking sheet. Leave 1 inch (2.5 cm) between each. Bake 15 minutes or until golden brown. Cool 5 minutes.

Yield: 8 servings

Per serving: 23 g water; 192 calories (45% from fat, 10% from protein, 45% from carb); 5 g protein; 10 g total fat; 6 g saturated fat; 3 g monounsaturated fat; 1 g polyunsaturated fat; 22 g carbohydrate; 3 g fiber; 2 g sugar; 142 mg phosphorus; 89 mg calcium; 1 mg iron; 115 mg sodium; 147 mg potassium; 342 IU vitamin A; 92 mg vitamin E; 0 mg vitamin C; 49 mg cholesterol

Oatmeal Raisin Scones

I've learned to like scones in recent years. This version not only tastes great, but is healthy too.

2 cups (240 g) whole wheat pastry flour

3 tablespoons (45 g) brown sugar

1 teaspoon baking powder

$^1/_2$ teaspoon baking soda

$^1/_2$ cup (112 g) unsalted butter, chilled

1$^1/_2$ cups (120 g) rolled oats

$^1/_2$ cup (75 g) raisins

1 cup (235 ml) buttermilk

2 tablespoons cinnamon

2 tablespoons (26 g) sugar

Preheat oven to 375°F (190°C, gas mark 5). Combine flour, brown sugar, baking powder, and baking soda. Cut in butter until mixture resembles coarse crumbs. Stir in oats and raisins. Add buttermilk and mix with a fork until dough forms a ball. Turn out on lightly floured board and knead 6 to 8 minutes. Pat dough into $^1/_2$-inch (1-cm) thickness.

Cut 8 to 10 rounds or wedges and place them on ungreased baking sheet. Sprinkle with sugar and cinnamon. Bake 20 to 25 minutes.

Yield: 10 servings

Per serving: 29 g water; 273 calories (34% from fat, 9% from protein, 57% from carb); 6 g protein; 11 g total fat; 6 g saturated fat; 3 g monounsaturated fat; 1 g polyunsaturated fat; 41 g carbohydrate; 5 g fiber; 13 g sugar; 185 mg phosphorus; 97 mg calcium; 2 mg iron; 80 mg sodium; 262 mg potassium; 296 IU vitamin A; 78 mg vitamin E; 1 mg vitamin C; 25 mg cholesterol

Whole Grain Scones

The mornings we have these for breakfast, I forgo my usual coffee for a cup of tea.

1 egg

$1/2$ cup (100 g) sugar

5 tablespoons (75 ml) canola oil

$1/8$ teaspoon lemon peel

$1/2$ cup (40 g) rolled oats

$1/4$ cup (25 g) wheat bran

$1 1/2$ cups (180 g) whole wheat pastry flour

2 tablespoons poppyseeds

1 tablespoon baking powder

$1/2$ teaspoon cinnamon

$1/2$ cup (120 ml) skim milk

Lemon Topping:

3 tablespoons (45 ml) lemon juice

$1/4$ cup (25 g) confectioners' sugar

Preheat oven to 375°F (190°C, gas mark 5). Whisk the egg, sugar, and oil together in a bowl. Mix the lemon peel and all of the dry ingredients together in a separate bowl and stir with a wooden spoon until all of them are evenly dispersed throughout. Slowly add the dry ingredients into the egg, sugar, and oil, and mix to create a thick dough. Add the milk and mix well. Coat a baking sheet with nonstick vegetable oil spray. Scoop up tablespoons of the dough and drop them one by one in mounds onto the baking sheet, leaving 2 inches (5 cm) of space between. Bake for 15 to 20 minutes, just until the crust is barely golden brown and the dough is dry. Remove from the oven and let cool for 10 minutes. With a fork, mix the lemon topping ingredients until the sugar is completely melded in. Drizzle 1 tablespoon ever each scone.

Yield: 10 servings

Per serving: 21 g water; 218 calories (36% from fat, 8% from protein, 56% from carb); 5 g protein; 9 g total fat; 1 g saturated fat; 5 g monounsaturated fat; 3 g polyunsaturated fat; 32 g carbohydrate; 3 g fiber; 14 g sugar; 165 mg phosphorus; 138 mg calcium; 1 mg iron; 164 mg sodium; 152 mg potassium; 61 IU vitamin A; 16 mg vitamin E; 2 mg vitamin C; 21 mg cholesterol

Holiday Scones

I created this recipe one year when I was looking for a use for leftover candied fruit from the Christmas baking season. I'd only had scones a few times and they'd struck me as kind of dry and nor very exciting, but this version turned out really well.

2 cups (240 g) whole wheat pastry flour

$1/3$ cup (67 g) sugar

1 tablespoon baking powder

6 tablespoons (85 g) unsalted butter

$^3/_4$ cup candied fruit

1 egg

$^1/_2$ cup (120 ml) skim milk

$^1/_2$ teaspoon lemon peel

$^3/_4$ cup (75 g) confectioners' sugar

2 tablespoons (30 ml) lemon juice

In a medium bowl stir together the first three ingredients. With a pastry blender, cut in butter until mixture resembles coarse crumbs. Stir in fruit. Stir together egg, milk, and lemon peel. Add to dry ingredients, stir until just moistened. On a floured surface, knead dough 5 or 6 times until it forms a ball. Place dough on baking sheet coated with nonstick vegetable oil spray, spread to 8-inch (20-cm) circle, about 1 inch (2.5 cm) thick. Cut into 8 wedges. Separate wedges slightly. Bake at 400°F (200°C, gas mark 6) for 15 to 20 minutes or until light golden brown and center is set. Combine confectioners' sugar and lemon juice. Mix well. Drizzle over warm scones.

Yield: 8 servings

Per serving: 33 g water; 325 calories (27% from fat, 7% from protein, 66% from carb); 6 g protein; 10 g total fat; 6 g saturated fat; 3 g monounsaturated fat; 1 g polyunsaturated fat; 57 g carbohydrate; 5 g fiber; 20 g sugar; 190 mg phosphorus; 148 mg calcium; 2 mg iron; 210 mg sodium; 335 mg potassium; 862 IU vitamin A; 92 mg vitamin E; 3 mg vitamin C; 49 mg cholesterol

Apple Pinwheels

These little apple rolls are another good weekend breakfast—sweet, but low in fat.

2 cups (250 g) sifted flour

4 teaspoons (18.4 g) baking powder

4 tablespoons (56 g) unsalted butter, divided

$^3/_4$ cup (180 ml) skim milk

4 cups (600 g) apple, peeled and sliced

1 teaspoon (2.3 g) cinnamon

$1^1/_4$ cups (285 g) brown sugar, divided

Preheat oven to 425°F (220°C, or gas mark 7). Sift flour with baking powder. Cut in 2 tablespoons (28 g) butter with two spatulas or a pastry blender. Add milk, mixing quickly and lightly. Turn onto a lightly floured surface. Roll into an oblong sheet $^1/_4$-inch (0.6-cm) thick. Melt remaining 2 tablespoons (28 g) butter and brush over dough. Cover with apples. Mix together cinnamon and 1 cup (225 g) of the brown sugar and sprinkle over the apple. Roll up like a jelly roll. Cut into 12 slices. Sprinkle remaining $^1/_4$ cup (60 g) brown sugar over baking sheet sprayed with nonstick vegetable oil spray. Place rolls, cut sides down, on pan. Bake for 25 minutes.

Yield: 12 servings

Per serving: 221 calories (16% from fat, 5% from protein, 79% from carbohydrate); 3 g protein; 4 g total fat; 3 g saturated fat; 1 g monounsaturated fat; 0 g polyunsaturated fat; 44 g carbohydrate; 1 g fiber; 26 g sugar; 83 mg phosphorus; 140 mg calcium; 2 mg iron; 181 mg sodium; 165 mg potassium; 214 IU vitamin A; 45 mg ATE vitamin E; 2 mg vitamin C; 10 mg cholesterol; 49 g water

Banana Sticky Buns

Am I the only one that seems to always have bananas at that use-or-throw-away stage? I hate throwing things away, so I went looking for a different recipe to use bananas and found this one.

$^3/_4$ cup (75 g) unsalted pecans

$^1/_4$ cup (56 g) unsalted butter

$^1/_3$ cup (75 g) plus $^1/_4$ cup (60 g) brown sugar, divided

2 cups (250 g) flour

1 tablespoon (13.8 g) baking powder

6 tablespoons (90 ml) applesauce

$^2/_3$ cup (150 g) mashed bananas

Preheat oven to 375°F (190°C, or gas mark 5). Divide pecans, butter, and $^1/_3$ cup (75 g) brown sugar between 12 muffin cups. Bake for 5 minutes, or until butter is melted. Combine flour and baking powder. Stir in applesauce and banana until mixture forms a soft dough. On a lightly floured surface, knead dough a few times until it holds together. Roll or press dough into a 9 x12-inch (23 × 30-cm) rectangle. Spread remaining $^1/_4$ cup (60 g) brown sugar over dough. Roll up from long side. Slice into 12 rolls. Place each in a muffin cup. Bake for 12 to 15 minutes, or until golden. Allow to cool 1 minute before inverting onto a serving platter.

Yield: 12 servings

Per serving: 212 calories (37% from fat, 6% from protein, 58% from carbohydrate); 3 g protein; 9 g total fat; 6 g saturated fat; 2 g monounsaturated fat;02 g polyunsaturated fat; 31 g carbohydrate; 2 g fiber; 13 g sugar; 75 mg phosphorus; 89 mg calcium; 2 mg iron; 168 mg sodium; 142 mg potassium; 214 IU vitamin A; 46 mg ATE vitamin E; 1 mg vitamin C; 12 mg cholesterol; 20 g water

Whole Wheat Coffee Cake

A nice whole wheat coffee cake with a crunchy filling.

$1^3/_4$ cups (210 g) whole wheat pastry flour

1 teaspoon baking powder

1 teaspoon baking soda

$^1/_2$ cup (112 g) unsalted butter, softened

$^2/_3$ cup (133 g) sugar

2 eggs

1 teaspoon vanilla extract

1 cup (230 g) sour cream

Bran Nut Filling:

$^1/_3$ cup (75 g) packed brown sugar

$^1/_2$ cup bran flakes (20 g) cereal

$^1/_2$ cup (60 g) chopped walnuts

1 teaspoon cinnamon

Mix flour, baking powder, and baking soda; set aside. In large bowl beat butter, sugar, eggs, and vanilla until light and fluffy. At low speed stir in sour cream alternately with flour mixture until blended. To make the bran nut filling, combine all filling ingredients in a small bowl. To assemble the cake, spread one-third of the sour cream mixture in 9-inch (23-cm) square pan coated with nonstick vegetable oil spray. Sprinkle on about $^1/_2$ cup filling. Repeat layering twice. Bake in preheated 350°F (180°C, gas mark 4) oven for 30 to 45 minutes. Cool slightly.

Yield: 12 servings

Per serving: 27 g water; 275 calories (45% from fat, 8% from protein, 46% from carb); 6 g protein; 14 g total fat; 7 g saturated fat; 4 g monounsaturated fat; 2 g polyunsaturated fat; 33 g carbohydrate; 3 g fiber; 17 g sugar; 148 mg phosphorus; 68 mg calcium; 2 mg iron; 85 mg sodium; 174 mg potassium; 451 IU vitamin A; 97 mg vitamin E; 1 mg vitamin C; 68 mg cholesterol

Apple Coffee Cake

The kind of coffee cake you can find in old-fashioned bakeries, if you can find an old-fashioned bakery.

$2^1/_2$ cups (300 g) whole wheat pastry flour

2 teaspoons sugar

2 teaspoons baking powder

1 cup (225 g) unsalted butter

1 egg

$^1/_4$ cup (60 ml) skim milk

6 apples, sliced

Topping:

$1^1/_2$ cups (300 g) sugar

1 tablespoon flour

$^1/_2$ teaspoon cinnamon

Combine first three ingredients. Cut in butter with a pastry blender until crumbly, then add egg and milk; beat and blend. Spread evenly on foil-lined 10 × 15-inch (25 × 37-cm) jelly-roll pan and up the sides. Put sliced apples in rows, overlapping them slightly with pointed edges down. Combine topping ingredients and sprinkle over apples. Bake at 375°F (190°C, gas mark 5) about 25 minutes, until crust is golden brown.

Yield: 15 servings

Per serving: 55 g water; 291 calories (39% from fat, 5% from protein, 56% from carb); 4 g protein; 13 g total fat; 8 g saturated fat; 3 g monounsaturated fat; 1 g polyunsaturated fat; 43 g carbohydrate; 3 g fiber; 26 g sugar; 103 mg phosphorus; 58 mg calcium; 1 mg iron; 76 mg sodium; 144 mg potassium; 430 IU vitamin A; 110 mg vitamin E; 2 mg vitamin C; 47 mg cholesterol

Oatmeal Breakfast Cake

Serve with warm milk and cinnamon.

1 cup (235 ml) canola oil

$1^1/_2$ cups (300 g) sugar

4 eggs, beaten

2 cups (475 ml) skim milk

4 teaspoons (18 g) baking powder

6 cups (480 g) rolled oats

1 teaspoon cinnamon

1 cup (86 g) dried apples

1 cup (110 g) slivered almonds

Thoroughly mix all ingredients together. Pour into 10 × 13-inch (25 × 33-cm) pan. Bake 30 minutes at 350°F (180°C, gas mark 4).

Yield: 12 servings

Per serving: 60 g water; 377 calories (61% from fat, 6% from protein, 32% from carb); 6 g protein; 27 g total fat; 2 g saturated fat; 16 g monounsaturated fat; 7 g polyunsaturated fat; 31 g carbohydrate; 2 g fiber; 29 g sugar; 168 mg phosphorus; 185 mg calcium; 1 mg iron;

206 mg sodium; 185 mg potassium; 178 IU vitamin A; 51 mg vitamin E; 0 mg vitamin C; 80 mg cholesterol

Tip: This recipe freezes well and is excellent to make ahead of time.

Banana Bread

Another good recipe for using up bananas. This makes a great breakfast or snack.

1³/₄ cups (215 g) flour

1¹/₄ teaspoons (5.8 g) baking powder

1 teaspoon (4.6 g) baking soda

²/₃ cup (133 g) sugar

¹/₄ cup (56 g) unsalted butter

2 eggs

¹/₄ cup (60 ml) skim milk

1 cup (225 g) mashed banana

¹/₄ cup (30 g) chopped pecans

Preheat oven to 350°F (180°C, or gas mark 4). Stir together flour, baking powder, and baking soda. In a mixing bowl, cream sugar and butter with an electric mixer until light and fluffy. Add eggs and milk, beating until smooth. Add dry ingredients and banana alternately, beating until smooth after each addition. Stir in pecans. Pour batter into lightly greased 9 × 4 × 2-inch (23 × 10 × 5-cm) loaf pan. Bake for 60 to 65 minutes, or until a knife inserted near the center comes out clean. Cool 10 minutes before removing from pan.

Yield: 12 servings

Per serving: 187 calories (28% from fat, 8% from protein, 64% from carbohydrate); 4 g protein; 6 g total fat; 5 g saturated fat; 1 g monounsaturated fat; 0 g polyunsaturated fat; 30 g carbohydrate; 1 g fiber; 14 g sugar; 61 mg phosphorus; 49 mg calcium; 1 mg iron; 219 mg sodium; 145 mg potassium; 261 IU vitamin A; 49 mg ATE vitamin E; 2 mg vitamin C; 45 mg cholesterol; 30 g water

Cranberry Bread

Reader Miguel sent me this recipe that gets rid of your leftover cranberry sauce. I don't know about your house, but that is the one thing that never seems to be completely finished here after Thanksgiving, so I was really grateful. The flavor is excellent. I used the jellied cranberry sauce, but I don't see any reason why the whole berry sauce wouldn't work just as well.

¹/₂ cup (120 ml) applesauce

1 cup (200 g) sugar

2 eggs

1 teaspoon (5 ml) vanilla

2 cups (250 g) flour

1 teaspoon (4.6 g) baking soda

¹/₃ cup (80 g) orange juice

1 cup (150 g) apples, peeled and chopped

1 cup (277 g) cranberry sauce

1 cup (125 g) chopped walnuts

Preheat oven to 350°F (180°C, or gas mark 4). Cream together the applesauce and sugar until light and fluffy. Beat in eggs and vanilla. Combine flour and baking soda. Add dry ingredients alternately with orange juice to egg mixture, beating just until blended. Fold in apples, cranberry sauce, and walnuts. Lightly coat two 7¹/₂ × 3³/₄ × 2¹/₄-inch (18.8 × 9.4 × 5.6-cm) loaf pans with nonstick vegetable oil spray. Pour batter into prepared pans and bake for 50 minutes, or until a wooden pick inserted in the center comes out clean.

Yield: 24 servings

Per serving: 133 calories (22% from fat, 9% from protein, 69% from carbohydrate); 3 g protein; 3 g total fat; 0 g saturated fat; 1 g monounsaturated fat; 2 g polyunsaturated fat; 23 g carbohydrate; 1 g fiber; 14 g sugar; 46 mg phosphorus; 9 mg calcium; 1 mg iron; 66 mg sodium; 73 mg potassium; 31 IU vitamin A; 0 mg ATE vitamin E; 2 mg vitamin C; 17 mg cholesterol; 24 g water

Whole Wheat Pineapple Zucchini Bread

The pineapple adds flavor and moistness to a great breakfast bread.

3 eggs

1 cup (235 ml) applesauce

2 cups (400 g) sugar

2 teaspoons (10 ml) vanilla

2 cups (250 g) shredded zucchini

8 ounces (225 g) crushed pineapple, drained

2 cups (250 g) flour

1 cup (125 g) whole wheat flour

2 teaspoons (9.2 g) baking soda

$^1/_2$ teaspoon (2.3 g) baking powder

$1^1/_2$ teaspoons (3.5 g) cinnamon

$^3/_4$ teaspoon (1.7 g) nutmeg

Preheat oven to 350°F (180°C, or gas mark 4). Grease two 9 × 5-inch (12.5 × 23-cm) loaf pans. Combine eggs, applesauce, sugar, and vanilla in a large bowl. Mix well. Add zucchini and pineapple and mix well. Combine flours, baking soda, baking powder, cinnamon, and nutmeg. Stir into zucchini mixture until just moistened. Pour into prepared loaf pans. Bake for 1 hour, or until knife inserted near center comes out clean.

Yield: 24 servings

Per serving: 139 calories (3% from fat, 8% from protein, 89% from carbohydrate); 3 g protein; 1 g total fat; 0 g saturated fat; 0 g monounsaturated fat; 0 g polyunsaturated fat; 31 g carbohydrate; 1 g fiber; 19 g sugar; 46 mg phosphorus; 18 mg calcium; 1 mg iron; 131 mg sodium; 104 mg potassium; 56 IU vitamin A; 0 mg ATE vitamin E; 3 mg vitamin C; 50 mg cholesterol; 35 g water

Pumpkin Bread

If you have some leftover pumpkin when you make pumpkin pie, you can make it into pumpkin bread. This makes a great breakfast without even needing any toppings on it.

3 cups (600 g) sugar

1 cup (235 ml) applesauce

4 eggs

16 ounces canned or cooked fresh pumpkin

$3^1/_2$ cups (438 g) flour

4 teaspoons (18.4 g) baking soda

1 teaspoon (4.6 g) baking powder

2 teaspoons (4.6 g) cinnamon

1 teaspoon (1.8 g) ground ginger

$^2/_3$ cup (160 ml) water

Preheat oven to 350°F (180°C, or gas mark 4). Cream sugar and applesauce. Add eggs and pumpkin; mix well. Sift together flour, baking soda, baking powder, cinnamon, and ginger. Add to pumpkin mixture alternately with water. Mix well after each addition. Divide batter evenly between two well-greased and floured glass 9 × 5-inch (23 × 12.5-cm) loaf pans. Bake for 1$^1/_2$ hours, or until knife inserted near center comes out clean. Let stand for 10 minutes. Remove from pans to cool.

Yield: 24 servings

Per serving: 184 calories (3% from fat, 7% from protein, 90% from carbohydrate); 3 g protein; 1 g total fat; 0 g saturated fat; 0 g monounsaturated fat; 0 g polyunsaturated fat; 42 g carbohydrate; 1 g fiber; 27 g sugar; 44 mg phosphorus; 28 mg calcium; 1 mg iron; 250 mg sodium; 103 mg potassium; 2983 IU vitamin A; 0 mg ATE vitamin E; 1 mg vitamin C; 35 mg cholesterol; 43 g water

Nut Bread

Another good use for recipe bananas, this provides grab-and-go breakfast for most of the week when I make it.

1$^3/_4$ cups (210 g) whole wheat pastry flour

1$^1/_4$ teaspoons baking powder

1 teaspoon baking soda

$^2/_3$ cup (133 g) sugar

$^1/_2$ cup (112 g) unsalted butter

2 eggs

2 tablespoons (28 ml) skim milk

1 cup (225 g) mashed banana

$^1/_4$ cup (28 g) chopped pecans

Stir together flour, baking powder, and baking soda. In a mixing bowl, cream sugar and butter with electric mixer until light. Add eggs and milk, beating until smooth. Add dry ingredients and banana alternately, beating until smooth after each addition. Stir in pecans. Turn batter into 9 × 4 × 2-inch (23 × 10 × 5-cm) loaf pan coated with nonstick vegetable oil spray. Bake at 350°F (180°C, gas mark 4) for 60 to 65 minutes until knife inserted near center comes out clean. Cool 10 minutes before removing from pan.

Yield: 12 servings

Per serving: 27 g water; 218 calories (42% from fat, 7% from protein, 51% from carb); 4 g protein; 11 g total fat; 5 g saturated fat; 3 g monounsaturated fat; 1 g polyunsaturated fat; 29 g carbohydrate; 3 g fiber; 14 g sugar; 104 mg phosphorus; 48 mg calcium; 1 mg iron; 67 mg sodium; 167 mg potassium; 302 IU vitamin A; 78 mg vitamin E; 2 mg vitamin C; 60 mg cholesterol

21

Yeast Breads

would have to say that the bread machine is probably the most useful tool or appliance I have had in maintaining a low-sodium lifestyle. Bread is one of those sneaky sodium things. Each slice does not have a *lot*, maybe 200 to 300 mg. But before you know it if you aren't careful you've added 1000 mg to your diet in one day. If you make your own bread you have control over the other ingredients like the kind of fat used and whether it's refined or whole grain.

I got my current bread machine for Christmas five years ago. It was not a terribly expensive model, around $80 at the time, but even so it has a lot of capabilities that I never use. The one nice feature I do like is that it has an automatic dispenser for adding things like fruit and nuts at the right time.

Making bread in a bread machine is incredibly simple and almost foolproof. You dump the ingredients in, turn it on, and come back a couple of hours later to freshly baked bread. The only other things you may have to do are add other ingredients about 20 minutes into the cycle, if your machine doesn't have the automatic dispenser I mentioned, and check the consistency of the dough about 5 to 7 minutes after you start it. If you are really pressed for time, you can skip that last step, but you do run the risk of ending up with bread that does not have the ideal texture.

Flour from wheat grown in different locations can require variations in the flour-to-water ratio.

The time of year you use flour can also affect this ratio; flour tends to be drier and need more water in the winter. The dough should form a smooth ball and not be sticky (too little flour) or lumpy (too little liquid). I've sometimes had to add as much as $^{1}/_{4}$ cup (30 g) of additional flour or (60 ml) water until it looks right.

All the recipes in this chapter were made using a bread machine and instant yeast, also known as bread machine yeast. If you are using active dry yeast it's best to activate it with warm water as described below. Any of these recipes can also be made without a bread machine. You'll have the same delicious, healthy bread, but you'll have to spend more time mixing, kneading, and shaping. The following general procedures should get you started.

Bread machines generally have you put all the liquid ingredients in, then all the dry, although some do it the other way around. Most keep the yeast separate from the liquid until the kneading. When making bread by hand, however, start with the yeast, liquid, and sugar, then add the other ingredients except the flour, and finally add the flour. Most recipes not designed for a bread machine give you a range of flour; sometimes you need more, sometimes less. So you might want to start with $^{1}/_{4}$ to $^{1}/_{2}$ cup (30 to 60 g) less than the recipe calls for and then add more until the dough reaches the right consistency.

Start with warm water or whatever liquid the recipe calls for. Around 85°F (29°C) is about right. The idea is to get the liquid warm enough so the yeast grows, but not so warm that it kills it. Mix the wet ingredients and yeast together with a spoon. Stir in the flour until it gets too stiff to stir. Dump it out onto a floured counter and knead until the surface is smooth, adding more flour if the dough is too sticky.

Grease a large bowl. Grease the top of the dough by placing it into the greased bowl, then turning it over so the greased part is on top and the ungreased part is on the bottom. Cover with a cloth and put someplace warm to rise until doubled in size.

When the dough has doubled, punch it down, form into a loaf by kneading and shaping it, then put in a greased loaf pan or on a greased baking sheet. Let rise until almost doubled in size, then place in a preheated 375°F (190°C, or gas mark 5) oven and bake until done, usually when the loaf sounds hollow when tapped on the bottom.

This, of course, is just one way to make bread by hand. It follows the traditional way of doing it. You can find many other methods, including some that reduce the amount of kneading by combining some of the ingredients with a mixer or food processor. Generally speaking, you can use any recipe or method that you like, simply substituting the ingredients.

Oatmeal Bread

Wonderful slightly sweet flavor. Great toasted for breakfast or for sandwiches.

1 cup (80 g) quick-cooking oats

$^2/_3$ cup (157 ml) skim milk

$^1/_3$ cup (78 ml) water

1 tablespoon unsalted butter

$^1/_2$ cup (60 g) whole wheat flour

2 cups (274 g) bread flour

3 tablespoons (45 g) brown sugar

1 teaspoon yeast

Spread the oats in a baking pan and toast in a 350°F (180°C, gas mark 4) oven until lightly browned, about 15 minutes, stirring occasionally. Place ingredients in bread machine in order specified by manufacturer. Process on whole wheat cycle.

Yield: 12 servings

Per serving: 24 g water; 178 calories (12% from fat, 14% from protein, 74% from carb); 6 g protein; 2 g total fat; 1 g saturated fat; 1 g monounsaturated fat; 1 g polyunsaturated fat; 33 g carbohydrate; 3 g fiber; 3 g sugar; 128 mg phosphorus; 35 mg calcium; 2 mg iron; 11 mg sodium; 143 mg potassium; 58 IU vitamin A; 16 mg vitamin E; 0 mg vitamin C; 3 mg cholesterol

Oatmeal Bread to Live For

This is a sturdy loaf, very nourishing. Great with salads, soups, as sandwiches, or toasted with jam . . . in the winter, spring, summer, fall.

1$^1/_4$ cups (295 ml) water

2 teaspoons (10 ml) canola oil

1 tablespoon (15 g) brown sugar

1 cup (80 g) quick-cooking oats

2$^1/_4$ cups (270 g) whole wheat flour, divided

1 tablespoon vital wheat gluten

1$^1/_4$ teaspoons yeast

1 tablespoon sunflower seeds

Put water, oil, and sugar in the bread machine. Add the oats and let it sit for 5 minutes. Add 2 cups (240 g) of flour and the gluten. Make a well in the middle of the flour for the yeast. Turn on the bread machine. (Use a setting for 1$^1/_2$-pound [680 g] loaf, dark if you have it.) If the dough seems too sticky, add additional flour as required. Add the sunflower seeds at the beep.

Yield: 12 servings

Per serving: 28 g water; 146 calories (14% from fat, 16% from protein, 70% from carb); 6 g protein; 2 g total fat; 0 g saturated fat; 1 g monounsaturated fat; 1 g polyunsaturated fat; 27 g carbohydrate; 4 g fiber; 1 g sugar; 159 mg phosphorus; 17 mg calcium; 2 mg iron; 3 mg sodium; 165 mg potassium; 2 IU vitamin A; 0 mg vitamin E; 0 mg vitamin C; 0 mg cholesterol

Maple Oatmeal Bread

A slightly sweet bread with maple flavor, this one is just made for breakfast. It seems to me it would be perfect for French toast.

1 3/4 teaspoons yeast

2/3 cup (157 ml) warm water

2 1/2 cups (342 g) bread flour

1/2 cup (60 g) whole wheat flour

1/3 cup (27 g) rolled oats

1/3 cup (80 ml) maple syrup

1/4 cup (17 g) nonfat dry milk

2 tablespoons (28 g) unsalted butter, room temperature

Add ingredients to the bread machine in the order specified by manufacturer. Process on sweet bread or whole wheat cycle.

Yield: 12 servings

Per serving: 21 g water; 178 calories (14% from fat, 12% from protein, 74% from carb); 6 g protein; 3 g total fat; 1 g saturated fat; 1 g monounsaturated fat; 0 g polyunsaturated fat; 33 g carbohydrate; 2 g fiber; 6 g sugar; 89 mg phosphorus; 32 mg calcium; 2 mg iron; 11 mg sodium; 129 mg potassium; 94 IU vitamin A; 26 mg vitamin E; 0 mg vitamin C; 5 mg cholesterol

Old-Fashioned Oatmeal Bread

The molasses gives this bread a nice, sweet flavor, perfect for sandwiches with simple meats like sliced chicken or turkey.

1 cup (235 ml) water

1/4 cup (60 ml) molasses

2 tablespoons (28 g) unsalted butter

3 cups (375 g) bread flour

1/2 cup (40 g) quick-cooking oats

2 tablespoons (15 g) nonfat dry milk powder

2 teaspoons (8 g) yeast

Place all ingredients in the bread machine pan in the order specified by the manufacturer. Process on the white bread cycle.

Yield: 12 servings

Per serving: 178 calories (14% from fat, 12% from protein, 75% from carbohydrate); 5 g protein; 3 g total fat; 2 g saturated fat; 1 g monounsaturated fat; 0 g polyunsaturated fat; 33 g carbohydrate; 1 g fiber; 4 g sugar; 68 mg phosphorus; 33 mg calcium; 2 mg iron; 29 mg sodium; 177 mg potassium; 117 IU vitamin A; 28 mg ATE vitamin E; 0 mg vitamin C; 6 mg cholesterol; 27 g water

Hearty Oatmeal Bread

This has a wonderful, slightly sweet flavor that is great toasted for breakfast or for sandwiches.

1 cup (80 g) quick-cooking oats

2/3 cup (160 ml) skim milk

1/3 cup (80 ml) water

1 tablespoon (14 g) unsalted butter

2 1/2 cups (310 g) bread flour

3 tablespoons (45 g) brown sugar

1 teaspoon (4 g) yeast

Preheat oven to 350°F (180°C, or gas mark 4). Spread the oats in a baking pan and toast in the oven for 15 minutes, or until lightly browned, stirring occasionally. Place all ingredients in the bread machine pan in the order specified by the manufacturer. Process on the whole-grain cycle.

Yield: 12 servings

Per serving: 157 calories (11% from fat, 13% from protein, 76% from carbohydrate); 5 g protein; 2 g total fat; 2 g saturated fat; 0 g monounsaturated fat; 0 g polyunsaturated fat; 29 g carbohydrate; 1 g fiber; 3 g sugar; 81 mg phosphorus; 31 mg calcium; 2 mg iron; 21 mg sodium; 97 mg potassium; 78 IU vitamin A; 20 mg ATE vitamin E; 0 mg vitamin C; 5 mg cholesterol; 23 g water

Rustic Italian Bread

This is a recipe that we've been using for a while, and it's our favorite for Italian bread. I use the bread machine to make my dough and then bake it in the oven to get that traditional look.

1 cup (235 ml) water

2 tablespoons (30 ml) olive oil

3 cups (375 g) bread flour

2 teaspoons (8 g) sugar

2 teaspoons (8 g) active dry yeast

2 tablespoons (18 g) cornmeal, for baking sheet

1 egg white, slightly beaten

Add water, oil, flour, sugar, and yeast to your bread machine pan according to the manufacturer's instructions. Set on the dough setting. When the cycle is done, remove dough from the machine. Sprinkle cornmeal onto a baking sheet. Punch dough down and form into a long or oval loaf. Cover and let rise for 25 more minutes, or until doubled again. Preheat oven to 375°F (190°C, or gas mark 5). Uncover dough and slash the top with a sharp knife or razor. Brush all over with the beaten egg white. Bake for 25 to 35 minutes, or until it sounds hollow when tapped on the bottom.

Yield: 12 servings

Per serving: 156 calories (17% from fat, 12% from protein, 71% from carbohydrate); 5 g protein; 3 g total fat; 0 g saturated fat; 2 g monounsaturated fat; 0 g polyunsaturated fat; 27 g carbohydrate; 1 g fiber; 1 g sugar; 44 mg phosphorus; 6 mg calcium; 2 mg iron; 6 mg sodium; 55 mg potassium; 4 IU vitamin A; 0 mg ATE vitamin E; 0 mg vitamin C; 0 mg cholesterol; 27 g water

Italian Wheat Bread

This great bread recipe came from subscriber Pat. This could also be taken out of the machine at the end of the dough cycle and shaped into a more traditional Italian loaf.

3 tablespoons (45 ml) olive oil

1 cup (235 ml) warm water

1 1/2 cups (185 g) whole wheat flour

1 1/2 cups (185 g) bread flour

1 1/2 teaspoons (6 g) yeast

Place all ingredients in the bread machine pan in the order specified by the manufacturer. Process on the white or French bread cycle.

Yield: 12 servings

Per serving: 144 calories (24% from fat, 12% from protein, 64% from carbohydrate); 4 g protein; 4 g total

fat; 1 g saturated fat; 3 g monounsaturated fat; 1 g polyunsaturated fat; 23 g carbohydrate; 2 g fiber; 0 g sugar; 75 mg phosphorus; 9 mg calcium; 1 mg iron; 2 mg sodium; 88 mg potassium; 2 IU vitamin A; 0 mg ATE vitamin E; 0 mg vitamin C; 0 mg cholesterol; 24 g water

Whole Wheat French Bread

This is particularly good with soup or a bean dish. You can bake it either in the bread machine or in the oven, as I do here.

$^3/_4$ teaspoon (3 g) yeast

1 tablespoon (15 ml) honey

1 cup (235 ml) water

2 cups (250 g) whole wheat flour

$1^1/_2$ cups (185 g) bread flour

Place all ingredients in the bread machine pan in the order specified by the manufacturer. Process on the dough cycle. Remove the dough from the machine. Shape into a tapered loaf. Place on a greased baking sheet, cover with a towel, and let rise until doubled, about 30 minutes. Preheat oven to 400°F (200°C, or gas mark 6). Cut diagonal slices about $^1/_4$ inch (0.4 cm) long across the top of the loaf with a sharp knife. Brush with cold water. Bake for 15 to 20 minutes, or until done.

Yield: 12 servings

Per serving: 136 calories (4% from fat, 14% from protein, 82% from carbohydrate); 5 g protein; 1 g total fat; 0 g saturated fat; 0 g monounsaturated fat; 0 g polyunsaturated fat; 28 g carbohydrate; 3 g fiber; 2 g

sugar; 89 mg phosphorus; 10 mg calcium; 2 mg iron; 2 mg sodium; 104 mg potassium; 2 IU vitamin A; 0 mg ATE vitamin E; 0 mg vitamin C; 0 mg cholesterol; 24 g water

100% Whole Wheat Bread

This recipe is a variation of one that came with my bread machine. It makes a reasonably light, very tasty bread, good for sandwiches.

$1^1/_4$ cups (295 ml) water

2 tablespoons (28 g) unsalted butter

3 cups (360 g) whole wheat flour

$^1/_4$ cup (60 g) brown sugar

$1^3/_4$ teaspoons yeast

1 tablespoon vital wheat gluten

Place ingredients in bread machine in order specified by manufacturer. Process on whole wheat cycle.

Yield: 12 servings

Per serving: 28 g water; 140 calories (15% from fat, 13% from protein, 72% from carb); 5 g protein; 2 g total fat; 0 g saturated fat; 1 g monounsaturated fat; 1 g polyunsaturated fat; 27 g carbohydrate; 4 g fiber; 5 g sugar; 113 mg phosphorus; 16 mg calcium; 1 mg iron; 4 mg sodium; 150 mg potassium; 87 IU vitamin A; 18 mg vitamin E; 0 mg vitamin C; 0 mg cholesterol

Crunchy Honey Wheat Bread

This makes a nice bread with soup or for sandwiches. It has a lot of flavor, and the nuts add texture.

1¼ cups (285 ml) water

3 tablespoons (45 ml) honey

2 tablespoons (28 g) unsalted butter

2 cups (250 g) whole wheat flour

1½ cups (185 g) bread flour

½ cup (60 g) sliced almonds, toasted

1¼ teaspoons (5 g) yeast

Place all ingredients in the bread machine pan in the order specified by the manufacturer. Process on the whole wheat cycle.

Yield: 12 servings

Per serving: 199 calories (24% from fat, 12% from protein, 63% from carbohydrate); 6 g protein; 6 g total fat; 4 g saturated fat; 2 g monounsaturated fat; 0 g polyunsaturated fat; 33 g carbohydrate; 4 g fiber; 5 g sugar; 122 mg phosphorus; 25 mg calcium; 2 mg iron; 25 mg sodium; 153 mg potassium; 103 IU vitamin A; 23 mg ATE vitamin E; 0 mg vitamin C; 10 mg cholesterol; 31 g water

Wheat Bread

This recipe is lighter than a lot of homemade breads and just sweet enough. I can't help but wonder if the lower-than-usual amount of yeast had anything to do with that. I'd been experimenting by reducing the yeast in some recipes, but not usually this low. Time for some more experimentation—I may be on to something here!

1 cup (235 ml) plus 1 tablespoon (15 ml) water

1½ tablespoons (21 g) unsalted butter

¼ cup (60 ml) honey

1½ cups (185 g) bread flour

1½ cups (185 g) whole wheat flour

1 tablespoon (7.5 g) nonfat dry milk powder

1 teaspoon (4 g) yeast

Place all ingredients in the bread machine pan in the order specified by the manufacturer. Process on the whole wheat cycle.

Yield: 12 servings

Per serving: 149 calories (12% from fat, 12% from protein, 77% from carbohydrate); 4 g protein; 2 g total fat; 2 g saturated fat; 0 g monounsaturated fat; 0 g polyunsaturated fat; 29 g carbohydrate; 2 g fiber; 6 g sugar; 77 mg phosphorus; 14 mg calcium; 1 mg iron; 19 mg sodium; 96 mg potassium; 85 IU vitamin A; 20 mg ATE vitamin E; 0 mg vitamin C; 4 mg cholesterol; 26 g water

Sunflower Honey Wheat Bread

This makes a nice bread with soup or for sandwiches. It has a lot of flavor, and the seeds add texture.

1¼ cups (295 ml) water

3 tablespoons (60 g) honey

2 tablespoons (28 g) unsalted butter

2 cups (240 g) whole wheat flour

1 1/2 cups (187 g) bread flour

1 tablespoon vital wheat gluten

1/2 cup (72 g) sunflower seeds, toasted

1 1/4 teaspoons yeast

Place ingredients in bread machine in order specified by manufacturer. Process on whole wheat cycle.

Yield: 12 servings

Per serving: 30 g water; 197 calories (23% from fat, 13% from protein, 64% from carb); 7 g protein; 5 g total fat; 2 g saturated fat; 1 g monounsaturated fat; 2 g polyunsaturated fat; 33 g carbohydrate; 4 g fiber; 5 g sugar; 154 mg phosphorus; 15 mg calcium; 2 mg iron; 3 mg sodium; 155 mg potassium; 62 IU vitamin A; 16 mg vitamin E; 0 mg vitamin C; 5 mg cholesterol

Whole Wheat Beer Bread

This bread is good with soups and chili and makes excellent toast. The flavor of the bread will change, depending on type of beer used.

1 1/2 cups (187 g) all-purpose flour

1 1/2 cups (180 g) whole wheat flour

4 1/2 teaspoons (20 g) baking powder

1 tablespoon baking soda

1/3 cup (75 g) brown sugar

12 ounces (355 ml) beer

Preheat oven to 350°F (180°C, gas mark 4). Coat a 9 × 5-inch (23 × 13-cm) loaf pan with nonstick vegetable oil spray. In a large mixing bowl, combine all-purpose flour, whole wheat flour, baking powder, baking soda, and brown sugar. Pour in beer; stir until a stiff batter is formed. It may be necessary to mix dough with your hands. Scrape dough into prepared loaf pan. Bake in preheated oven for 50 to 60 minutes, until a toothpick inserted into center of the loaf comes out clean.

Yield: 12 servings

Per serving: 30 g water; 140 calories (3% from fat, 11% from protein, 86% from carb); 4 g protein; 0 g total fat; 0 g saturated fat; 0 g monounsaturated fat; 0 g polyunsaturated fat; 30 g carbohydrate; 2 g fiber; 6 g sugar; 111 mg phosphorus; 115 mg calcium; 2 mg iron; 187 mg sodium; 105 mg potassium; 1 IU vitamin A; 0 mg vitamin E; 0 mg vitamin C; 0 mg cholesterol

Sesame Wheat Bread

A good sandwich bread, with a little crunch and the flavor of sesame seeds.

1 1/2 cups (355 ml) water

2 tablespoons (28 g) unsalted butter

1 1/2 cups (185 g) bread flour

1 1/2 cups (185 g) whole wheat flour

1 cup (187 g) uncooked multigrain cereal

1/4 cup (30 g) sesame seeds

3 tablespoons (45 g) brown sugar

1 1/2 teaspoons (6 g) yeast

Place all ingredients in the bread machine pan in the order specified by the manufacturer. Process on the whole wheat cycle.

Yield: 12 servings

Per serving: 211 calories (15% from fat, 12% from protein, 73% from carbohydrate); 6 g protein; 4 g total fat; 3 g saturated fat; 1 g monounsaturated fat; 0 g polyunsaturated fat; 39 g carbohydrate; 3 g fiber; 3 g sugar; 105 mg phosphorus; 39 mg calcium; 2 mg iron; 25 mg sodium; 127 mg potassium; 102 IU vitamin A; 23 mg ATE vitamin E; 0 mg vitamin C; 10 mg cholesterol; 35 g water

Buttermilk Wheat Bread

Another great bread with a nice hot bowl of soup or stew for dinner. The buttermilk gives it an almost sourdough flavor. It's also good toasted.

1 cup (235 ml) buttermilk

$^1/_4$ cup (60 ml) water

1 tablespoon (14 g) unsalted butter

$1^1/_2$ cups (185 g) whole wheat flour

$1^1/_2$ cups (185 g) bread flour

1 tablespoon (13 g) sugar

1 teaspoon (4 g) yeast

Place all ingredients in the bread machine in the order specified by the manufacturer. Process on the whole wheat cycle.

Yield: 12 servings

Per serving: 134 calories (11% from fat, 14% from protein, 74% from carbohydrate); 5 g protein; 2 g total fat; 2 g saturated fat; 0 g monounsaturated fat; 0 g polyunsaturated fat; 25 g carbohydrate; 2 g fiber; 2 g

sugar; 92 mg phosphorus; 32 mg calcium; 1 mg iron; 33 mg sodium; 117 mg potassium; 57 IU vitamin A; 13 mg ATE vitamin E; 0 mg vitamin C; 4 mg cholesterol; 27 g water

Onion and Garlic Wheat Bread

Looking for a bread with a little more flavor to stand up to some of your spicier meals? This may be just the one.

$^1/_2$ cup (80 g) finely chopped onion

$^1/_2$ teaspoon finely chopped garlic

1 tablespoon sugar

$^1/_2$ cup (60 g) whole wheat flour

$2^1/_2$ cups (342 g) bread flour

$1^1/_2$ tablespoons nonfat dry milk

$1^1/_2$ teaspoons yeast

$^3/_4$ cup (175 ml) water

$1^1/_2$ tablespoons (21 g) unsalted butter

Place ingredients in bread machine in order specified by manufacturer. Process on white bread cycle.

Yield: 12 servings

Per serving: 25 g water; 143 calories (13% from fat, 13% from protein, 74% from carb); 5 g protein; 2 g total fat; 1 g saturated fat; 0 g monounsaturated fat; 0 g polyunsaturated fat; 27 g carbohydrate; 2 g fiber; 2 g sugar; 59 mg phosphorus; 15 mg calcium; 2 mg iron; 5 mg sodium; 79 mg potassium; 58 IU vitamin A; 16 mg vitamin E; 1 mg vitamin C; 4 mg cholesterol

Rich Granola Bread

This makes a wonderful breakfast bread, either plain or with a little cream cheese.

$^1/_2$ cup (112 g) unsalted butter, softened

$^1/_4$ cup (85 g) molasses

1 egg

$1^3/_4$ cups (210 g) whole wheat pastry flour

1 teaspoon baking powder

1 teaspoon baking soda

1 cup (230 g) plain fat-free yogurt

$^1/_4$ cup (60 g) brown sugar

$1^1/_4$ cups (105 g) granola

Coat 1 loaf pan generously with nonstick vegetable oil spray. Preheat oven to 350°F (180°C, gas mark 4). In a large bowl, beat together butter, molasses, and egg. Sift together the flour, baking powder, and baking soda, then add in batches to butter mixture alternately with the yogurt and brown sugar, blending well. Mix in granola and turn batter into the prepared loaf pan. Bake for 1 hour or until done.

Yield: 12 servings

Per serving: 24 g water; 226 calories (35% from fat, 8% from protein, 57% from carb); 5 g protein; 9 g total fat; 5 g saturated fat; 3 g monounsaturated fat; 1 g polyunsaturated fat; 33 g carbohydrate; 3 g fiber; 15 g sugar; 128 mg phosphorus; 83 mg calcium; 1 mg iron; 98 mg sodium; 258 mg potassium; 274 IU vitamin A; 73 mg vitamin E; 0 mg vitamin C; 39 mg cholesterol

Debbie's Multigrain Bread

This recipe was sent to me by newsletter subscriber Debbie. Unlike most of our recipes, this is a hand-mixed and kneaded bread, rather than a bread machine one. I tried it that way, and it's got a great flavor.

1 cup (235 ml) lukewarm water

$4^1/_2$ teaspoons (10.5 g) yeast (2 packages)

$^1/_4$ cup (60 ml) molasses

5 cups (625 g) whole wheat flour, divided

$^1/_4$ cup (56 g) unsalted butter

$^1/_2$ cup wheat germ

$^1/_2$ cup flaxseed

$^1/_2$ cup oat bran

$^1/_4$ cup brown sugar

1 cup (235 ml) boiling water

Preheat oven to 375°F (190°C, or gas mark 5). Dissolve the yeast in the lukewarm water, add the molasses, and let stand for 5 minutes. Beat in 2 cups (250 g) of the whole wheat flour, cover, and let rise for 30 to 60 minutes. This will create a "sponge."

Meanwhile, in a large bowl, combine the remaining ingredients, except the 3 cups (375 g) of whole wheat flour. Let stand 30 to 60 minutes. Add the risen sponge to the oat bran mixture and then stir in the remaining 3 cups (375 g) of whole wheat flour. Knead to make an elastic dough. Cover and let rise until doubled in bulk (1 to $1^1/_2$ hours). Divide dough in 2 pieces and shape into loaves. Place in greased loaf pans and let rise for 1 hour. Bake for 25 to 30 minutes, or until crust is as brown as you prefer.

Yield: 24 servings

Per serving: 154 calories (23% from fat, 13% from protein, 64% from carbohydrate); 5 g protein; 4 g total fat; 3 g saturated fat; 1 g monounsaturated fat; 0 g polyunsaturated fat; 26 g carbohydrate; 5 g fiber; 5 g sugar; 153 mg phosphorus; 32 mg calcium; 2 mg iron; 30 mg sodium; 233 mg potassium; 114 IU vitamin A; 26 mg ATE vitamin E; 0 mg vitamin C; 6 mg cholesterol; 24 g water

Seven-Grain Bread

You should be able to find seven-grain cereal in most large grocery stores. This makes a good sandwich bread and also toasts well.

1 1/3 cups (315 ml) water

1 1/2 tablespoons (21 g) unsalted butter

1 1/4 cups (155 g) bread flour

1 cup (125 g) whole wheat flour

2 tablespoons (26 g) sugar

3/4 cup (87 g) seven-grain cereal

1 1/2 tablespoons (11.3 g) nonfat dry milk powder

1 1/2 teaspoons (6 g) yeast

Add all ingredients to the bread machine pan in the order suggested by the manufacturer. Process on the white bread cycle.

Yield: 12 servings

Per serving: 150 calories (11% from fat, 12% from protein, 76% from carbohydrate); 5 g protein; 2 g total fat; 3 g saturated fat; 0 g monounsaturated fat; 0 g polyunsaturated fat; 29 g carbohydrate; 2 g fiber; 2 g sugar; 71 mg phosphorus; 16 mg calcium; 2 mg iron;

20 mg sodium; 86 mg potassium; 89 IU vitamin A; 21 mg ATE vitamin E; 0 mg vitamin C; 6 mg cholesterol; 31 g water

15-Grain Bread

This makes a fairly heavy loaf, good for sandwiches or with a soup and salad–type meal.

1 cup (235 ml) plus 2 tablespoons (30 ml) water

2 tablespoons (28 g) unsalted butter

1 1/3 cups (166 g) bread flour

1 cup (125 g) whole wheat flour

1/4 cup (29 g) 15-grain cereal

3 tablespoons (45 g) brown sugar

2 1/4 teaspoons (5.3 g) yeast

Place all ingredients in the bread machine in the order specified by the manufacturer. Process on the whole wheat cycle.

Yield: 12 servings

Per serving: 131 calories (16% from fat, 12% from protein, 72% from carbohydrate); 4 g protein; 2 g total fat; 2 g saturated fat; 0 g monounsaturated fat; 0 g polyunsaturated fat; 24 g carbohydrate; 2 g fiber; 3 g sugar; 71 mg phosphorus; 11 mg calcium; 1 mg iron; 4 mg sodium; 98 mg potassium; 86 IU vitamin A; 18 mg ATE vitamin E; 0 mg vitamin C; 4 mg cholesterol; 26 g water

Cornmeal Bread

An alternative to cornbread, this makes good sandwiches as well as a great accompaniment to a soup or chili meal.

1 cup (235 ml) water

$^1/_4$ cup (60 ml) olive oil

1 egg

2 tablespoons (26 g) sugar

1 cup (140 g) cornmeal

2 cups (250 g) bread flour

$1^1/_2$ teaspoons (6 g) yeast

Place all ingredients in the bread machine pan in the order specified by the manufacturer. Process on the white bread cycle.

Yield: 12 servings

Per serving: 185 calories (26% from fat, 10% from protein, 64% from carbohydrate); 5 g protein; 5 g total fat; 1 g saturated fat; 3 g monounsaturated fat; 1 g polyunsaturated fat; 29 g carbohydrate; 1 g fiber; 2 g sugar; 49 mg phosphorus; 8 mg calcium; 2 mg iron; 12 mg sodium; 70 mg potassium; 48 IU vitamin A; 0 mg ATE vitamin E; 0 mg vitamin C; 17 mg cholesterol; 29 g water

German Dark Bread

To me this is almost purely a sandwich bread. Other than maybe a pork-chops-and-cabbage meal, I can't picture it for anything else. But it's perfect with mild-flavored fillings like chicken, turkey, or egg salad.

1 cup (235 ml) water

$^1/_4$ cup (85 g) molasses

1 tablespoon unsalted butter

2 cups (274 g) bread flour

$1^1/_4$ cups (160 g) rye flour

2 tablespoons cocoa powder

$1^1/_2$ teaspoons yeast

1 tablespoon vital wheat gluten

Place ingredients in bread machine in order specified by the manufacturer. Process on whole wheat cycle.

Yield: 12 servings

Per serving: 25 g water; 156 calories (9% from fat, 11% from protein, 79% from carb); 5 g protein; 2 g total fat; 1 g saturated fat; 0 g monounsaturated fat; 0 g polyunsaturated fat; 31 g carbohydrate; 3 g fiber; 4 g sugar; 58 mg phosphorus; 22 mg calcium; 2 mg iron; 4 mg sodium; 175 mg potassium; 30 IU vitamin A; 8 mg vitamin E; 0 mg vitamin C; 3 mg cholesterol

Brown Bread

A hearty bread, great with full-flavored soups or chili. It also makes great toast.

1 egg

1 cup (235 ml) water

2 tablespoons (28 g) unsalted butter

2 tablespoons (30 ml) molasses

1 tablespoon (15 g) brown sugar

$1^1/_2$ cups (185 g) bread flour

1 cup (125 g) whole wheat flour

$^1/_2$ cup (40 g) oats, rolled or quick-cooking

$^1/_3$ cup (47 g) cornmeal

$1^1/_2$ teaspoons (6 g) yeast

Place all ingredients in the bread machine pan in the order specified by the manufacturer. Process on the whole wheat cycle.

Yield: 12 servings

Per serving: 174 calories (16% from fat, 13% from protein, 71% from carbohydrate); 6 g protein; 3 g total fat; 2 g saturated fat; 1 g monounsaturated fat; 0 g polyunsaturated fat; 31 g carbohydrate; 3 g fiber; 3 g sugar; 105 mg phosphorus; 23 mg calcium; 2 mg iron; 34 mg sodium; 177 mg potassium; 130 IU vitamin A; 23 mg ATE vitamin E; 0 mg vitamin C; 23 mg cholesterol; 30 g water

Tomato Sandwich Bread

The perfect bread for tomato sandwiches.

1 tablespoon (15 ml) water

3 cups (375 g) bread flour

$^1/_4$ teaspoon (0.8 g) garlic powder

2 tablespoons (26 g) sugar

$1^1/_2$ teaspoons (1 g) dried basil

2 teaspoons (8 g) yeast

$^1/_3$ cup (37 g) oil-packed sun-dried tomatoes

Place all ingredients except tomatoes in the bread machine pan in the order specified by the manufacturer. Process on the white bread cycle. Add the tomatoes at the beep, or 5 minutes before the end of the kneading cycle.

Yield: 12 servings

Per serving: 141 calories (7% from fat, 13% from protein, 80% from carbohydrate); 5 g protein; 1 g total fat; 0 g saturated fat; 0 g monounsaturated fat; 0 g polyunsaturated fat; 28 g carbohydrate; 1 g fiber; 2 g sugar; 47 mg phosphorus; 9 mg calcium; 2 mg iron; 9 mg sodium; 99 mg potassium; 48 IU vitamin A; 0 mg ATE vitamin E; 3 mg vitamin C; 0 mg cholesterol; 8 g water

Whole Wheat Zucchini Bread

Most zucchini bread is the sweet, quick bread variety. This one is a hearty yeast loaf that goes very well with soup for dinner.

1 cup (235 ml) warm water

2 teaspoons (10 ml) honey

1 tablespoon (15 ml) canola oil

$^3/_4$ cup (95 g) shredded zucchini

$^3/_4$ cup (90 g) whole wheat flour

2 cups (250 g) bread flour

$^1/_2$ teaspoon (0.4 g) dried basil

2 teaspoons (5.4 g) sesame seeds

$1^1/_2$ teaspoons (6 g) yeast

Place all ingredients in the bread machine in the order specified by the manufacturer. Process on the wheat or whole-grain cycle.

Yield: 12 servings

Per serving: 124 calories (12% from fat, 13% from protein, 75% from carbohydrate); 4 g protein; 2 g total fat; 0 g saturated fat; 0 g monounsaturated fat; 1 g polyunsaturated fat; 23 g carbohydrate; 2 g fiber; 1 g sugar; 58 mg phosphorus; 9 mg calcium; 1 mg iron; 3 mg sodium; 85 mg potassium; 19 IU vitamin A; 0 mg ATE vitamin E; 1 mg vitamin C; 0 mg cholesterol; 31 g water;

Whole Grain Veggie Focaccia Bread

I just happened to see a loaf of foccacia bread in the bakery section of a local supermarket that was decorated this way. It looks great and tastes pretty good too.

³/₄ cup (180 ml) water

2 tablespoons (28 ml) olive oil

1¹/₂ cups (205 g) bread flour

¹/₂ cup (60 g) whole wheat flour

1 tablespoon vital wheat gluten

1 tablespoon sugar

1¹/₂ tablespoons (16 g) yeast

¹/₂ cup (80 g) sliced onion

¹/₂ cup (75 g) sliced green bell pepper

¹/₂ cup (75 g) sliced red bell pepper

2 tablespoons grated Parmesan cheese

Place first 7 ingredients in bread machine in order specified by manufacturer. Process on dough cycle. Remove the dough from machine when cycle ends. Pat into 8 × 12-inch (20 × 30-cm) rectangle on baking sheet sprayed with nonstick vegetable oil spray. Cover and let rise until doubled, about 30 minutes. Thinly slice onion and separate into rings. Thinly slice bell peppers into rings. Place onion and pepper on top of dough. Sprinkle cheese over top. Bake at 400°F (200°C, gas mark 6) until done, 15 to 18 minutes.

Yield: 6 servings

Per serving: 71 g water; 239 calories (22% from fat, 14% from protein, 63% from carb); 9 g protein; 6 g total fat; 1 g saturated fat; 4 g monounsaturated fat; 1 g polyunsaturated fat; 38 g carbohydrate; 3 g fiber; 4 g sugar; 131 mg phosphorus; 40 mg calcium; 3 mg iron; 37 mg sodium; 205 mg potassium; 446 IU vitamin A; 2 mg vitamin E; 27 mg vitamin C; 2 mg cholesterol

Soft Breadsticks

I went to my recipe software to find a nice yeast breadstick to have with a seafood stew and to my surprise there wasn't a one. So I started digging through other files and came up with this one. You might want to try it with some of the soups and stews too.

1 cup warm water

3 tablespoons brown sugar

¹/₄ cup canola oil

3 cups bread flour

2¹/₂ teaspoons yeast

Make dough using your favorite method: bread machine, mixer, or by hand. Roll out into a 10 × 12-inch rectangle. Cut into strips about 1 inch wide. Give each strip a twist and place on a greased cookie sheet. Let rise for at least 20 minutes. Bake at 375°F for 10 to 15 minutes.

Yield: 12 servings

Per serving: 179 calories (26% from fat, 10% from protein, 64% from carb); 4 g protein; 5 g total fat; 1 g saturated fat; 1 g monounsaturated fat; 3 g polyunsaturated fat; 30 g carb; 1 g fiber; 3 g sugar; 45 mg phosphorus; 9 mg calcium; 3 mg sodium; 63 mg potassium; 1 IU vitamin A; 0 mg vitamin E; 0 mg vitamin C; 0 mg cholesterol

Whole Wheat Flatbread

Make your own flatbread for roll-ups or other filled sandwiches.

1$^1/_2$ teaspoons yeast

$^3/_4$ cup (180 ml) water, warm (100–110°F or 38–43°C)

1$^1/_2$ cups (205 g) bread flour

1$^1/_2$ cups (180 g) whole wheat flour

2 tablespoons (28 g) unsalted butter, melted

In small bowl dissolve yeast in warm water. Let stand 5 minutes. Place flours in bowl of food processor. Turn on machine and slowly add yeast-water mixture. Keep machine running until dough just forms a ball. Place ball in bowl coated with nonstick vegetable oil spray. Cover with towel and let rise 1 hour in warm place. Punch down dough and turn out on lightly floured surface. Roll dough into a log about 1$^1/_2$ inches (4 cm) thick. Cut log vertically into 12 equal pieces. Roll each piece into a 6-inch (15-cm) circle. In large cast-iron or heavy skillet over high heat, cook breads one at a time, 1 to 2 minutes until they begin to form bubbles. With tongs, turn and cook other side 1 to 2 minutes, until golden brown. Brush with melted butter. Store tightly wrapped in the refrigerator for 1 week. To reheat, cook in microwave on high 1 minute on microwave-safe dish lightly covered with plastic wrap.

Yield: 12 servings

Per serving: 19 g water; 131 calories (17% from fat, 13% from protein, 70% from carb); 4 g protein; 3 g total fat; 1 g saturated fat; 1 g monounsaturated fat; 0 g polyunsaturated fat; 23 g carbohydrate; 2 g fiber; 0 g sugar; 76 mg phosphorus; 9 mg calcium; 1 mg iron; 2 mg sodium; 89 mg potassium; 61 IU vitamin A; 16 mg vitamin E; 0 mg vitamin C; 5 mg cholesterol

Potato Rolls

We like these for Thanksgiving. They are tender and flavorful and the leftovers are just right for a small turkey sandwich for lunch the next day.

$^1/_2$ cup prepared mashed potatoes

$^1/_4$ cup skim milk

$^1/_4$ cup canola oil

1 egg

$^1/_4$ cup sugar

4 cups bread flour

2$^1/_4$ teaspoons yeast

Place ingredients in bread machine in order specified by manufacturer. Process on dough cycle. When done, remove from bread machine pan and punch down. Separate into 15 balls. Place rolls in 12 × 17-inch baking pan or on cookie sheet. Cover with towel and allow to rise until doubled, about $^1/_2$ hour. Bake at 350°F (175°C) until golden brown, about 20 minutes.

Yield: 15 servings

Per serving: 16 g water; 195 calories (24% from fat, 11% from protein, 65% from carb); 5 g protein; 5 g total fat; 1 g saturated fat; 3 g monounsaturated fat; 1 g polyunsaturated fat; 32 g carbohydrate; 1 g fiber; 4 g sugar; 57 mg phosphorus; 15 mg calcium; 0 mg iron; 10 mg sodium; 81 mg potassium; 41 IU vitamin A; 11 mg vitamin E; 0 mg vitamin C; 15 mg cholesterol

Wheat Germ Rolls

Wheat germ adds a little flavor and nutritional value to these rolls. They make nice sandwich rolls, but you can shape them into 16 smaller dinner rolls if you prefer.

1 cup water

2 teaspoons canola oil

1 egg

3 cups bread flour

$^1/_4$ cup sugar

$^1/_2$ cup wheat germ

$1^1/_2$ teaspoons yeast

Place ingredients in bread machine in the order specified by manufacturer. Process on dough cycle. Remove dough and shape into 10 rolls. Place on greased baking sheet. Cover and let rise until doubled, about 30 minutes. Bake at 375°F until golden, about 20 minutes.

Yield: 10 servings

Per serving: 10 g water; 220 calories (17% from fat, 13% from protein, 70% from carb); 7 g protein; 4 g total fat; 1 g saturated fat; 1 g monounsaturated fat; 2 g polyunsaturated fat; 38 g carbohydrate; 5 g fiber; 4 g sugar; 104 mg phosphorus; 13 mg calcium; 0 mg iron; 14 mg sodium; 125 mg potassium; 136 IU vitamin A; 0 mg vitamin E; 0 mg vitamin C; 0 mg cholesterol

Rye Rolls

Another good sandwich roll. I like roast beef on rye, personally.

1 cup (235 ml) skim milk

$1^1/_2$ tablespoons (21 g) unsalted butter

1 egg

$1^1/_2$ cups (205 g) bread flour

2 cups (256 g) rye flour

$^1/_4$ cup (50 g) sugar

1 tablespoon caraway seed

2 tablespoons (24 g) yeast

Place all ingredients in bread machine in order specified by manufacturer. Process on dough cycle. At end of cycle, remove to a floured board. Pull into 10 pieces. Shape each into a rounded, flattened roll and place on baking sheet coated with nonstick vegetable oil spray. Cover and let rise until double, about 30 minutes. Bake in preheated 375°F (190°C, gas mark 5) oven 12 to 15 minutes or until golden brown.

Yield: 10 servings

Per serving: 30 g water; 212 calories (14% from fat, 13% from protein, 73% from carb); 7 g protein; 3 g total fat; 1 g saturated fat; 1 g monounsaturated fat; 0 g polyunsaturated fat; 39 g carbohydrate; 4 g fiber; 5 g sugar; 132 mg phosphorus; 52 mg calcium; 2 mg iron; 26 mg sodium; 177 mg potassium; 139 IU vitamin A; 38 mg vitamin E; 0 mg vitamin C; 26 mg cholesterol

Focaccia Rolls

These rolls makes marvelous sandwiches. I particularly like them with egg and Swiss cheese for breakfast.

$^3/_4$ cup (180 ml) water

2 tablespoons (28 ml) olive oil

2 cups (274 g) bread flour

1 tablespoon sugar

1 1/2 tablespoons (16 g) yeast

1 tablespoon basil

1 teaspoon rosemary

2 tablespoons grated Parmesan cheese

Place first 5 ingredients in bread machine in order specified by manufacturer. Process on dough cycle. Remove the dough from machine when cycle ends. Pat into 8 × 12-inch (20 × 30-cm) rectangle on a floured board. Cut into six 4-inch (10-cm) squares. Place on baking sheet sprayed with nonstick vegetable oil spray. Cover and let rise until doubled, about 30 minutes. Make depressions in top at 1-inch (2.5-cm) intervals with finger. Sprinkle herbs and cheese over top. Bake at 400°F (200°C, gas mark 6) until done, 15 to 18 minutes.

Yield: 6 servings

Per serving: 36 g water; 230 calories (23% from fat, 13% from protein, 64% from carb); 7 g protein; 6 g total fat; 1 g saturated fat; 4 g monounsaturated fat; 1 g polyunsaturated fat; 37 g carbohydrate; 2 g fiber; 2 g sugar; 97 mg phosphorus; 38 mg calcium; 3 mg iron; 32 mg sodium; 120 mg potassium; 47 IU vitamin A; 2 mg vitamin E; 0 mg vitamin C; 1 mg cholesterol

Whole Wheat Hamburger Buns

Slightly sweet and quite light for homemade bread, these are my favorite sandwich rolls.

1 cup (235 ml) water

2 tablespoons (28 g) unsalted butter

1 egg

2 cups (250 g) bread flour

1 1/4 cups (155 g) whole wheat flour

1/4 cup (50 g) sugar

1 tablespoon (12 g) yeast

Place all the ingredients in the bread machine pan in the order specified by the manufacturer. Process on the dough cycle. At the end of the cycle, remove dough to a floured board. Pull into 10 pieces. Shape each into a rounded, flattened roll and place on greased baking sheet. Cover and let rise until doubled, about 30 minutes. Preheat oven to 375°F (190°C, or gas mark 5) and bake for 12 to 15 minutes, or until golden brown.

Yield: 10 servings

Per serving: 198 calories (15% from fat, 13% from protein, 72% from carbohydrate); 7 g protein; 3 g total fat; 2 g saturated fat; 1 g monounsaturated fat; 0 g polyunsaturated fat; 36 g carbohydrate; 3 g fiber; 5 g sugar; 103 mg phosphorus; 16 mg calcium; 2 mg iron; 38 mg sodium; 136 mg potassium; 144 IU vitamin A; 27 mg ATE vitamin E; 0 mg vitamin C; 25 mg cholesterol; 35 g water

Whole Wheat Onion Rolls

If you are looking for a roll with flavor to use for sandwiches with things like roast beef or meat loaf, you might want to give these a try. I used an envelope of Goodman's low sodium onion soup mix for the flavoring (available in the kosher section of the international aisle in my local Safeway), but you could get much the same taste with 4 tablespoons (24 g) low sodium beef bouillon, 1 teaspoon (3 g) of onion powder, and 2 tablespoons of dried minced onion.

$^3/_4$ cup (180 ml) flat beer

$^1/_2$ cup (120 ml) water

1 tablespoon (14 g) unsalted butter

4 ounces (115 g) low sodium onion soup mix

2 cups (250 g) bread flour

$1^1/_4$ cups (155 g) whole wheat flour

4 teaspoons (16 g) sugar

$1^3/_4$ teaspoons (7 g) yeast

Place all the ingredients in the bread machine pan in the order specified by the manufacturer. Process on the dough cycle. Remove the dough from the machine and separate into 10 balls. Shape each into a round, flattened roll. Place on a baking sheet sprayed with nonstick vegetable oil spray. Cover and let rise until doubled, about 30 minutes. Preheat oven to 375°F (190°C, or gas mark 5) and bake for 12 to 15 minutes, or until lightly browned.

Yield: 10 servings

Per serving: 183 calories (10% from fat, 13% from protein, 77% from carbohydrate); 6 g protein; 2 g total fat; 2 g saturated fat; 0 g monounsaturated fat; 0 g polyunsaturated fat; 35 g carbohydrate; 3 g fiber; 2 g sugar; 91 mg phosphorus; 17 mg calcium; 2 mg iron; 95 mg sodium; 108 mg potassium; 62 IU vitamin A; 14 mg ATE vitamin E; 0 mg vitamin C; 4 mg cholesterol; 34 g water

Seven-Grain Sesame Seed Rolls

These are a nice, crunchy, chewy sort of roll, perfect for mild-flavored fillings like turkey or chicken salad.

$1^1/_4$ cups (285 ml) water

3 tablespoons (23 g) nonfat dry milk powder

$1^1/_2$ tablespoons (22 ml) canola oil

3 tablespoons (45 ml) molasses

$2^1/_2$ cups (310 g) bread flour

1 cup (116 g) seven-grain cereal

2 teaspoons (8 g) yeast

3 tablespoons (24 g) sesame seeds

Add all ingredients to the bread machine pan in the order specified by the manufacturer. Process on the dough cycle. Remove dough from the bread machine at the end of the cycle, form into rolls, cover, and let rise until doubled. Preheat oven to 375°F (190°C, or gas mark 5) and bake for 15 minutes, or until golden brown.

Yield: 10 servings

Per serving: 218 calories (13% from fat, 12% from protein, 75% from carbohydrate); 7 g protein; 3 g total fat; 0 g saturated fat; 1 g monounsaturated fat; 1 g polyunsaturated fat; 41 g carbohydrate; 3 g fiber; 5 g sugar; 112 mg phosphorus; 39 mg calcium; 2 mg iron; 13 mg sodium; 234 mg potassium; 34 IU vitamin A; 9 mg ATE vitamin E; 0 mg vitamin C; 0 mg cholesterol; 37 g water

Sun-Dried Tomato Wheat Rolls

These have a great flavor for sandwiches. We made them originally for sliced pork subs, but they would also be good with something simple like chicken salad or a burger. The leftover ones became breakfast sandwiches for me several days one week.

1 cup (235 ml) skim milk

1/4 cup (60 g) fat-free sour cream

1 tablespoon (13 g) sugar

2 cups (250 g) bread flour

1 cup (125 g) whole wheat flour

1/4 cup oil-packed sun-dried tomatoes, chopped

2 1/2 teaspoons (10 g) yeast

Place all ingredients in the bread machine pan in the order specified by the manufacturer. Process on the dough cycle. At the end of the cycle, remove dough to a floured board. Pull into 10 pieces (or fewer if making sub rolls). Shape each into a rounded, flattened roll and place on a greased baking sheet. Cover and let rise until doubled, about 1 hour. Preheat oven to 350°F (180°C, or gas mark 4) and bake for 20 to 25 minutes, or until golden brown.

Yield: 10 servings

Per serving: 172 calories (6% from fat, 16% from protein, 78% from carbohydrate); 7 g protein; 1 g total fat; 0 g saturated fat; 0 g monounsaturated fat; 0 g polyunsaturated fat; 32 g carbohydrate; 2 g fiber; 1 g sugar; 118 mg phosphorus; 52 mg calcium; 2 mg iron; 26 mg sodium; 192 mg potassium; 109 IU vitamin A; 21 mg ATE vitamin E; 3 mg vitamin C; 3 mg cholesterol; 33 g water

Whole Wheat Pizza Dough

We used this dough to make a pizza full of fresh vegetables from the garden, but you could use it with any toppings you desire.

2 teaspoons (8 g) active dry yeast

2 cups (250 g) bread flour

1 1/2 cups (185 g) whole wheat flour

1 tablespoon (13 g) sugar

2 tablespoons (30 ml) olive oil

1 1/2 cups (355 ml) water

Place all ingredients in the bread machine pan in the order specified by the manufacturer and process on the dough cycle. Turn out the dough onto a floured board. At this point you may form the pizzas or refrigerate the dough for several hours, well wrapped in plastic so it won't dry out. Makes enough dough for two 12-inch (30-cm) pizzas, or two 10-inch (25-cm) thick-crust pizzas. Preheat oven to 400°F (200°C, or gas mark 6). Bake for 15 minutes, or until lightly browned around the edges. Top as desired and return to oven for 5 to 10 minutes, or until cheese is melted and crust is browned.

Yield: 16 servings

Per serving: 119 calories (16% from fat, 12% from protein, 71% from carbohydrate); 4 g protein; 2 g total fat; 0 g saturated fat; 1 g monounsaturated fat; 0 g polyunsaturated fat; 22 g carbohydrate; 2 g fiber; 1 g sugar; 62 mg phosphorus; 7 mg calcium; 1 mg iron; 2 mg sodium; 73 mg potassium; 1 IU vitamin A; 0 mg ATE vitamin E; 0 mg vitamin C; 0 mg cholesterol; 26 g water

Whole Wheat Bagels

Bagels really aren't as difficult to make as they sound. This recipe produces big, soft bagels that are crispy on the outside and just a little chewy on the inside, like what is typically called New York–style. They are good cold for sandwiches, toasted, or warm right out of the oven.

$1^{1}/_{2}$ cups (355 ml) warm water

2 tablespoons (30 ml) honey

1 tablespoon (15 ml) vinegar

2 cups (250 g) whole wheat flour

$1^{1}/_{4}$ cups (155 g) bread flour

$1^{1}/_{2}$ tablespoons (22 ml) olive oil

2 teaspoons (8 g) yeast

Place all ingredients in the bread machine pan in the order specified by the manufacturer. Process on the dough cycle. At the end of the cycle, separate dough into 8 pieces. Shape each into a flattened ball, then use your thumbs to pull a hole in the center of each and stretch into a doughnut shape. Place on a greased baking sheet, cover, and let rise until doubled, about 30 minutes. While dough is rising, bring about 2 inches (5 cm) of water to boil in a large pan and preheat oven to 350°F (180°C, or gas mark 4). Drop bagels a few at a time into boiling water and boil for 1 minute, turning once. Remove with a slotted spoon or pancake turner and return to baking sheet. When all bagels have been boiled, bake for 20 to 25 minutes, or until golden brown.

Yield: 8 servings

Per serving: 221 calories (14% from fat, 12% from protein, 74% from carbohydrate); 7 g protein; 3 g total fat; 1 g saturated fat; 2 g monounsaturated fat; 1 g polyunsaturated fat; 42 g carbohydrate; 4 g fiber; 5 g sugar; 138 mg phosphorus; 16 mg calcium; 2 mg iron; 4 mg sodium; 167 mg potassium; 3 IU vitamin A; 0 mg ATE vitamin E; 0 mg vitamin C; 0 mg cholesterol; 53 g water

Raisin Bread

Great for breakfast; sweet enough that it doesn't need anything added.

$1^{1}/_{4}$ cups (295 ml) water

2 tablespoons (28 g) unsalted butter, softened

$2^{1}/_{2}$ cups (342 g) bread flour

$^{3}/_{4}$ cup (90 g) whole wheat flour

$^{1}/_{4}$ cup (50 g) sugar

$1^{1}/_{2}$ teaspoons yeast

2 teaspoons cinnamon

$^{3}/_{4}$ cup (110 g) raisins

Place all ingredients except raisins in bread machine in order specified by manufacturer. Bake on sweet bread or white bread cycle. Add raisins at the beep or after first kneading.

Yield: 12 servings

Per serving: 31 g water; 195 calories (12% from fat, 10% from protein, 78% from carb); 5 g protein; 3 g total fat; 1 g saturated fat; 1 g monounsaturated fat; 0 g polyunsaturated fat; 39 g carbohydrate; 2 g fiber; 10 g sugar; 71 mg phosphorus; 18 mg calcium; 2 mg iron; 3 mg sodium; 149 mg potassium; 61 IU vitamin A; 16 mg vitamin E; 0 mg vitamin C; 5 mg cholesterol

Banana Raisin Bread

This makes a great breakfast bread. I like it with toasted with a little peanut butter and a drizzle of honey, but I'll leave it up to you how (and if) to make it more tasty and less healthy.

$^3/_4$ (175 ml) cup + 2 tablespoons (28 ml) water

$^1/_2$ cup (112 g) mashed banana

3 cups (411 g) bread flour

2 tablespoons (30 g) brown sugar

1 teaspoon cinnamon

2 teaspoons yeast

$^1/_2$ cup (75 g) raisins

Place all ingredients except raisins in bread machine in order specified by manufacturer. Process on white bread cycle. Add raisins at the beep or 5 minutes before the end of the kneading cycle.

Yield: 12 servings

Per serving: 30 g water; 164 calories (4% from fat, 11% from protein, 85% from carb); 5 g protein; 1 g total fat; 0 g saturated fat; 0 g monounsaturated fat; 0 g polyunsaturated fat; 35 g carbohydrate; 2 g fiber; 8 g sugar; 51 mg phosphorus; 14 mg calcium; 2 mg iron; 3 mg sodium; 142 mg potassium; 7 IU vitamin A; 0 mg vitamin E; 1 mg vitamin C; 0 mg cholesterol

Banana Chip Bread

A sweet bread, good for breakfast. I don't know about you, but we always seem to have a couple bananas at that stage where you'd prefer they not be quite as ripe, so I'm always on the lookout for ways to use them. This particular recipe was a big hit.

$^1/_2$ cup (120 ml) orange juice

$1^1/_4$ cups (281 g) mashed banana

2 tablespoons (28 ml) oil

$^1/_4$ cup (85 g) honey

1 teaspoon orange peel

$3^1/_2$ cups (479 g) bread flour

1 cup (80 g) coconut

$1^1/_2$ teaspoons yeast

$^3/_4$ cup (75 g) crushed banana chips

Place all ingredients except banana chips in bread machine in order specified by manufacturer. Process on sweet bread cycle. Add the banana chips at the beep or 5 minutes before the end of kneading.

Yield: 12 servings

Per serving: 35 g water; 266 calories (22% from fat, 8% from protein, 69% from carb); 6 g protein; 7 g total fat; 4 g saturated fat; 1 g monounsaturated fat; 2 g polyunsaturated fat; 47 g carbohydrate; 2 g fiber; 10 g sugar; 61 mg phosphorus; 11 mg calcium; 2 mg iron; 3 mg sodium; 204 mg potassium; 29 IU vitamin A; 0 mg vitamin E; 6 mg vitamin C; 0 mg cholesterol

Diet Soda Bread

A newsletter subscriber sent me this bread recipe, which uses diet soda instead of beer. She says she's also tried it with tangerine soda, and it came out great that way too.

12 ounces (355 ml) diet cola

1 cup (80 g) quick-cooking oats

3 cups (411 g) bread flour

$2^3/_4$ teaspoons yeast

Place all ingredients in bread machine in order directed by manufacturer and set for 1¹/₂-pound (710 g) loaf, light or regular setting, white bread.

Yield: 12 servings

Per serving: 34 g water; 177 calories (8% from fat, 15% from protein, 77% from carb); 7 g protein; 2 g total fat; 0 g saturated fat; 0 g monounsaturated fat; 1 g polyunsaturated fat; 34 g carbohydrate; 2 g fiber; 0 g sugar; 116 mg phosphorus; 14 mg calcium; 2 mg iron; 4 mg sodium; 111 mg potassium; 1 IU vitamin A; 0 mg vitamin E; 0 mg vitamin C; 0 mg cholesterol

Caramel Apple Bread

A good breakfast bread. Also great for French toast.

1 cup (235 ml) water

2 tablespoons (28 g) unsalted butter

3 cups (375 g) bread flour

¹/₄ cup (60 g) brown sugar

³/₄ teaspoon (1.7 g) cinnamon

2 teaspoons (8 g) yeast

¹/₃ cup (40 g) pecans, chopped and toasted

¹/₂ cup (75 g) apple, coarsely chopped

Place all ingredients except apple and pecans in the bread machine pan in the order specified by the manufacturer. Process on the sweet bread or white bread cycle. Add pecans and apple at the beep or after the first kneading.

Yield: 12 servings

Per serving: 183 calories (23% from fat, 10% from protein, 67% from carbohydrate); 5 g protein; 5 g total fat; 3 g saturated fat; 2 g monounsaturated fat; 0 g polyunsaturated fat; 31 g carbohydrate; 1 g fiber; 5 g sugar; 53 mg phosphorus; 16 mg calcium; 2 mg iron; 24 mg sodium; 83 mg potassium; 105 IU vitamin A; 23 mg ATE vitamin E; 0 mg vitamin C; 10 mg cholesterol; 29 g water

Three-Apple Bread

This makes a nice breakfast bread—just sweet enough without jelly.

¹/₂ cup (120 ml) apple juice

¹/₂ cup (120 ml) unsweetened applesauce

3 cups (375 g) bread flour

1¹/₂ tablespoons (21 g) unsalted butter

¹/₂ cup (75 g) apple, peeled and chopped

¹/₂ teaspoon (1.2 g) cinnamon

¹/₄ teaspoon (0.6 g) nutmeg

1¹/₂ teaspoons (6 g) yeast

Place all the ingredients in the bread machine pan in the order specified by the manufacturer. Process on the light crust setting. Allow to cool 1 hour before slicing.

Yield: 12 servings

Per serving: 149 calories (12% from fat, 12% from protein, 76% from carbohydrate); 4 g protein; 2 g total fat; 2 g saturated fat; 0 g monounsaturated fat; 0 g polyunsaturated fat; 28 g carbohydrate; 1 g fiber; 2 g sugar; 43 mg phosphorus; 9 mg calcium; 2 mg iron; 17 mg sodium; 71 mg potassium; 81 IU vitamin A; 17 mg ATE vitamin E; 2 mg vitamin C; 4 mg cholesterol; 27 g water

Tip: Use apple cider instead of juice for an even deeper flavor.

22

Cookies

Who doesn't like cookies? They are almost the perfect dessert, just a little bit of something sweet at the end of a meal. The cookies in this chapter are, of course, healthier than most. They contain things like whole grain, fruits (and a few veggies) and nuts containing omega-3 fatty acids. So indulge yourself and have a cookie.

Chocolate Chip Cookies

These are lighter than most chocolate chip cookies, owing to the beaten egg white. But the taste will satisfy any cookie lover.

$2^1/_4$ cups (280 g) flour

1 teaspoon (4.6 g) baking powder

$^3/_4$ cup (170 g) brown sugar, packed

2 tablespoons (28 g) unsalted butter

1 teaspoon (5 ml) vanilla extract

4 large egg whites, room temperature

$^1/_2$ cup (100 g) sugar

$^1/_3$ cup (80 ml) light corn syrup

$1^1/_4$ cups (220 g) semisweet chocolate chips

Preheat oven to 375°F (190°C, or gas mark 5). Lightly spoon flour into dry measuring cups and level with a knife. Combine flour and baking powder. Beat brown sugar, butter, and vanilla extract with an electric mixer on medium speed for 5 minutes, or until well-blended. Beat egg whites until foamy using clean, dry beaters. Gradually add sugar, 1 tablespoon at a time; beat until soft peaks form. Add corn syrup; beat until stiff peaks form. Fold brown sugar mixture into egg white mixture. Add flour mixture and stir to combine. Add chocolate chips. Drop dough by level tablespoons 1 inch (2.5 cm) apart onto baking sheets coated with nonstick vegetable oil spray. Bake for 10 minutes, or until golden. Remove from the oven and let stand 5 minutes. Remove cookies from pans, and cool on wire racks. Store loosely covered.

Yield: 48 servings

Per serving: 76 calories (21% from fat, 6% from protein, 73% from carbohydrate); 1 g protein; 2 g total fat; 2 g saturated fat; 0 g monounsaturated fat; 0 g polyunsaturated fat; 15 g carbohydrate; 0 g fiber; 8 g sugar; 16 mg phosphorus; 12 mg calcium; 0 mg iron; 23 mg sodium; 39 mg potassium; 25 IU vitamin A; 6 mg ATE vitamin E; 0 mg vitamin C; 3 mg cholesterol; 4 g water

Whole Wheat Chocolate Chip Cookies

What's not to like about chocolate chip cookies?

1 cup (225 g) unsalted butter

$^1/_4$ cup (64 g) peanut butter

1 cup (340 g) honey

2 eggs

$1^1/_2$ cups (180 g) whole wheat pastry flour

1 teaspoon baking soda

2 cups (160 g) rolled oats

2 cups (350 g) chocolate chips

1 cup (110 g) chopped pecans

Cream together first 4 ingredients. Add next 5 ingredients and mix well. Add additional flour if needed to form a stiff dough. Drop by teaspoon on baking sheet. Bake at 375°F (190°C, gas mark 5) for 10 minutes.

Yield: 48 servings

Per serving: 6 g water; 194 calories (52% from fat, 7% from protein, 41% from carb); 3 g protein; 12 g total fat; 5 g saturated fat; 4 g monounsaturated fat; 1 g

polyunsaturated fat; 21 g carbohydrate; 2 g fiber; 13 g sugar; 80 mg phosphorus; 28 mg calcium; 1 mg iron; 22 mg sodium; 107 mg potassium; 191 IU vitamin A; 51 mg vitamin E; 0 mg vitamin C; 29 mg cholesterol

Good-for-You Chocolate Chip Cookies

Oatmeal chocolate chip cookies that you'll never suspect have been made more healthy.

$^1/_4$ cup (55 g) unsalted butter

$^2/_3$ cup (150 g) packed brown sugar

$^1/_4$ cup (85 g) honey

1 egg

1 teaspoon vanilla extract

$^1/_4$ cup (60 ml) skim milk

1 teaspoon baking soda

$^1/_2$ teaspoon baking powder

1 cup (82 g) granola

$^3/_4$ cup (60 g) quick-cooking oats

2 cups (240 g) whole wheat pastry flour

1 cup (175 g) chocolate chips

Cream together butter and brown sugar. Mix in honey, egg, vanilla, and milk. Then mix in baking soda and baking powder. Add granola, oats, and flour. Mix all ingredients. Stir in chocolate chips. Place on nonstick baking sheet by teaspoons. Bake at 325°F (170°C, gas mark 3) for 10 minutes.

Yield: 36 servings

Per serving: 4 g water; 100 calories (28% from fat, 8% from protein, 64% from carb); 2 g protein; 3 g total fat; 2 g saturated fat; 1 g monounsaturated fat; 0 g polyunsaturated fat; 17 g carbohydrate; 1 g fiber; 9 g sugar; 54 mg phosphorus; 24 mg calcium; 1 mg iron; 25 mg sodium; 78 mg potassium; 61 IU vitamin A; 16 mg vitamin E; 0 mg vitamin C; 10 mg cholesterol

White Chocolate–Cranberry Cookies

These were inspired by cookies that were served as a snack at a training session I had at work. I was looking for a soft cookie with white chocolate chips and dried cranberries.

$^1/_2$ cup (112 g) shortening

1 cup (225 g) brown sugar

1 egg

1 teaspoon vanilla extract

$1^3/_4$ cups (210 g) whole wheat pastry flour

1 teaspoon baking soda

$^1/_4$ cup (60 ml) buttermilk

$^1/_2$ cup (87 g) white chocolate chips

$^1/_2$ cup (60 g) dried cranberries

Beat shortening until light. Add sugar and beat until fluffy. Beat in egg and vanilla. Stir together dry ingredients. Add alternately with buttermilk. Beat until smooth. Stir in chips and cranberries. Drop about 2 inches (5 cm) apart on baking sheet coated with nonstick vegetable oil spray. Bake at 375°F (190°C, gas mark 5) 8 to 10 minutes, until lightly browned.

Yield: 36 servings

Per serving: 4 g water; 91 calories (37% from fat, 5% from protein, 57% from carb); 1 g protein; 4 g total fat; 1 g saturated fat; 2 g monounsaturated fat; 1 g polyunsaturated fat; 13 g carbohydrate; 1 g fiber; 9 g sugar; 33 mg phosphorus; 15 mg calcium; 0 mg iron; 9 mg sodium; 75 mg potassium; 14 IU vitamin A; 4 mg vitamin E; 0 mg vitamin C; 6 mg cholesterol

Tip: If you like softer cookies like these, replace the butter with shortening like butter-flavored Crisco and the white sugar with brown in your favorite recipes.

Chocolate Peanut Cookies

This a quick and easy treat. It only makes 6 cookies, but the nonbake method makes it possible to stir up a batch whenever you want them. (I've found you can cheat on the 30 minutes and take them out of the freezer a little early too.)

1^5/$_8$ ounces (45 g) chocolate candy bar

4 tablespoons (64 g) crunchy peanut butter

1 cup (60 g) lightly sweetened bran cereal, such as Fiber One

Melt the chocolate bar and peanut butter in microwave until smooth, checking at 30-second intervals. Be careful not to burn. Stir to mix melted chocolate and peanut butter. Add cereal and gently toss until coated. Drop on waxed paper or foil, making 6 cookies. Freeze for 30 minutes, then put in resealable plastic bags and refrigerate.

Yield: 6 servings

Per serving: 1 g water; 124 calories (49% from fat, 10% from protein, 41% from carb); 4 g protein; 8 g total fat;

2 g saturated fat; 4 g monounsaturated fat; 2 g polyunsaturated fat; 15 g carbohydrate; 6 g fiber; 5 g sugar; 100 mg phosphorus; 53 mg calcium; 2 mg iron; 93 mg sodium; 169 mg potassium; 17 IU vitamin A; 4 mg vitamin E; 2 mg vitamin C; 2 mg cholesterol

Oat Bran Cookies

The old favorite oatmeal raisin cookies updated to be even healthier with the addition of oat bran.

1 cup (235 ml) canola oil

1 teaspoon (5 ml) vanilla

2 eggs

1^1/$_2$ cups (340 g) packed brown sugar

2 cups (160 g) quick-cooking or rolled oats

2 cups (200 g) oat bran

1 cup (125 g) flour

^{1}/$_2$ teaspoon (2.3 g) baking soda

1 cup (165 g) raisins

Preheat oven to 350°F (180°C, or gas mark 4). Mix oil, vanilla, eggs, and sugar together in a large bowl. Combine dry ingredients and stir into sugar mixture. Stir in raisins. Drop onto a baking sheet coated with nonstick vegetable oil spray. Bake for 15 minutes, or until lightly browned.

Yield: 48 servings

Per serving: 122 calories (39% from fat, 6% from protein, 55% from carbohydrate); 2 g protein; 5 g total fat; 0 g saturated fat; 3 g monounsaturated fat; 2 g polyunsaturated fat; 17 g carbohydrate; 1 g fiber; 9 g sugar; 55 mg phosphorus; 16 mg calcium; 1 mg iron; 28 mg sodium; 97 mg potassium; 28 IU vitamin A; 6 mg ATE vitamin E; 0 mg vitamin C; 6 mg cholesterol; 4 g water

Mudball Cookies

The name may not sound too appetizing, but wait until you taste them.

1 cup (80 g) quick-cooking oats

$^1/_2$ cup (55 g) broken pecans

$^1/_2$ cup (45 g) instant cocoa mix

$^1/_2$ cup (130 g) peanut butter

$^1/_2$ cup (170 g) honey

1 cup (72 g) graham cracker crumbs

Mix oats, nut pieces, and instant cocoa mix in a large bowl. Add peanut butter and honey. Mix everything in the bowl until it looks like mud. Place graham cracker crumbs on a sheet of waxed paper. Take 1 teaspoon of cookie mixture at a time and roll in your hands to make a ball. Roll the cookie balls in the cracker crumbs and place on a paper plate or baking sheet. Store in the refrigerator.

Yield: 24 servings

Per serving: 2 g water; 111 calories (41% from fat, 8% from protein, 51% from carb); 2 g protein; 5 g total fat; 1 g saturated fat; 2 g monounsaturated fat; 1 g polyunsaturated fat; 15 g carbohydrate; 1 g fiber; 9 g sugar; 49 mg phosphorus; 12 mg calcium; 1 mg iron; 78 mg sodium; 73 mg potassium; 2 IU vitamin A; 0 mg vitamin E; 0 mg vitamin C; 0 mg cholesterol

Whole Wheat Sunflower Seed Cookies

Crunchy sweet nuggets of goodness.

4 tablespoons (55 g) unsalted butter

$^1/_2$ cup (170 g) honey

$1^1/_2$ cups (180 g) whole wheat pastry flour

1 cup (68 g) nonfat dry milk

$^1/_2$ teaspoon baking soda

2 tablespoons (28 ml) water

2 eggs

$^1/_2$ teaspoon vanilla extract

1 cup (175 g) chocolate chips

$^1/_2$ cup (72 g) sunflower seeds

$^1/_4$ cup (37 g) chopped peanuts

Combine all ingredients. Drop by teaspoon onto baking sheet coated with nonstick vegetable oil spray. Bake in 350°F (180°C, gas mark 4) oven for 12 minutes.

Yield: 48 servings

Per serving: 4 g water; 68 calories (39% from fat, 11% from protein, 50% from carb); 2 g protein; 3 g total fat; 1 g saturated fat; 1 g monounsaturated fat; 1 g polyunsaturated fat; 9 g carbohydrate; 1 g fiber; 6 g sugar; 55 mg phosphorus; 28 mg calcium; 0 mg iron; 17 mg sodium; 70 mg potassium; 81 IU vitamin A; 23 mg vitamin E; 0 mg vitamin C; 13 mg cholesterol

Graham Cracker Praline Cookies

An easy sort of toffee cookie.

24 graham crackers

1 cup (225 g) unsalted butter

1 cup (225 g) packed dark brown sugar

1 cup (110 g) chopped pecans

Place crackers on ungreased baking sheet with an edge. Melt butter and sugar. Bring to a boil. Add pecans and boil 2 minutes, no longer. Pour over graham crackers and bake in 275°F (140°C, gas mark 1) oven for 10 minutes. Remove, let cool slightly, and cut into fingers while still warm.

Yield: 48 servings

Per serving: 1 g water; 86 calories (61% from fat, 3% from protein, 37% from carb); 1 g protein; 6 g total fat; 3 g saturated fat; 2 g monounsaturated fat; 1 g polyunsaturated fat; 8 g carbohydrate; 1 g fiber; 6 g sugar; 12 mg phosphorus; 4 mg calcium; 0 mg iron; 29 mg sodium; 17 mg potassium; 120 IU vitamin A; 32 mg vitamin E; 0 mg vitamin C; 10 mg cholesterol

Granola Cookies

Tasty treats for breakfast or a snack. And healthy besides.

1 cup (145 g) firmly packed dates

1 cup (260 g) apple juice concentrate

3 tablespoons (48 g) peanut butter

3 tablespoons (60 g) honey

1 teaspoon vanilla extract

1 tablespoon (20 g) molasses

1 tablespoon chopped walnuts

$^1/_2$ cup (40 g) coconut

$^1/_2$ cup (75 g) raisins

$2^1/_3$ cups (280 g) whole wheat flour

2 cups (160 g) quick-cooking oats

Blend dates and apple juice until smooth. Add peanut butter, honey, vanilla, and molasses. Blend well and place in mixing bowl. Add nuts, coconut, raisins, and flour and mix well. Add oats and blend, with hands if needed. Spoon onto nonstick baking sheet; press with wet fork or fingers until $^1/_4$ inch (0.5 cm) thick. Bake at 300°F (150°C, gas mark 2) about 20 minutes.

Yield: 36 servings

Per serving: 5 g water; 91 calories (15% from fat, 10% from protein, 75% from carb); 2 g protein; 2 g total fat; 0 g saturated fat; 0 g monounsaturated fat; 0 g polyunsaturated fat; 18 g carbohydrate; 2 g fiber; 8 g sugar; 61 mg phosphorus; 11 mg calcium; 1 mg iron; 9 mg sodium; 135 mg potassium; 1 IU vitamin A; 0 mg vitamin E; 3 mg vitamin C; 0 mg cholesterol

High-Fiber Cookies

These tasty cookies get extra bran and flavor from two kinds of cereal.

1 cup (100 g) oat bran

1 cup (80 g) rolled oats

1 cup (60 g) lightly sweetened bran cereal, such as Fiber One

1 cup (40 g) bran flakes cereal

1 cup (145 g) raisins

1 cup (120 g) chopped walnuts

$^3/_4$ cup (150 g) sugar

$^3/_4$ cup (170 g) brown sugar

1 cup (225 g) unsalted butter

1 egg

2 teaspoons vanilla extract

2 cups (240 g) whole wheat pastry flour

1 teaspoon baking powder

1 teaspoon baking soda

$^1/_2$ cup (120 ml) water, room temperature

Place oat bran, rolled oats, bran cereal, bran flakes, raisins, and walnuts in a bowl. Mix lightly and set aside. Place sugars and butter in mixing bowl and mix at medium speed until light and fluffy. Add egg and vanilla and mix lightly, scraping the bowl before and after adding the egg. In a separate bowl, combine the flour, baking powder, and baking soda and mix at low speed about 30 seconds to blend well. Add flour mixture and water to sugar mixture and mix at medium speed only until flour is moistened. Add bran mixture and mix at medium speed until well blended. Drop by heaping tablespoons onto a baking sheet that has been sprayed with nonstick vegetable oil spray or lined with aluminum foil. Bake at 375°F (190°C, gas mark 5) for 12 to 14 minutes or until lightly browned. Remove from oven and let sit for 1 minute. Remove cookies to wire rack and cool to room temperature.

Yield: 48 servings

Per serving: 6 g water; 120 calories (41% from fat, 7% from protein, 52% from carb); 2 g protein; 6 g total fat; 3 g saturated fat; 2 g monounsaturated fat; 1 g polyunsaturated fat; 17 g carbohydrate; 2 g fiber; 9 g sugar; 64 mg phosphorus; 23 mg calcium; 1 mg iron; 28 mg sodium; 97 mg potassium; 171 IU vitamin A; 47 mg vitamin E; 2 mg vitamin C; 15 mg cholesterol

Molasses Cookies

Perfect cookie dough for making gingerbread men.

1 cup (225 g) unsalted butter, softened

1 cup (200 g) sugar

1 cup (340 g) molasses

$^1/_3$ cup (78 ml) water, boiling

1 tablespoon (15 ml) vinegar

5 cups (600 g) whole wheat pastry flour

2 teaspoons baking soda

1 teaspoon ginger

1 teaspoon cinnamon

Cream butter and sugar. Add molasses, water, and vinegar. Combine dry ingredients. Beat into creamed mixture. Cover and chill for at least 3 hours. On a lightly floured surface, roll dough to $^1/_4$-inch (0.5-cm) thickness. Cut out cookies with cookie cutter or glass dipped in flour. Place on baking sheets coated with nonstick vegetable oil spray. Bake at 375°F (190°C, gas mark 5) for 8 minutes or until edges are lightly browned.

Yield: 72 servings

Per serving: 4 g water; 75 calories (31% from fat, 6% from protein, 63% from carb); 1 g protein; 3 g total fat; 2 g saturated fat; 1 g monounsaturated fat; 0 g polyunsaturated fat; 12 g carbohydrate; 1 g fiber; 5 g sugar; 31 mg phosphorus; 14 mg calcium; 1 mg iron; 3 mg sodium; 104 mg potassium; 80 IU vitamin A; 21 mg vitamin E; 0 mg vitamin C; 7 mg cholesterol

Oat and Wheat Cookies

A simple and easy-to-make cookie. But don't let the simplicity fool you, I find them to be just the little bit of sweetness I want after dinner.

$^3/_4$ cup (165 g) unsalted butter

$^1/_2$ cup (130 g) peanut butter

$^2/_3$ cup (150 g) brown sugar

1$^1/_4$ cups (150 g) whole wheat pastry flour

1 teaspoon baking soda

1$^1/_4$ cups (100 g) rolled oats

Mix all ingredients. Drop by rounded teaspoons onto ungreased baking sheet. Bake at 375°F (190°C, gas mark 5) for 10 to 12 minutes or until golden brown. Cool on baking sheet 1 minute, then cool on racks.

Yield: 36 servings

Per serving: 2 g water; 95 calories (53% from fat, 8% from protein, 39% from carb); 2 g protein; 6 g total fat; 3 g saturated fat; 2 g monounsaturated fat; 1 g polyunsaturated fat; 10 g carbohydrate; 1 g fiber; 4 g sugar; 41 mg phosphorus; 9 mg calcium; 0 mg iron; 20 mg sodium; 69 mg potassium; 119 IU vitamin A; 32 mg vitamin E; 0 mg vitamin C; 10 mg cholesterol

Oat Bran Ginger Cookies

Similar to gingersnaps, these cookies still offer the health effects of oat bran.

$^3/_4$ cup (170 g) packed brown sugar

$^1/_2$ cup (120 ml) light corn syrup

8 tablespoons (112 g) unsalted butter, softened

1 egg

3 cups (300 g) oat bran

$^3/_4$ cup (90 g) flour

2 teaspoons (3.6 g) ground ginger

1 teaspoon (2.3 g) cinnamon

1 teaspoon (4.6 g) baking soda

$^1/_4$ cup (50 g) sugar

Preheat oven to 350°F (180°C, or gas mark 4). Beat brown sugar, corn syrup, and butter until light and fluffy. Add egg and beat until well blended. In a large bowl combine the oat bran, flour, ginger, cinnamon, and baking soda. Gradually add the oat bran mixture to the brown sugar mixture. Mix well. Shape into 1-inch (2.5-cm) balls. Roll in sugar. Place 2 inches (5 cm) apart on ungreased baking sheet. Flatten to 2-inch (5-cm) diameter. Bake for 12 minutes, or until light golden brown.

Yield: 42 servings

Per serving: 72 calories (29% from fat, 4% from protein, 66% from carbohydrate); 1 g protein; 2 g total fat; 2 g saturated fat; 0 g monounsaturated fat; 0 g polyunsaturated fat; 12 g carbohydrate; 0 g fiber; 7 g sugar; 22 mg phosphorus; 12 mg calcium; 1 mg iron; 49 mg sodium; 37 mg potassium; 133 IU vitamin A; 30 mg ATE vitamin E; 0 mg vitamin C; 7 mg cholesterol; 3 g water

Oat Bran Peanut Cookies

Another old favorite updated to include oat bran. Just one more tasty way to get your daily helping (and not feel guilty about eating a little something sweet).

1/2 cup (120 ml) canola oil

1 cup (260 g) reduced-sodium peanut butter

2 eggs

1/2 cup (115 g) packed brown sugar

1/2 cup (100 g) sugar

2 cups (200 g) oat bran

1 cup (125 g) flour

1 teaspoon (4.6 g) baking powder

1 teaspoon (4.6 g) baking soda

Preheat oven to 350°F (180°C, or gas mark 4). In a large bowl combine the oil, peanut butter, and eggs until well blended. Mix in the brown sugar, then the remaining ingredients. Refrigerate overnight. Form into 1-inch (2.5-cm) balls and place on an ungreased baking sheet. Press down on the tops of the cookies with a fork to form the typical crisscross pattern. Bake for 15 minutes, or until lightly browned.

Yield: 24 servings

Per serving: 180 calories (51% from fat, 9% from protein, 39% from carbohydrate); 4 g protein; 10 g total fat; 1 g saturated fat; 5 g monounsaturated fat; 3 g polyunsaturated fat; 18 g carbohydrate; 1 g fiber; 10 g sugar; 71 mg phosphorus; 30 mg calcium; 2 mg iron; 119 mg sodium; 135 mg potassium; 55 IU vitamin A; 11 mg ATE vitamin E; 0 mg vitamin C; 17 mg cholesterol; 5 g water

Oatmeal Spice Cookies

A subscriber contributed this excellent recipe for oatmeal cookies. They have become family favorites.

1 cup (145 g) raisins

1 cup (235 ml) water

1/2 cup (112 g) unsalted butter, softened

1/4 cup (60 ml) vegetable oil

1 1/2 cups (300 g) sugar

2 eggs

1 teaspoon vanilla extract

2 1/2 cups (300 g) whole wheat pastry flour

1/2 teaspoon baking powder

1 teaspoon baking soda

2 teaspoons cinnamon

1/4 teaspoon nutmeg

2 cups (160 g) quick-cooking oats

1/2 cup (60 g) chopped walnuts

Preheat oven to 350°F (180°C, gas mark 4). Simmer raisins and water in saucepan on low until plump, approximately 20 minutes. Drain liquid into measuring cup and add water to make 1/2 cup liquid. Cream butter, oil, and sugar. Add eggs and vanilla. Stir in raisin liquid. Sift flour and spices; add to sugar mixture. Add oats, nuts, and raisins. Drop by rounded teaspoons onto ungreased baking sheet. Flatten slightly, then bake 8 to 10 minutes or until slightly brown.

Yield: 48 servings

Per serving: 9 g water; 120 calories (33% from fat, 9% from protein, 58% from carb); 3 g protein; 5 g total fat; 2 g saturated fat; 1 g monounsaturated fat; 1 g polyunsaturated fat; 18 g carbohydrate; 2 g fiber; 8 g sugar; 72 mg phosphorus; 14 mg calcium; 1 mg iron; 10 mg sodium; 90 mg potassium; 72 IU vitamin A; 19 mg vitamin E; 0 mg vitamin C; 15 mg cholesterol

Trail Mix Cookies

This was an experiment that went right. The nutritional information will vary somewhat depending on the ingredients of the trail mix you find.

³/₄ cup (165 g) unsalted butter

³/₄ cup (150 g) sugar

1 egg

1 teaspoon vanilla extract

2 cups (240 g) whole wheat pastry flour

1 teaspoon baking soda

1 teaspoon cinnamon

¹/₄ teaspoon nutmeg

³/₄ cup (175 ml) skim milk

1³/₄ cups (140 g) quick-cooking oats

1¹/₂ cups (200 g) trail mix

Cream together butter and sugar. Add egg and vanilla and beat well. Stir together dry ingredients (except oats and trail mix). Add to mixture alternately with milk, mixing well. Stir in oats and trail mix. Drop by tablespoons on a baking sheet covered with nonstick vegetable oil spray. Bake at 400°F (200°C, gas mark 6) until lightly browned, 8 to 10 minutes.

Yield: 60 servings

Per serving: 5 g water; 82 calories (42% from fat, 10% from protein, 49% from carb); 2 g protein; 4 g total fat; 2 g saturated fat; 1 g monounsaturated fat; 1 g polyunsaturated fat; 10 g carbohydrate; 1 g fiber; 3 g sugar; 56 mg phosphorus; 13 mg calcium; 1 mg iron; 4 mg sodium; 69 mg potassium; 84 IU vitamin A; 22 mg vitamin E; 0 mg vitamin C; 10 mg cholesterol

Raisin-Granola Cookies

Good-tasting snacks that you can feel good about.

1³/₄ (145 g) cups granola

1¹/₂ cups (180 g) whole wheat pastry flour

1 cup (225 g) unsalted butter, softened

³/₄ cup (150 g) sugar

³/₄ cup (170 g) packed dark brown sugar

1 teaspoon baking soda

1 teaspoon vanilla extract

1 egg

1¹/₂ cups (220 g) raisins

Preheat oven to 375°F (190°C, gas mark 5). Coat baking sheets with nonstick vegetable oil spray. Into large bowl measure all ingredients except raisins. With mixer at low speed, beat ingredients just until mixed. Increase speed to medium and beat 2 minutes, occasionally scraping bowl with rubber spatula. Stir in raisins until mixture is well blended. Drop dough by heaping teaspoons about 2 inches (5 cm) apart on baking sheets. Bake 12 to 15 minutes until cookies are lightly browned around edges. Remove to wire racks and allow to cool. Store cookies in a tightly covered container up to 1 week.

Yield: 48 servings

Per serving: 3 g water; 97 calories (39% from fat, 4% from protein, 57% from carb); 1 g protein; 4 g total fat; 3 g saturated fat; 1 g monounsaturated fat; 0 g polyunsaturated fat; 14 g carbohydrate; 1 g fiber; 9 g sugar; 29 mg phosphorus; 6 mg calcium; 0 mg iron; 19 mg sodium; 53 mg potassium; 126 IU vitamin A; 34 mg vitamin E; 0 mg vitamin C; 15 mg cholesterol

Apple Cookies

A nice, soft, chewy cookie . . . and it includes things that are good for you.

2 cups (240 g) whole wheat pastry flour

1 teaspoon baking soda

1 teaspoon cinnamon

$^1/_2$ teaspoon cloves

$^1/_2$ teaspoon nutmeg

$^1/_2$ cup (112 g) unsalted butter

1$^1/_4$ cups (210 g) firmly packed brown sugar

1 egg

1 cup (110 g) chopped pecans

1 cup (125 g) finely chopped apple

1 cup (145 g) raisins

$^1/_4$ cup (60 ml) skim milk

Sift flour with baking soda, cinnamon, cloves, and nutmeg. In a large mixing bowl, cream butter and brown sugar; beat in egg until well-blended. Stir in half of flour and spice mixture, then stir in pecans, apple, and raisins. Blend in milk, then remaining flour mixture. Drop by rounded tablespoons of dough, about 2 inches (5 cm) apart, onto baking sheets coated with nonstick vegetable oil spray. Bake at 375°F (190°C, gas mark 5) for 12 to 15 minutes, or until done.

Yield: 36 servings

Per serving: 8 g water; 114 calories (38% from fat, 5% from protein, 56% from carb); 2 g protein; 5 g total fat; 2 g saturated fat; 2 g monounsaturated fat; 1 g polyunsaturated fat; 17 g carbohydrate; 1 g fiber; 11 g sugar; 44 mg phosphorus; 18 mg calcium; 1 mg iron; 7 mg sodium; 110 mg potassium; 94 IU vitamin A; 24 mg vitamin E; 0 mg vitamin C; 13 mg cholesterol

Crunchy Orange Cookies

A different kind of oatmeal cookie, with a nice, unexpected orange flavor.

1 cup (225 g) unsalted butter

1 cup (200 g) sugar

2 eggs

$^1/_4$ cup (60 ml) orange juice

1 teaspoon vanilla extract

2 teaspoons grated orange peel

2 cups (240 g) whole wheat pastry flour

1 teaspoon baking soda

2 cups (160 g) quick-cooking oats

1 cup (145 g) raisins

$^1/_2$ cup (55 g) chopped pecans

Cream butter and sugar until light. Beat in eggs, juice, vanilla, and orange peel. Add dry ingredients and mix well. Stir in by hand oats, raisins, and pecans. Drop by teaspoon on baking sheet coated with nonstick vegetable oil spray. Bake at 375°F (190°C, gas mark 5) for 10 to 15 minutes.

Yield: 42 servings

Per serving: 6 g water; 117 calories (44% from fat, 7% from protein, 49% from carb); 2 g protein; 6 g total fat; 3 g saturated fat; 2 g monounsaturated fat; 1 g polyunsaturated fat; 15 g carbohydrate; 1 g fiber; 7 g sugar; 52 mg phosphorus; 10 mg calcium; 1 mg iron; 5 mg sodium; 80 mg potassium; 151 IU vitamin A; 40 mg vitamin E; 1 mg vitamin C; 23 mg cholesterol

Fruit Cookies

Pick your favorite fruit or fruits to make these cookies your own. My personal favorites are cranberries, cherries, and pineapple.

1 $^1/_2$ cups (337 g) mashed banana

$^1/_3$ cup (80 ml) canola oil

1 teaspoon vanilla extract

1 $^1/_2$ cups (120 g) rolled oats

$^1/_2$ cup (50 g) oat bran

1 $^1/_2$ cups (240 g) mixed dried fruits, coarsely chopped

$^1/_2$ cup (60 g) chopped walnuts

Preheat oven to 350°F (180°C, gas mark 4). Coat 2 baking sheets with nonstick vegetable oil spray. Mash bananas in a large bowl until smooth. Stir in oil and vanilla. Add oats, oat bran, mixed fruits, and walnuts. Stir well to combine. Drop by rounded teaspoons on baking sheets about 1 inch (2.5 cm) apart. Flatten slightly with back of a spoon. Bake 20 to 25 minutes or until bottom and edges are lightly brown. Cool completely; refrigerate.

Yield: 24 servings

Per serving: 23 g water; 115 calories (38% from fat, 6% from protein, 56% from carb); 2 g protein; 5 g total fat; 0 g saturated fat; 2 g monounsaturated fat; 2 g polyunsaturated fat; 17 g carbohydrate; 2 g fiber; 9 g sugar; 49 mg phosphorus; 8 mg calcium; 1 mg iron; 4 mg sodium; 139 mg potassium; 28 IU vitamin A; 3 mg vitamin E; 3 mg vitamin C; 0 mg cholesterol

Apricot Pecan Balls

No-bake cookies with great apricot flavor.

1 $^1/_2$ cups crushed vanilla wafers

1 cup (110 g) chopped pecans

$^1/_2$ cup (50 g) confectioners' sugar

$^1/_2$ cup (65 g) chopped dried apricots

$^1/_4$ cup (60 ml) light corn syrup

2 tablespoons (28 ml) apricot brandy

$^1/_2$ cup (50 g) confectioners' sugar, sifted

In a bowl stir together vanilla wafers, pecans, confectioners' sugar, and the apricots. Stir in corn syrup and brandy. Using 1 level tablespoon for each cookie, shape mixture into balls. Roll each ball in sifted confectioners' sugar. Store in a covered container.

Yield: 36 servings

Per serving: 4 g water; 60 calories (41% from fat, 3% from protein, 56% from carb); 0 g protein; 3 g total fat; 0 g saturated fat; 1 g monounsaturated fat; 1 g polyunsaturated fat; 9 g carbohydrate; 1 g fiber; 6 g sugar; 13 mg phosphorus; 5 mg calcium; 0 mg iron; 13 mg sodium; 22 mg potassium; 65 IU vitamin A; 2 mg vitamin E; 0 mg vitamin C; 2 mg cholesterol

Low Fat Pumpkin Cookies

These cookies sometimes end up being eaten for breakfast around our house. They are almost like muffins, only smaller.

2 cups (250 g) flour

1 teaspoon (4.6 g) baking powder

$^1/_2$ teaspoon (2.3 g) baking soda

1 teaspoon (2.3 g) cinnamon

$^1/_2$ teaspoon (0.9 g) ground ginger

1 teaspoon (1.9 g) ground allspice

$^1/_4$ cup (60 ml) canola oil

1 cup (225 g) packed brown sugar

1 egg

1 cup (225 g) canned or cooked fresh pumpkin

1 teaspoon (5 ml) vanilla

Preheat oven to 350°F (180°C, or gas mark 4). In a medium bowl, combine flour, baking powder, baking soda, cinnamon, ginger, and allspice. In a large bowl beat oil, brown sugar, egg, pumpkin, and vanilla. Stir flour mixture into wet ingredients until just combined. Drop spoonfuls of dough about 1 inch (2.5 cm) apart on an ungreased baking sheet. Bake for 12 to 14 minutes.

Yield: 30 servings

Per serving: 81 calories (23% from fat, 7% from protein, 70% from carbohydrate); 1 g protein; 2 g total fat; 0 g saturated fat; 1 g monounsaturated fat; 1 g polyunsaturated fat; 14 g carbohydrate; 1 g fiber; 7 g sugar; 21 mg phosphorus; 22 mg calcium; 1 mg iron; 46 mg sodium; 63 mg potassium; 1283 IU vitamin A; 0 mg ATE vitamin E; 0 mg vitamin C; 9 mg cholesterol; 11 g water

Zucchini Cookies

No one will ever guess the secret ingredient in these supermoist cookies.

$^1/_2$ cup (112 g) unsalted butter, softened

$^3/_4$ cup (150 g) sugar

1 egg

$^1/_2$ teaspoon vanilla extract

$1^1/_2$ cups (187 g) flour

1 teaspoon cinnamon

$^1/_2$ teaspoon baking soda

1 cup (80 g) quick-cooking oats

$1^1/_2$ cups (169 g) shredded zucchini

1 cup (82 g) granola

12 ounces (340 g) chocolate chips

Mix all ingredients in a large bowl. Drop by heaping teaspoons onto baking sheet. Bake in 350°F (180°C, gas mark 4) oven for 10 to 12 minutes.

Yield: 48 servings

Per serving: 6 g water; 97 calories (40% from fat, 6% from protein, 53% from carb); 2 g protein; 4 g total fat; 2 g saturated fat; 2 g monounsaturated fat; 0 g polyunsaturated fat; 13 g carbohydrate; 1 g fiber; 7 g sugar; 36 mg phosphorus; 18 mg calcium; 1 mg iron; 15 mg sodium; 54 mg potassium; 86 IU vitamin A; 21 mg vitamin E; 1 mg vitamin C; 11 mg cholesterol

Thumbprint Cookies

These are wonderful cookies that no one will ever know are low in fat.

$^1/_4$ cup (56 g) unsalted butter, softened

$^1/_2$ cup (115 g) packed brown sugar

1 egg

1 teaspoon (5 ml) vanilla

$1^1/_2$ cups (185 g) flour

6 tablespoons (90 ml) raspberry jam

Preheat oven to 350°F (180°C, or gas mark 4). In a large bowl, cream butter and brown sugar together using an electric mixer. Add egg and vanilla, and mix until blended. Gradually add flour and mix, forming a large ball. Form 1-inch (2.5-cm) balls and place them 1 inch (2.5-cm) apart on a baking sheet, making a deep thumbprint in the center of each. Bake for 10 minutes. Remove from oven. After 1 minute, place on a wire rack to cool. Place 1 teaspoon (5 ml) of raspberry jam in the center of each cookie.

Yield: 24 servings

Per serving: 79 calories (23% from fat, 6% from protein, 71% from carbohydrate); 1 g protein; 2 g total fat; 2 g saturated fat; 0 g monounsaturated fat; 0 g polyunsaturated fat; 14 g carbohydrate; 0 g fiber; 7 g sugar; 14 mg phosphorus; 8 mg calcium; 1 mg iron; 8 mg sodium; 38 mg potassium; 93 IU vitamin A; 18 mg ATE vitamin E; 0 mg vitamin C; 9 mg cholesterol; 5 g water

Meringue Cookies

These might just be the ultimate in fat-free cookies. They are such crunchy, sweet little nuggets that you won't even miss the fat.

3 egg whites

$^1/_4$ teaspoon (0.8 g) cream of tartar

$^3/_4$ cup (150 g) superfine sugar

Preheat oven to 225°F (110°C). Beat egg whites with an electric mixer on medium speed until foamy. Add cream of tartar and continue beating egg whites until soft peaks form. Gradually add sugar, beating well after each addition. Mix until all the sugar has been added and the egg whites are stiff and glossy.

Drop by the tablespoon onto a baking sheet. Bake for 1 hour. Switch off oven, and leave in the oven for 2 to 3 hours

Yield: 24 servings

Per serving: 17 calories (1% from fat, 11% from protein, 89% from carbohydrate); 0 g protein; 0 g total fat; 0 g saturated fat; 0 g monounsaturated fat; 0 g polyunsaturated fat; 4 g carbohydrate; 0 g fiber; 4 g sugar; 1 mg phosphorus; 0 mg calcium; 0 mg iron; 7 mg sodium; 12 mg potassium; 0 IU vitamin A; 0 mg ATE vitamin E; 0 mg vitamin C; 0 mg cholesterol; 4 g water

Tip: Superfine sugar is more finely pulverized than regular sugar, making it dissolve more easily. Many large grocery stores have it in the baking aisle, but if you can't find it you can substitute regular sugar that has been processed in a blender or food processor until powdery.

Poppyseed Cookies

If you like poppyseeds, you'll love these. If you don't like poppyseeds, you still may . . .

$^1/_2$ cup (112 g) unsalted butter, softened

$^3/_4$ cup (170 g) packed brown sugar

2 eggs, beaten

$^1/_2$ teaspoon vanilla extract

$^1/_2$ teaspoon lemon peel

$^1/_3$ cup poppyseeds

2 cups (240 g) whole wheat pastry flour

2 teaspoons baking powder

Cream together butter and sugar. Beat until light. Add eggs and vanilla. Beat until creamy. Combine remaining ingredients. Add and stir until well mixed.

Drop by teaspoons on baking sheet. Bake at 350°F (180°C, gas mark 4) until lightly browned, about 10 minutes.

Yield: 30 servings

Per serving: 5 g water; 89 calories (42% from fat, 8% from protein, 50% from carb); 2 g protein; 4 g total fat; 2 g saturated fat; 1 g monounsaturated fat; 1 g polyunsaturated fat; 12 g carbohydrate; 1 g fiber; 6 g sugar; 57 mg phosphorus; 51 mg calcium; 1 mg iron; 41 mg sodium; 69 mg potassium; 113 IU vitamin A; 31 mg vitamin E; 0 mg vitamin C; 24 mg cholesterol

Almond Crunch Cookies

I love the almond and butter brickle taste of these cookies. The inch-and-a-half balls make pretty big cookies. You could make them smaller if you like.

1 cup (200 g) sugar

1 cup (100 g) confectioners' sugar, sifted

1 cup (225 g) unsalted butter, softened

1 cup (235 ml) canola oil

2 eggs

2 teaspoons almond extract

4$^1/_2$ cups (540 g) whole wheat pastry flour

1 teaspoon baking soda

1 teaspoon cream of tartar

2 cups (220 g) chopped almonds

6 ounces (170 g) Heath Bar chips

Combine sugar, confectioners' sugar, butter, and oil in a large mixing bowl; beat at medium speed with electric mixer until blended. Add eggs and almond extract, beating well. Combine flour, soda, and cream of tartar; gradually add to creamed mixture, beating just until blended after each addition. Stir in almonds and chips. Chill dough 3 to 4 hours. Shape dough into 1$^1/_2$-inch (4-cm) balls and place at least 3 inches (7.5 cm) apart on ungreased baking sheets. Flatten cookies with a fork dipped in sugar, making a crisscross pattern. Bake at 350°F (180°C, gas mark 4) for 14 to 15 minutes or until lightly browned. Transfer to racks to cool.

Yield: 48 servings

Per serving: 4 g water; 197 calories (58% from fat, 7% from protein, 36% from carb); 3 g protein; 13 g total fat; 4 g saturated fat; 6 g monounsaturated fat; 2 g polyunsaturated fat; 18 g carbohydrate; 2 g fiber; 9 g sugar; 76 mg phosphorus; 22 mg calcium; 1 mg iron; 15 mg sodium; 109 mg potassium; 139 IU vitamin A; 35 mg vitamin E; 0 mg vitamin C; 21 mg cholesterol

Pecan Cookies

Full of pecans and other good things, these are another cookie that you can eat with a little less guilt than usual.

1 cup (110 g) chopped pecans

$^1/_2$ cup (40 g) coconut

$^1/_4$ cup (36 g) sesame seeds

$^1/_2$ cup (112 g) unsalted butter

$^1/_2$ cup (100 g) sugar

1 egg

1 teaspoon vanilla extract

$^1/_4$ cup (60 ml) skim milk

1 cup (120 g) whole wheat pastry flour

$^1/_2$ teaspoon baking soda

1 cup (82 g) granola

$^1/_2$ cup (75 g) raisins

Combine pecans, coconut, and sesame seeds. Heat at 350°F (180°C, gas mark 4) until lightly toasted. Cream butter and sugar. Beat in egg, vanilla, and milk. Sift together flour and baking soda. Stir into egg mixture until blended. Stir in granola, pecan mixture, and raisins. Drop by spoonfuls onto baking sheets coated with nonstick vegetable oil spray. Bake at 375°F (190°C, gas mark 5) for 15 to 20 minutes until lightly browned.

Yield: 36 servings

Per serving: 4 g water; 95 calories (54% from fat, 6% from protein, 40% from carb); 1 g protein; 6 g total fat; 2 g saturated fat; 2 g monounsaturated fat; 1 g polyunsaturated fat; 10 g carbohydrate; 1 g fiber; 5 g sugar; 41 mg phosphorus; 19 mg calcium; 0 mg iron; 13 mg sodium; 64 mg potassium; 94 IU vitamin A; 25 mg vitamin E; 0 mg vitamin C; 13 mg cholesterol

Peanut-Granola Cookies

These make a nice, soft, chewy cookie with a great granola flavor.

1$^3/_4$ cups (145 g) granola

1$^1/_2$ cups (180 g) whole wheat pastry flour

1 cup (225 g) unsalted butter, softened

$^3/_4$ cup (150 g) sugar

$^3/_4$ cup (170 g) packed dark brown sugar

1 teaspoon baking soda

1 teaspoon vanilla extract

1 egg

1 cup (145 g) peanuts, unsalted, coarsely chopped

Preheat oven to 375°F (190°C, gas mark 5). Coat baking sheets with nonstick vegetable oil spray. Measure all ingredients into a large bowl except peanuts. With mixer at low speed, beat ingredients just until mixed. Increase speed to medium and beat 2 minutes. Stir in peanuts until well blended. Drop dough by heaping teaspoons, about 2 inches (5 cm) apart. Bake 12 to 15 minutes until lightly browned around edges. Remove to rack and cool completely. Store in container with tight lid.

Yield: 48 servings

Per serving: 3 g water; 97 calories (39% from fat, 4% from protein, 57% from carb); 1 g protein; 4 g total fat; 3 g saturated fat; 1 g monounsaturated fat; 0 g polyunsaturated fat; 14 g carbohydrate; 1 g fiber; 9 g sugar; 29 mg phosphorus; 6 mg calcium; 0 mg iron; 19 mg sodium; 53 mg potassium; 126 IU vitamin A; 34 mg vitamin E; 0 mg vitamin C; 15 mg cholesterol

Fudgy Brownies

Quick brownie recipe, with a fiber boost not just from the whole wheat flour, but from the cocoa.

1 cup (225 g) unsalted butter

$^1/_2$ cup (45 g) cocoa powder

2 cups (400 g) sugar

4 eggs

2 teaspoons vanilla extract

1 cup (120 g) whole wheat pastry flour

Heat oven to 350°F (180°C, gas mark 4). In microwave, melt butter and cocoa together, stirring once or twice. When melted, add sugar, eggs, and vanilla. Stir to mix well, then add flour. Pour into 13 × 9-inch (33 × 23-cm) pan coated with nonstick vegetable oil spray. Bake 25 minutes.

Yield: 18 servings

Per serving: 13 g water; 224 calories (46% from fat, 5% from protein, 49% from carb); 3 g protein; 12 g total fat; 7 g saturated fat; 3 g monounsaturated fat; 1 g polyunsaturated fat; 29 g carbohydrate; 2 g fiber; 23 g sugar; 67 mg phosphorus; 15 mg calcium; 1 mg iron; 20 mg sodium; 84 mg potassium; 376 IU vitamin A; 102 mg vitamin E; 0 mg vitamin C; 80 mg cholesterol

Granola Bars

You can add unsalted nuts to this if you want or substitute chocolate chips or other dried fruit for the raisins to vary the flavor.

3 cups (240 g) quick-cooking oats

$^1/_2$ cup (115 g) brown sugar

$^1/_4$ cup (28 g) wheat germ

$^1/_2$ cup (112 g) unsalted butter

$^1/_4$ cup (60 ml) corn syrup

$^1/_4$ cup (85 g) honey

$^1/_2$ cup (75 g) raisins

$^1/_2$ cup (40 g) sweetened coconut

Combine the oats, sugar, and wheat germ. Cut in the butter until the mixture is crumbly. Stir in the corn syrup and honey. Add the raisins and coconut. Press into a 9-inch (23-cm) square pan coated with

nonstick vegetable oil spray. Bake in a 350°F (180°C, gas mark 4) oven for 20 to 25 minutes. Let cool 10 minutes, then cut into bars.

Yield: 27 servings

Per serving: 4 g water; 153 calories (30% from fat, 8% from protein, 61% from carb); 3 g protein; 5 g total fat; 3 g saturated fat; 1 g monounsaturated fat; 1 g polyunsaturated fat; 24 g carbohydrate; 2 g fiber; 10 g sugar; 107 mg phosphorus; 17 mg calcium; 1 mg iron; 9 mg sodium; 129 mg potassium; 105 IU vitamin A; 28 mg vitamin E; 0 mg vitamin C; 9 mg cholesterol

Zucchini Bars

Sweet and moist, these are almost perfect, in my humble opinion.

3 eggs

2 cups (400 g) sugar

1 cup (225 g) unsalted butter, melted

2 cups (226 g) grated zucchini

1 tablespoon vanilla extract

3 cups (360 g) whole wheat pastry flour

1 teaspoon baking soda

$^1/_2$ teaspoon baking powder

1 tablespoon cinnamon

1 cup (120 g) chopped walnuts

Topping:

$^1/_2$ cup (56 g) wheat germ

$^1/_2$ cup (115 g) brown sugar

1 teaspoon cinnamon

Beat eggs until light and foamy. Add sugar, butter, zucchini, and vanilla. Combine flour, baking soda, baking powder, and cinnamon. Add to egg-zucchini mixture. Stir until well blended; add walnuts. Pour into a 13 × 9 × 2-inch (33 × 23 × 5-cm) baking pan coated with nonstick vegetable oil spray. To make the topping: Mix wheat germ, brown sugar, and cinnamon together and sprinkle over batter. Bake in a 350°F (180°C, gas mark 4) oven for 15 to 20 minutes. Cool on rack. Cut into bars.

Yield: 18 servings

Per serving: 25 g water; 342 calories (40% from fat, 8% from protein, 52% from carb); 7 g protein; 16 g total fat; 7 g saturated fat; 4 g monounsaturated fat; 3 g polyunsaturated fat; 46 g carbohydrate; 4 g fiber; 29 g sugar; 171 mg phosphorus; 42 mg calcium; 2 mg iron; 33 mg sodium; 224 mg potassium; 397 IU vitamin A; 98 mg vitamin E; 3 mg vitamin C; 67 mg cholesterol

Trail Bars

No-bake bars make a great grab-and-go breakfast or snack.

1 cup (235 ml) light corn syrup

$^1/_2$ cup (115 g) packed brown sugar

$1^1/_2$ cups (390 g) crunchy peanut butter

1 teaspoon vanilla extract

1 cup (68 g) nonfat dry milk

1 cup (82 g) granola

1 cup (40 g) bran flakes cereal

1 cup (145 g) raisins

1 cup (175 g) chocolate chips

Line 9 × 13-inch (23 × 33-cm) pan with waxed paper. In heavy saucepan (or large bowl in microwave) combine syrup and sugar; bring to boil. Remove from heat; stir in peanut butter and vanilla. Add remaining ingredients except chocolate; cool slightly. Add chocolate pieces; press into prepared pan. Refrigerate 30 minutes; cut into bars. Store in refrigerator.

Yield: 24 servings

Per serving: 5 g water; 241 calories (37% from fat, 10% from protein, 54% from carb); 6 g protein; 10 g total fat; 2 g saturated fat; 5 g monounsaturated fat; 2 g polyunsaturated fat; 34 g carbohydrate; 2 g fiber; 20 g sugar; 123 mg phosphorus; 67 mg calcium; 1 mg iron; 143 mg sodium; 284 mg potassium; 169 IU vitamin A; 23 mg vitamin E; 1 mg vitamin C; 2 mg cholesterol

Johnny Appleseed Squares

Apple snack bars with lots of flavor and nutrition too.

$1^1/_2$ cups (180 g) whole wheat pastry flour

$^1/_2$ teaspoon baking soda

$1^1/_2$ cups (120 g) rolled oats

1 cup (225 g) brown sugar

2 eggs

$^1/_2$ cup (112 g) unsalted butter, melted

2 cups (250 g) chopped apples

1 tablespoon (15 ml) lemon juice

$^1/_3$ cup (50 g) raisins

$^1/_3$ cup (37 g) chopped pecans

Mix together flour and baking soda. Stir in oats and brown sugar. Gradually add eggs and butter, stirring with fork until crumbly. Firmly press half of mixture into bottom of 9-inch (23-cm) square pan coated with nonstick vegetable oil spray. Mix apples and lemon juice; stir in raisins and pecans. Place apple mixture in even layer over crumb base. Roll remaining oats mixture between 2 sheets of waxed paper to form a 9-inch (23-cm) square. Remove top of waxed paper and invert dough over filling, pressing dough down lightly. Remove paper. Bake in 375°F (190°C, gas mark 5) oven for 30 minutes. Drizzle confectioners' sugar over top, if desired.

Yield: 12 servings

Per serving: 29 g water; 284 calories (36% from fat, 7% from protein, 57% from carb); 5 g protein; 12 g total fat; 6 g saturated fat; 4 g monounsaturated fat; 1 g polyunsaturated fat; 42 g carbohydrate; 4 g fiber; 23 g sugar; 139 mg phosphorus; 39 mg calcium; 2 mg iron; 23 mg sodium; 239 mg potassium; 292 IU vitamin A; 76 mg vitamin E; 1 mg vitamin C; 60 mg cholesterol

Peanut Bars

These bar cookies are super easy to make and very good to eat.

$^1/_2$ cup (112 g) unsalted butter

$^1/_2$ cup (115 g) brown sugar

$^1/_2$ cup (100 g) sugar

1 egg

$^1/_2$ teaspoon vanilla extract

1$^1/_2$ cups (120 g) quick-cooking oats

$^3/_4$ cup (90 g) whole wheat pastry flour

$^1/_2$ teaspoon baking soda

1 cup (260 g) crunchy peanut butter

$^1/_2$ cup (75 g) raisins

Combine all ingredients and mix well. Pat mixture evenly into a 9-inch (23-cm) square baking dish coated with nonstick vegetable oil spray. Bake at 350°F (180°C, gas mark 4) for 30 minutes. Cool in pan. Cut into bars.

Yield: 18 servings

Per serving: 5 g water; 236 calories (48% from fat, 9% from protein, 43% from carb); 6 g protein; 13 g total fat; 5 g saturated fat; 5 g monounsaturated fat; 3 g polyunsaturated fat; 26 g carbohydrate; 3 g fiber; 16 g sugar; 108 mg phosphorus; 22 mg calcium; 1 mg iron; 79 mg sodium; 212 mg potassium; 177 IU vitamin A; 47 mg vitamin E; 0 mg vitamin C; 25 mg cholesterol

23

Fruit Desserts

The fruit desserts in this chapter run the gamut from light refreshing things perfect for a hot summer evening to cobblers and apple dumplings that could be a meal in themselves. And then there's the fruit soup and fruit pizza. In any case it's hard to go wrong when you start with the nutrition of fresh fruit and you may find that your family appreciates something a little different.

Apple Cobbler

A newsletter subscriber sent me this recipe originally. And as she pointed out, for those of us who don't like to peel apples, it doesn't take as many as a "real" apple pie. (I'm still hoping for an apple peeler for Christmas some year.)

4 apples, peeled

1 teaspoon cinnamon

1 egg

$^3/_4$ cup (165 g) unsalted butter, melted

$^1/_2$ cup (100 g) + 1 tablespoon sugar, divided

$^1/_2$ teaspoon baking powder

1 cup (120 g) whole wheat pastry flour

Slice the apples and place in a bowl. Add cinnamon and 1 tablespoon sugar and mix well. Dump into a 10-inch (25-cm) glass pie plate that has been sprayed with nonstick vegetable oil spray. In the same bowl, beat the egg. Add melted butter, $^1/_2$ cup (100 g) sugar, baking powder, and flour. Pour over apples (it'll be thick, so I actually put little spoonfuls all over to make sure it all gets covered). Bake at 350°F (180°C, gas mark 4) for 40 to 45 minutes until golden brown and a toothpick inserted comes out clean.

Yield: 8 servings

Per serving: 65 g water; 301 calories (53% from fat, 4% from protein, 43% from carb); 3 g protein; 19 g total fat; 11 g saturated fat; 5 g monounsaturated fat; 1 g polyunsaturated fat; 34 g carbohydrate; 3 g fiber; 21 g sugar; 82 mg phosphorus; 37 mg calcium; 1 mg iron; 45 mg sodium; 134 mg potassium; 600 IU vitamin A; 154 mg vitamin E; 3 mg vitamin C; 72 mg cholesterol

Tip: Golden Delicious apples work well for this.

Apple Crunch

A tasty apple dessert with a crunchy topping.

$^1/_2$ cup (50 g) sugar

5 tablespoons (40 g) flour, divided

$^1/_2$ teaspoon cinnamon

$^1/_4$ teaspoon nutmeg

5 cups (550 g) sliced apples

1 tablespoon unsalted butter

2 cups (164 g) granola

$^1/_2$ cup (115 g) brown sugar, packed

$^1/_3$ cup (75 g) unsalted butter, softened

Coat a 9-inch-square (23-cm) pan with nonstick vegetable oil spray. Mix sugar, 3 tablespoons (24 g) flour, cinnamon, and nutmeg. Stir in apples and turn into pan. Dot with butter. Mix remaining ingredients; sprinkle over apples. Bake at 350°F (180°C, gas mark 4) for 25 to 30 minutes.

Yield: 12 servings

Per serving: 43 g water; 208 calories (29% from fat, 3% from protein, 68% from carb); 2 g protein; 7 g total fat; 4 g saturated fat; 2 g monounsaturated fat; 0 g polyunsaturated fat; 37 g carbohydrate; 1 g fiber; 26 g sugar; 50 mg phosphorus; 19 mg calcium; 1 mg iron; 56 mg sodium; 117 mg potassium; 205 IU vitamin A; 50 mg vitamin E; 2 mg vitamin C; 16 mg cholesterol

Tip: Serve warm with milk poured over.

Apple Dumplings

I remember having apple dumplings for dinner occasionally when I was young. But when I went looking for recipes, most were nothing like what I remember, which was a whole apple wrapped in pastry. Many seem to call for chopping the apples, and most include a sugar syrup that my mother never made. This one is a compromise, downsized to half an apple to make it more appropriate for dessert. I'd serve them warm with milk.

3 cups (360 g) whole wheat pastry flour

2 teaspoons baking powder

$^1/_4$ cup (56 g) shortening

$^3/_4$ cup (175 ml) milk

3 apples (Winesap, York, or other baking apples)

2 tablespoons (28 g) unsalted butter, divided

1 tablespoon sugar

$1^1/_2$ teaspoons cinnamon

Combine first 2 ingredients. Cut in shortening with pastry blender until mixture resembles coarse meal; gradually add milk, stirring to make a soft dough. Roll dough on lightly floured surface to $^1/_4$-inch (0.5-cm) thickness, shaping into a 21×14-inch (53×36-cm) rectangle. Cut dough with a pastry cutter into six 7-inch (18-cm) squares. Peel and core apples, cut in half, place 1 apple half on each pastry square; dot each with 1 teaspoon butter. Sprinkle each with $^1/_2$ teaspoon sugar and $^1/_4$ teaspoon cinnamon. Moisten edges of each dumpling with water, bringing corners to middle and pinching edges to seal. Place the dumplings in a $12 \times 8 \times 2$-inch ($30 \times 20 \times 5$-cm) baking dish coated with nonstick vegetable oil spray and bake in a 375°F (190°C, gas mark 5) oven for 35 minutes.

Yield: 6 servings

Per serving: 90 g water; 364 calories (32% from fat, 10% from protein, 58% from carb); 9 g protein; 14 g total fat; 5 g saturated fat; 5 g monounsaturated fat; 3 g polyunsaturated fat; 56 g carbohydrate; 8 g fiber; 10 g sugar; 281 mg phosphorus; 160 mg calcium; 3 mg iron; 179 mg sodium; 353 mg potassium; 212 IU vitamin A; 50 mg vitamin E; 3 mg vitamin C; 11 mg cholesterol

Crumb Topped Apples

An easy-to-put-together apple dessert that satisfies without having too much fat.

For Apples:

4 apples, peeled, cored, and chopped

$^1/_2$ cup (100 g) sugar

1 teaspoon (2.3 g) cinnamon

1 tablespoon (14 g) unsalted butter

For Topping:

$^1/_2$ cup (60 g) flour

$^1/_2$ cup (100 g) sugar

1 teaspoon (4.6 g) baking powder

1 egg

$^1/_2$ cup (100 g) sugar

1 tablespoon (14 g) unsalted butter

To make the apples: Preheat oven to 350°F (180°C, or gas mark 4). Mix apples, sugar, and cinnamon; pour into a greased 8×8-inch (20×20-cm) baking dish. Dot with butter.

To make the topping: Mix topping ingredients and pour over apples. Bake for 30 to 35 minutes.

Yield: 6 servings

Per serving: 317 calories (12% from fat, 3% from protein, 85% from carbohydrate); 3 g protein; 4 g total fat; 3 g saturated fat; 1 g monounsaturated fat; 0 g polyunsaturated fat; 70 g carbohydrate; 2 g fiber; 59 g sugar; 53 mg phosphorus; 65 mg calcium; 1 mg iron; 141 mg sodium; 130 mg potassium; 271 IU vitamin A; 46 mg ATE vitamin E; 4 mg vitamin C; 41 mg cholesterol; 85 g water

Apple Tapioca

My wife has been looking for the apple tapioca recipe that used to be on the Minute™ brand tapioca box for years. This is the closest one we've found so far, even though it's a slow cooker one rather than the original stovetop recipe.

4 cups (600 g) apples, peeled and sliced

$^{1}/_{2}$ cup (115 g) brown sugar

$^{3}/_{4}$ teaspoon (1.7 g) cinnamon

2 tablespoons (1 g) tapioca

2 tablespoons (30 ml) lemon juice

1 cup (235 ml) boiling water

In a medium bowl, toss apples with brown sugar, cinnamon, and tapioca until evenly coated. Place apples in a slow cooker. Pour lemon juice over the top. Pour in boiling water. Cook on high for 3 to 4 hours.

Yield: 4 servings

Per serving: 176 calories (1% from fat, 1% from protein, 98% from carbohydrate); 0 g protein; 0 g total fat; 0 g saturated fat; 0 g monounsaturated fat; 0 g polyunsaturated fat; 46 g carbohydrate; 2 g fiber; 38 g sugar; 19 mg phosphorus; 37 mg calcium; 1 mg iron; 13 mg sodium; 207 mg potassium; 44 IU vitamin A; 0 mg ATE vitamin E; 8 mg vitamin C; 0 mg cholesterol; 162 g water

Apple Tart

This makes a nice apple pie–like dessert without the extra work and fat of the crust.

4 apples, peeled and sliced

1 teaspoon (2.3 g) cinnamon

$^{1}/_{2}$ cup (100 g) + 1 tablespoon (13 g) sugar, divided

1 egg

$^{1}/_{4}$ cup (56 g) unsalted butter, melted

$^{1}/_{2}$ teaspoon (2.3 g) baking powder

1 cup (125 g) flour

Preheat oven to 350°F (180°C, or gas mark 4). Place the apples in a bowl. Add cinnamon and 1 tablespoon (13 g) sugar and mix well. Pour into a 10-inch (25-cm) glass pie plate coated with nonstick vegetable oil spray. In the same bowl beat the egg. Add melted butter, the remaining $^{1}/_{2}$ cup (100 g) sugar, baking powder, and flour. Pour over apples. Bake for 40 to 45 minutes, or until golden brown and a wooden pick inserted in the center comes out clean.

Yield: 8 servings

Per serving: 200 calories (27% from fat, 5% from protein, 68% from carbohydrate); 3 g protein; 6 g total fat; 4 g saturated fat; 2 g monounsaturated fat; 02 g polyunsaturated fat; 35 g carbohydrate; 1 g fiber; 21 g sugar; 41 mg phosphorus; 31 mg calcium; 1 mg iron; 45 mg sodium; 104 mg potassium; 306 IU vitamin A; 54 mg ATE vitamin E; 3 mg vitamin C; 22 mg cholesterol; 65 g water

Apple Topping

You can use this on pancakes or as a topping for ice cream or even a side dish with pork.

3 apples, peeled, cored, and chopped

$1/4$ cup (85 g) honey

1 teaspoon cinnamon

Combine ingredients in a microwave-safe bowl. Microwave on high until apples are soft, about 5 minutes

Yield: 4 servings

Per serving: 87 g water; 112 calories (1% from fat, 1% from protein, 98% from carb); 0 g protein; 0 g total fat; 0 g saturated fat; 0 g monounsaturated fat; 0 g polyunsaturated fat; 30 g carbohydrate; 2 g fiber; 27 g sugar; 12 mg phosphorus; 13 mg calcium; 0 mg iron; 1 mg sodium; 100 mg potassium; 38 IU vitamin A; 0 mg vitamin E; 4 mg vitamin C; 0 mg cholesterol

Baked Apples

A simple dessert, but one that is sure to please. Serve with a little milk or low fat ice cream, if you desire.

6 apples

$1/4$ cup (60 g) brown sugar

$1/2$ cup (80 g) raisins

$1/2$ teaspoon (1.2 g) cinnamon

$1/4$ teaspoon (0.6 g) nutmeg

1 tablespoon (14 g) unsalted butter

Preheat oven to 350°F (180°C, or gas mark 4). Wash and core apples; place in a shallow baking dish. Combine brown sugar, raisins, cinnamon, and nutmeg in a small bowl. Fill the center of each apple with brown sugar mixture and dot with $1/2$ teaspoon (2 g) of the butter. Add just enough water to the baking dish to cover the bottom; bake, uncovered, for 30 minutes, or until apples are tender, basting with juices occasionally.

Yield: 6 servings

Per serving: 155 calories (11% from fat, 2% from protein, 87% from carbohydrate); 1 g protein; 2 g total fat; 2 g saturated fat; 0 g monounsaturated fat; 0 g polyunsaturated fat; 36 g carbohydrate; 2 g fiber; 30 g sugar; 31 mg phosphorus; 25 mg calcium; 1 mg iron; 26 mg sodium; 253 mg potassium; 149 IU vitamin A; 23 mg ATE vitamin E; 6 mg vitamin C; 3 mg cholesterol; 114 g water

Chocolate Caramel Apples

Decadence defined. Yes, coating an apple with both caramel and chocolate is overdoing it a bit. But it sure tastes good.

5 apples

5 wooden craft sticks

14 ounces (400 g) caramels, individual candies unwrapped

2 tablespoons (28 ml) water

7 ounces (200 g) chocolate candy bar, broken into pieces

1 tablespoon shortening

Bring a large pot of water to a boil. Dip apples into boiling water briefly, using a slotted spoon, to remove any wax that may be present. Wipe dry and set aside to cool. Insert sticks into the apples through the cores. Line a baking sheet with waxed paper and coat with nonstick vegetable oil spray. Place the unwrapped caramels into a microwave-safe medium bowl along with 2 tablespoons (28 ml) of water. Cook on high for 2 minutes, then stir and continue cooking and stirring at 1-minute intervals until caramel is melted and smooth. Hold apples by the stick and dip into the caramel to coat. Set on waxed paper; refrigerate for about 15 minutes to set. Heat the chocolate with the shortening in a microwave-safe bowl until melted and smooth. Dip apples into the chocolate to cover the layer of caramel. Return to the waxed paper to set.

Yield: 5 servings

Per serving: 124 g water; 600 calories (30% from fat, 5% from protein, 65% from carb); 7 g protein; 21 g total fat; 8 g saturated fat; 8 g monounsaturated fat; 4 g polyunsaturated fat; 101 g carbohydrate; 3 g fiber; 85 g sugar; 187 mg phosphorus; 191 mg calcium; 1 mg iron; 226 mg sodium; 433 mg potassium; 151 IU vitamin A; 28 mg vitamin E; 5 mg vitamin C; 15 mg cholesterol

Cranberry Apple Crisp

Cranberry apple is a popular flavor combination. Here a can of cranberry sauce adds kick to an apple crisp.

2$^1/_2$ pounds (1 kg) apple, peeled, cored, and cut into $^1/_2$-inch (1-cm) chunks

16 ounces (455 g) whole berry cranberry sauce

2 tablespoons (30 ml) lemon juice

1 cup (80 g) rolled oats

$^1/_2$ cup (60 g) whole wheat pastry flour

$^1/_3$ cup (40 g) chopped walnuts

$^1/_4$ cup (60 g) packed brown sugar

$^1/_4$ cup (65 g) apple juice concentrate, thawed

1 tablespoon (15 ml) canola oil

Preheat oven to 350°F (180°C, gas mark 4). Combine apple, cranberry sauce, and lemon juice in a large bowl. Transfer to a 9$^1/_2$-inch (24-cm) deep-dish pie pan. Whisk oats, flour, walnuts, and brown sugar in a medium bowl. Whisk apple juice concentrate and oil in a small bowl until blended; drizzle over dry ingredients and mix with your fingers until moistened. Sprinkle over apples. Bake until apples are tender and top is golden, 40 to 45 minutes.

Yield: 8 servings

Per serving: 167 g water; 304 calories (16% from fat, 6% from protein, 78% from carb); 4 g protein; 6 g total fat; 0 g saturated fat; 2 g monounsaturated fat; 3 g polyunsaturated fat; 63 g carbohydrate; 5 g fiber; 45 g sugar; 123 mg phosphorus; 28 mg calcium; 1 mg iron; 22 mg sodium; 296 mg potassium; 81 IU vitamin A; 0 mg vitamin E; 15 mg vitamin C; 0 mg cholesterol

Crunchy Baked Apples

Granola adds crunch to these apples, while honey and apple and orange juice provide sweetness.

4 Granny Smith apples

$^1/_2$ cup (41 g) granola

2 cinnamon sticks, broken in half

$^1/_2$ cup (170 g) honey

1 cup (235 ml) apple juice

1 cup (235 ml) orange juice

Slice tops off apples. Seed and core. Do not cut off bottom of apple. Place apples in a baking dish. Fill opening with granola. Place cinnamon sticks in top of apples. Dribble honey over apples. Pour apple and orange juice in dish to cook the apples. Bake uncovered for 2 hours at 300°F (150°C, gas mark 2).

Yield: 4 servings

Per serving: 226 g water; 286 calories (3% from fat, 2% from protein, 95% from carb); 2 g protein; 1 g total fat; 0 g saturated fat; 0 g monounsaturated fat; 0 g polyunsaturated fat; 73 g carbohydrate; 2 g fiber; 58 g sugar; 55 mg phosphorus; 22 mg calcium; 1 mg iron; 45 mg sodium; 360 mg potassium; 97 IU vitamin A; 0 mg vitamin E; 26 mg vitamin C; 0 mg cholesterol

Easy Apple Dessert

The microwave preparation makes this especially quick and easy.

$^1/_2$ cup (42 g) graham crackers, crushed

5 apples, cored and peeled

$^1/_2$ teaspoon (1.2 g) cinnamon

$^1/_4$ teaspoon (0.5 g) allspice

$^1/_4$ cup (40 g) raisins

$^1/_3$ cup (80 ml) apple juice

Spray a microwave-safe pie plate with nonstick vegetable oil spray. Spread the cracker crumbs in the plate. Cover with apple slices. Sprinkle with cinnamon and allspice. Spread raisins over the top. Pour juice over. Cover and microwave for 15 minutes.

Yield: 6 servings

Per serving: 108 calories (7% from fat, 3% from protein, 90% from carbohydrate); 1 g protein; 1 g total fat; 0 g saturated fat; 0 g monounsaturated fat; 0 g polyunsaturated fat; 26 g carbohydrate; 2 g fiber; 18 g sugar; 27 mg phosphorus; 14 mg calcium; 1 mg iron; 44 mg sodium; 175 mg potassium; 42 IU vitamin A; 0 mg ATE vitamin E; 5 mg vitamin C; 0 mg cholesterol; 106 g water

Honey Grilled Apples

A great finish to your grilled meal. And the best part is that it cooks while you're eating the rest of the meal.

4 apples

1 tablespoon (15 ml) honey

2 tablespoons (30 ml) lemon juice

1 tablespoon (14 g) unsalted butter

Core apples and cut slices through the skin to make each apple resemble orange sections. Mix together the honey, lemon juice, and butter. Spoon mixture into apple cores. Wrap apples in greased heavy-duty aluminum foil, fold up, and seal. Grill until tender, about 20 minutes.

Yield: 4 servings

Per serving: 104 calories (23% from fat, 2% from protein, 75% from carbohydrate); 0 g protein; 3 g total fat; 2 g saturated fat; 1 g monounsaturated fat; 0 g polyunsaturated fat; 21 g carbohydrate; 2 g fiber; 17 g sugar; 17 mg phosphorus; 10 mg calcium; 0 mg iron; 31 mg sodium; 131 mg potassium; 200 IU vitamin A; 34 mg ATE vitamin E; 9 mg vitamin C; 6 mg cholesterol; 119 g water

Per serving: 152 g water; 239 calories (40% from fat, 13% from protein, 46% from carb); 8 g protein; 11 g total fat; 6 g saturated fat; 3 g monounsaturated fat; 1 g polyunsaturated fat; 29 g carbohydrate; 2 g fiber; 21 g sugar; 190 mg phosphorus; 225 mg calcium; 1 mg iron; 183 mg sodium; 211 mg potassium; 341 IU vitamin A; 75 mg vitamin E; 5 mg vitamin C; 30 mg cholesterol

Oat Baked Apple

Stick these in the oven before dinner and by the time you are finished, you'll have a great dessert waiting for you.

4 ounces (113 g) Cheddar cheese, divided

3 tablespoons quick-cooking oats

2 tablespoons (30 g) brown sugar

1 tablespoon oat bran

1 tablespoon coarsely chopped pecans

1 tablespoon raisins

$^1/_4$ teaspoon cinnamon

4 apples, cored

$^1/_2$ cup (120 ml) cold water

Preheat oven to 375°F (190°C, gas mark 5). Cut half of cheese into small cubes; shred remainder. Mix cheese cubes, oats, brown sugar, oat bran, pecans, raisins, and cinnamon until well blended. Place baking apples in 8-inch (20-cm) square pan; fill with oat mixture. Pour water in bottom of pan. Cover with foil; bake 30 minutes. Uncover and continue baking 15 minutes or until tender. Sprinkle with shredded cheese. Continue baking until cheese is melted.

Yield: 4 servings

Apple and Banana Fritters

A search for something for breakfast that would use up some overripe bananas was rewarded with the this recipe. They are incredibly light and very tasty. Sprinkle with confectioners' sugar or dip in honey if you don't mind adding a few more calories to the ones they already have.

1 cup (120 g) whole wheat pastry flour

1 tablespoon sugar

1 tablespoon baking powder

$^1/_2$ cup (120 ml) skim milk

1 egg

1 tablespoon (15 ml) canola oil

$^1/_2$ cup (75 g) chopped banana

$^1/_2$ cup (62 g) chopped apple

$^1/_2$ teaspoon nutmeg

Stir together flour, sugar, and baking powder. Combine the milk, egg, and oil. Add banana, apple, and nutmeg. Stir into dry ingredients, stirring until just moistened. Drop by tablespoons into hot oil. Fry for 2 to 3 minutes on a side until golden brown. Drain.

Yield: 4 servings

Per serving: 74 g water; 212 calories (23% from fat, 13% from protein, 64% from carb); 7 g protein; 6 g total fat; 1 g saturated fat; 3 g monounsaturated fat; 1 g polyunsaturated fat; 36 g carbohydrate; 5 g fiber; 8 g sugar; 249 mg phosphorus; 267 mg calcium; 2 mg iron; 405 mg sodium; 311 mg potassium; 157 IU vitamin A; 38 mg vitamin E; 3 mg vitamin C; 60 mg cholesterol

Fresh Fruit Compote

This makes a refreshing ending to just about any meal, especially in the spring when berries are in season.

2 peaches, sliced

2 cups (290 g) blueberries

2 cups (300 g) sliced banana

2 cups (290 g) strawberries, hulled and halved

$^1/_4$ cup (50 g) sugar

2 cups (460 g) plain fat-free yogurt

Combine fruit with sugar in a large bowl. Toss and transfer to a serving bowl. Serve with yogurt.

Yield: 4 servings

Per serving: 378 g water; 309 calories (3% from fat, 12% from protein, 85% from carb); 10 g protein; 1 g total fat; 0 g saturated fat; 0 g monounsaturated fat; 0 g polyunsaturated fat; 70 g carbohydrate; 7 g fiber; 52 g sugar; 257 mg phosphorus; 270 mg calcium; 1 mg iron; 97 mg sodium; 1012 mg potassium; 341 IU vitamin A; 2 mg vitamin E; 67 mg vitamin C; 2 mg cholesterol

Berry Cobbler

You could use any kind of berry that happens to be available for this dessert. I prefer either blackberries or raspberries, but blueberries or strawberries would work too.

2 tablespoons (16 g) cornstarch

$^1/_2$ cup (120 ml) water, divided

$1^1/_2$ cups (300 g) sugar, divided

1 tablespoon (15 ml) lemon juice

4 cups (580 g) blackberries

1 cup (125 g) flour

1 teaspoon (4.6 g) baking powder

3 tablespoons (42 g) unsalted butter

Preheat oven to 400°F (200°C, or gas mark 6). In a saucepan, stir together the cornstarch and $^1/_4$ cup (60 ml) cold water until cornstarch is completely dissolved. Add 1 cup (200 g) sugar, lemon juice, and blackberries; combine gently. In a bowl, combine the flour, remaining sugar, and baking powder. Blend in the butter until the mixture resembles coarse meal. Boil the remaining $^1/_4$ cup (60 ml) water and stir into the flour mixture until it just forms a dough. Transfer the blackberry mixture to a $1^1/_2$-quart (1.4-L) baking dish. Drop spoonfuls of the dough carefully onto the berries, and bake the cobbler on a baking sheet in the middle of the oven for 20 to 25 minutes, or until the topping is golden.

Yield: 8 servings

Per serving: 280 calories (15% from fat, 4% from protein, 82% from carbohydrate); 3 g protein; 5 g total fat; 3 g saturated fat; 1 g monounsaturated fat; 0 g polyunsaturated fat; 59 g carbohydrate; 4 g fiber; 41 g sugar; 48 mg phosphorus; 61 mg calcium; 1 mg iron; 109 mg sodium; 142 mg potassium; 379 IU vitamin A; 52 mg ATE vitamin E; 16 mg vitamin C; 6 mg cholesterol; 83 g water

Red and Blue Berry Cobbler

With a little vanilla ice cream or whipped topping, you can have a quick red, white, and blue American dessert.

2 cups strawberries, halved

2 cups (290 g) blueberries

$^1/_2$ cup (120 ml) raspberry jam

2 tablespoons (8 g) cornstarch

1 cup (125 g) flour

2 tablespoons (26 g) plus $^1/_2$ teaspoon (2 g) sugar, divided

2 teaspoons (9.2 g) baking powder

2 tablespoons (28 g) unsalted butter

2 tablespoons (30 ml) skim milk

1 egg

Preheat oven to 425°F (220°C, or gas mark 7). Grease 1$^1/_2$-quart baking dish. In large bowl, combine berries, jam, and cornstarch. Mix gently. Spread in prepared baking dish. Bake for 15 to 20 minutes, or until berries begin to bubble. Meanwhile, in a large bowl, combine flour, 2 tablespoons (26 g) sugar, and baking powder. Mix well. With a pastry blender or two forks, cut in butter until crumbly. In a small bowl, combine milk and egg; beat well. Stir into flour mixture until stiff dough forms, adding additional milk if necessary. On a lightly floured surface, roll out dough to $^1/_2$-inch (1.3-cm) thickness. With a cookie cutter, cut out stars or other shapes. Stir hot fruit mixture; top with dough cutouts. Sprinkle cutouts with remaining $^1/_2$ teaspoon (2 g) sugar. Bake for 10 to 20 minutes, or until fruit bubbles around edges and biscuits are light golden brown

Yield: 8 servings

Per serving: 208 calories (15% from fat, 7% from protein, 78% from carbohydrate); 4 g protein; 4 g total fat; 3 g saturated fat; 1 g monounsaturated fat; 0 g polyunsaturated fat; 41 g carbohydrate; 2 g fiber; 19 g sugar; 87 mg phosphorus; 95 mg calcium; 1 mg iron; 215 mg sodium; 160 mg potassium; 211 IU vitamin A; 37 mg ATE vitamin E; 28 mg vitamin C; 21 mg cholesterol; 85 g water

Raspberry Cobbler

Raspberries are one of the higher-fiber fruits available, so this is a good choice when they are in season.

2 tablespoons (16 g) cornstarch

$^1/_4$ cup (60 ml) cold water

1$^1/_2$ cups (300 g) sugar, divided

1 tablespoon (15 ml) lemon juice

4 cups (500 g) raspberries

1 cup (120 g) whole wheat pastry flour

1 teaspoon baking powder

6 tablespoons (85 g) unsalted butter

$^1/_4$ cup (60 ml) boiling water

In a saucepan, stir together the cornstarch and cold water until cornstarch is completely dissolved. Add 1 cup (200 g) sugar, lemon juice, and raspberries; combine gently. In a bowl, combine the flour, remaining sugar, and baking powder. Blend in the butter until the mixture resembles coarse meal. Add the boiling water and stir the mixture until it just forms a dough. Bring the raspberry mixture to a boil, stirring. Transfer to a 1$^1/_2$-quart (1.5-L) baking dish.

Drop spoonfuls of the dough carefully onto the mixture, and bake the cobbler on a baking sheet in the middle of a preheated 400°F (200°C, gas mark 6) oven for 20 to 25 minutes or until the topping is golden. Serve warm with vanilla ice cream or whipped cream.

Yield: 8 servings

Per serving: 73 g water; 314 calories (26% from fat, 4% from protein, 71% from carb); 3 g protein; 9 g total fat; 6 g saturated fat; 2 g monounsaturated fat; 1 g polyunsaturated fat; 58 g carbohydrate; 6 g fiber; 41 g sugar; 85 mg phosphorus; 58 mg calcium; 1 mg iron; 64 mg sodium; 160 mg potassium; 288 IU vitamin A; 71 mg vitamin E; 17 mg vitamin C; 23 mg cholesterol

Strawberry Pie

This comes from my mother, who sent it to me when she heard we'd been berry picking.

3 cups (510 g) strawberries, sliced

one prepared piecrust

1 cup (235 ml) water

2 tablespoons (16 g) cornstarch

$^1/_2$ cup (100 g) sugar

one 3-ounce (85 g) box sugar-free strawberry gelatin

Put sliced berries in piecrust. Combine water, cornstarch, and sugar. Heat until sugar is melted and mixture is clear. Stir in gelatin and pour over berries. Chill until set.

Yield: 8 servings

Per serving: 79 calories (2% from fat, 5% from protein, 93% from carbohydrate); 1 g protein; 0 g total fat;

0 g saturated fat; 0 g monounsaturated fat; 0 g polyunsaturated fat; 19 g carbohydrate; 1 g fiber; 15 g sugar; 30 mg phosphorus; 10 mg calcium; 0 mg iron; 4 mg sodium; 88 mg potassium; 7 IU vitamin A; 0 mg ATE vitamin E; 34 mg vitamin C; 0 mg cholesterol; 82 g water

Tip: The sugar-free gelatin has quite a bit less sodium than the regular.

Strawberry Rhubarb Pie Filling

Great pie filling, or use as a topping for ice cream or pudding. (Or pancakes, if it's time for breakfast.)

2 cups chopped rhubarb

2 cups (340 g) slightly chopped strawberries

$^1/_2$ cup (100 g) sugar

3 tablespoons (24 g) cornstarch

Place fruit and sugar in bowl and let stand 15 minutes, stirring occasionally. Stir in cornstarch. Cook and stir until mixture is thickened and bubbly.

Yield: 8 servings

Per serving: 79 g water; 86 calories (1% from fat, 2% from protein, 96% from carb); 1 g protein; 0 g total fat; 0 g saturated fat; 0 g monounsaturated fat; 0 g polyunsaturated fat; 22 g carbohydrate; 2 g fiber; 15 g sugar; 12 mg phosphorus; 35 mg calcium; 0 mg iron; 3 mg sodium; 170 mg potassium; 56 IU vitamin A; 0 mg vitamin E; 25 mg vitamin C; 0 mg cholesterol

Cranberry Orange Ring

A molded dessert or salad that goes well with chicken, turkey, or ham.

2 oranges

6 ounces (170 g) strawberry-flavored gelatin, such as Jell-O

1¹/₂ cups (355 ml) boiling water

1¹/₂ cups (415 g) jellied cranberry sauce

1 tablespoon orange peel

²/₃ cup (74 g) chopped pecans

Section oranges. Finely dice and drain sections. Dissolve gelatin in boiling water. Stir cranberry sauce until smooth; blend into gelatin with orange peel. Chill until slightly thick, then fold in diced oranges and pecans. Pour into 5-cup ring mold. Chill until firm. Unmold.

Yield: 8 servings

Per serving: 117 g water; 245 calories (23% from fat, 5% from protein, 72% from carb); 3 g protein; 7 g total fat; 1 g saturated fat; 4 g monounsaturated fat; 2 g polyunsaturated fat; 46 g carbohydrate; 3 g fiber; 43 g sugar; 65 mg phosphorus; 30 mg calcium; 0 mg iron; 115 mg sodium; 138 mg potassium; 134 IU vitamin A; 0 mg vitamin E; 27 mg vitamin C; 0 mg cholesterol

Pear Pie

Delicious as is or with a little dollop of whipped topping.

1¹/₃ cup whole wheat flour

¹/₃ cup canola oil

2 tablespoons cold water

¹/₂ cup (100 g) sugar

3 tablespoons (24 g) flour

1 teaspoon cinnamon

1 teaspoon lemon peel

5 cups pears, peeled and sliced

1 tablespoon unsalted butter

1 tablespoon (15 ml) lemon juice

Add oil to flour and mix well with fork. Sprinkle water over and mix well. With hands press into ball and flatten. Roll between two pieces in waxed paper. Remove top waxed paper, invert over pan, and remove other paper. Press into place. Combine sugar, flour, cinnamon, and lemon peel in mixing bowl. Arrange pears in layers in the prepared crust, sprinkling sugar mixture over each layer. Dot with butter. Sprinkle with lemon juice. Bake at 450°F (230°C) for 10 minutes. Reduce temperature to 350°F (175°C), and bake for an additional 35 to 40 minutes.

Yield: 8 servings

Per serving: 80 g water; 281 calories (34% from fat, 5% from protein, 62% from carb); 3 g protein; 11 g total fat; 2 g saturated fat; 6 g monounsaturated fat; 3 g polyunsaturated fat; 4 g carbohydrate; 6 g fiber; 23 g sugar; 84 mg phosphorus; 216 mg calcium; 0 mg iron; 2 mg sodium; 212 mg potassium; 71 IU vitamin A; 12 mg vitamin E; 6 mg vitamin C; 4 mg cholesterol

Crumb-Topped Cherry Cobbler

A quick and easy cobbler recipe, low in fat.

21-ounce (595-g) can cherry pie filling

2 tablespoons (28 g) unsalted butter

$^1/_2$ cup (40 g) quick-cooking oats

$^1/_4$ cup (30 g) flour

$^1/_2$ cup (100 g) sugar

2 tablespoons (16 g) chopped pecans

Preheat oven to 350°F (180°C, or gas mark 4). Spray a 2-quart (1.9-L) casserole dish with nonstick vegetable oil spray. Pour cherry pie filling into prepared dish. Mix butter, oats, flour, sugar, and pecans. Crumble over cherry pie filling. Bake for 20 to 25 minutes.

Yield: 8 servings

Per serving: 205 calories (19% from fat, 3% from protein, 77% from carbohydrate); 2 g protein; 4 g total fat; 3 g saturated fat; 1 g monounsaturated fat; 0 g polyunsaturated fat; 40 g carbohydrate; 1 g fiber; 13 g sugar; 46 mg phosphorus; 15 mg calcium; 1 mg iron; 44 mg sodium; 111 mg potassium; 303 IU vitamin A; 34 mg ATE vitamin E; 3 mg vitamin C; 6 mg cholesterol; 55 g water

Ambrosia

A lighter dessert, the sort of refreshing end you might want with a heavy meal or something like a spicy curry. But it still contains 5 grams of fiber per serving.

4 cups orange slices

2 cups (300 g) sliced banana

1 cup (110 g) coarsely chopped pecans

2 ounces (57 g) coconut

In a large glass bowl, arrange alternate layers of orange slices, banana, pecans, and coconut. Sprinkle a small amount of orange juice between layers if desired. Repeat layers. Chill several hours.

Yield: 8 servings

Per serving: 122 g water; 218 calories (47% from fat, 5% from protein, 48% from carb); 3 g protein; 12 g total fat; 3 g saturated fat; 6 g monounsaturated fat; 3 g polyunsaturated fat; 28 g carbohydrate; 5 g fiber; 16 g sugar; 70 mg phosphorus; 49 mg calcium; 1 mg iron; 2 mg sodium; 443 mg potassium; 246 IU vitamin A; 0 mg vitamin E; 53 mg vitamin C; 0 mg cholesterol

Hawaiian Fruit Salad

The little extras in the dressing for this salad, like lime juice and crystallized ginger, are what really make it special.

2 cups (310 g) diced pineapple

1 cup (170 g) diced honeydew melon

1 cup (175 g) diced mango

2 tablespoons (28 ml) lime juice

2 tablespoons (40 g) honey

1 tablespoon chopped fresh cilantro

1 tablespoon minced crystallized ginger

$^1/_2$ cup (75 g) minced red bell pepper

1 tablespoon sesame seeds

Mix all ingredients except sesame seeds in large bowl. Let stand 10 minutes for flavors to blend. Divide fruit mixture among wine glasses and sprinkle with sesame seeds.

Yield: 6 servings

Per serving: 139 g water; 110 calories (8% from fat, 4% from protein, 88% from carb); 1 g protein; 1 g total fat; 0 g saturated fat; 0 g monounsaturated fat; 0 g polyunsaturated fat; 27 g carbohydrate; 2 g fiber; 24 g sugar; 27 mg phosphorus; 34 mg calcium; 1 mg iron; 8 mg sodium; 256 mg potassium; 679 IU vitamin A; 0 mg vitamin E; 37 mg vitamin C; 0 mg cholesterol

Tropical Twist

A light, but still satisfying, dessert full of fruit and other good things.

2 oranges

2 cups (300 g) sliced banana

2 kiwifruits, peeled, sliced

10 ounces (280 g) miniature marshmallows

1 $^1/_2$ cups (345 g) sour cream

$^1/_4$ cup (85 g) honey

$^1/_2$ teaspoon vanilla extract

$^1/_3$ cup (27 g) coconut, toasted

$^1/_4$ cup (27 g) slivered almonds

From 1 orange, grate $^1/_2$ teaspoon peel and section oranges. Place in large bowl with banana and kiwifruit. Stir in next 4 ingredients; toss to coat well. Spoon into 4 dessert bowls. Top with coconut and almonds.

Yield: 8 servings

Per serving: 146 g water; 332 calories (23% from fat, 5% from protein, 72% from carb); 4 g protein; 9 g total fat; 5 g saturated fat; 3 g monounsaturated fat; 1 g polyunsaturated fat; 63 g carbohydrate; 4 g fiber; 43 g sugar; 97 mg phosphorus; 90 mg calcium; 1 mg iron; 49 mg sodium; 464 mg potassium; 328 IU vitamin A; 45 mg vitamin E; 51 mg vitamin C; 18 mg cholesterol

Winter Fruit Bowl

Great blending of fruit flavors, with the tartness of the grapefruit and cranberries offset by the sweetness of the banana and marmalade.

2 grapefruits

$^1/_2$ cup (100 g) sugar

$^1/_4$ cup (75 g) orange marmalade

1 cup (100 g) cranberries, fresh or frozen

1 $^1/_2$ cups (225 g) sliced banana

Section grapefruit. Reserve juice and add water to make 1 cup (235 ml). Combine juice with sugar and marmalade. Heat to boiling. Stir to dissolve sugar. Add cranberries; cook and stir until skins pop, 5 to 8 minutes. Cool. Add grapefruit, cover, and chill. Add sliced banana just before serving.

Yield: 5 servings

Per serving: 180 g water; 295 calories (2% from fat, 2% from protein, 96% from carb); 2 g protein; 1 g total fat; 0 g saturated fat; 0 g monounsaturated fat; 0 g polyunsaturated fat; 77 g carbohydrate; 5 g fiber; 63 g sugar; 28 mg phosphorus; 28 mg calcium; 0 mg iron; 10 mg sodium; 442 mg potassium; 1284 IU vitamin A; 0 mg vitamin E; 52 mg vitamin C; 0 mg cholesterol

Creamy Fruit Salad

Easy to prepare . . . and fruit salads are always enjoyed.

14 ounces (397 g) pineapple chunks, in juice

11 ounces (310 g) mandarin oranges, undrained

1 cup (150 g) sliced banana

1 cup (145 g) halved strawberries

³/₄ cup (113 g) halved seedless green grapes

1 cup (145 g) blueberries, fresh or frozen and thawed

3¹/₂ ounces (100 g) instant vanilla pudding mix

¹/₂ cup (41 g) granola

Drain chunk pineapple and orange segments, reserving liquid in small bowl. In large bowl, combine banana, strawberries, grapes, and blueberries. Sprinkle pudding mix into reserved liquid; mix until combined and slightly thickened. Fold into fruit until well combined. Spoon into serving dishes. Garnish with granola.

Yield: 8 servings

Per serving: 142 g water; 144 calories (4% from fat, 4% from protein, 93% from carb); 1 g protein; 1 g total fat; 0 g saturated fat; 0 g monounsaturated fat; 0 g polyunsaturated fat; 36 g carbohydrate; 3 g fiber; 28 g sugar; 121 mg phosphorus; 22 mg calcium; 1 mg iron; 201 mg sodium; 291 mg potassium; 390 IU vitamin A; 0 mg vitamin E; 33 mg vitamin C; 0 mg cholesterol

Brandied Fruit

The flavor of this develops more and more over time. Use over ice cream, pound cake, or just as a little special snack.

15 ounces (425 g) pineapple chunks, drained

16 ounces (455 g) canned sliced peaches, drained

16 ounces (455 g) canned apricot halves, drained

10 ounces (280 g) maraschino cherries, drained

1¹/₄ cups (250 g) sugar

1¹/₄ cups (295 ml) brandy

Combine all ingredients in a clean, nonmetal bowl; stir gently. Cover and let stand at room temperature for 3 weeks, stirring fruit twice a week. Serve fruit over ice cream or pound cake, reserving at least 1 cup starter at all times. To replenish starter, add 1 cup sugar and 1 of the first 4 ingredients every 1 to 3 weeks, alternating fruits each time; stir gently. Cover and let stand at room temperature 3 days before using.

Yield: 12 servings

Per serving: 126 g water; 224 calories (1% from fat, 2% from protein, 98% from carb); 1 g protein; 0 g total fat; 0 g saturated fat; 0 g monounsaturated fat; 0 g polyunsaturated fat; 43 g carbohydrate; 2 g fiber; 41 g sugar; 17 mg phosphorus; 25 mg calcium; 0 mg iron; 4 mg sodium; 161 mg potassium; 807 IU vitamin A; 0 mg vitamin E; 6 mg vitamin C; 0 mg cholesterol

Pumpkin Custard

This is basically a pumpkin pie without the crust. This recipe is also a little less sweet than most pies.

2 eggs

1 tablespoon sugar

1 cup (235 ml) skim milk

2 cups (490 g) pumpkin, cooked or canned

1 teaspoon cinnamon

1 teaspoon ginger

Beat the eggs and combine with the sugar. Add the milk and pumpkin and mix well. Add the spices and pour into an 8-inch (20-cm) pie pan. Bake in a moderate oven for 50 to 60 minutes. Test by inserting a knife near the edge. When it comes out clean, the custard is finished. Cut into 6 equal portions when chilled. This custard will keep the pie-wedge shape without a crust.

Yield: 6 servings

Per serving: 125 g water; 81 calories (23% from fat, 23% from protein, 54% from carb); 5 g protein; 2 g total fat; 1 g saturated fat; 1 g monounsaturated fat; 0 g polyunsaturated fat; 11 g carbohydrate; 3 g fiber; 5 g sugar; 111 mg phosphorus; 94 mg calcium; 2 mg iron; 55 mg sodium; 271 mg potassium; 12885 IU vitamin A; 51 mg vitamin E; 4 mg vitamin C; 80 mg cholesterol

Sweet Potato Pie

You'll be hard pressed to tell the difference between this and pumpkin pie.

For Crust:

$1/3$ cup (80 ml) canola oil

$1^1/3$ cups (165 g) flour

2 tablespoons (30 ml) cold water

For Filling:

2 cups (650 g) cooked and mashed sweet potatoes

$3/4$ cup (150 g) sugar

$1/2$ teaspoon (0.9 g) ground ginger

$1/2$ teaspoon (1.1 g) nutmeg

$1/2$ teaspoon (1.2 g) cinnamon

2 eggs

$1^1/2$ cups (355 ml) fat-free evaporated milk

1 teaspoon (5 ml) vanilla

Preheat oven to 400°F (200°C, or gas mark 6).

To make the crust: Add oil to flour and mix well with a fork. Sprinkle water over and mix well. With your hands, press dough into a ball and flatten. Roll between two pieces of waxed paper. Remove the top piece of waxed paper, invert over pie plate, and remove the other piece of waxed paper. Press into place.

To make the filling: Combine sweet potatoes, sugar, ginger, nutmeg, and cinnamon in a mixing bowl. Add eggs and mix well. Add milk and vanilla and combine. Pour into pie shell. Bake for 45 to 50 minutes, or until knife inserted near the center comes out clean.

Yield: 8 servings

Per serving: 345 calories (26% from fat, 10% from protein, 64% from carbohydrate); 9 g protein; 10 g total fat; 1 g saturated fat; 3 g monounsaturated fat; 5 g polyunsaturated fat; 55 g carbohydrate; 3 g fiber; 29 g sugar; 162 mg phosphorus; 175 mg calcium; 2 mg iron; 106 mg sodium; 426 mg potassium; 13153 IU vitamin A; 57 mg ATE vitamin E; 11 mg vitamin C; 52 mg cholesterol; 123 g water

Sweet Potato Pudding

Coconut milk gives this pudding its unique flavor. You should be able to find it in the baking aisle of many large supermarkets.

4 cups (1.3 kg) cooked and mashed sweet potatoes

$3/4$ cup (150 g) sugar

2 eggs, beaten

$1/2$ cup (120 ml) coconut milk

1 tablespoon (15 ml) lime juice

$1/4$ cup (60 ml) rum

$1/2$ teaspoon (2.3 g) baking powder

$1/2$ teaspoon (1.2 g) cinnamon

$1/4$ cup (40 g) raisins

Preheat oven to 350°F (180°C, or gas mark 4). To mashed potatoes, alternate adding sugar and eggs, mixing well after each addition. Add coconut milk. Blend well. Mix in lime juice and rum. Mix well. Combine baking powder and cinnamon and add to potato mixture, along with raisins. Mix well. Pour mixture into a greased tube cake or Bundt pan and bake for 50 minutes, or until done.

Yield: 8 servings

Per serving: 271 calories (13% from fat, 7% from protein, 80% from carbohydrate); 5 g protein; 4 g total fat; 3 g saturated fat; 0 g monounsaturated fat; 0 g polyunsaturated fat; 53 g carbohydrate; 4 g fiber; 31 g sugar; 97 mg phosphorus; 77 mg calcium; 2 mg iron; 105 mg sodium; 502 mg potassium; 25871 IU vitamin A; 0 mg ATE vitamin E; 22 mg vitamin C; 25 mg cholesterol; 162 g water

Ribbon Fruit Mold

This makes a mold that is not only tasty, but very pretty with its different-colored layers.

Raspberry Layer:

1 cup (235 ml) boiling water

3 ounces (85 g) raspberry gelatin

10 ounces (284 g) frozen raspberries

Orange Layer:

1 cup (235 ml) boiling water

3 ounces (85 g) orange gelatin

8 ounces (225 g) cream cheese, softened

11 ounces (310 g) mandarin oranges

Lime Layer:

1 cup (235 ml) boiling water

3 ounces (85 g) lime gelatin

1 cup (155 g) crushed pineapple with syrup

Raspberry layer: Pour boiling water on raspberry gelatin in large bowl. Stir until gelatin is dissolved. Stir in frozen raspberries. Chill until thickened. Pour into 9 × 13 × 2-inch (23 × 33 × 5-cm) baking pan.

Chill until almost firm. Orange layer: Pour boiling water on orange gelatin in large bowl. Stir until gelatin is dissolved. Stir gradually into cream cheese. Chill until thickened slightly. Mix in orange segments (with syrup). Pour evenly on raspberry layer. Chill. Lime layer: Pour boiling water on lime gelatin in a large bowl. Stir until gelatin is dissolved. Stir in pineapple (with syrup). Chill slightly. Pour over orange layer. Chill until firm.

Yield: 8 servings

Per serving: 196 g water; 270 calories (33% from fat, 8% from protein, 60% from carb); 5 g protein; 10 g total fat; 6 g saturated fat; 3 g monounsaturated fat; 1 g polyunsaturated fat; 42 g carbohydrate; 3 g fiber; 37 g sugar; 91 mg phosphorus; 44 mg calcium; 1 mg iron; 238 mg sodium; 175 mg potassium; 737 IU vitamin A; 102 mg vitamin E; 25 mg vitamin C; 31 mg cholesterol

Dessert Pizza

We've made this several times for kids' parties, and it is always one of the most popular items. By the way, grown-ups seem to like it too.

$^1/_2$ cup (112 g) unsalted butter

$^3/_4$ cup (170 g) brown sugar

1 egg yolk

1 teaspoon (5 ml) vanilla

$1^1/_2$ cups (185 g) flour

$1^1/_4$ cups (220 g) chocolate chips

$1^1/_2$ cups (75 g) miniature marshmallows

$^1/_2$ cup (75 g) dry-roasted peanuts, chopped

Preheat oven to 350°F (180°C, or gas mark 4). Beat the butter in a large mixing bowl with an electric mixer on medium-high speed for 30 seconds. Add brown sugar and beat until combined. Beat in egg yolk and vanilla until combined. Beat in as much of the flour as you can with the mixer. Stir in any remaining flour with a wooden spoon. Spread dough in a lightly greased 12-inch (30-cm) pizza pan. Bake for 25 minutes, or until golden. Sprinkle hot crust with the chocolate chips. Let stand for 1 to 2 minutes to soften. Spread chocolate over crust. Sprinkle with marshmallows and nuts. Bake for 3 minutes more or until marshmallows are puffed and beginning to brown. Cool in pan on a wire rack.

Yield: 16 servings

Per serving: 247 calories (44% from fat, 6% from protein, 50% from carbohydrate); 4 g protein; 12 g total fat; 7 g saturated fat; 3 g monounsaturated fat; 0 g polyunsaturated fat; 32 g carbohydrate; 1 g fiber; 20 g sugar; 67 mg phosphorus; 44 mg calcium; 1 mg iron; 81 mg sodium; 135 mg potassium; 338 IU vitamin A; 79 mg ATE vitamin E; 0 mg vitamin C; 26 mg cholesterol; 4 g water

Fruit Soup

A cool, refreshing soup. This is another of those recipes where you can pick and choose the ingredients to get your favorites.

24 ounces (709 ml) grapefruit juice

16 ounces (455 g) plums

16 ounces (455 g) canned apricots, drained

20 ounces (567 g) frozen raspberries

$^1/_4$ cup (38 g) quick-cooking tapioca

2 cinnamon sticks

6 whole cloves

3 cups (450 g) sliced banana

In a large pan, combine all ingredients except banana. Cook slowly 30 minutes or until heated through. Can be served hot or cold. Ladle soup into bowls. Top with sliced banana or strawberries.

Yield: 16 servings

Per serving: 87 g water; 70 calories (4% from fat, 6% from protein, 90% from carb); 1 g protein; 0 g total fat; 0 g saturated fat; 0 g monounsaturated fat; 0 g polyunsaturated fat; 17 g carbohydrate; 4 g fiber; 10 g sugar; 25 mg phosphorus; 14 mg calcium; 0 mg iron; 2 mg sodium; 251 mg potassium; 518 IU vitamin A; 0 mg vitamin E; 14 mg vitamin C; 0 mg cholesterol

Baked Stuffed Peaches

The coconut-almond flavor of macaroons just seems to go with peaches. So here we combine the two in a treat of a dessert.

6 peaches, peeled and halved

$1/2$ cup (100 g) sugar

$1/2$ pound (225 g) macaroons, crushed (about 2 cups crumbs)

4 egg yolks

Scoop out about 1 teaspoon of the center pulp of each peach half. Mash pulp; mix with sugar, macaroon crumbs, and egg yolks. Place halves close together, cut side up, in baking dish, about 8 × 12

inches (20 × 30 cm), coated with nonstick vegetable oil spray. Spoon macaroon mixture into center of each. Bake in a slow 300°F (150°C, gas mark 2) oven for 30 minutes, or until peaches are tender.

Yield: 6 servings

Per serving: 141 g water; 329 calories (26% from fat, 8% from protein, 66% from carb); 7 g protein; 10 g total fat; 6 g saturated fat; 2 g monounsaturated fat; 1 g polyunsaturated fat; 57 g carbohydrate; 3 g fiber; 55 g sugar; 106 mg phosphorus; 29 mg calcium; 1 mg iron; 156 mg sodium; 351 mg potassium; 647 IU vitamin A; 59 mg vitamin E; 9 mg vitamin C; 140 mg cholesterol

Tip: Serve these stuffed peaches warm. You might offer cream for those who don't count calories.

Fruit Pizza

A great dessert for a kids' party, but also popular with older people.

20 ounces (570 g) sugar cookie dough

8 ounces (225 g) cream cheese

$1/3$ cup (67 g) sugar

$1/2$ teaspoon vanilla extract

2 cups (300 g) sliced banana

3 kiwifruits, sliced

1 pound (455 g) strawberries, sliced

1 cup (145 g) blueberries

$1/2$ cup (160 g) peach preserves

2 tablespoons (28 ml) water

Freeze dough for 1 hour. Line a 14-inch (36-cm) pizza pan with foil. Slice dough $1/8$ inch (0.3 cm) thick and line pan; overlap slices but don't flatten into pan. Bake at 375°F (190°C, gas mark 5) for 12 minutes or until browned. Cool completely. Invert crust onto another pan, remove foil, and put on serving plate. Combine cream cheese, sugar, and vanilla until blended. Spread on crust; arrange fruit. Put preserves and water in bowl and stir to glaze-like consistency. Pour over fruit; chill.

Yield: 14 servings

Per serving: 99 g water; 341 calories (37% from fat, 4% from protein, 59% from carb); 4 g protein; 14 g total fat; 6 g saturated fat; 6 g monounsaturated fat; 1 g polyunsaturated fat; 51 g carbohydrate; 3 g fiber; 27 g sugar; 110 mg phosphorus; 62 mg calcium; 1 mg iron; 224 mg sodium; 322 mg potassium; 280 IU vitamin A; 63 mg vitamin E; 42 mg vitamin C; 30 mg cholesterol

Fruit with Amaretto Cream

For those times when you are looking for something a little fancier for dessert.

1 1/2 tablespoons Amaretto liqueur

2 tablespoons (30 g) packed brown sugar

1/2 cup (115 g) sour cream

1 cup (145 g) strawberries, halved

1 cup (145 g) blueberries

1 cup (150 g) seedless green grapes

In small mixing bowl, combine Amaretto and brown sugar. Add sour cream and mix well. Prepare at least 2 hours before serving; stir occasionally to dissolve

brown sugar. Put fruit into sherbet glasses or small soufflé dishes. Drizzle with sauce.

Yield: 4 servings

Per serving: 111 g water; 134 calories (32% from fat, 5% from protein, 63% from carb); 2 g protein; 5 g total fat; 3 g saturated fat; 1 g monounsaturated fat; 0 g polyunsaturated fat; 21 g carbohydrate; 2 g fiber; 17 g sugar; 49 mg phosphorus; 50 mg calcium; 0 mg iron; 22 mg sodium; 195 mg potassium; 196 IU vitamin A; 40 mg vitamin E; 27 mg vitamin C; 15 mg cholesterol

Date Apple Waldorf Salad

Another fruity, sweet dessert. This is the kind of thing that kids love (and older people, too).

1 orange

2 cups (300 g) diced unpeeled apple

1/2 cup (75 g) dates, snipped

1/2 cup (50 g) chopped celery

1/3 cup (40 g) chopped walnuts

1/4 cup (60 g) mayonnaise

1 tablespoon sugar

3/4 cup (56 g) whipped dessert topping (such as Cool-Whip), thawed

Peel orange; section over bowl to catch juices. Halve sections and reserve 1 tablespoon juice. In medium bowl, combine apple, dates, celery, walnuts, and orange sections. Blend together mayonnaise, sugar, and reserved orange juice. Fold in the whipped dessert topping; combine with date mixture.

Yield: 6 servings

Per serving: 76 g water; 211 calories (53% from fat, 5% from protein, 42% from carb); 3 g protein; 13 g total fat; 2 g saturated fat; 3 g monounsaturated fat; 6 g polyunsaturated fat; 24 g carbohydrate; 3 g fiber; 19 g sugar; 64 mg phosphorus; 37 mg calcium; 0 mg iron; 69 mg sodium; 258 mg potassium; 202 IU vitamin A; 21 mg vitamin E; 18 mg vitamin C; 9 mg cholesterol

24

Grain, Nut, and Legume Desserts

Sometimes you want a "real" dessert, say cake or pie. This chapter has a number of cakes, featuring lower fat versions of some traditional favorites. It also contains some healthier recipes for piecrusts and some puddings and rice dishes. And then there are the bean pies. Yes, it is a pie whose filling is made primarily from navy beans. You need to try it, because it's the kind of thing that just reading about doesn't do justice to.

Apple Cake

Everyone wants something sweet every once in a while. But that doesn't mean that it can't still be good for you. Whole wheat flour and apples bump up the nutrition and fiber levels of this cake, but the taste just says "good."

2¼ cups (270 g) whole wheat pastry flour

1 cup (200 g) sugar

¾ cup (170 g) packed brown sugar

1 tablespoon cinnamon

2 teaspoons baking powder

½ teaspoon baking soda

¾ cup (175 ml) canola oil

1 teaspoon vanilla extract

3 eggs

2 cups (250 g) finely chopped apple

1 cup (120 g) chopped walnuts

¼ cup (25 g) confectioners' sugar, sifted

Generously grease and flour a 10-inch (25-cm) fluted tube pan; set aside. In a large mixing bowl combine the flour, sugars, cinnamon, baking powder, and baking soda. Add oil, vanilla, and the eggs; beat until well mixed. Stir in the chopped apple and walnuts. Spoon batter evenly into prepared pan. Bake in a 350°F (180°C, gas mark 4) oven for 45 to 50 minutes, or until cake tests done. Cool in pan 12 minutes; invert cake onto a wire rack. Cool thoroughly. Sprinkle with confectioners' sugar.

Yield: 16 servings

Per serving: 22 g water; 317 calories (45% from fat, 7% from protein, 48% from carb); 6 g protein; 17 g total fat; 1 g saturated fat; 8 g monounsaturated fat; 6 g polyunsaturated fat; 40 g carbohydrate; 3 g fiber; 26 g sugar; 135 mg phosphorus; 65 mg calcium; 2 mg iron; 81 mg sodium; 174 mg potassium; 62 IU vitamin A; 15 mg vitamin E; 1 mg vitamin C; 44 mg cholesterol

Applesauce Date Cake

Further proof that something sweet and delicious can still have significant nutritional value. This cake keeps well and is great for snacks or with lunches.

2 cups (240 g) whole wheat pastry flour

2 teaspoons baking soda

1 teaspoon cinnamon

½ teaspoon allspice

½ teaspoon nutmeg

¼ teaspoon cloves

2 eggs

1 cup (225 g) packed brown sugar

½ cup (112 g) unsalted butter, softened

2 cups applesauce, divided

1 cup (145 g) chopped dates

¾ cup (84 g) coarsely chopped pecans

Preheat oven to 350°F (180°C, gas mark 4). Spray a 9 × 9 × 2-inch (23 × 23 × 5-cm) pan with nonstick vegetable oil spray. Stir together flour, baking soda, and spices. Add eggs, brown sugar, butter, and 1 cup applesauce. Beat at low speed just until the ingredients are combined. At medium speed, beat 2 minutes longer, occasionally scraping the side of the bowl. Add remaining applesauce, dates, and pecans; beat 1 minute. Pour batter into pan. Bake 50 minutes or until knife inserted in center comes out clean. Cool 10 minutes in pan.

Yield: 12 servings

Per serving: 48 g water; 341 calories (35% from fat, 6% from protein, 59% from carb); 5 g protein; 14 g total fat; 6 g saturated fat; 5 g monounsaturated fat; 2 g polyunsaturated fat; 53 g carbohydrate; 5 g fiber; 35 g sugar; 125 mg phosphorus; 45 mg calcium; 2 mg iron; 24 mg sodium; 313 mg potassium; 295 IU vitamin A; 76 mg vitamin E; 1 mg vitamin C; 60 mg cholesterol

Chocolate Cherry Cake

This is a great special occasion cake (Valentine's Day comes immediately to mind).

2 cups (240 g) whole wheat pastry flour

$1^{1}/_{2}$ cups (300 g) sugar

$1^{1}/_{4}$ teaspoons baking soda

1 teaspoon baking powder

3 tablespoons nonfat dry milk powder

$^{2}/_{3}$ cup (135 g) shortening

$^{1}/_{3}$ cup (30 g) cocoa powder

1 can cherry pie filling

2 eggs

1 teaspoon almond extract

Combine all ingredients. Pour into greased and floured 13 × 9-inch (33 × 23-cm) pan. Bake at 350°F (180°C, gas mark 4) until done, about 30 minutes.

Yield: 16 servings

Per serving: 34 g water; 260 calories (33% from fat, 5% from protein, 62% from carb); 4 g protein; 10 g total fat; 3 g saturated fat; 4 g monounsaturated fat; 2 g polyunsaturated fat; 42 g carbohydrate; 3 g fiber; 19 g sugar; 98 mg phosphorus; 42 mg calcium; 1 mg iron; 52 mg sodium; 151 mg potassium; 131 IU vitamin A; 15 mg vitamin E; 1 mg vitamin C; 30 mg cholesterol

Irish Apple Cake

I was searching for Irish dessert recipes last St. Patrick's Day and came across one similar to this one. It's like a half cake/half pie and absolutely delicious.

$^{1}/_{4}$ pound (113 g) unsalted butter

$1^{3}/_{4}$ cups (210 g) whole wheat pastry flour

$^{1}/_{4}$ teaspoon baking powder

$^{1}/_{2}$ cup (100 g) sugar

1 egg, beaten

$^{1}/_{2}$ cup (120 ml) skim milk

2 apples

1 tablespoon sugar

$^{1}/_{2}$ teaspoon ground cloves

Cut butter into flour and baking powder to make dry crumbs. Add sugar, beaten egg, and enough milk to make a soft dough. Divide dough in two. Roll one half into a circle to fit an ovenproof plate coated with nonstick vegetable oil spray. Peel and core apples. Slice them onto the dough and add sugar and cloves. Roll out the remaining pastry and fit on top. Press the sides together; cut a slit through the lid. Bake at 350°F (180°C, gas mark 4) about 40 minutes, or until apples are cooked through and the pastry is nicely browned.

Yield: 6 servings

Per serving: 69 g water; 370 calories (40% from fat, 7% from protein, 53% from carb); 7 g protein; 17 g total fat; 10 g saturated fat; 4 g monounsaturated fat; 1 g polyunsaturated fat; 51 g carbohydrate; 5 g fiber; 23 g sugar; 176 mg phosphorus; 65 mg calcium; 2 mg iron; 50 mg sodium; 237 mg potassium; 580 IU vitamin A; 152 mg vitamin E; 2 mg vitamin C; 81 mg cholesterol

Low Fat Apple Cake

This recipe originally came from my mother. It was one of my favorites for years. I reduced the fat by replacing the oil in the original recipe with applesauce.

1 cup (235 ml) applesauce

2 cups (400 g) sugar

3 eggs

2$^1/_2$ cups (310 g) flour

2 teaspoons (9.2 g) baking powder

1 teaspoon (4.6 g) baking soda

$^1/_2$ teaspoon (1.2 g) cinnamon

$^1/_2$ teaspoon (1.1 g) nutmeg

1 teaspoon (5 ml) vanilla

3 cups (450 g) apples, peeled and chopped

Preheat oven to 350°F (180°C, or gas mark 4). Mix applesauce and sugar together, add eggs. Sift together flour, baking powder, baking soda, cinnamon, and nutmeg; add to sugar mixture. Stir in vanilla; fold in apples. Pour into 9 × 13-inch (23 × 33-cm) pan. Bake for 1 to 1$^1/_2$ hours, or until knife

inserted in center comes out clean. Dust top with powdered sugar, if desired.

Yield: 24 servings

Per serving: 131 calories (3% from fat, 7% from protein, 90% from carbohydrate); 2 g protein; 0 g total fat; 0 g saturated fat; 0 g monounsaturated fat; 0 g polyunsaturated fat; 30 g carbohydrate; 1 g fiber; 19 g sugar; 34 mg phosphorus; 30 mg calcium; 1 mg iron; 107 mg sodium; 61 mg potassium; 37 IU vitamin A; 0 mg ATE vitamin E; 1 mg vitamin C; 25 mg cholesterol; 29 g water

Low Fat Cranberry Cake

When I first came across a version of this recipe it sounded so good that I had to try it. Of course, the original was full of fat and sodium, but we've solved that problem with no loss of taste.

2 cups (220 g) cranberries

1$^3/_4$ cups (350 g) sugar, divided

$^1/_2$ cup (120 ml) water

1 cup (125 g) flour

1$^1/_2$ teaspoons (7 g) baking powder

$^1/_2$ cup (120 ml) applesauce

1 egg

$^1/_4$ cup (60 ml) skim milk

$^1/_4$ cup (60 ml) orange juice

1 teaspoon (1.7 g) orange peel, grated

$^1/_2$ teaspoon (3 ml) vanilla

Preheat oven to 375°F (190°C, or gas mark 5). Spray bottom and sides of a 9-inch (23-cm) round baking pan with nonstick vegetable oil spray. Combine cranberries, 1 cup (200 g) sugar, and water in a large saucepan. Bring to a boil. Reduce heat and simmer for 10 minutes, or until slightly thickened to a syrupy consistency. Pour into prepared pan. Cool to room temperature. Sift together flour, remaining $^3/_4$ cup (150 g) sugar, and baking powder into a large bowl. In another bowl, stir applesauce, egg, milk, orange juice, orange peel, and vanilla until blended. Stir into dry ingredients just until blended. Pour over cranberry mixture. Bake for 25 to 30 minutes, or until a wooden pick inserted in the center comes out clean. Let cake cool in pan about 5 minutes. Loosen cake around edges of pan. Place inverted serving platter over cake and turn both upside down. Shake gently, then remove pan. Serve warm.

Yield: 12 servings

Per serving: 232 calories (2% from fat, 3% from protein, 94% from carbohydrate); 2 g protein; 1 g total fat; 0 g saturated fat; 0 g monounsaturated fat; 0 g polyunsaturated fat; 57 g carbohydrate; 2 g fiber; 44 g sugar; 39 mg phosphorus; 49 mg calcium; 1 mg iron; 75 mg sodium; 64 mg potassium; 35 IU vitamin A; 3 mg ATE vitamin E; 2 mg vitamin C; 17 mg cholesterol; 37 g water

Honey Oatmeal Cake

A great breakfast or snack cake. Of course, I happen to be very fond of the flavor of honey.

1$^1/_4$ cups (295 ml) water, boiling

1 cup (80 g) rolled oats

$^1/_2$ cup (112 g) unsalted butter, softened

1$^1/_2$ cups (510 g) honey

2 eggs

1 teaspoon vanilla extract

1$^3/_4$ cups (210 g) whole wheat pastry flour

1 teaspoon baking soda

1 teaspoon ground cinnamon

$^1/_4$ teaspoon ground nutmeg

Combine first 3 ingredients in a large bowl; stir well. Set aside for 20 minutes. Add honey, eggs, and vanilla; stir well. Combine whole wheat flour and remaining ingredients; gradually add to honey mixture. Pour into a greased and floured 13 × 9 × 2-inch (33 × 23 × 5-cm) baking pan. Bake at 350°F (180°C, gas mark 4) for 30 to 40 minutes or until toothpick comes out clean. Cool in pan. Frost if desired or sprinkle with confectioners' sugar.

Yield: 15 servings

Per serving: 35 g water; 238 calories (27% from fat, 6% from protein, 67% from carb); 4 g protein; 8 g total fat; 4 g saturated fat; 2 g monounsaturated fat; 1 g polyunsaturated fat; 42 g carbohydrate; 2 g fiber; 28 g sugar; 92 mg phosphorus; 18 mg calcium; 1 mg iron; 14 mg sodium; 107 mg potassium; 227 IU vitamin A; 61 mg vitamin E; 0 mg vitamin C; 48 mg cholesterol

Low Fat Devil's Food Cake

This makes a fairly heavy, very moist cake, almost like brownies or bars.

2 cups (250 g) flour

1³/₄ cups (350 g) sugar

¹/₂ cup (43 g) unsweetened cocoa powder

1 tablespoon (13.8 g) baking soda

²/₃ cup (160 ml) applesauce

¹/₃ cup (80 ml) buttermilk

2 tablespoons (30 ml) canola oil

1 cup (235 ml) coffee

Preheat oven to 350°F (180°C, or gas mark 4). Spray a 9 × 13-inch (23 × 33-cm) pan with nonstick vegetable oil spray and then dust with flour, shaking out the excess. In a large bowl, mix together flour, sugar, cocoa, and baking soda. Stir in applesauce, buttermilk, and oil. Heat coffee to boiling and stir into batter. Batter will be thin. Pour into prepared pan. Bake for 35 to 40 minutes, or until a wooden pick inserted in the center comes out clean.

Yield: 24 servings

Per serving: 116 calories (12% from fat, 5% from protein, 83% from carbohydrate); 2 g protein; 2 g total fat; 0 g saturated fat; 1 g monounsaturated fat; 0 g polyunsaturated fat; 25 g carbohydrate; 1 g fiber; 16 g sugar; 28 mg phosphorus; 8 mg calcium; 1 mg iron; 162 mg sodium; 55 mg potassium; 2 IU vitamin A; 0 mg ATE vitamin E; 0 mg vitamin C; 0 mg cholesterol; 20 g water

Lower-Fat Carrot Cake

This is lighter than most carrot cakes, but the flavor is very close to the traditional one.

¹/₄ cup (60 ml) canola oil

³/₄ cup (180 ml) applesauce

¹/₂ cup (120 ml) skim milk

1¹/₂ cups (300 g) sugar

3 eggs

2 cups (250 g) flour

4 teaspoons (18.4 g) baking soda

2¹/₂ teaspoons (5.8 g) cinnamon

¹/₂ teaspoon (1.1 g) nutmeg

¹/₂ teaspoon (1.2 g) ground cloves

1¹/₂ teaspoons (8 ml) vanilla

2 cups (260 g) shredded carrot

¹/₂ cup (60 g) chopped walnuts

¹/₂ cup (80 g) raisins

8 ounces (225 g) crushed pineapple, undrained

Preheat oven to 350°F (180°C, or gas mark 4). Coat a rectangular 9 × 13-inch (23 × 33-cm) cake pan with nonstick vegetable oil spray. In one bowl, beat together oil, applesauce, milk, sugar, and eggs. In another bowl, stir together flour, baking soda, cinnamon, nutmeg, and cloves. Combine both sets of ingredients and beat, mixing in vanilla. Add carrots, walnuts, raisins, and pineapple, mixing well after each addition. Bake for 1 hour, or until done. Cool and remove from pan.

Yield: 16 servings

Per serving: 239 calories (24% from fat, 8% from protein, 68% from carbohydrate); 5 g protein; 7 g total fat; 1 g saturated fat; 3 g monounsaturated fat; 3 g polyunsaturated fat; 42 g carbohydrate; 2 g fiber; 27 g sugar; 73 mg phosphorus; 37 mg calcium; 1 mg iron; 353 mg sodium; 206 mg potassium; 2757 IU vitamin A; 5 mg ATE vitamin E; 3 mg vitamin C; 45 mg cholesterol; 55 g water

Orange Zucchini Cake

Moist and sweet, this makes a great snack cake.

1 cup (120 g) whole wheat pastry flour

1 teaspoon baking powder

$^1/_2$ teaspoon baking soda

1 teaspoon ground cinnamon

$^1/_2$ teaspoon ground nutmeg

$^3/_4$ cup (150 g) sugar

$^1/_2$ cup (120 ml) canola oil

2 eggs

$^1/_2$ cup (30 g) all-bran cereal

$1^1/_2$ teaspoons grated orange peel

1 teaspoon vanilla extract

1 cup (113 g) grated zucchini

$^1/_2$ cup (55 g) chopped pecans

$^3/_4$ cup (110 g) raisins

Combine flour, baking powder, baking soda, cinnamon, and nutmeg. Set aside. In large bowl, beat sugar, oil, and eggs until well combined. Stir in cereal, orange peel, and vanilla. Add flour mixture, zucchini, pecans, and raisins. Mix well. Spread evenly in 10 × 6-inch (25 × 15-cm) baking dish coated with nonstick vegetable oil spray. Bake at 325°F (170°C, gas mark 3) for 35 minutes or until wooden pick inserted near center comes out clean. Cool completely.

Yield: 12 servings

Per serving: 20 g water; 252 calories (47% from fat, 6% from protein, 47% from carb); 4 g protein; 14 g total fat; 1 g saturated fat; 8 g monounsaturated fat; 4 g polyunsaturated fat; 31 g carbohydrate; 3 g fiber; 20 g sugar; 118 mg phosphorus; 54 mg calcium; 1 mg iron; 63 mg sodium; 205 mg potassium; 116 IU vitamin A; 27 mg vitamin E; 3 mg vitamin C; 39 mg cholesterol

Pineapple Upside-Down Cake

I hadn't had one of these in many years when I recently made this. Having had the first warm slice, I wondered why.

6 tablespoons (85 g) unsalted butter, divided

$^1/_2$ cup (115 g) dark brown sugar

5 slices pineapple

5 maraschino cherries

$^1/_2$ cup (120 ml) skim milk

1 egg

1 teaspoon vanilla extract

$1^1/_4$ cups (150 g) whole wheat pastry flour

$^1/_2$ cup (100 g) sugar

2 teaspoons baking powder

Preheat the oven to 375°F (190°C, gas mark 5). Melt half of the butter in a heavy cast-iron skillet or ovenproof pan. Add the brown sugar and stir well. Whisk in 2 teaspoons (10 ml) of water. Remove from the heat and add a single layer of pineapple slices. Place a cherry in the middle of each. Set aside. Melt the rest of the butter. Whisk in the milk, egg, and vanilla. Combine the flour, sugar, and baking powder in a separate mixing bowl. Beat the milk mixture into the flour mixture until a smooth batter forms. Pour over the pineapple in the skillet. Bake for 30 to 35 minutes or until the center is firm. Allow to cool for 10 minutes. Invert the pan onto a serving plate. Serve warm or at room temperature.

Yield: 8 servings

Per serving: 49 g water; 278 calories (31% from fat, 6% from protein, 63% from carb); 4 g protein; 10 g total fat; 6 g saturated fat; 3 g monounsaturated fat; 1 g polyunsaturated fat; 45 g carbohydrate; 3 g fiber; 30 g sugar; 124 mg phosphorus; 108 mg calcium; 1 mg iron; 145 mg sodium; 149 mg potassium; 354 IU vitamin A; 92 mg vitamin E; 2 mg vitamin C; 49 mg cholesterol

Red Velvet Cake

This is one of those old-time traditional cakes, updated to provide a little extra fiber by using whole wheat flour.

2$^{1}/_{2}$ cups (300 g) whole wheat pastry flour

1$^{1}/_{2}$ cups (300 g) sugar

2 teaspoons cocoa powder

1 teaspoon baking soda

2 eggs

$^{1}/_{2}$ cup (120 ml) canola oil

$^{1}/_{2}$ cup (120 ml) buttermilk

2 tablespoons (28 ml) red food coloring

1 teaspoon vanilla extract

Icing:

$^{1}/_{4}$ cup (55 g) unsalted butter

4 cups (400 g) confectioners' sugar

$^{1}/_{2}$ teaspoon vanilla extract

8 ounces (225 g) cream cheese

1 cup (110 g) chopped pecans

Mix together the first four ingredients in a large bowl. Blend eggs with a fork, add oil, and blend again. Add the dry ingredients and mix with whisk till smooth. Add and blend in buttermilk, food coloring, and vanilla. Pour into 3 greased and floured 8-inch (20-cm) cake pans. Bake at 350°F (180°C, gas mark 4) for 30 minutes. Cool for 10 minutes and gently remove from pan. Icing: Mix ingredients until light and fluffy.

Yield: 16 servings

Per serving: 23 g water; 457 calories (39% from fat, 6% from protein, 55% from carb); 7 g protein; 20 g total fat; 6 g saturated fat; 9 g monounsaturated fat; 4 g polyunsaturated fat; 65 g carbohydrate; 3 g fiber; 49 g sugar; 137 mg phosphorus; 40 mg calcium; 1 mg iron; 63 mg sodium; 184 mg potassium; 317 IU vitamin A; 85 mg vitamin E; 0 mg vitamin C; 53 mg cholesterol

Easy Pumpkin Cupcakes

Use a cake mix and canned pumpkin pie filling to make these tasty cupcakes quick and easy to prepare.

1 package yellow cake mix

2 cups (490 g) pumpkin pie mix

2 eggs

6 ounces (170 g) butterscotch chips

Mix all ingredients together and place in greased or lined cupcake pan. Bake at 350°F (180°C, gas mark 4) for 15 to 20 minutes.

Yield: 24 servings

Per serving: 20 g water; 65 calories (12% from fat, 5% from protein, 83% from carb); 1 g protein; 1 g total fat; 0 g saturated fat; 0 g monounsaturated fat; 0 g polyunsaturated fat; 14 g carbohydrate; 2 g fiber; 7 g sugar; 19 mg phosphorus; 14 mg calcium; 0 mg iron; 93 mg sodium; 38 mg potassium; 1897 IU vitamin A; 8 mg vitamin E; 1 mg vitamin C; 20 mg cholesterol

Whole Wheat Piecrust

I find this oil-based piecrust easier to work with than crusts with solid shortening. And it seems to stay flaky through more handling.

$^1/_3$ cup (80 ml) canola oil

$1^1/_3$ cups (160 g) whole wheat pastry flour

2 tablespoons (28 ml) water, cold

Add oil to flour and mix well with fork. Sprinkle water over and mix well. With hands press into ball and flatten. Roll between 2 pieces of waxed paper. Remove top waxed paper, invert over pan, and remove other paper. Press into place. For pies that do not require a baked filling, bake at 400°F (200°C, gas mark 6) until lightly browned, about 12 to 15 minutes.

Yield: 8 servings

Per serving: 6 g water; 150 calories (56% from fat, 7% from protein, 37% from carb); 3 g protein; 10 g total fat; 1 g saturated fat; 6 g monounsaturated fat; 3 g polyunsaturated fat; 15 g carbohydrate; 2 g fiber; 0 g sugar; 69 mg phosphorus; 7 mg calcium; 1 mg iron; 1 mg sodium; 81 mg potassium; 2 IU vitamin A; 0 mg vitamin E; 0 mg vitamin C; 0 mg cholesterol

High-Fiber Piecrust

A really simple piecrust with 4 grams of fiber. You can add sugar or other sweeteners or spices like cinnamon depending on the final flavor you want.

1 cup (60 g) lightly sweetened bran cereal, such as Fiber One

$^1/_2$ cup (120 ml) water, approximately

Crush cereal to a powder in a resealable plastic bag. Add any sweetener or spice desired to taste here and shake together. Dump evenly into a 9-inch (23-cm) springform or pie plate. Drizzle a little water at a time just to moisten the crumbs. Spread and press crust evenly. Use as stated in recipe, either baking before or simply pouring filling in, then baking or refrigerating.

Yield: 8 servings

Per serving: 15 g water; 15 calories (8% from fat, 7% from protein, 85% from carb); 1 g protein; 0 g total fat; 0 g saturated fat; 0 g monounsaturated fat; 0 g polyunsaturated fat; 6 g carbohydrate; 4 g fiber; 0 g sugar; 38 mg phosphorus; 25 mg calcium; 1 mg iron; 27 mg sodium; 45 mg potassium; 3 IU vitamin A; 0 mg vitamin E; 2 mg vitamin C; 0 mg cholesterol

Bean Pie

Bean pies were something I'd never heard of until I started looking for ways to add fiber to my diet. It turns out a bean pie is a sweet custard pie whose filling consists of mashed beans, usually navy beans, sugar, butter, milk, and spices. It is similar to a pumpkin pie. Bean pies are commonly associated with soul food or southern cuisine. They are also associated with the Nation of Islam movement: its leader, Elijah Muhammad, encouraged their consumption in lieu of richer foods associated with African American cuisine, and the followers of his community commonly sell bean pies as part of their fund-raising efforts.

3 cups (531 g) cooked great northern beans, drained

3 eggs

1$^{1}/_{4}$ cups (250 g) sugar

$^{1}/_{4}$ cup (55 g) unsalted butter, melted

1 teaspoon vanilla extract

1 teaspoon ground cinnamon

1 teaspoon ground nutmeg

$^{1}/_{4}$ teaspoon ground allspice

1 teaspoon baking powder

$^{1}/_{3}$ cup (80 ml) fat-free evaporated milk

1 piecrust, 9 inch (23 cm), baked, cooled

In mixing bowl with electric mixer, beat the drained beans until smooth. Beat in eggs, sugar, butter, vanilla, cinnamon, nutmeg, and allspice. In a separate bowl, combine baking powder and milk. Add to bean mixture. Beat mixture well to blend; pour into the cooled pie shell. Bake the pie in preheated 350°F (180°C, gas mark 4) oven for 50 minutes, or until set. Let pie cool before slicing.

Yield: 8 servings

Per serving: 99 g water; 441 calories (32% from fat, 11% from protein, 57% from carb); 12 g protein; 16 g total fat; 6 g saturated fat; 6 g monounsaturated fat; 3 g polyunsaturated fat; 64 g carbohydrate; 6 g fiber; 33 g sugar; 224 mg phosphorus; 137 mg calcium; 3 mg iron; 224 mg sodium; 429 mg potassium; 323 IU vitamin A; 89 mg vitamin E; 2 mg vitamin C; 105 mg cholesterol

Pinto Bean Pecan Pie

Like a pecan pie, but with the added fiber boost of a secret ingredient, pinto beans. You won't believe it unless you try it.

$^{1}/_{3}$ cup (75 g) unsalted butter

1 cup (200 g) sugar

$^{2}/_{3}$ cup (150 g) packed brown sugar

3 eggs, slightly beaten

1 cup (171 g) pinto beans, cooked and mashed

$^{1}/_{3}$ cup (37 g) chopped pecans

1 piecrust, unbaked

Preheat oven to 350°F (180°C, gas mark 4). Cream together butter, sugars, and eggs. Add beans and nuts, mix well, and pour into unbaked pie shell. Bake for 35 to 40 minutes.

Yield: 8 servings

Per serving: 25 g water; 493 calories (37% from fat, 8% from protein, 55% from carb); 10 g protein; 21 g total fat; 8 g saturated fat; 8 g monounsaturated fat; 4 g polyunsaturated fat; 69 g carbohydrate; 5 g fiber; 44 g sugar; 173 mg phosphorus; 62 mg calcium; 3 mg iron; 211 mg sodium; 463 mg potassium; 341 IU vitamin A; 93 mg vitamin E; 2 mg vitamin C; 109 mg cholesterol

Lemon Biscotti

These make a nice snack or a quick breakfast with whatever your favorite breakfast beverage is. The double baking gives them the traditional crunchiness.

2¹/₂ cups (310 g) flour

1 teaspoon (4.6 g) baking powder

1 teaspoon (4.6 g) baking soda

4 eggs

³/₄ cup (150 g) sugar

1 tablespoon (5 g) lemon zest

1¹/₂ teaspoons (8 ml) lemon juice

Preheat oven to 325°F (170°C, or gas mark 3). Sift together flour, baking powder, and baking soda. In another bowl, beat eggs and sugar together, then beat in lemon zest and lemon juice. Add flour mixture to egg mixture and stir until well mixed. On a floured surface, knead dough for 2 minutes. Divide dough in half and shape into 2 logs, about 1 inch (2.5 cm) high and 4 inches (10 cm) wide. Bake for 30 minutes, or until golden brown. Remove from oven and cool. Reduce oven temperature to 300°F (150°C, or gas mark 2). Slice logs diagonally into ¹/₂-inch (1.3-cm) thick slices and put slices back on baking sheet, cut side down. Bake for another 20 minutes.

Yield: 24 servings

Per serving: 81 calories (5% from fat, 13% from protein, 82% from carbohydrate); 3 g protein; 0 g total fat; 0 g saturated fat; 0 g monounsaturated fat; 0 g polyunsaturated fat; 16 g carbohydrate; 0 g fiber; 6 g sugar; 31 mg phosphorus; 19 mg calcium; 1 mg iron; 92 mg sodium; 49 mg potassium; 38 IU vitamin A; 0 mg ATE vitamin E; 0 mg vitamin C; 35 mg cholesterol; 11 g water

Tip: If you're not into dunking and want a softer cookie, reduce the second baking time to 10 minutes.

Brown Rice Pudding

Quick rice pudding recipe that uses leftover rice. (I tend to make a lot of rice when I cook it so I can use it in all these recipes calling for leftovers.)

2 cups (440 g) cooked brown rice

1¹/₂ cups (355 ml) skim milk

¹/₂ cup (170 g) honey

1 cup (145 g) golden raisins

1 tablespoon unsalted butter

1 teaspoon cinnamon

In medium saucepan, combine rice, milk, honey, and raisins and bring to boil. Reduce heat and simmer 20 minutes, stirring frequently. Remove from heat and stir in butter and cinnamon.

Yield: 4 servings

Per serving: 168 g water; 426 calories (8% from fat, 7% from protein, 85% from carb); 8 g protein; 4 g total fat; 2 g saturated fat; 1 g monounsaturated fat; 0 g polyunsaturated fat; 96 g carbohydrate; 4 g fiber; 60 g sugar; 235 mg phosphorus; 174 mg calcium; 2 mg iron; 66 mg sodium; 543 mg potassium; 277 IU vitamin A; 80 mg vitamin E; 3 mg vitamin C; 9 mg cholesterol

Cool Rice

A kind of instant rice pudding and similar to the dish served at many family get-togethers during my childhood.

¹/₂ pound (225 g) brown rice

6 ounces (170 g) nondairy whipped topping, such as Cool Whip

1/4 cup (50 g) sugar

1 teaspoon vanilla extract

10 ounces (284 g) crushed pineapple

5 maraschino cherries, halved

Cook rice according to package directions and cool. Combine all ingredients in large bowl.

Yield: 5 servings

Per serving: 106 g water; 217 calories (33% from fat, 4% from protein, 63% from carb); 2 g protein; 8 g total fat; 5 g saturated fat; 2 g monounsaturated fat; 0 g polyunsaturated fat; 35 g carbohydrate; 1 g fiber; 22 g sugar; 72 mg phosphorus; 50 mg calcium; 0 mg iron; 47 mg sodium; 132 mg potassium; 257 IU vitamin A; 63 mg vitamin E; 4 mg vitamin C; 26 mg cholesterol

Cranberry Rice

An alternative to cranberry sauce . . . or just a nice sweet dish for your holiday. This can be used either as a side dish or as a dessert.

2 cups (475 ml) water, divided

1 1/3 cups (267 g) sugar, divided

2 cups (200 g) cranberries

1 1/3 cups (292 g) cooked, cooled brown rice

1/4 teaspoon cinnamon

1 apple, peeled and sliced

In a saucepan combine 1/2 cup (120 ml) of the water and 1 cup (200 g) of the sugar. Bring to boil. Add cranberries, return to boil, reduce heat, and simmer 10 minutes or until most of the berries have popped.

Add rice, cinnamon, and the remaining water and sugar. Bring to boil. Reduce heat, cover, and simmer 5 minutes. Remove from heat and stir in apple. Cover and let stand for 10 minutes.

Yield: 6 servings

Per serving: 161 g water; 249 calories (2% from fat, 2% from protein, 96% from carb); 1 g protein; 0 g total fat; 0 g saturated fat; 0 g monounsaturated fat; 0 g polyunsaturated fat; 62 g carbohydrate; 3 g fiber; 49 g sugar; 43 mg phosphorus; 12 mg calcium; 0 mg iron; 5 mg sodium; 71 mg potassium; 30 IU vitamin A; 0 mg vitamin E; 6 mg vitamin C; 0 mg cholesterol

Date Nut Loaf

A sweet bread that's great for either breakfast or dessert. I like it with a little bit of apple butter.

1 cup (235 ml) water, boiling

1 cup (145 g) chopped dates

1/4 cup (55 g) unsalted butter

1/2 cup (115 g) packed brown sugar

1/4 cup (50 g) sugar

1 egg

1 3/4 cups (210 g) whole wheat pastry flour

1/2 teaspoon baking soda

1/2 teaspoon baking powder

3/4 cup (84 g) coarsely chopped pecans

Preheat oven to 350°F (180°C, gas mark 4). Spray 8 × 4-inch (20 × 10-cm) loaf pan with nonstick vegetable oil spray. Pour boiling water over dates and let soften. Beat butter until creamy in large bowl. Gradually beat in the sugars and cream well; beat in the egg. Beat in the dates and their liquid (at lowest speed). Sift together flour, baking soda, and baking powder. Add gradually, on lowest speed, to the creamed mixture; stir in the pecans. Turn into loaf pan coated with nonstick vegetable oil spray. Bake 45 minutes, or until knife inserted in middle of loaf comes out clean. Cool loaf in pan on rack for 10 minutes and turn out on rack to cool.

Yield: 8 servings

Per serving: 43 g water; 361 calories (34% from fat, 6% from protein, 60% from carb); 6 g protein; 15 g total fat; 5 g saturated fat; 6 g monounsaturated fat; 3 g polyunsaturated fat; 57 g carbohydrate; 6 g fiber; 34 g sugar; 156 mg phosphorus; 59 mg calcium; 2 mg iron; 51 mg sodium; 353 mg potassium; 230 IU vitamin A; 59 mg vitamin E; 0 mg vitamin C; 42 mg cholesterol

Tip: This will keep for at least a week refrigerated. For longer storage, freeze.

Double Apricot Bread

A great bread for those mornings when you want a little something sweet. It doesn't require anything on it, but you could add a little apricot jam and make it a triple.

16 ounces (455 g) canned apricots, drained

2^1/$_2$ cups (300 g) whole wheat pastry flour

1^1/$_4$ cups (250 g) sugar

3^1/$_2$ teaspoons (16 g) baking powder

^{1}/$_2$ teaspoon pumpkin pie spice

2 eggs, beaten

^{1}/$_2$ cup (120 ml) skim milk

3 tablespoons (45 ml) canola oil

1 cup (130 g) chopped dried apricots

In a blender container or food processor bowl, blend or process canned apricot halves until smooth. Set aside. In a large bowl combine flour, sugar, baking powder, and pumpkin pie spice. In another bowl combine eggs, the apricot puree, milk, and oil. Add to flour mixture, stirring just until combined. Stir in dried apricots. Pour into two 8 × 4 × 2-inch (20 × 10 × 5-cm) loaf pans coated with nonstick vegetable oil spray. Bake in a 350°F (180°C, gas mark 4) oven 45 to 50 minutes or until a toothpick inserted near center comes out clean. Cool in pans 10 minutes. Remove from pans. Cool completely. Slice and serve.

Yield: 16 servings

Per serving: 41 g water; 195 calories (16% from fat, 8% from protein, 75% from carb); 4 g protein; 4 g total fat; 0 g saturated fat; 2 g monounsaturated fat; 1 g polyunsaturated fat; 39 g carbohydrate; 3 g fiber; 23 g sugar; 120 mg phosphorus; 89 mg calcium; 1 mg iron; 124 mg sodium; 241 mg potassium; 824 IU vitamin A; 14 mg vitamin E; 2 mg vitamin C; 30 mg cholesterol

Peanut Butter Burritos

These make great snacks for kids, and adults seem to like them too.

6 whole wheat tortillas, 6 inch (15 cm)

^{3}/$_4$ cup (195 g) crunchy peanut butter

1 cup (145 g) raisins

1 cup (175 g) chocolate chips

Spread each tortilla with 2 tablespoons peanut butter. Sprinkle with raisins and chocolate chips. Roll up tortillas.

Yield: 6 servings

Per serving: 14 g water; 516 calories (45% from fat, 10% from protein, 45% from carb); 13 g protein; 27 g total fat; 7 g saturated fat; 13 g monounsaturated fat; 5 g polyunsaturated fat; 61 g carbohydrate; 5 g fiber; 34 g sugar; 226 mg phosphorus; 120 mg calcium; 3 mg iron; 373 mg sodium; 597 mg potassium; 49 IU vitamin A; 13 mg vitamin E; 1 mg vitamin C; 6 mg cholesterol

Tip: Vary the flavor by adding nuts, candies, mini marshmallows, or other flavors of baking chips.

25

Cooking Terms, Weights and Measurements, and Gadgets

Cooking Terms

Confused about a term I used in one of the recipes? Take a look at the list here and see if there might be an explanation. I've tried to include anything that I thought might raise a question.

Al dente

"To the tooth," in Italian. The pasta is cooked just enough to maintain a firm, chewy texture.

Bake

To cook in the oven. Food is cooked slowly with gentle heat, concentrating the flavor.

Baste

To brush or spoon liquid, fat, or juices over meat during roasting to add flavor and to prevent it from drying out.

Beat

To smooth a mixture by briskly whipping or stirring it with a spoon, fork, wire whisk, rotary beater, or electric mixer.

Blend

To mix or fold two or more ingredients together to obtain equal distribution throughout the mixture.

Boil

To cook food in heated water or other liquid that is bubbling vigorously.

Braise

A cooking technique that requires browning meat in oil or other fat and then cooking slowly in liquid. The effect of braising is to tenderize the meat.

Bread

To coat the food with crumbs (usually with soft or dry bread crumbs), sometimes seasoned.

Broil

To cook food directly under the heat source.

Broth or stock

A flavorful liquid made by gently cooking meat, seafood, or vegetables (and/or their by-products, such as bones and trimmings) often with herbs and vegetables, in liquid, usually water.

Brown

A quick sautéing, pan/oven broiling, or grilling done either at the beginning or end of meal preparation, often to enhance flavor, texture, or visual appeal.

Brush

Using a pastry brush to coat a food such as meat or bread with melted butter, glaze, or other liquid.

Chop

To cut into irregular pieces.

Coat

To evenly cover food with flour, crumbs, or a batter.

Combine

To blend two or more ingredients into a single mixture.

Core

To remove the inedible center of fruits such as pineapples.

Cream

To beat butter or margarine, with or without sugar, until light and fluffy. This process traps in air bubbles, later used to create height in cookies and cakes.

Cut in

To work margarine or butter into dry ingredients.

Dash

A measure approximately equal to $1/16$ teaspoon.

Deep fry

To completely submerge the food in hot oil. It's a quick way to cook some food and, as a result, this method often seems to seal in the flavors of food better than any other technique.

Dice

To cut into cubes.

Direct heat

Heat waves radiate from a source and travel directly to the item being heated with no conductor between them. Examples are grilling, broiling, and toasting.

Dough

Used primarily for cookies and breads. Dough is a mixture of shortening, flour, liquid, and other ingredients that maintains its shape when placed on a flat surface, although it will change shape through the leavening process once baked.

Dredge

To coat lightly and evenly with sugar or flour.

Dumpling

A batter or soft dough that is formed into small mounds that are then steamed, poached, or simmered.

Dust

To sprinkle food lightly with spices, sugar, or flour for a light coating.

Fold

To cut and mix lightly with a spatula to keep as much air in the mixture as possible.

Fritter

Sweet or savory foods coated with or mixed into batter, then deep-fried.

Fry

To cook food in hot oil, usually until a crisp brown crust forms.

Glaze

A liquid that gives an item a shiny surface. Examples are fruit jams that have been heated, or chocolate that has been thinned.

Grease

To coat a skillet or baking sheet with a thin layer of oil or butter.

Grill

To cook over the heat source (traditionally over wood coals) in the open air.

Grind

To mechanically cut a food into small pieces.

Hull

To remove the leafy parts of soft fruits such as strawberries or blackberries.

Knead

To work dough with the heels of your hands in a pressing and folding motion until it becomes smooth and elastic.

Marinate

To soak food in aromatic ingredients to add flavor.

Mince

To chop food into tiny irregular pieces.

Mix

To beat or stir two or more foods together until they are thoroughly combined.

Pan fry

To cook in a hot pan with a small amount of hot oil, butter, or other fat, turning the food over once or twice.

Poach

To simmer food in a liquid.

Pot roast

A large piece of meat, usually browned in fat and cooked in a covered pan.

Purée

Food that has been mashed or processed in a blender or food processor.

Reduce

To cook liquids down so that some of the water content evaporates.

Roast

To cook uncovered in the oven.

Sauté

To cook with a small amount of hot oil, butter, or other fat, tossing the food around over high heat.

Sear

To brown a food quickly on all sides using high heat to seal in the juices.

Shred

To cut into fine strips.

Simmer

To cook slowly in a liquid over low heat.

Skim

To remove the surface layer (of impurities, scum, or fat) from liquids such as stocks and jams while cooking. This is usually done with a flat slotted spoon.

Smoke

To expose foods to wood smoke to enhance their flavor and help preserve and/or evenly cook them.

Steam

To cook in steam by suspending foods over boiling water in a steamer or covered pot.

Stew

To cook food in liquid for a long time until tender, usually in a covered pot.

Stir

To mix ingredients with a utensil.

Stir-fry

To cook quickly over high heat with a small amount of oil by constantly stirring. This technique often employs a wok.

Toss

To mix ingredients lightly by lifting and dropping them using two utensils.

Whip

To beat an item to incorporate air, augment volume, and add substance.

Zest

To finely grate the thin, brightly colored outer part of the rind of citrus fruits. It contains volatile oils, used as a flavoring.

Weights and Measurements

Here is a quick refresher on measurements.

3 teaspoons = 1 tablespoon
2 tablespoons = 1 fluid ounce
4 tablespoons = 2 fluid ounces = $^1/_4$ cup
5$^1/_3$ tablespoons = 16 teaspoons = $^1/_3$ cup
8 tablespoons = 4 fluid ounces = $^1/_2$ cup
16 tablespoons = 8 fluid ounces = 1 cup
2 cups = 1 pint
4 cups = 2 pints = 1 quart
16 cups = 8 pints = 4 quarts = 1 gallon

Metric Conversions

One of the questions that my newsletter readers have raised is whether I could also publish recipes with metric measurements. This would certainly be a good idea, because most of the world uses the metric system. Unfortunately, the software I use doesn't have a way to automatically convert from U.S. to metric measurements. There are some measurements that I can give you an easy conversion for, such as Fahrenheit to Celsius oven temperatures. Other things are not so easy. The information below is intended to be helpful to readers who use the metric system of weights and measures.

Measurements of Liquid Volume

The following measures are approximate, but close enough for most, if not all, of the recipes in this book.

1 quart = 1 liter
1 cup = 250 milliliters
$^3/_4$ cup = 200 milliliters

$^1/_2$ cup = 125 milliliters

$^1/_3$ cup = 105 milliliters

$^1/_4$ cup = 60 milliliters

1 fluid ounce = 30 milliliters

1 tablespoon = 15 milliliters

1 teaspoon = 5 milliliters

Measurements of Weight

Much of the world measures dry ingredients by weight, rather than by volume, as is done in the United States. There is no easy conversion for this, because each item is different. However, the following conversions may be useful.

1 ounce = 28.4 grams

1 pound = 454 grams (about half a kilo)

Oven Temperatures

Finally, we come to one that is relatively straightforward, the Fahrenheit to Celsius conversion.

100°F = 38°C

150°F = 66°C

200°F = 95°C

225°F = 110°C

250°F = 120°C

275°F = 140°C

300°F = 150°C

325°F = 165°C

350°F = 180°C

375°F = 190°C

400°F = 205°C

425°F = 220°C

450°F = 230°C

475°F = 240°C

500°F = 260°C

Gadgets

The following are some of the tools that I use in cooking. Some are used very often and some very seldom, but all help make things a little easier or quicker. Why are some things here and others not? No reason, except that most of these are things I considered a little less standard than a stove, an oven, a grill, and a mixer.

Blender

Okay, so everyone has a blender. And it's a handy little tool for blending and puréeing things. I don't really think I need to say any more about that.

Bread Machine

When I went on a low-sodium diet I discovered that one of the biggest single changes you can make to reduce your sodium intake is to make your own bread. Most commercial bread has well over 100 mg per slice. Many rolls and specialty breads are in the 300 to 400 mg range. A bread machine can reduce the amount of effort required to make your own bread to a manageable level. It takes at most 10 minutes to load it and turn it on. You can even set it on a timer to have your house filled with the aroma of fresh bread when you come home. Even if you're not watching your sodium, there is nothing like the smell of bread baking and the taste right out of the "oven."

Canning Kettle

If you are planning on making large batches of things like pickles and salsa so you don't have to go through the process of making them every couple of weeks, then you are going to need a way to preserve food. Most items can be frozen of course, if that is your preference. But some things just seem to work better in jars. What you need is a kettle big enough to make sure the jars can be covered by water when being processed in a boiling water bath. There are also racks to sit the jars in and special tongs to make lifting them in and out of the water easier. I had a porcelain-covered kettle that I used for this for many years, and it also doubled as a stockpot, before I got the one described below. It's better for canning than for soup because the relatively thin walls allow the water to heat faster (and the soup to burn).

Deep Fryer

Obviously, if you are watching your fat intake, this should not be one of your most often used appliances. I don't use it nearly as often as I used to, but it still occupies a place in the appliance garage in the corner of the kitchen counter. It's a Fry Daddy, big enough to cook a batch of fries or fish for three or four people at a time.

Food Processor

I'm a real latecomer to the food processor world. It always seemed like a nice thing to have, but something I could easily do without. We bought one to help shred meat and other things for my wife's mother, who was having some difficulty swallowing large chunks of food. I use it now all the time to grind bread into crumbs or chop the peppers and onions that seem to go into at least three meals a week. It's a low-end model that doesn't have the power to grind meat or complete some of the heavier tasks, but I've discovered it's a real timesaver for a number of things.

Grill

The George Foreman models are the most popular example of this item. My son's girlfriend gave me this for Christmas a few years ago. (And he didn't have the good sense to hang on to her . . . but that's a different story.) I use it fairly often. When we built our house we included a Jenn-Air cooktop with a built-in grill and for years that was used regularly. It still is for some things; I much prefer the way it does burgers or steak when it's too cold to grill them outside, but it's difficult to clean and doesn't do nearly as nice a job as the Foreman at things like grilled veggies and fish. And the design allows the fat to drain away, giving you a healthier, lower fat meal.

Grinder

Many years ago we bought an Oster Kitchen Center. It was one of those all-in-one things that included a stand mixer, blender (the one we still use), food chopper, and grinder attachment. The grinder was never a big deal that got any use . . . until I started experimenting with sausage recipes. Since then, I've discovered that grinding your own meat can save you both money and fat. Buying a beef or pork roast on sale, trimming it of most fat, and grinding it yourself can give you hamburger or sausage meat that is well over 90 percent lean and still less expensive than the fattier stuff you buy at the store. So now the grinder gets fairly regular use.

Hand Chopper

My daughter got this gem at a Wal-Mart in North Carolina while she was in school there. It was from one of those guys with the podium and the auctioneer's delivery and the extra free gifts if you buy it within the next 10 minutes. Neither of us has ever seen one like it since. The food processor has taken over some of its work, but it still does a great job chopping things like onions as fine as you could want without liquefying them.

Pasta Maker

I bought this toy after seeing it on a Sunday morning TV infomercial. It's a genuine Ronco/Popiel "As Seen on TV" special, but try not to hold that against it. Unlike the pasta cutters that merely slice rolled dough into flat noodles, this one mixes the whole mess, then extrudes it through dies with various-shaped holes in them. The recipes say you can use any kind of flour, but I've found that buying the semolina flour that is traditionally used for pasta gives you dough that's easier to work with, as well as having better texture and flavor. The characterization of it as a "toy" is pretty accurate. There aren't really any nutritional advantages over store-bought pasta. If you buy the semolina, the cost is probably about the same as some of the more expensive imported pastas. But it's fun to play with, it makes a great conversation piece, and the pasta tastes good.

SaladShooter

We seem to end up with a lot of these gadgets, don't we? This is another one that's been around for a while, but it's still my favorite implement for shredding potatoes for hash browns or cabbage for coleslaw.

Sausage Stuffer

This is really an addition to the Kitchen Center grinder. I found it at an online appliance repair site. It is really just a series of different-sized tubes that fit on the end of the grinder to stuff your ground meat into casings. I do this occasionally to make link sausage, but most of the time I just make patties or bulk sausage.

Slicer

This was a close-out floor model that I bought years ago. Before going on the low-sodium diet, I used to buy deli meat in bulk and slice it myself. Now it's most often used to slice a roast or smoked piece of meat for sandwiches.

Slow Cooker

I've tried to avoid calling it a Crock-Pot, which is a trademark of Rival. Anyway, whatever the brand, no kitchen should be without one.

Smoker

This was another pre-diet purchase that has been used even more since. I started with a Brinkman model that originally used charcoal. Then I bought an add-on electric heat source for it that works a lot better in cold weather. A few years ago the family gave me a fancy MasterChef electric one that seals like an oven and has a thermostat to hold the temperature. Not only do I like the way it does ribs and other traditional smoked foods, but we also use it fairly regularly to smoke a beef or pork roast or turkey breast to use for sandwiches.

Springform Pan

A round, straight-sided pan. The sides are formed into a hoop that can be unclasped and detached from its base.

Steamer (Rice Cooker)

I use this primarily for cooking rice, but it's really a Black & Decker Handy Steamer Plus that does a great job steaming vegetables, too. It does make excellent rice, perfect every time. So I guess the bottom line is that those of you who have trouble making rice like me (probably because like me you can't follow the instructions not to peek) should consider getting one of these or one of the Japanese-style rice cookers.

Stockpot

The key here is to spend the extra money to get a heavy-gauge one (another thing I eventually learned from personal experience). The lighter weight ones will not only dent and not sit level on the stove, but they will also burn just about everything you put in them. Mine also has a heavy glass lid that seals the moisture in well.

Turbo Cooker

Another infomercial sale. It is a large, dome-lidded fry pan with racks that fit inside it. You can buy them at many stores too, but mine is the "Plus" model that has two steamer racks and a timer. It really will cook a whole dinner quickly, "steam frying" the main course and steaming one or two more items. The only bad news is most of the recipes involve additions and changes every few minutes, so even if you only take a half hour to make dinner, you spend that whole time at the stove.

Waffle maker

I don't use this often, but waffles are a nice change of pace for breakfast or dinner.

Wok

A round-bottomed pan popular in Asian cooking.

About the Author

DICK LOGUE is the author of several cookbooks and founder of the website www.lowsodiumcooking.com. After being diagnosed with congestive heart failure more than ten years ago, Dick threw himself into the process of creating healthy versions of his favorite recipes. A cook since the age of twelve, he grows his own vegetables, bakes his own bread, and cans a variety of foods. He is the author of *500 Low-Sodium Recipes*, *500 Low-Cholesterol Recipes*, *500 High-Fiber Recipes*, *500 Low-Glycemic-Index Recipes*, *500 Heart-Healthy Slow Cooker Recipes*, *500 400-Calorie Recipes*, and *500 15-Minute Low-Sodium Recipes*. He lives in La Plata, Maryland.

Index